Clinical
Investigations
at a Glance

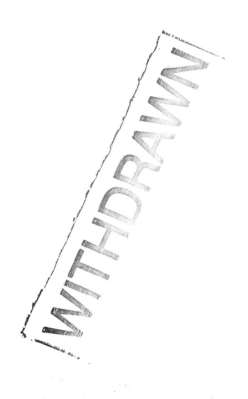

This book is dedicated to Adam.
He knows why.

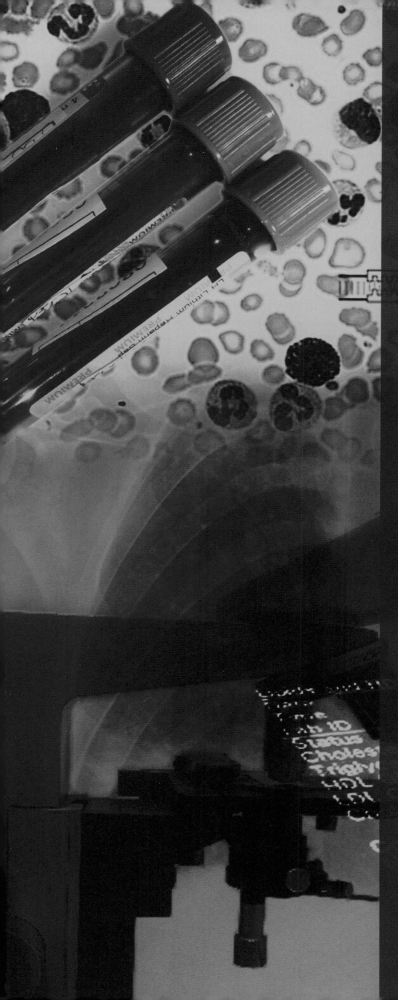

Clinical Investigations at a Glance

Jonathan Gleadle
MA, DPhil, BM, BCh, FRCP(UK), FRACP
Professor of Medicine
Flinders University
and Consultant Nephrologist
Flinders Medical Centre, Adelaide, Australia

Jordan Li
MBBS, FRACP
Senior Lecturer
Flinders University
and Consultant Physician
Flinders Medical Centre, Adelaide, Australia

Tuck Yong
MBBS, FRACP
Consultant Physician
Adelaide, Australia

WILEY Blackwell

Registered office:	John Wiley & Sons, Ltd, The Atrium, Southern Gate, Chichester, West Sussex, PO19 8SQ, UK
Editorial offices:	9600 Garsington Road, Oxford, OX4 2DQ, UK
	The Atrium, Southern Gate, Chichester, West Sussex, PO19 8SQ, UK
	350 Main Street, Malden, MA 02148-5020, USA

For details of our global editorial offices, for customer services and for information about how to apply for permission to reuse the copyright material in this book please see our website at www.wiley.com/wiley-blackwell

Library of Congress Cataloging-in-Publication Data

Names: Gleadle, Jonathan, author. | Li, Jordan, author. | Yong, Tuck, author.
Title: Clinical investigations at a glance / Jonathan Gleadle, Jordan Li, Tuck Yong.
Other titles: At a glance series (Oxford, England)
Description: Chichester, West Sussex : John Wiley & Sons, Ltd.,
   2017. | Series: At a glance series | Includes bibliographical references and index.
Identifiers: LCCN 2016009162 (print) | LCCN 2016011193 (ebook) | ISBN
   9781118759325 (pbk.) | ISBN 9781118759301 (pdf) | ISBN 9781118759318 (epub)
Subjects: | MESH: Diagnostic Techniques and Procedures | Handbooks
Classification: LCC RC71.3 (print) | LCC RC71.3 (ebook) | NLM WB 39 | DDC
   616.07/5—dc23
LC record available at http://lccn.loc.gov/2016009162

A catalogue record for this book is available from the British Library.

Wiley also publishes its books in a variety of electronic formats. Some content that appears in print may not be available in electronic books.

Cover image: ©David Heinrich

Set in Minion Pro 9.5/11.5 by Aptara
Printed and bound in Singapore by Markono Print Media Pte Ltd

1   2017

Contents

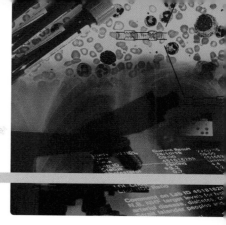

Part 3

Conditions   117

Cardiovascular disease

Respiratory disease and sleep disorders

Gastroenterology and hepatology

Nephrology and urology

Preface

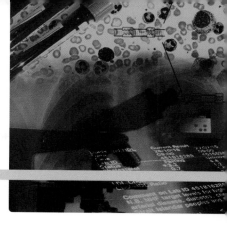

We have written this book to try to improve the understanding of clinical investigations in medicine. It has arisen as a response to many students asking "What test should I do?" "What do I do about this incidental finding?" "Why was this test wrong?" Our patients asking "What is this test for?" "What does this test mean?" "Will it hurt?" And our medical colleagues referring patients with "The scan has shown a cyst, what do I do now?"

It was also written in part because of the growing recognition that many people are overdiagnosed, undergo too many tests and are overtreated for a wide range of conditions. There are a bewildering and growing array of tests that doctors can request in attempting to establish diagnosis and prognosis. Whilst many have provided powerful improvements in the accuracy of diagnosis, many carry with them the risk of incidental findings, significant cost and potential for harm. Understanding the role of such tests, their interpretation and how to deal with such asymptomatic discoveries is an increasing part of modern medical practice. Screening the general population for disease with tests is an increasingly difficult area and it is essential to consider whether patients are likely to benefit and whether any test will affect the patient's outcome or management.

All clinical investigations are an adjunct to thorough clinical history and examination but not a substitute, and nor do they treat patients. Investigations should be ordered if they are of benefit in diagnosis, management, prevention and prognosis. This book is intended to assist clinicians develop evidence-based use of clinical investigations and interpret results of these investigations properly. We hope that this book will contribute to the better use of clinical investigations, improve diagnostic accuracy and reduce unnecessary tests or harm.

Jonathan Gleadle
Jordan Li
Tuck Yong

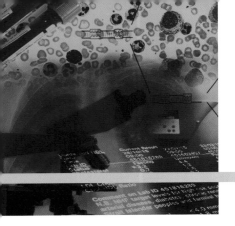

Acknowledgements

We are grateful to the many colleagues and students who have improved this book, provided images or edited the text and would particularly like to thank Elizabeth Johnston for helping to initiate this project.

We would like to thank the following for their expert reviews and provision of images.

Dr Marc Agazarian
Consultant Radiologist
Department of Medical Imaging
Flinders Medical Centre

Dr Justin Ardill
Consultant Cardiologist
Department of Cardiology
Flinders Medical Centre

Dr Virginia Au
Consultant Radiologist
Department of Medical Imaging
Flinders Medical Centre

Dr Jir-Ping Boey
Senior Registrar
Department of Haematology
Flinders Medical Centre

Dr Jeff Bowden
Consultant Respiratory Physician
Department of Respiratory and Sleep medicine
Flinders Medical Centre & Flinders University

Lynn Brown
Chief Cardiac Sonographer
Department of Cardiology
Flinders Medical Centre

Dr Joseph Frasca
Consultant Neurologist
Department of Neurology
Flinders Medical Centre

Ashley Gaw
Medical student
School of Medicine, Flinders University

Dr Zbigniew Gieroba
Consultant Geriatrician
Department of Aged Care
Flinders Medical Centre

Professor David Gordon
Consultant Infectious Disease Physician
Department of Microbiology & Infectious Diseases
Flinders Medical Centre & Flinders University

Lucy I-Ning Huang
Medical student
School of Medicine, Flinders University

Dr Neil Jones
Consultant Radiologist
Department of Medical Imaging
Flinders Medical Centre

Associate Professor Sonja Klebe
Consultant Surgical Pathologist
SA Pathology
Flinders Medical Centre & Flinders University

Dr Su Yin Lau
Senior Registrar
Department of Gastroenterology and Hepatology
Flinders Medical Centre

Jonathon Jing-Ping Liu
Medical student
School of Medicine, Flinders University

Dr Anand Rose
Consultant Respiratory Physician
Department of Respiratory and Sleep Medicine
Flinders Medical Centre & Flinders University

Dr Mark Siddins
Consultant Urologist
Flinders Private Hospital

Dr Magdalena Sobieraj-Teague
Consultant Haematologist
Department of Haematology and Genetic Pathology
Flinders Medical Centre & Flinders University

Dr Chrismin Tan
Senior Registrar
Department of Medical Imaging
Flinders Medical Centre

Dr Tilenka Thynne
Consultant Endocrinologist and Clinical Pharmacologist
Departments of Endocrinology and Clinical Pharmacology
Flinders Medical Centre & Flinders University

Dr Yew Toh Wong
Consultant Vascular Surgeon
Department of Vascular surgery
Flinders Medical Centre & Flinders University

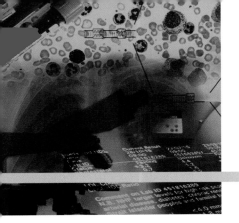

Abbreviations

AAA	abdominal aortic aneurysm
ABG	arterial blood gas
ABI	ankle–brachial index
ACE	angiotensin converting enzyme
ACR	albumin : creatinine ratio
ACS	acute coronary syndrome
ADA	adenosine deaminase
ADH	antidiuretic hormone
AFB	acid-fast bacillus
AFP	α-fetoprotein
AHI	apnoea–hypopnoea index
AIDS	acquired immunodeficiency syndrome
AKI	acute kidney injury
AKP	alkaline phosphatase
ALT	alanine aminotransferase
ALP	alkaline phosphatase
AMI	acute myocardial infarction
AML	acute myeloid leukaemia
ANA	antinuclear antibody
ANCA	antineutrophil cytoplasmic antibody
Anti-CCP	anticyclic citrullinated peptide antibodies
APC	activated protein C
APS	antiphospholipid syndrome
APTT	activated partial thromboplastin time
AS	ankylosing spondylitis
AST	aspartate aminotransferase
AUC	area under the concentration curve
AVM	arteriovenous malformation
AXR	abdominal X-ray
BAEP	brainstem auditory evoked potential
BAL	bronchoalveolar lavage
BCC	basal cell carcinoma
BCG	bacillus Calmette–Guérin
β-hCG	beta subunit of human chorionic gonadotropin
BMC	bone mineral content
BMD	bone mineral density
BMI	body mass index
BNP	brain natriuretic peptide
BP	blood pressure
BPH	benign prostate hyperplasia
BPPV	benign positional paroxysmal vertigo
BGL	blood glucose level
C1-INH	C1 esterase inhibitor
CABG	coronary artery bypass grafting
CAD	coronary artery disease
CAP	community acquired pneumonia
CBD	common bile duct
CCF	congestive cardiac failure
CD	Crohn's disease
CEA	carcinoembryonic antigen
CIDP	chronic inflammatory demyelinating polyneuropathy
CIN	contrast induced nephropathy
CK	creatine kinase
CKD	chronic kidney disease
CHL	conductive hearing loss
CLL	chronic lymphocytic leukaemia
CML	chronic myeloid leukaemia
CMR	cardiac magnetic resonance imaging
CMT	Charcot–Marie–Tooth (disease)
CMV	cytomegalovirus
CNS	central nervous system
COPD	chronic obstructive pulmonary disease
CPPD	calcium pyrophosphate deposition disease
CRBSI	catheter-related bloodstream infection
CRH	corticotropin-releasing hormone
CRC	colorectal cancer
CRP	C-reactive protein
CSA	central sleep apnoea
CSF	cerebrospinal fluid
CT	computed tomography
CTA	CT angiography
CTE	enteroclysis combined with CT
CTEPH	chronic thromboembolic pulmonary hypertension
CTG	cardiotocography
CTPA	computed tomography pulmonary angiography
CUP	cancer of unknown primary
CVP	central venous pressure
CXR	chest X-ray
DAT	direct antiglobulin test
DCIS	ductal carcinoma in situ
DcSSc	diffuse cutaneous scleroderma
DEXA	dual-energy X-ray absorptiometry
DHEA-S	dehydroepiandrosterone sulphate
DI	diabetes insipidus
DIC	disseminated intravascular coagulopathy
DIF	direct immunofluorescence

DIP	distal interphalangeal	GPA	granulomatosis with polyangiitis
DKA	diabetic ketoacidosis	GRA	glucocorticoid remediable hyperaldosteronism
DPL	diagnostic peritoneal lavage	H&E	haematoxylin and eosin
DRE	digital rectal examination	HAART	highly active antiretroviral therapy
DSA	digital subtraction angiography	HAE	hereditary angioedema
ds-DNA	double-stranded DNA	HAP	hospital-acquired pneumonia
DVT	deep vein thrombosis	Hb	haemoglobin
DWI	diffusion-weighted imaging	HCC	hepatocellular carcinoma
EBV	Epstein–Barr virus	hCG	human chorionic gonadotrophin
ECF	extracellular fluid	HD	Huntington's disease
ECG	electrocardiogram	HDL	high-density lipoprotein
EDS	excessive daytime sleepiness	HER	human epidermal growth factor receptor
EEG	electroencephalogram	HF	heart failure
EF	ejection fraction	HIT	heparin-induced thrombocytopenia
eGFR	estimated glomerular filtration rate	HIV	human immunodeficiency virus
EGFR	epidermal growth factor receptor	HL	Hodgkin's lymphoma
EIA	enzyme immunoassay	HPV	human papillomavirus
ELISA	enzyme-based immunosorbent assay	HRCT	high-resolution computed tomography
EMG	electromyography	HRM	high-resolution manometry
ENA	extractable nuclear antigen	HSV	herpes simplex virus
EPS	electrophysiological study	HUS	haemolytic uremic syndrome
ERCP	endoscopic retrograde cholangiopancreatography	IBD	inflammatory bowel disease
ESR	erythrocyte sedimentation rate	IBS	irritable bowel syndrome
EST	exercise stress test	ICT	immunochromatographic test
ET	endotracheal	ICP	intracranial pressure
EUC	electrolytes, urea and creatinine	IDA	iron deficiency anaemia
EUS	endoscopic ultrasound	IE	infective endocarditis
FAI	free androgen index	Ig	immunoglobulin
FAST	focused abdominal sonography for trauma	IGF	insulin-like growth factor
FBC	full blood count	IGRA	interferon gamma release assay
FDG	fluoro-2-deoxy-D-glucose	IHD	ischaemic heart disease
FEV1	forced expiratory volume in 1 second	IIF	indirect immunofluorescence assay
FH	familial hypercholesterolaemia	ILD	interstitial lung disease
FHH	familial hypocalciuric hypercalcaemia	INR	international normalised ratio
FLAIR	fluid-attenuated inversion recovery	IPH	idiopathic pulmonary hypertension
FLC	free light chain	IPI	International Prognostic Index
FMD	fibromuscular dysplasia	IPSS	International Prognostic Scoring System
FNA	fine-needle aspiration	ITP	immune thrombocytopenic purpura
FOBT	faecal occult blood test	ITT	insulin tolerance test
FPG	fasting plasma glucose	IUGR	intrauterine growth retardation
FSGS	focal and segmental glomerulosclerosis	KCR	potassium : creatinine ratio
FSH	follicle-stimulating hormone	KUB	kidney, ureter and bladder (X-ray)
FT3	free triiodothyronine	LBBB	left bundle branch block
FT4	free thyroxine	LBO	large bowel obstruction
FTA-Abs	fluorescent treponemal antibody absorption	LBP	low back pain
FVC	forced vital capacity	LCR	ligase chain reaction
G6PD	glucose-6-phosphate dehydrogenase	LcSSc	limited cutaneous scleroderma
GAT	granulocyte agglutination test	LDH	lactate dehydrogenase
GBS	Guillain–Barré syndrome	LDL	low-density lipoprotein
GCA	giant cell arteritis	LFTs	liver function tests
GCS	Glasgow coma scale	LH	luteinising hormone
GFR	glomerular filtration rate	LP	lumbar puncture
GGT	gamma glutamyl transferase	LRTI	lower respiratory tract infection
GH	growth hormone	LTBI	latent tuberculosis infection
GHRH	growth hormone releasing hormone	MAHA	microangiopathic haemolytic anaemia
GI	gastrointestinal	MCD	minimal change disease
GIFT	granulocyte immunofluorescence test	MCP	metacarpophalangeal
GORD	gastroesophageal reflux disease	MCS	microbiology culture and sensitivity

MCV	mean corpuscular volume	**PTLD**	post-transplant lymphoproliferative disorders
MDS	myelodysplastic syndromes	**PUD**	peptic ulcer disease
MELD	model for end-stage liver disease	**PUO**	pyrexia of unknown origin
MEN	multiple endocrine neoplasia	**PV**	polycythaemia vera
MGUS	monoclonal gammopathy of undetermined significance	**PVD**	peripheral vascular disease
MIBG	metaiodobenzylguanidine	**RA**	rheumatoid arthritis
MM	multiple myeloma	**RAS**	renal artery stenosis
MMSE	mini-mental state examination	**RBC**	red blood cell
MPA	microscopic polyangiitis	**RCC**	renal cell carcinoma
MRA	magnetic resonance angiography	**RDI**	respiratory disturbance index
MRI	magnetic resonance imaging	**REM**	rapid-eye movement
MRSA	methicillin-resistant *Staphylococcus aureus*	**RF**	rheumatoid factor
MRV	magnetic resonance venography	**RLS**	restless leg syndrome
MRCP	magnetic resonance cholangiopancreatography	**RNS**	repetitive nerve stimulation
MS	multiple sclerosis	**RPR**	rapid plasma reagin
MSCC	metastatic spinal cord compression	**RTA**	renal tubular acidosis
MTC	medullary thyroid cancer	**SAAG**	serum-ascites albumin gradient
NAAT	nucleic acid amplification test	**SAH**	subarachnoid haemorrhage
NASH	non-alcoholic steatohepatitis	**SBO**	small bowel obstruction
NCS	nerve conduction study	**SCC**	squamous cell carcinoma
NHL	non-Hodgkin's lymphoma	**SFEMG**	single-fibre electromyography
NPV	negative predictive value	**SHBG**	sex hormone-binding globulin
NSAID	non-steroidal anti-inflammatory drug	**SIADH**	syndrome of inappropriate antidiuretic hormone secretion
OAE	oto-acoustic emission	**SLE**	systemic lupus erythematosus
OCT	optical coherence tomography	**SLN**	sentinel lymph node
OGTT	oral glucose tolerance	**SLNB**	sentinel lymph node biopsy
OSA	obstructive sleep apnoea	**SNHL**	sensorineural hearing loss
PAD	peripheral arterial disease	**SOHL**	sudden onset of hearing loss
PAH	pulmonary arterial hypertension	**SOT**	solid organ transplant
PAN	polyarteritis nodosa	**SPECT**	single-photon emission computed tomography
pANCA	perinuclear antineutrophil cytoplasmic antibody	**SPN**	solitary pulmonary nodule
PAOP	pulmonary artery occlusion pressure	**SSEP**	somatosensory evoked potential
PAP	pulmonary artery pressure	**SSRI**	selective serotonin reuptake inhibitor
PCOS	polycystic ovary syndrome	**STD**	sexually transmitted disease
PCR	polymerase chain reaction; protein-to-creatinine ratio	**STEMI**	ST elevation myocardial infarction
PCV	packed cell volume	**SUI**	stress urinary incontinence
PDU	penile Doppler ultrasound	**TB**	tuberculosis
PE	pulmonary embolism	**TCC**	transitional cell carcinoma
PEFR	peak expiratory flow rate	**TDM**	therapeutic drug monitoring
PET	positron emission tomography	**TFT**	thyroid function tests
PFT	pulmonary function test	**TG**	thyroglobulin
PH	pulmonary hypertension	**TIA**	transient ischaemic attack
PHA	primary hyperaldosteronism	**TIBC**	total iron binding capacity
PID	pelvic inflammatory disease	**TLCO**	carbon monoxide transfer factor
PIP	proximal interphalangeal	**TOE**	transoesophageal echocardiography
PLED	paroxysmal lateral epileptiform discharge	**TPHA**	treponema pallidum haemagglutination
PMR	polymyalgia rheumatica	**TPO**	thyroid peroxidase
PPI	proton pump inhibitor	**TPPA**	*Treponema pallidum* particle agglutination
PSA	prostate-specific antigen	**TSH**	thyroid-stimulating hormone
PSG	polysomnography	**TST**	tuberculin skin testing
PSI	pneumonia severity index	**TTE**	transthoracic echocardiography
PT	prothrombin time	**TTP**	thrombotic thrombocytopenic purpura
PTC	percutaneous transhepatic cholangiography	**UC**	ulcerative colitis
PTH	parathyroid hormone	**UGI**	upper gastrointestinal
PTHrP	PTH-related protein	**UGB**	upper gastrointestinal bleeding
		USS	ultrasound scan
		UTI	urinary tract infection

UUI	urgency urinary incontinence	**VT**	ventricular tachycardia
VA	visual acuity	**VTE**	venous thromboembolism
VATS	video-assisted thoracic surgery	**VWD**	von Willebrand disease
VCE	video capsule endoscopy	**VWF**	von Willebrand factor
VDRL	Venereal Disease Research Laboratory (test)	**VZV**	varicella zoster virus
VEP	visual evoked potential	**WBC**	white blood cell
VHL	von Hippel–Lindau	**WHO**	World Health Organization
V/Q	ventilation–perfusion	**WHR**	waist-to-hip ratio
VRE	vancomycin-resistant enterococcus	**WPW**	Wolff–Parkinson–White (syndrome)

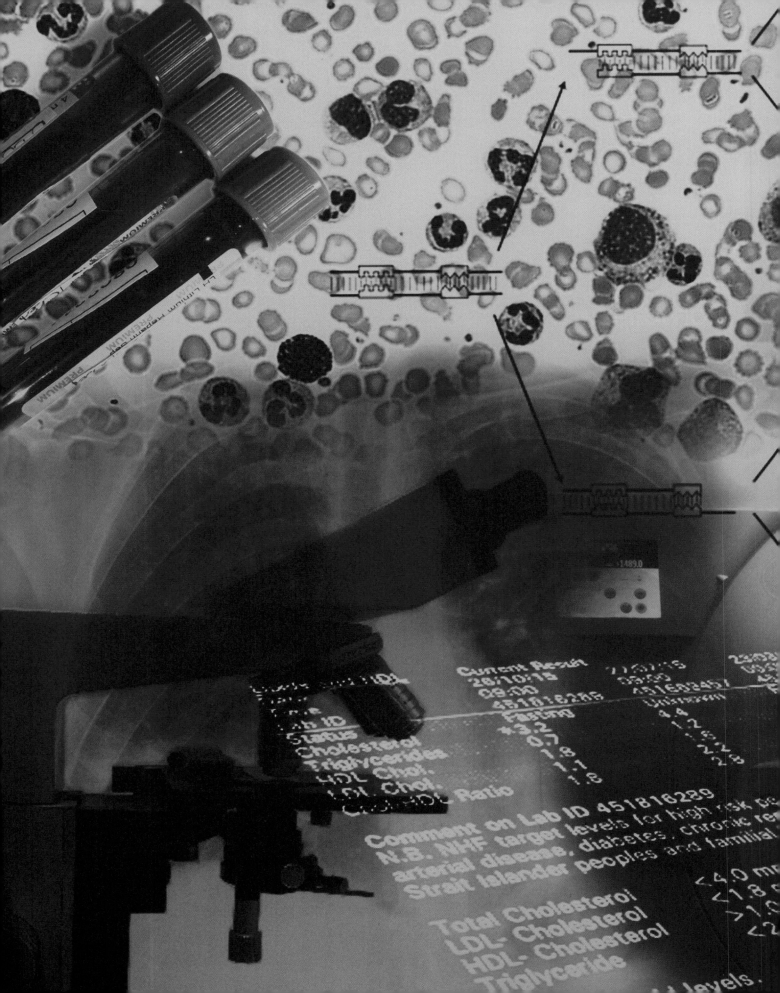

Overview of tests

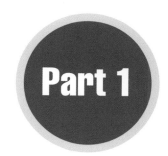

Part 1

Chapters

1 Investigations and interpreting tests

Box 1.1   What is the reason for investigations?

- To confirm the diagnosis or to exclude other diagnoses
- To obtain detailed information for a particular diagnosis
- To investigate the complication of disease
- To monitor the progress of disease and the results of treatment
- To detect evidence of disease before clinical manifestation

Remember:
- Patient's identity
- Accurate request form
- What is the purpose of this test?
- Any risks
- Any alternative investigations
- Confidentiality
- How you and patient will receive the results

Figure 1.1   Blood tests

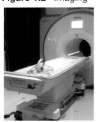

Figure 1.2   Imaging

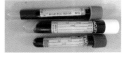
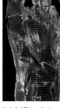

(a) MRI scan

(b) MRI of the right foot

How will this test affect me?

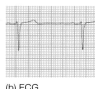

Figure 1.3   Tests utilising electrical activity

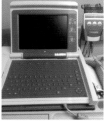

(a) ECG machine

(b) ECG

Figure 1.4   Biopsies

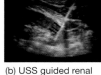
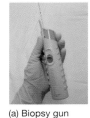

(a) Biopsy gun

(b) USS guided renal biopsy

(c) Renal biopsy H&E histopathology examination

Figure 1.5   Urine analysis

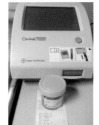

Figure 1.6   Genetic tests

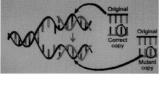

Figure 1.7   Joint aspiration culture grew mycoplasma

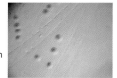

	Use	Definition	Formula
Accuracy	Ability of a test to correctly detect the presence or absence of a disease		
Sensitivity	Ability of a test to correctly detect the presence of a condition	Sensitivity is the probability that a test will indicate 'disease' among those with the disease	Sensitivity=A/(A+C)x100
Specificity	Ability of a test to correctly detect the absence of a condition	Specificity is the fraction of those without disease who will have a negative test result	Specificity=D/(D+B)x100
Positive predictive value	Frequency of positive initial diagnosis confirmed by gold standard test	Positive predictive value is the proportion of patients with positive test results who are correctly diagnosed	Positive Predictive Value =A/(A+B) × 100
Negative predictive value	Frequency of negative initial diagnosis confirmed by gold standard test	Negative predictive value is the proportion of patients with negative test results who are correctly diagnosed	Negative Predictive Value =D/(D+C) × 100

	Disease	Non disease	Total number
Positive test	A (True positive)	B (false positive)	Total number of test positive
Negative test	C (False negative)	D (True negative)	Total number of test negative
Total number	Total number of subjects with disease	Total number of subjects without disease	Total

The perfect investigation:
- 100% specificity
- 100% sensitivity
- No risks, adverse effects
- Cheap and easy to perform
- Provides definite information about patients' diagnosis, prognosis and management

Clinical Investigations at a Glance, First Edition. Jonathan Gleadle, Jordan Li and Tuck Yong. © 2017 John Wiley & Sons, Ltd. Published 2017 by John Wiley & Sons, Ltd.

Investigations are tests to determine more about a person's health, illness or prognosis. A variety of types of investigations can be undertaken, including: blood tests (e.g. biochemistry, haematology, immunology – Figure 1.1), radiology (e.g. plain X-rays, CT scans, ultrasounds, nuclear medicine tests, MRI scans – Figure 1.2), tests utilising electrical activity (e.g. ECG, EEG or nerve conduction – Figure 1.3), biopsies (tissue obtained for histological and cytological analysis – Figure 1.4), analysis of other biological fluids/specimens (e.g. urine, stool, cerebrospinal fluid – Figure 1.5), genetic testing (e.g. analysing for a DNA mutation that might cause disease – Figure 1.6) and tests for infection (e.g. attempts to culture an organism, detect DNA or an antibody response – Figure 1.7).

Investigations may be undertaken during an acute illness to contribute to making a diagnosis (e.g. a CT scan of the head in someone who is unconscious) or as a screening test in a well individual (e.g. a mammogram) to look for asymptomatic disease. Sometimes tests are undertaken to exclude particular diagnoses, especially if symptoms or signs of that illness can be subtle or nonspecific.

Prior to undertaking investigations in non-emergency settings, a detailed history and physical examination should be performed. Information obtained will often lead to selecting the most appropriate investigations.

When undertaking an investigation it is essential to ensure that it is done on the right person. Identification can be helped by accurate completion of request forms, verification of identity with questions about name, address, date of birth and examination of wrist bands. The use of sticky labels can improve the amount of information on a tube or a request form, but it is easy to mistakenly stick the wrong label on the wrong tube.

The person should have an appropriate understanding of the reason for the test, with consent that includes potential risks and consequences, the possible outcomes of the test and its implications.

The result

When requesting a test, consider how you (or other health professionals) will receive/check/chase the result and how the result will be communicated to the patient (and other relevant health professionals involved in care).

Confidentiality

Remember that all test results (and, indeed, even the fact that a patient is undergoing a test) should be regarded as confidential, restricted to the patient or professionals directly involved in their care and only shared with relatives and friends with the patient's explicit permission and understanding. Similarly, test results and images should be stored in a confidential manner.

Repeating tests

In some situations it may be helpful to repeat a test; for example, when following change in an incidentally noted pulmonary nodule on CT scanning or repeating urea, creatinine and electrolytes to monitor response to rehydration. However, be wary of repeating tests too frequently or at too short an interval. Recognise that some abnormalities may take days or weeks to resolve following treatment and that the levels of some blood tests have prolonged half-lives. It is important to recognise that there will be variation in any test because of inter-individual variation and analytical variation.

Specificity and sensitivity

A perfect diagnostic test would be positive in every patient who has the disease (i.e. have no false negatives). This is the sensitivity of the test. The ideal test would also not be positive in any patient without the disease (i.e. have no false positives). This is the specificity. Diagnostic sensitivity is the proportion of individuals with disease who have a positive test associated with that disease. Diagnostic specificity refers to the proportion of individuals without disease who yield a negative test. A 'perfect' test would have both 100% diagnostic sensitivity and specificity. A test with 50% sensitivity and specificity is no better than tossing a coin.

For any test result one can compare the probability of getting that result if the patient truly had the condition with the probability if they were healthy. The ratio of these probabilities is the likelihood ratio (LR), calculated as sensitivity/$(1 - \text{specificity})$.

Receiver operator characteristic curves

A receiver operator characteristic curve plots the false-positive rate (FPR = $1 -$ specificity) versus the true-positive rate (TPR = sensitivity). They assess the diagnostic accuracy of any test. The area under the curve (range: 0.5–1.0) is a quantitative representation of test accuracy, where values from 0.5 to 0.7 represent low accuracy, from 0.7 to 0.9 represent tests that are useful for some purposes, and >0.9 represent tests with high accuracy.

Measures of disease probability

No test is perfect, and after every test the true disease state of the patient remains uncertain. Quantitating this residual uncertainty can be done with Bayes' theorem. This provides a mathematical way to calculate the post-test probability of disease from three parameters: the pre-test probability of the disease, the test sensitivity and test specificity. Pre-test probability: can be estimated using population prevalence of disease or more patient-specific data.

$$\text{Post-test probability} = \frac{\text{Pre-test probability} \times \text{test sensitivity}}{\begin{array}{c}\text{Pre-test probability} \times \text{test sensitivity} +\\ (1 - \text{disease prevalence}) \times \text{test false-positive rate}\end{array}}$$

Normal range

When interpreting tests it is important to examine the test value with the normal range for that patient. These reference ranges are often derived from a population of 'normal' individuals and reflect the prediction interval within which 95% of values fall such that 2.5% of values will be less than the lower limit of this interval and 2.5% of the time it will be greater. However, this assumes a normal distribution of values and may not account for changes with age, gender and other physiological or pathological changes, such as impaired renal function. For some tests, because a large proportion of the 'normal' population have values associated with disease risk, a healthy or recommended range is quoted (e.g. vitamin D or cholesterol).

Incidental findings: none of us are 'normal'

Incidental findings are results that you were not looking for. With increasingly sophisticated testing, very large number of healthy individuals can be found to have 'abnormalities' detected. Examples include benign cysts in the liver, detected with CT scans or ultrasounds, and small pulmonary nodules. The interpretation of such incidental findings can be difficult but should be grounded in the pre-test probability, any symptoms or signs and the incidence of such findings in healthy individuals.

2 Screening tests

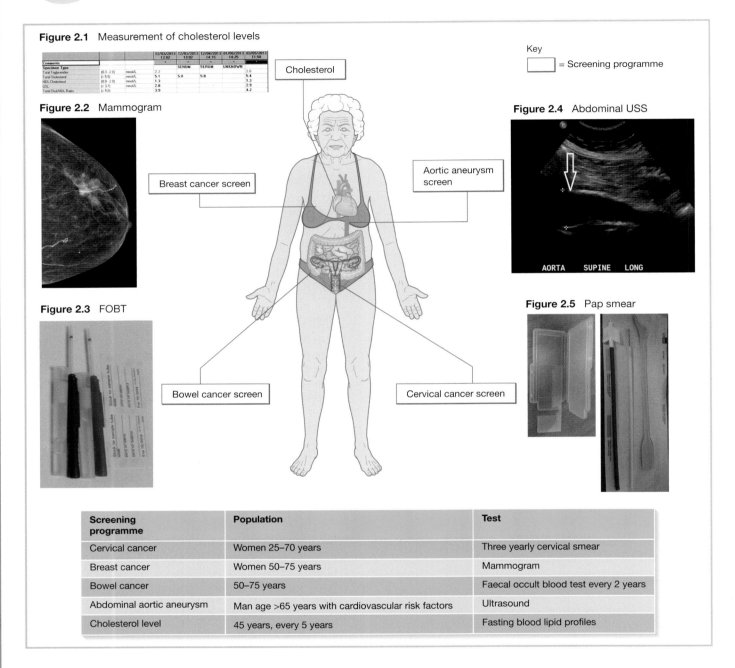

Figure 2.1 Measurement of cholesterol levels

Figure 2.2 Mammogram

Figure 2.3 FOBT

Figure 2.4 Abdominal USS

Figure 2.5 Pap smear

Key

☐ = Screening programme

Cholesterol

Breast cancer screen

Aortic aneurysm screen

Bowel cancer screen

Cervical cancer screen

Screening programme	Population	Test
Cervical cancer	Women 25–70 years	Three yearly cervical smear
Breast cancer	Women 50–75 years	Mammogram
Bowel cancer	50–75 years	Faecal occult blood test every 2 years
Abdominal aortic aneurysm	Man age >65 years with cardiovascular risk factors	Ultrasound
Cholesterol level	45 years, every 5 years	Fasting blood lipid profiles

Screening tests are tests designed to detect disease in asymptomatic individuals. Often they are designed to detect disease at an early and readily treatable stage. For a screening test to be successful the following should be considered.

The condition
- This should have a relatively high prevalence in the population to be screened.
- This should be an important health problem, usually with a latent or pre-symptomatic stage.
- The epidemiology and natural history of the condition should be adequately understood.

The screening test
- This should be a simple, safe, precise, acceptable, sensitive, specific and well-validated screening test.
- The distribution of test values in the target population should be known and a suitable cut-off level defined.
- There should be an agreed policy on the further diagnostic investigation of individuals with a positive test result and on the choices available to those individuals.
- This should have no or low adverse effects.

The treatment
- There should be an effective treatment or intervention for patients identified through early detection, with evidence of early treatment leading to better outcomes than late treatment.

The screening programme
- There should be evidence from high-quality randomised controlled trials that the screening programme is effective in reducing mortality or morbidity.
- The benefit from the screening programme should outweigh the physical and psychological harm (caused by the test, diagnostic procedures and treatment).
- Facilities for diagnosis and treatment should be readily available for the screened population.
- Should be cost effective.
- The population to be screened should have reasonable life expectancy.
- Case finding should be a continuing process and not a 'once and for all' project.

For some screening tests robust evidence exists for their capacity to reduce mortality. However, other screening programmes lack such clear evidence of benefit. For example, annual screening with chest radiograph did not reduce lung cancer mortality compared with usual care (no screening).

What is case finding?

Case finding occurs when a patient presents with symptoms, risk factors or concerns about a particular condition. It enables the targeting of resources to individuals or groups at high risk of a disease. It is often applied to the identification of contacts of people with specific infectious diseases.

Examples of screening tests
These include:
- cervical smear (Figure 2.5) or liquid-based cytology to detect potentially precancerous lesions and prevent cervical cancer;
- mammography to detect breast cancer (Figure 2.2);
- colonoscopy and faecal occult blood test (Figure 2.3) to detect colorectal cancer;
- ultrasound scan for abdominal aortic aneurysm (Figure 2.4);
- oral glucose challenge screening test for gestational diabetes;
- screening for diabetes and hypercholesterolaemia (Figure 2.1).

Examples of conditions where screening is controversial or lacking in definite evidence of benefit
- Prostate-specific antigen (PSA) testing to detect prostate cancer.
- Screening for diabetes and hypercholesterolaemia.

Examples of conditions where population screening is not generally recommended
- Hypertension
- Depression
- Osteoporosis
- Kidney disease.

Limitations of screening
- As for any test, the screening test may miss patients with the condition (false negatives) or erroneously detect patients with the condition (false positives).
- The screening may have adverse effects from the screening itself (e.g. the irradiation of mammography), from the subsequent confirmatory tests or treatments (e.g. an unnecessary biopsy) or from generating anxiety. It might also produce a misplaced sense of security from a false-negative test. In some situations patients may be detected with the condition that would never lead to symptomatic disease (e.g. PSA screening in elderly men). There are also important cost considerations.

3 Consent for investigations

When undertaking tests it is important that the patient consents to the test

The consent process should ensure patients understand:
- what the test will involve
- what are the potential benefits and information gained by the test
- what the potential adverse outcomes of the test are
- what are the potential implications of a positive or negative result.

Do not make assumptions about a patient's understanding of risk or the implications of the test.

Adverse outcomes of a test include:
- side effects
- complications
- failure of the investigation to achieve a desired result (e.g. failure of an attempted pleural aspirate to yield fluid)
- false-negative or false-positive result
- implication for employment, insurance, immigration, army service.

Questions that patients and doctors may need to address around any test
What is the test?
Why is it needed?
What might it show?
What will happen if I don't have the test?
What alternatives are there?
What are the risks of the test?
Am I at particular risk?
What will happen if the test is positive or negative?
How can the test go wrong?
How much radiation will I be exposed to?

Clinical Investigations at a Glance, First Edition. Jonathan Gleadle, Jordan Li and Tuck Yong. © 2017 John Wiley & Sons, Ltd. Published 2017 by John Wiley & Sons, Ltd.

Consenting to investigations

When undertaking tests it is important that the patient consents to the test. This consent should be fully informed, meaning that they understand what the test will involve, what are the potential benefits and information gained by the test, what the potential adverse outcomes of the test are and what are the potential implications of a positive or negative result. Communicate the reason, possible benefits and risks of any investigation in clear, straightforward language tailored to the understanding and responses of the patient. The amount of information about risk that you share with patients will depend on the individual patient and what they want or need to know. Explore the consequences of not undertaking a particular investigation and any appropriate alternatives. Do not make assumptions about a patient's understanding of risk or the importance they attach to different outcomes.

Implicit, assumed, oral or written consent?

For many simple or straightforward tests, such as a blood test for anaemia, consent is implicit and assumed. For others, with greater complexity and potential hazard (e.g. coronary angiography), greater explanation and written consent may be required. The considerations around consent for investigations are similar to those for consent to treatment.

Before accepting a patient's consent, you must consider whether they have been given the information they want or need, and whether they understand the details and implications of what is proposed. Patients can give consent orally or in writing, or may imply consent by complying with the proposed investigation; for example, by rolling up their sleeve to have their blood taken. In the case of minor or routine investigations or treatments, it is usually sufficient to have oral or implied consent. In cases that involve higher risk, it is important to get the patient's written consent. This is so that everyone involved understands what was explained and agreed.

You should also get written consent from a patient if the investigation or treatment is complex or involves significant risks, if there may be significant consequences for the patient's employment, health or social or personal life, or if the investigation has a research purpose. The consent should be documented in a consent form and/or in the medical notes and should include the information discussed, any specific requests by the patient, any written, visual or audio information given to the patient, and details of any decisions that are made.

If it is not possible to get written consent then in an emergency oral consent may be appropriate, but you must still give the patient the information they want and need and the consent should be clearly documented in medical notes.

It is important that consent is voluntary; patients may be put under pressure by employers, insurers, relatives or others, to accept a particular investigation or treatment. You should be aware of this and other situations in which patients may be vulnerable. Such situations may include if they are resident in a care home, subject to mental health legislation, detained by the police or immigration services, or in prison.

You must respect a patient's decision to refuse an investigation, even if you think their decision is wrong or irrational.

Consent from surrogate decision-makers

In some situations, such as patients with mental incapacity or children, consent needs to be obtained from the next of kin, a guardian or parents.

Request forms

When completing a request form, ensure all information about identity is completed accurately and legibly. Many investigations will be interpreted by specialists (e.g. radiologists and pathologists) whose interpretation will be substantially improved by full clinical details. Consider whether there are any particular cautions that should be noted on the request (e.g. abnormal kidney function in a patient to receive contrast, metallic implant in patients undergoing MRI, problems with mobility or potential difficulties with communication).

How will the test affect the patient?

It may be helpful to consider the following questions when contemplating an investigation:
- Why is the test being ordered?
- What would be the consequences of not ordering the test?
- How good is the test at discriminating between health and disease?
- How will the test influence patient management and outcome?
- What are the risks associated with the test (particularly if it is invasive)?
- How will incidental findings affect the patient?

Consequences of test results

The results of some tests may have major long-term health and other implications. This includes viral serology for tests such as HIV or hepatitis B. A positive result might have profound implications for long-term health, insurance or family members, and counselling around the potential consequences of a positive (or negative) test is necessary. Genetic testing of an individual may also have implications for relatives and may need exploration; for example, non-paternity might become apparent.

Adverse outcomes of a test include side effects, complications and failure of the investigation to achieve a desired result (e.g. failure of an attempted pleural aspirate to yield fluid or no diagnostic tissue obtained with a renal biopsy). Such risks are not fixed but will vary dramatically depending upon the patient's circumstances and other health issues.

Further testing

Sometimes there may be uncertainty about a diagnosis that can only be resolved by investigations which were not specifically ordered as part of the original request for testing. If these investigations fall outside the scope of the original consent given by the patient, the treating doctor should establish whether further discussion with, and consent from, the patient is necessary before proceeding.

4 Risks of tests

Table 4.1 Relative radiation doses

Investigation	Dose (mSv)	Number of CXR	Cancer risk
Extremity X-ray	0.01	0.5	1 in 2,000,000
Chest X-ray	0.02	1	1 in 1,000,000
Abdominal X-ray	0.14	7	1 in 150,000
V/Q scan	0.7	50	1 in 20,000
Lumbar spine X-ray	1.3	65	1 in 15,000
Head CT	2	100	1 in 10,000
Bone scan	4	200	1 in 5000
Barium enema	7	350	1 in 3000
Chest CT	8	400	1 in 2500
Standard PET scan	8	400	1 in 2500
Abdominal CT	10–15	500–750	1 in 1500

Figure 4.1 Peripheral limb ischaemia due to cholesterol embolisation

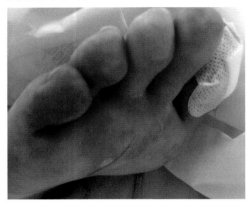

Figure 4.2 Renal biopsy shows show intravascular cholesterol crystals, which are seen as cholesterol clefts in histologically processed biopsies

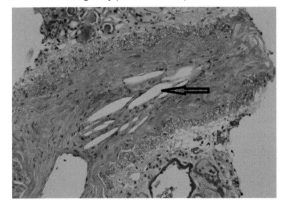

Clinical Investigations at a Glance, First Edition. Jonathan Gleadle, Jordan Li and Tuck Yong. © 2017 John Wiley & Sons, Ltd. Published 2017 by John Wiley & Sons, Ltd.

Radiation

Always consider whether the potential benefits of a test clearly outweigh its risks. Many radiological tests use ionising **radiation** (e.g. X-rays). This has potential risks, most notably the promotion of cancer. The risk of such tests is usually linked to the dose of radiation that each test exposes a patient to and varies according to the test (see Table 4.1). For many tests the dose of radiation received is not substantially elevated above background radiation, so that the risk to the patient is low. However, for some individuals, multiple high-exposure tests may pose a significant risk, and greater precautions need be taken for young patients, the foetus in utero and for particularly vulnerable organs (e.g. testes and ovaries).

MRI and ultrasound scans appear to have no or low risk of radiation-associated risks. However, for MRI, precautions need to be considered or the test avoided for those with particular metallic implants.

Contrast

Iodinated radiographic contrast may cause renal failure. Patients at particular risk include those with impaired renal function, those systemically unwell, those taking other potentially nephrotoxic medications and those with dehydration or hypotension. If it is essential that at-risk patients undergo a test that includes the administration of contrast, then the patient should be optimally hydrated, often including the administration of intravenous saline, and some centres administer *N*-acetylcysteine.

Gadolinium contrast for MRI carries a rare risk in patients with renal impairment of a skin condition called nephrogenic systemic fibrosis (or nephrogenic fibrosing dermopathy). Whilst this condition is rare, the use of gadolinium is contraindicated in patients with stage 4 or 5 CKD (eGFR <30 mL/min/ 1.73m^2).

Blood tests and needles

Venepuncture to obtain blood for tests is relatively safe with very rare risks. In patients with profound abnormalities of coagulation, large bruises can be produced. Errors may arise from misinterpretation of haemolysed samples, laboratory errors or misidentification of samples or patients. Arterial punctures to obtain arterial blood gases or to access the arterial tree for imaging studies carry greater risk of local bleeding, bruising and false aneurysms, particularly in patients with coagulation problems, and risk increases with the size of needle used. Infections at the site of needle insertion or introduction of bacteria into the circulation are rare but can occur. Specific measures such as bed rest, compression devices or sutures may be used to reduce the occurrence of bleeding. The insertion of catheters into the vascular tree can lead to arterial dissection, the displacement or generation of emboli and a syndrome called **cholesterol embolisation**. This is a condition most commonly seen after invasive vascular procedures such as coronary angiography, in which there is embolisation containing cholesterol crystals and other material, which can lead to renal impairment or failure, peripheral limb ischaemia (Figure 4.1), a livedo reticularis rash and sometimes an inflammatory response that includes eosinophilia and an elevated CRP. Biopsies of affected tissues, such as skin, gut or kidney, can show intravascular cholesterol crystals, which are seen as cholesterol clefts in histologically processed biopsies (Figure 4.2).

Endoscopic investigations

Gastrointestinal endoscopies, bronchoscopy, cystoscopy and hysteroscopy are frequently performed investigations that carry a small risk of bleeding and perforation. Antiplatelet agents or anticoagulants may need to be withheld prior to these procedures and sometimes after, depending on interventions performed to reduce the risk of bleeding. Colonoscopy involves bowel preparation, which can rarely result in volume depletion and electrolyte disturbances. Transbronchial biopsy performed during bronchoscopy is associated with the risk of pneumothorax.

Biopsies

Biopsies of organs or lumps are associated with significant risks of bleeding, and of damage to other neighbouring structures. Biopsies of lesions may be associated with sampling error depending on the approach used to obtain the sample, which can lead to false-negative results. Optimisation of blood clotting, including the cessation of antiplatelet agents (such as aspirin) or anticoagulation, may be required to reduce such risks. Blood pressure should be controlled and post-biopsy protocols often include a period of bed rest and close observations of the biopsy site, pulse and blood pressure.

Tests may lead to the identification of asymptomatic or incidental findings. This may lead to substantial worry or to further tests, such as biopsies or resection, which can be associated with considerable harm.

It is important to remember that tests may be wrong. Hyperkalaemia might be due to haemolysis, a low haemoglobin might be due to dilution in blood taken from a drip arm, an X-ray could be mislabelled with the wrong identity, a low oxygen tension could be because venous blood was sampled rather than arterial blood. If a result is surprising, question it; consider a repeat or an independent method of confirmation.

Tests are not treatments

If a patient is unwell, treat the patient. Do not wait for the result of a test. If a patient has meningism and you suspect bacterial meningitis, give antibiotics; do not wait 2 hours for a CT scan of the head, another hour to do a lumbar puncture and two more hours before the cerebrospinal fluid microscopy result is available to you.

5 Genetic tests

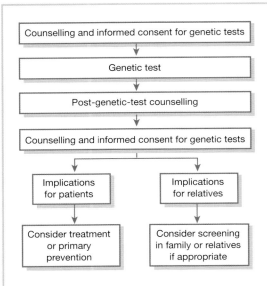

Counselling and informed consent for genetic tests

↓

Genetic test

↓

Post-genetic-test counselling

↓

Counselling and informed consent for genetic tests

↓

Implications for patients | Implications for relatives

Consider treatment or primary prevention | Consider screening in family or relatives if appropriate

Cautions about genetic testing
- Many current testing methods do not detect all mutations that might occur in a gene.
- Genetic testing may not produce a clinically useful result if a variant of unknown clinical significance is identified.
- Genetic tests usually provide probabilistic, not deterministic, information and do not definitively predict a clinical outcome.
- There may be a number of different genes that can cause a disease; some of these genes may not have been identified as yet.
- A mutation in one gene can cause different diseases.
- In a single tumour there may be a wide range of tumour associated mutations which vary between the different cells making up a cancer
- The technologies involved in genetic testing are wide ranging and rapidly evolving and include light microscopic examination of chromosomes to visualise chromosomal aberrations, PCR tests for specific mutations, DNA sequencing of specific genes, gene expression studies utilising microarrays and 'next generation' sequencing of all expressed exomes or even whole genomes.

Table 5.1 Common genetic test in clinical practice

Genetic disorder	Indications for genetic tests	Gene involved	Clinical usage
Cystic fibrosis	Diagnosis	*GFTR*	Diagnosis and drug metabolism
Haemochromatosis	Family history, especially siblings, with hereditary haemochromatosis	*HFE* mutation *C282Y*, especially homozygotes	Risk prediction, primary prevention for cirrhosis; counselling for genetic testing among asymptomatic people
Familial hypercholesterolemia (FH)	Family history of premature coronary artery disease	DNA testing and low-density lipoprotein cholesterol level measurement	Primary prevention; cascade testing of relatives of people diagnosed with FH
Huntington disease	Family history of Huntington disease	Mutations in the *HTT* gene cause Huntington disease	Risk prediction and counselling
Factor V Leiden thrombophilia	Spontaneous venous thromboembolism (VTE)	Mutation in the F5 gene causes factor V Leiden thrombophilia	VTE risk prediction and primary prevention
Breast cancer	Family history of breast/ovarian or other types of *BRCA*-related cancer	*BRCA1* and *BRCA2* genes	Risk prediction for referral for BRCA genetic counselling, chemoprevention
Colon cancer	Newly diagnosed colorectal cancer or known Lynch syndrome in family	Mutation of *MLH1, MSH2, MSH6, PMS2* or *EPCAM* gene increases the risk of developing Lynch syndrome	Diagnostic test and screening, cascade testing of relatives

Clinical Investigations at a Glance, First Edition. Jonathan Gleadle, Jordan Li and Tuck Yong. © 2017 John Wiley & Sons, Ltd. Published 2017 by John Wiley & Sons, Ltd.

A genetic test is 'the analysis of human DNA, RNA, chromosomes, proteins, and certain metabolites in order to detect heritable disease-related genotypes, mutations, phenotypes, or karyotypes for clinical purposes'. Genetic testing has had an increasing role in the diagnosis and management of many diseases as the understanding of the genetic contributions to disease have expanded and the technologies for genetic tests have become more sophisticated.

Counselling and informed consent around such tests may be particularly important, and written consent is often appropriate. Genetic counselling involves information-giving by specifically trained professionals with discussion and exploration of the implications for the individual and their family in a framework that is unique for each person. Genetic counselling is usually required before and after predictive genetic tests, following a positive genetic carrier test and following an abnormal result on a prenatal diagnostic or screening test and for decision-making about tests likely to provide uncertain results and/or to have significant implications for the patient and their family. Genetic testing may have profound diagnostic, prognostic and social implications, including the potential demonstration of non-paternity or non-maternity. In younger individuals in whom consent may be complicated it may be appropriate to defer predictive genetic testing until the individual is older and able to make their own informed decisions around testing.

An individual's ethnic background may provide important clues to their chances of inheriting particular genetic disorders; for example, the high prevalence of thalassaemia in parts of the world where malaria was or is endemic.

Many common diseases, such as diabetes, dementia, hypertension, osteoarthritis and obesity, are multifactorial with important genetic contributions. Large-scale genome-wide association studies involving thousands of subjects and thousands of DNA markers (single nucleotide polymorphisms) are identifying some of the genes associated with these diseases. However, most of these discoveries are not yet helpful for definitely predicting disease risk, and the interactions of multiple genetic variants (many with modest relative risk) with environmental effects are likely to make accurate predictions for any individual difficult.

Tests may be diagnostic and help to provide a diagnosis in an affected individual or predictive and attempt to determine the chances of an individual or a relative being affected in the future. There are different types of genetic test that may be used clinically:

- **Somatic cell genetic testing** involves testing tissue such as cancer for non-heritable mutations. This may be for diagnostic purposes or to assist in selecting treatment for a known cancer (e.g. testing for *K-Ras* mutations in colorectal cancer to guide treatment with anti-epidermal-growth-factor receptor treatments).
- **Diagnostic testing for heritable mutations** involves testing an affected person to identify the underlying mutation(s) responsible for the disease. This may involve testing one or more genes for a heritable mutation (Table 5.1). Sometimes it may be difficult to distinguish a disease causing mutation from a polymorphism.
- **Predictive testing for heritable mutations** involves testing an unaffected person for a germline mutation identified in relatives. The risk of disease may vary according to the gene, the mutation, its pattern of inheritance and the family history.
- **Carrier testing for heritable mutations** involves testing for the presence of a mutation that does not place the person at increased risk of developing the disease, but does increase the risk of having an affected child developing the disease.
- **Pharmacogenetic testing** for a genetic variant that alters the way a drug is metabolised.

There are many genetic tests that are used in clinical practice. Commonly used examples are summarised in Table 5.1.

6 Principles of radiological investigations

Figure 6.1 **X-ray** of left ankle shows no evidence of fracture

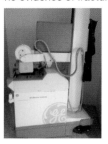 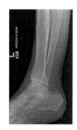

Advantages

Easily accessible
Inexpensive
Quick to perform

Disadvantages

Do not provide much anatomical details
Expose the patient to ionising radiation

Figure 6.2 Abdominal **CT** shows gas within the bladder and renal pelvis of the transplant kidney due to emphysematous cystitis

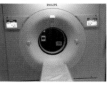 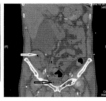

Advantages

Non-invasive
Provides excellent anatomical detail not hindered by bowel gas or obesity

Disadvantages

High ionising radiation
Higher cost compared to ultrasound
Possible contrast reaction
Significant detection of incidental anomalies

Figure 6.3 **MRI** of the left ankle shows no osteomyelitis but a fluid collection in anteromedial distal shin

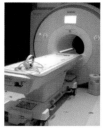 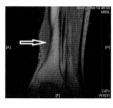

Advantages

No radiation exposure
High sensitivity to a wide range of pathologies
Functional imaging and metabolic imaging

Disadvantages

Lengthy scanning times and expensive
Contraindicated in patients with a pacemaker, defibrillator

Figure 6.4 **Ultrasound** of left shin shows a demarcated area of subcutaneous collection

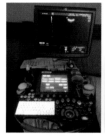 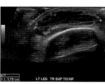

Advantages

No ionising radiation exposure
Can be used to follow up patient's progression
Non-invasive
Relatively inexpensive
Safe in obstetric use
Can be performed at the bedside for critical ill patient

Disadvantages

Operator-dependence
Imaging being limited by obesity, scarring, bowel gas and bone
Can be time-consuming especially to perform a Doppler ultrasound

Figure 6.5 **Transthoracic echocardiogram** shows no vegetation

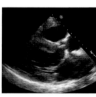 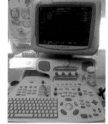

Figure 6.6 **Radionuclide** (Sestamibi) exercise cardiac perfusion scan shows no reversible ischaemia

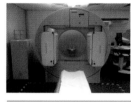 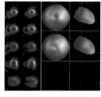

Advantages

Standardised technique
High sensitivity
Provide functional and anatomical assessment of organs

Disadvantages

Images have poor spatial resolution
Require injection of radiopharmaceutical

Table 6.2 Contraindications to MRI

Absolute contraindications	Relative contraindications
• Cardiac pacemaker or defibrillator	• Stents
• Metallic foreign body in eye	• Stapes implant
• Deep brain stimulator	• Drug-infusion pump
• Ferrous aneurysm clips	• Neuro- or bone-growth stimulator
• Gunshot close to vital structures	• Ocular prosthesis
• Cochlear implant	• Penile prosthesis
• Drug infusion devices	• Any implant or mechanical device
• Swan-Ganz catheters	
• Some dental implants	

Plain X-ray

X-rays are part of the high-energy end of the electromagnetic spectrum. X-rays are able to ionise atoms and break molecular bonds as they penetrate tissues, and hence are called ionising radiation. An X-ray picture is a result of the interaction of ionising radiation with different tissues as it passes through the body (Figure 6.1). As a result, X-rays moving through tissues of different densities are displayed distinctly depending on the amount of radiation absorbed. In plain X-rays, there are four distinct densities: gas, fat, soft tissue and fluid, and calcified structures. Air absorbs the least amount of X-rays and appears black, whereas calcified structures (e.g. bone) absorb the most, leading to a white density. Soft tissue and fluid have intermediate absorptive capacity and therefore appear grey.

CT

An X-ray tube emits focused X-ray beams as it rotates around the patient. Variable amounts of X-rays are registered by detectors, depending on the tissue composition. This information is transformed into a cross-sectional image using mathematical algorithms (Figure 6.2). Spiral or helical CT enables continuous scanning as the body is moved quickly through the gantry allowing a larger volume of tissue data to be recorded.

Pregnancy and a previous adverse reaction to contrast medium are contraindications to CT. If contrast is required, renal impairment is a relative contraindication.

Ultrasound

A transducer transmits a short pulse of ultrasound into the body and, depending on the tissue characteristics and interfaces, the beam is partially reflected, absorbed or transmitted. An image is generated based on the reflected ultrasound beam (Figure 6.4). Doppler ultrasound is based on the frequency alteration of the reflected ultrasound beam by moving blood, and the blood flow velocity can be calculated to assess a vascular stenosis. In colour Doppler ultrasound, the information is colour coded for velocity and direction. It can also be used to guide biopsy of a lesion or drainage of fluid collections.

Echocardiography

Echocardiography uses ultrasound in the 2–7 MHz range to provide detailed information about the structure and function of the heart. Using two-dimensional ultrasound, cardiac chambers and major blood vessels can be measured (Figure 6.5). Function of the left and right ventricles and motion of cardiac valves may be assessed. The integration of Doppler ultrasound techniques allows additional information from estimation of blood flow velocities within the heart. Colour Doppler can be useful to demonstrate patterns of flow and is particularly useful for valvular regurgitation. Windows for ultrasound of the heart within the thorax can be limited. Air within the lung conducts ultrasound poorly, ribs can obscure views and body habitus can affect image quality.

Radionuclide scans

Radionuclide scans use short-lived isotopes to image specific body systems. A functional image is obtained from detecting radioactive emissions and based on the concentration and distribution of the radioactive tracer (Figure 6.6). Mathematical analysis of activity can be performed and reported as half-clearance times, ejection fractions and relative perfusion.

Pregnancy is a relative contraindication.

MRI

MRI utilises strong magnetic fields and radiofrequency pulses to generate sectional images of the body in any plane (Figure 6.3). The image generated is determined by the density of protons or water molecules within the tissue and other physical characteristics of the tissue. Two sequences, T1- and T2-weighted, are usually obtained based on the rate of return to equilibrium of perturbed protons. Fat and subacute haemorrhage have high signal intensity (white) on T1-weighted images. Watery media such as cerebrospinal fluid (CSF) and oedematous tissue have low signal intensity (black) on T1 images but high signal intensity (white) on T2-weighted images. T1 images are used for anatomical definition and tissue characterisation, while T2 images are useful to evaluate pathology. The common sequences are listed in Table 6.1.

Table 6.1 Common MRI sequences

MRI sequence	Main indications
T1-weighted imaging	Good for showing anatomy; fluid (CSF) showing low signal intensity (black), muscle showing intermediate signal intensity (grey), fat showing high signal intensity (white), brain grey matter showing intermediate signal intensity (grey) white matter showing hyperintensity (white)
T2-weighted imaging	Good for showing pathology; fluid (CSF) showing high signal intensity (white), muscle showing intermediate signal intensity (grey), fat showing high signal intensity (white), brain grey matter showing intermediate signal intensity (grey), white matter showing hypointensity (dark)
Proton density imaging	Good for showing both anatomy and pathology. This provides excellent distinction between fluid and cartilage, ideal in the assessment of joints
Fat saturation	The signal from fat is suppressed; good to highlight structure on T1-weighted imaging
Short tau inversion recovery (STIR)	This suppresses fat signal more effectively than fat saturation. It is excellent for showing fluid, such as bone oedema
Fluid attenuation inversion recovery (FLAIR)	This suppresses fluid signal (CSF); good for showing cerebral lesions, such as multiple sclerosis plaques
Diffusion-weighted imaging (DWI)	This shows water diffusion patterns and can reveal microscopic details about tissue architecture, good for showing ischaemic stroke, active demyelination, encephalitis
Apparent diffusion coefficient (ADC)	This sequence measures diffusion; good for showing early ischaemia, the age of lesions.

Contraindications

Table 6.2 shows some of the common absolute and relative contraindications to MRI. Gadolinium-based contrast is contraindicated in advanced chronic kidney disease (eGFR <30 mL/min/1.73 m^2). It is also contraindicated in morbid obesity when the patient's girth and weight exceed the limits of the scanner.

7 Cytology and histopathology tests

The main goals of histopathology tests:
- make a diagnosis
- differentiate benign and malignant lesions
- assist monitoring disease progression
- guide management, especially in the management of malignancy
- screen a disease such as cervical smear
- classify the future risk of the disease.

Table 7.1 The types of specimen used for histopathology examination

- Larger specimens include whole organs or parts, which are removed during surgical operations.
- Small pieces of tissue are removed as biopsies, which include excision biopsies, or a core biopsy.
- Individual cells rather than groups of cells can be obtained via a fine-needle aspiration (FNA). This is performed using a thinner needle than that used in a core biopsy, but with a similar technique.

Table 7.2 Common cytology in clinical practice

- Cervical cytology
- Sputum cytology
- Bronchoscopy washing and brushing
- Urine cytology
- Pleural fluid cytology
- Ascitic fluid cytology
- Breast lump FNA
- Thyroid and salivary FNA
- Cerebrospinal fluid cytology

Figure 7.3 Perls' Prussian blue stain

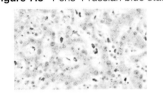

Figure 7.1 H&E stain shows a normal glomerulus

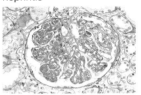

Figure 7.2 PAS stain shows mesangial deposits in lupus nephritis

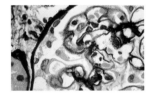

Figure 7.4 Silver stain shows epimembranous spikes in a patient with membranous nephropathy

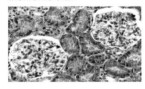

Figure 7.5 Masson's trichrome stain

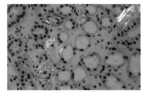

Table 7.3 The list of common special stains

Stain	Highlighted tissues	Utility
Periodic acid Schiff (PAS) (Figure 7.2)	Stain structures containing a high proportion of carbohydrates, such as glycogen, glycoproteins, proteoglycans typically found in connective tissues, mucus and basement membranes	Stain kidney and liver biopsies
Perls' Prussian blue (Figure 7.3)	Detect ferric iron (Fe^{3+}) in tissue preparations, blood or bone marrow smears	Abnormal amounts of iron in bone marrow can indicate haemochromatosis and haemosiderosis
Gomori methenamine silver stain (Figures 7.4)	Identify fungi, basement membrane and pneumocystis carinii in tissue specimens	Kidney and lung biopsies
Ziehl Neelsen stain	Detect and identify acid-fast bacilli in tissue	Identify tuberculosis in lung tissue
Masson's trichrome (Figure 7.5)	Display collagenous connective tissue fibres in tissue specimens	Differentiates collagen and smooth muscle in tumours
Congo red (Figures 7.6 and 7.7)	Stain amyloid by hydrogen bonding and other tissue components by electrochemical bonds	Amyloidosis

Figure 7.7 Congo red stain with birefringence

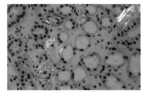

Table 7.4 Application of immunohistochemistry

- Diagnosis of primary malignant tumours as some tumours are so poorly differentiated that their histogenesis is not apparent on routine H&E-stained sections
- Determining the likely site of origin of metastatic tumours
- Categorisation of leukaemias and lymphomas (T and B cell markers)
- Detection of molecules that have prognostic or therapeutic significance; e.g. oestrogen and progesterone, HER2 receptor
- Detection of minimal disease or small volume residual tumour – highlighting small numbers of tumour cells, which may be difficult to appreciate on routine sections

Figure 7.6 Congo red stain in a kidney biopsy with amyloidosis

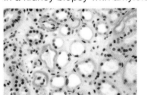

Figure 7.8 Immunofluorescent microscopy shows IgG granular capillary wall deposit pattern

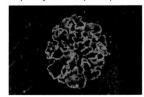

Figure 7.9 EM shows effacement of foot process consistent with minimal change disease

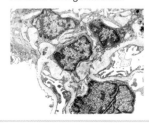

Clinical Investigations at a Glance, First Edition. Jonathan Gleadle, Jordan Li and Tuck Yong. © 2017 John Wiley & Sons, Ltd. Published 2017 by John Wiley & Sons, Ltd.

Histopathology is the examination of tissues (Table 7.1) from the body under a microscope to make a diagnosis and characterise disease.

Cytology and cytopathology

Cytology is the study of individual cells, and cytopathology is the study of individual cells in disease. Sampled fluid/tissue from a patient is smeared onto a slide and stained. This is then examined under the microscope to determine the number, type and characters of cells, which is useful in determining whether a disease is present and what is the likely diagnosis. Cytology is often used as a screening tool to look for disease and to decide whether or not more tests need to be performed (Table 7.2). The sampling techniques in cytology are: **exfoliative cytology** (the analysis of cells shed from body surfaces, such as cervical smear, urine and sputum cytology) and **aspiration cytology** (the analysis of cells from within a mass or organ). This involves a more invasive sampling procedure – FNA. A needle is inserted into the lesion usually under ultrasound or CT guidance to ensure that the suspicious area is being sampled. The cells retrieved are expressed onto a slide and prepared in a similar way to a cervical smear. If fluid is aspirated (e.g. from a thyroid cyst), it may be centrifuged so that the cell-containing sediment collects at the bottom of the tube, allowing the best material to be sampled for examination. Special stains are performed to highlight the cells and background material on the slide (see histopathology sections).

Frozen section histopathology

A frozen section is performed when immediate diagnosis is required during a surgical procedure because it will influence the type of surgery being performed. Time is crucial in performing a frozen section. The tissue will be examined on arrival by a pathologist who selects the area of most interest to be processed. It will be frozen using a cryostat or liquid nitrogen before sections are cut on a cooled microtome (cutting machine), mounted and stained. However, freezing results in some distortion of the tissue and a less satisfactory stain.

Usual histopathology

Prompt and adequate formalin fixation (with the exception of immunofluorescence (IF) and frozen-section specimens) is critical for histological samples.

Haematoxylin and eosin staining (H&E)

H&E staining (Figure 7.1) is used routinely in histopathology examination as it provides a very detailed view of the tissue by clearly staining cell structures, including the cytoplasm, nucleus, and organelles and extracellular components. This information is often sufficient to allow a disease diagnosis.

Special stains

Special stains can highlight specific tissue components to provide further characterisation (Table 7.3).

Immunohistochemistry staining

Immunohistochemistry staining combines anatomical, immunological and biochemical techniques for the identification of tissue components by means of a specific antigen–antibody reaction tagged with a visible label/dye. Immunohistochemistry makes it possible to visualise the distribution and localisation of specific cellular components within a cell or tissue on microscopic slides. The application of immunohistochemistry is listed in Table 7.4.

Immunofluorescence

Antibodies labelled with fluorescent dyes such as fluorescein isothiocyanate bind directly or indirectly to the antigen of interest (Figure 7.8). The fluorescence can then be quantified using a flow cytometer, array scanner or automated imaging instrument, or visualised using fluorescence or confocal microscopy.

Electron microscopy (EM)

EM utilises beams of electrons to magnify the cells and can magnify up to 2 million times, whereas the maximum power of a conventional light microscope is only 1000–2000 times. EM is helpful in diagnosing disease at this subcellular level (Figure 7.9). Examples include many types of kidney disease, such as minimal change disease or aggressive cancers that lose their normal proteins, making immunohistochemistry less useful in their identification.

The limitation of histopathology is the small sample size, the possibility of biopsy of adjacent non-pathological tissue, false-negative and false-positive staining, and the importance of expertise in analysis.

Molecular pathology and cytogenetics

Molecular pathology is the analysis of the genetic material (chromosomes and their DNA) of cells, and is an increasingly widely requested component of the pathology workup. Cytogenetics is the analysis of chromosomes. The two most commonly used techniques in molecular pathology and cytogenetics are fluorescence in-situ hybridisation (FISH) and direct sequencing of DNA.

FISH is a technique used to stain chromosomes to reveal areas where genes may have been deleted, duplicated or broken. Fluorescent labels to specific DNA sequences allow altered genes to be identified under a microscope. Direct sequencing of cell DNA is a way of looking at individual genes or groups of genes, to detect and characterise which mutation is present in a patient's tumour. This can be done traditionally (Sanger sequencing, capillary electrophoresis), or by next-generation sequencing.

For example, conventional histopathology can give a diagnosis of type of breast cancer, whether it has metastasised and whether it will respond to hormone and targeted therapies. Cytogenetics identify whether the patient has predisposing gene(s) mutation such as *BRCA1* and *BRCA2* that predisposed them to breast cancer, increase risk in the opposite breast and of developing other specific cancers (e.g. ovarian cancer). It also has implications for the patient's relatives and offspring. Did they inherit the faulty gene(s) and what are the chances that they will develop cancer in the future? By direct sequencing of the faulty gene, the close relatives of the patient can be screened for the mutation, after appropriate consent, allowing preventative steps to be taken.

8 Presenting at radiology and histopathology meetings

When presenting at a meeting it is important to ensure the following:

Identify the correct patient.
Succinct presentation of the clinical features.

Mrs Belinda Test is an 82-year-old woman. She was admitted from the emergency department last night with a 2-day history of worsening breathlessness and an episode of sharp right-sided chest pain the day before admission. She had recently been diagnosed to have lung cancer, treated with radiotherapy. She also has a history of ischaemic heart disease and congestive cardiac failure. Clinical examination revealed a sinus tachycardia and a temperature of 37.7 °C but no other abnormalities of note. Arterial blood gases showed hypoxaemia, the electrocardiogram showed T wave inversion in the inferior leads and she had a slightly elevated troponin T.

Formulate a differential diagnosis.

We made a provisional clinical diagnosis of pulmonary embolus, though our differential diagnosis also included pneumonia, progression of lung cancer and myocardial infarction with left ventricular failure.

Frame the question that the investigation is intended to address.

We would like to review her CXR and CTPA tests that were performed last night (Figures 8.1 and 8.2).

Mention previous test – e.g. old CXRs, CT scans, biopsies – that the current test should be compared against. Provide extra information that radiologist may ask.

We would like to compare with her pre-radiotherapy CXR (Figure 8.3).

Make a clear plan of who will inform the patients of the results, how that will occur and what is the plan for treatment, subsequent follow-up and the need for other tests.

Patient was informed of the results last night. She has been treated with low molecular weight heparin.

Ask radiologist questions.

Any evidence of right heart strain or failure given the mildly raised troponin T (Figure 8.4)?

Clinical Investigations at a Glance, First Edition. Jonathan Gleadle, Jordan Li and Tuck Yong. © 2017 John Wiley & Sons, Ltd. Published 2017 by John Wiley & Sons, Ltd.

Figure 8.1 (a) CXR shows reticular opacities in both lung fields in the upper/middle zones which are new compared with previous CXR. This may be radiation-induced changes. The right hilar/infrahilar soft-tissue opacity is stable (b) CXR lateral view

(a)

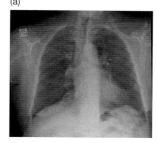

(b)

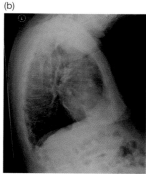

Figure 8.2 CTPA shows pulmonary arterial filling defects with non-occlusive thrombus in the segmental arteries

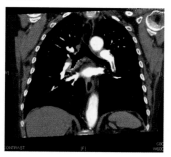

Figure 8.4 CTPA shows no reverse bowing of the interventricular septum to suggest right heart strain

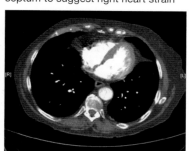

Figure 8.3 Previous CXR (8 weeks ago) shows volume loss involving the inferio-medial aspect of the right lower lobe with abnormal soft-tissue density in the right hilar/infrahilar region. The biopsy confirms lung squamous cell carcinoma

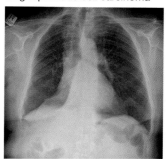

Many clinical units, particularly in hospitals, have regular meetings for the discussion of investigational tests. These commonly focus on the results of radiological or histological tests. There may be a review of all the X-rays undertaken the previous day or week or be the forum for planning further management, such as in the multidisciplinary meetings for cancer.

In such meetings, junior doctors or medical students are often expected to present the case followed by a discussion of the findings of the investigation by an expert pathologist or radiologist. When presenting at such meetings it is important to ensure that you:

• are discussing the correct patient and that the investigational findings refer to them;

• present the patient's case succinctly, focusing on the clinical features that are relevant to establishing a diagnosis;

• formulate a differential diagnosis;

• frame the question that the investigation is intended to address;

• mention any previous tests – such as old CXRs, CT scans, biopsies – that the current test should be compared against;

• are ready to answer follow-up questions about the patient's condition, other tests, response to treatment and so on;

• make a clear plan of who will inform the patient of the results, how that will occur and what the plan is for subsequent follow-up, need for other tests, treatment plan and so on.

9 Requesting tests

Requesting tests

Many clinical investigations require completion of a request form. It is essential that this is filled out accurately and completely.

The identity of the patient, their address, identification numbers, age, gender, date of birth and location (e.g. ward) must be completed accurately, legibly and completely.

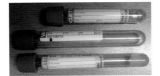

It is extremely important that specimen containers are correctly labelled with the correct information on the patient identification.

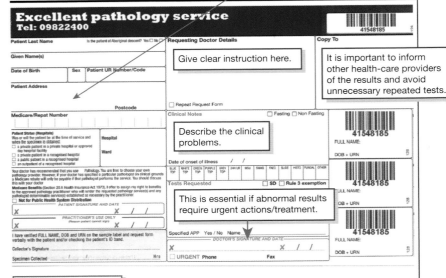

Give clear instruction here.

It is important to inform other health-care providers of the results and avoid unnecessary repeated tests.

Describe the clinical problems.

This is essential if abnormal results require urgent actions/treatment.

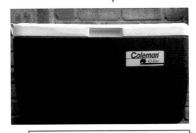

Ensure correct specimen handling and transportation.

How will the patient get to the testing facility?

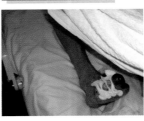

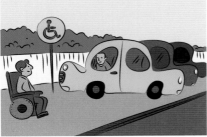

Do they need transport arranged? What is their mobility like?

Will they need particular assistance?

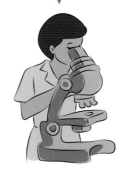

Request Form for Imaging

The identity of the patient, their address, identification numbers and age, gender, date of birth and location (e.g. ward) must be completed accurately, legibly and completely.

Describe the clinical problems.

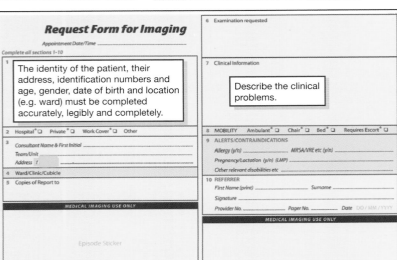

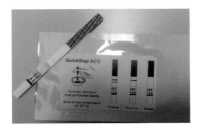

Other relevant conditions need to be indicated on the request form: obesity, claustrophobia, hearing impairment, visual impairment, colonisation with an antibiotic-resistant organism such as MRSA or VRE, seropositivity with blood-borne viruses such as HIV and hepatitis B or C. Does the patient need an interpreter present?

Clinical Investigations at a Glance, First Edition. Jonathan Gleadle, Jordan Li and Tuck Yong. © 2017 John Wiley & Sons, Ltd. Published 2017 by John Wiley & Sons, Ltd.

Many clinical investigations require completion of a request form. It is essential that this is filled out accurately and fully.

The **identity** of the patient, their address, identification numbers and age, gender, date of birth and location (e.g. ward) must be completed accurately, legibly and completely. Preprinted sticky labels or computer printouts may improve the accuracy of this information, but only if the correct patient's label is stuck onto the correct form.

Describe the clinical problem and the question the investigation is intended to address. More complete information is vital in guiding the correct investigation, interpretation and reporting of the test result. It may be appropriate to ask specific directed questions on the request form. Include the details of any previous relevant tests to which comparison should or could be made. If relevant, has the patient been fasting; the dose and timing of drug administration for drug levels should be given.

Whilst completing the request form it may be appropriate to consider if there are any contraindications or patient-specific risks involved in the testing (e.g. the risks of intravenous contrast worsening renal function in a patient with CKD). Does the patient have any relevant allergies to contrast, to other medications, to latex, and so on?

For some investigations, such as MRI, specific precautions and enquiry need to be directed to avoid patients with, for example, metallic implants being exposed to risk.

Other relevant conditions

It is important to consider whether the patient has any conditions or problems that might increase risk, require modifications to the test or particular precautions. These might include obesity, claustrophobia, hearing impairment, visual impairment, colonisation with an antibiotic-resistant organism such as methicillin-resistant *Staphylococcus aureus* (MRSA) or vancomycin-resistant enterococcus (VRE), seropositivity with blood-borne viruses such as HIV and hepatitis B or C. Indicate these clearly on the request form. Does the patient need an interpreter present?

If the patient is a woman of childbearing age, please consider whether she is or might be pregnant, especially if the studies will use ionising radiation.

Economic considerations

Financial issues can have both stimulatory and inhibitory influences on whether a particular investigation is undertaken. Restraint is required when requesting expensive tests, and these should be reserved for situations with a definite indication. The high cost of some investigations may limit their availability to specialised referral facilities (e.g. MRI and PET scans).

How will the patient get to the testing facility? Do they need transport arranged? What is their mobility like? Will they need particular assistance? Who will take the patient home?

Ensure the request form includes the **name** of the requesting doctor, signed if appropriate, that this is easily legible and a contact number. Consider how the test will be communicated to that doctor if a significant abnormality is detected or if clarification is needed.

Labelling specimen containers

It is extremely important that specimen containers are correctly labelled with the correct information, especially patient identification. Incorrect labelling, especially when another patient's identification sticker is used, can have potential deleterious consequences and significant medicolegal ramifications. This is particularly critical for important tests, such as blood typing.

Pre-investigation preparation

Some investigations require certain preparation. For example, an abdominal CT scan requires the patient to have oral contrast at a certain time prior to the examination. Some investigations may involve prior dietary restrictions.

Using the correct specimen containers and specimen handling

Ensure that the correct container is used. Under no circumstances should a specimen be transferred from one type of container to another (e.g. EDTA into heparin), nor should the cap of blood collection tubes be placed on the wrong tubes, as this may lead to erroneous results. Some investigations require specimen preservatives. If uncertain, always check with the local laboratory regarding the correct container to use so that the patient is not inconvenienced and resources are not wasted.

Some specimens should be delivered urgently to the laboratory to be processed, and some should not be left on the bench at room temperature for an extended period of time.

10 Therapeutic drug monitoring

Which drugs need monitoring?
- Drugs with marked pharmacokinetic variability
- Drugs with therapeutic and adverse effects related to drug concentration
- Drugs with a narrow therapeutic index
- Drugs where the desired therapeutic effect is difficult to monitor
- Drugs where undertreatment cannot be recognised clinically and can have significant consequences

Indications for drug monitoring
- After initiating treatment
- After adjusting dose
- Suboptimal response from the treatment
- Suspected non-compliance
- Starting or stopping a potentially interacting drug
- During pregnancy
- Developing renal or hepatic impairment
- To assess for drug toxicity or suspected overdose
- To confirm abstinence
- To assist diagnosis, as adverse drug effects may mimic disease state

Table 10.1 Drugs for which therapeutic monitoring is commonly required

Drug	Recommended therapeutic range	Sampling time	Half-life	Time to steady state (days)
Digoxin	0.5–2.0 µg/L	>8 h post-dose	36 hours	7–10
Amiodarone	1.0–2.5 mg/L	Pre-dose trough	40–55 days	N/A
Phenytoin	10–20 mg/L	Trough (any time once at steady state)	24 hours	5–7
Carbamazepine	5.0–12 mg/L	Pre-dose trough	10–17 hours	7–10
Sodium valproate	50–100 mg/L	Pre-dose trough	15 hours	3–5
Lamotrigine	1.5–3.0 mg/L	Pre-dose trough	24 hours	5
Lithium	0.6–1.2 mmol/L	Pre-dose trough	18–24 hours	3–7
Gentamicin	<0.5–2 µg/L	Pre-dose trough	1–3 hours	1
Vancomycin	10–20 mg/L	Pre-dose trough	3–8 hours	1–2

Record the time of last dose on the request form

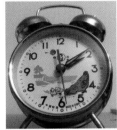

Use the correct collecting tube

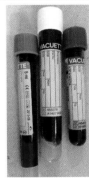

Figure 10.1 A sample of therapeutic monitoring AUC

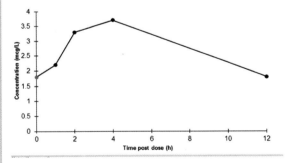

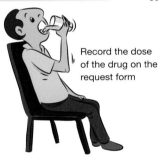

Record the dose of the drug on the request form

Information required for interpretation of drug concentration?
- Time of sample in relation to the last dose
- Duration of treatment with the current dose
- Dosing schedule
- Age and gender of patient
- Other drug therapy (potential for drug–drug interaction)
- Relevant medical history, especially liver and kidney disorders
- Reason for request (eg lack of effect, routine monitoring, suspected toxicity)

Therapeutic drug monitoring (TDM) refers to the individualisation of dosage by the measurement of plasma or blood concentrations of a medication to ensure plasma or blood drug concentrations are within a recommended therapeutic range. Variation in drug response between individuals can arise from two major sources: (a) dose and plasma concentration (pharmacokinetic variability) and (b) drug concentration at the receptor and the drug effect (pharmacodynamic variability).

Which drugs need monitoring?

Drugs that require therapeutic monitoring are those:
- with a marked pharmacokinetic variability;
- with therapeutic and adverse effects related to drug concentration;
- with a narrow therapeutic index;
- where the desired therapeutic effect is difficult to monitor;
- where undertreatment cannot be recognised clinically and can have significant consequences.

TDM is used in two important clinical situations: (a) in prevention of a condition such as seizures, arrhythmias or transplant rejection; (b) to avoid serious toxicity in drugs with a narrow therapeutic index, such as aminoglycosides and digoxin.

Examples of drugs that are commonly monitored are listed in Table 10.1.

Indications for therapeutic drug monitoring

For the majority of drugs, except immunosuppressants used in solid organ transplant, routine regular monitoring is not required. The common indications for TDM are listed on the opening page.

Sample collection

Usually, plasma or serum is used for drug assays, depending on the methods used. However, with cyclosporine, whole blood is assayed because of large shifts of drug between red cells and plasma with storage and temperature change. Some blood collecting tubes, especially those containing a gel to separate cells and plasma, may not be suitable for all drugs because of drug absorption by the gel or other components in the tube.

Timing of samples

The correct time of sampling is vital. Drug concentrations vary over the dosing interval and with duration of dosing in relation to achieving a steady state. The pre-dose or trough concentration is most often used as it is the least variable point in the dosing interval. For drugs with short half-lives in relation to the dosing interval, samples should be collected pre-dose. For drugs with long half-lives, such as phenytoin or amiodarone, samples collected at any point in the dosage interval can be satisfactory. For digoxin, any point after the distribution phase (i.e. after 6 hours post-dose) is acceptable. Therapeutic ranges are usually established using trough concentrations. Therefore, allowance will have to be made if samples were collected at other time points in the dosage interval.

Generally, it is best to take a blood sample for drug concentration measurement when a steady state has been reached unless there are concerns about toxicity. This does not apply to drugs with very long half-lives, such as amiodarone. If a sample is taken before steady state is reached, allowance needs to be made for this in interpreting the drug concentration.

The pharmacokinetic measurement most closely related to efficacy is the area under the concentration curve (AUC). AUC is a direct representation of total drug bioavailability and exposure during the time it takes for a drug to be excreted, and is calculated by dividing the amount of unchanged drug in circulation by the rate of clearance. A more simplified version of AUC known as abbreviated AUC, which only requires TDM during the first 4 hours after administration of a dose, can be used to simplify the monitoring requirements (Figure 10.1).

What information is required for interpretation of drug concentration?

Drug concentration needs to be interpreted in the context of the individual patient. Important information required for interpretation of a drug concentration is shown on the opening page.

Two other important factors need to be taken into consideration in interpreting drug concentrations: (a) protein binding and (b) active metabolites. Assays often measure total (bound and unbound) drug, whereas it is the unbound drug that produces a response. If binding is changed by disease states, displacement by another drug or nonlinearity in protein binding, the interpretation of total plasma or blood drug concentrations must be modified. Metabolites that may not be measured can contribute to the therapeutic response, and this needs to be taken into consideration with some drugs.

11 Investigations in resource-limited settings

Table 11.1 Recommended basic laboratory tests in resource-limited areas

Malaria microscopic evaluation
Haemoglobin, glucose measurement
Pulse oximetry
Urinalysis and microscopy examination
Microscopic evaluation of stool samples
Gram stain and cell count in cerebrospinal fluid samples
Acid-fast bacilli smear
Blood culture
HIV testing

Table 11.2 Common point-of-care tests

Blood glucose
Glycohaemoglobin (HbA1c)
Electrolytes
Urea and creatinine
Cardiac markers (troponin, BNP)
Coagulation study (INR)

Most clinical investigations and guidelines described in this textbook and other resources have been developed for clinicians practising in resource-rich developed countries, where advanced laboratory testing and imaging are readily available. However, these rarely take into consideration resource-constrained developing countries. Resource limitation may arise because of lack of accessibility, such as rural settings, patients' inability to pay for a service, or a low-income society/country where health resources are scarce.

In resource-limited settings, approaches to clinical investigations may vary; access to reliable diagnostic testing is severely limited and precise diagnosis more difficult. Allocation of resources to diagnostic laboratory testing has not usually been a priority for resource-limited health-care systems, but unreliable and inaccurate laboratory diagnostic testing leads to unnecessary expenditures. Uninvestigated deaths in developing countries are generally attributed to infectious diseases, most commonly tuberculosis, HIV infection and malaria, but the accuracy of these estimates remains uncertain in the absence of laboratory confirmation. Quality laboratory testing is needed to confirm clinical diagnoses, guide appropriate treatment, conduct accurate infectious disease surveillance and direct public health-care policy.

Clinical investigation in resource-limited settings

In resource-limited circumstances, clinicians can consider the following measures:
• Employ a thorough history-taking and physical examination to make a diagnosis or to narrow the diagnostic possibilities. Reliance on clinical diagnosis is attractive in resource-limited areas with a high prevalence of disease. It requires no extra cost and no special laboratory equipment or supplies; however, diagnoses based on clinical signs and symptoms can be nonspecific, unreliable and associated with increased mortality. Furthermore, in resource-limited situations it is particularly important to focus on whether an investigation can alter the patients' management or outcome.
• Use whatever basic investigations that are available to investigate and manage patients. Often, a resource-limited environment will make the clinician consider more carefully which investigation to perform and consider the factors that might influence the interpretation of the results. For example, if magnetic resonance imaging is not available in a rural health centre, the clinician will have to decide if the suspected diagnosis can be confirmed with other, more simple radiological investigations.
• The inability to collect patient samples results in missed opportunities to perform laboratory tests as an integral part of clinical care. This can be overcome by supplying consumables such as blood vacutainers, sterile urine-specimen containers and training personnel.

• Transport can be an obstacle. A courier, patient's carer/family member or ward personnel may help to transport the specimen.
• Monitor test quality routinely, establish systems for laboratory accreditation, implement standard written operating procedures (including quality-control procedures) and improve knowledge or skill of supervisors and technical personnel of laboratory.
• Develop affordable, simple, rapid diagnostic tests.

Set up basic simple tests in resource-limited area

In resource-limited areas, the basic tests listed in Table 11.1 should be guided by local disease prevalence but could include attempts to establish.

Utilisation of new technologies, such as non-culture-based methods (e.g. rapid malaria and HIV tests) for diagnosis of infectious diseases, offers the potential to overcome short-term logistical and educational barriers. These approaches allow more-widespread test availability and reproducibility without immediate infrastructure improvement.

Point-of-care testing

Recognising the needs within resource-limited areas, there are several point-of-care tests that can be used in clinical practice. Point-of-care testing can be defined as pathology testing performed on-site during the patient consultation. It allows a rapid test result to be generated and used to make an immediate, informed clinical decision.

There have been significant technological and analytical advances in point-of-care testing devices and reagent manufacture. An increasing range of tests (Table 11.2) can now be performed on very small sample volumes in less than 10 min. The analytical performance of these point-of-care tests can be equivalent to that of a laboratory test.

There is growing evidence to support the clinical, operational and economic effectiveness of point-of-care testing in resource-limited areas. Point-of-care testing can be helpful in improving diabetic control by reductions in HbA1c or increased time in therapeutic range for INR. In acute settings, the ability to perform tests such as potassium and blood gases by point-of-care testing in less than 5 min on an acutely ill patient can inform initial management. For example, being able to measure potassium levels in a patient presenting with severe vomiting or CKD in a remote health centre is particularly useful. Similarly, the ability to confirm suspected acute coronary syndrome using troponin point-of-care testing is extremely beneficial. These relate to reduced length of stay in emergency departments or reduced mortality through more rapid and effective risk stratification and treatment.

12 Tests for outpatient, inpatient and patients in intensive care

Investigation in intensive care unit

Figure 12.1 An indwelling arterial line enables monitoring of blood pressure

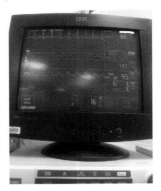

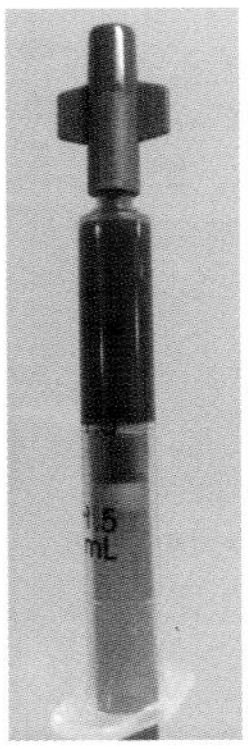

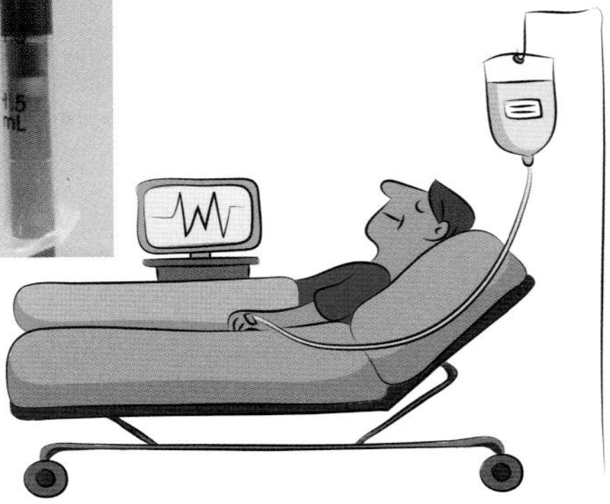

Figure 12.4 Ventilator

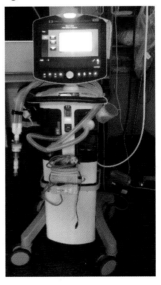

Figure 12.2 An arterial line provides ready access to samples of bloods for arterial blood gases test

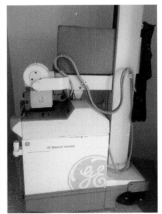

Daily determinations of:
- FBC
- electrolytes (including calcium, phosphate and magnesium)
- renal function
- liver function tests
- coagulation screen
- additional parameters related to nutrition if the patient is receiving total parenteral nutrition

Outpatient and inpatient tests
Why do we need this test?
What are we looking for?
Does the test require specific preparation, transport arrangements?
What are the possible results?
How will it affect the patient?
How and when will you know the result?
How and when will the result be communicated to the patient?
How often should the abnormal tests be repeated?

Figure 12.3 Automated arterial blood gas analyser

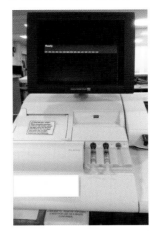

Figure 12.5 Bedside X-ray; daily CXR is needed in intubated and ventilated patients looking for ET tube placement, presence of pneumothoraces, pleural effusions and pulmonary infiltrates

Figure 12.8 Non-bedside investigations, such as CT and MRI

Figure 12.6 Bedside ultrasound

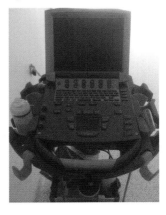

Figure 12.7 Bedside echocardiogram

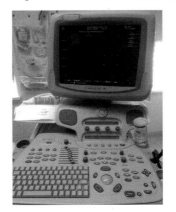

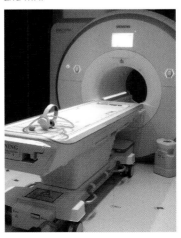

Clinical Investigations at a Glance, First Edition. Jonathan Gleadle, Jordan Li and Tuck Yong. © 2017 John Wiley & Sons, Ltd. Published 2017 by John Wiley & Sons, Ltd.

Intensive-care patients

Patients in intensive care will usually undergo a large number of frequent investigations ensuring that their diagnosis, response to treatment and complications are carefully monitored.

Regular investigations

Many patients will have an indwelling arterial line enabling monitoring of blood pressure and ready access to samples of bloods for arterial blood gases and other blood tests. It is important to be aware that whilst pulse oximetry can provide accurate information about the patient's oxygenation, blood gas testing is vital to ensure adequate ventilation with carbon dioxide clearance and to look for the development of acidosis or alkalosis. Many units will have protocols in place for the frequency of testing for arterial blood gases, glucose and other blood tests (Figures 12.1, 12.2 and 12.3). Daily determinations of FBC, electrolytes, renal function, liver function tests, calcium, phosphate, magnesium and coagulation screen are commonly undertaken. Additional parameters related to nutrition will also be monitored if the patient is receiving total parenteral nutrition. Many patients will undergo daily CXRs particularly when intubated and ventilated looking for endotracheal (ET) tube placement, presence of pneumothoraces, pleural effusions and pulmonary infiltrates (Figures 12.4 and 12.5).

Diagnostic tests

Whilst intensive-care patients undergo a lot of testing, history and examination are still crucial to accurate diagnosis and care. For example, a comprehensive history of the contents of a drug overdose or the circumstances preceding an unconscious collapse are central to achieving an accurate diagnosis. The development of a deep-vein thrombosis, a petechial rash or a pericardial rub may be crucial in managing the patient but require careful examination. Furthermore, impaired conscious level, sedation, ET tubes, neuropathies and analgesia may mask or prevent communication of problems. Some investigations, such as ultrasound, echocardiography or endoscopies, can take place 'at the bedside', but others, such as CT scanning and nuclear medicine tests, will require moving the patient to the relevant department and confers additional risks, particularly if the patient is receiving substantial ventilator or circulatory support (Figures 12.6, 12.7 and 12.8).

Complications

Many of the therapeutic interventions and intensive care can be associated with complications; for example, a pneumothorax or misplacement of a catheter or drain. The use of invasive devices, such as central lines, chest drains, urinary catheters and ET tubes combined with antibiotics and critical illness lead to particular vulnerabilities to infections that may require regular bacteriological surveillance of sputum, blood and urine with cultures. Colonisation and infection with antibiotic-resistant bacteria, such as methicillin-resistant *Staphylococcus aureus* and vancomycin-resistant enterococcus, can be a particular concern. The use of parenteral nutrition can lead to specific deficiencies that can be monitored with blood tests and guide replenishment. Drug handling is often perturbed by liver, renal or other dysfunctions, necessitating specific therapeutic drug monitoring to guide dose adjustments. Specific tests may be necessary, such as a CXR to confirm a correct pulmonary artery (PA) catheter placement and exclude complications such as a pneumothorax.

Monitoring

Many patients will undergo regular or continuous monitoring that overlaps with investigations. These include the determination of cardiac output using a PA catheter (Swan Ganz), regular surveillance of tracheal aspirates for infection, or daily 12-lead ECGs in coronary-care patients. For mechanically ventilated patients, continuous respiratory monitoring (e.g. PaO_2, $PaCO_2$, pulse oximetry, inspiratory to expiratory ratio) is performed to assure patient safety and ensure the intervention provided is appropriate. Neurological problems may require monitoring of intracranial pressure or an EEG.

As with all investigations, it is important to ensure careful completion of request forms and clear pathways for seeing and acting on the results.

Hospital inpatients

Inpatients may undergo a large volume of investigations and it is important that they are carefully considered. In patients who are deteriorating, immediately following major surgery with organ failure or unwell or receiving intravenous fluids, frequent (e.g. daily) determinations of electrolytes, renal function and FBC are often appropriate, However, frequent testing is unnecessary in stable patients.

If you do request a test, follow it up or ensure that one of your colleagues is going to do so, especially during shift changeovers. Just requesting a test does nothing for the patient; the test result needs to be seen, interpreted correctly and acted upon. This is particularly important when requesting cardiac markers for suspected acute coronary syndrome, electrolytes with potential clinically significant derangement (e.g. hyperkalaemia) or X-ray after an invasive pulmonary procedure. Not reviewing investigation results in a timely manner can lead to adverse patient outcomes and may also have medicolegal ramifications.

Outpatient testing

The results of tests in general practice or outpatients may occur immediately (e.g. 'point-of-care testing' of capillary blood glucose), but others usually will become available days or even weeks later. When requesting a test, make sure there is a clear plan that the patient understands when the results will be discussed with them and how. There are countless examples of patients erroneously assuming that no contact about a test result meant the test had been normal or worrying unnecessarily about an outcome.

Clinicians should ensure that there is a reliable system for all investigation results to be reviewed and followed up appropriately, especially for biopsy results and those that may have public health implications. In general, it is best to discuss the test results with the patient involved and done in person instead of through telephone, text-messaging or e-mail.

Many tests require specific preparation, such as fasting or a full bladder, may involve a potentially claustrophobic environment or require sedation. Ensure the patient understands what is involved and can comply, can travel to and from where the test is conducted and what the test involves.

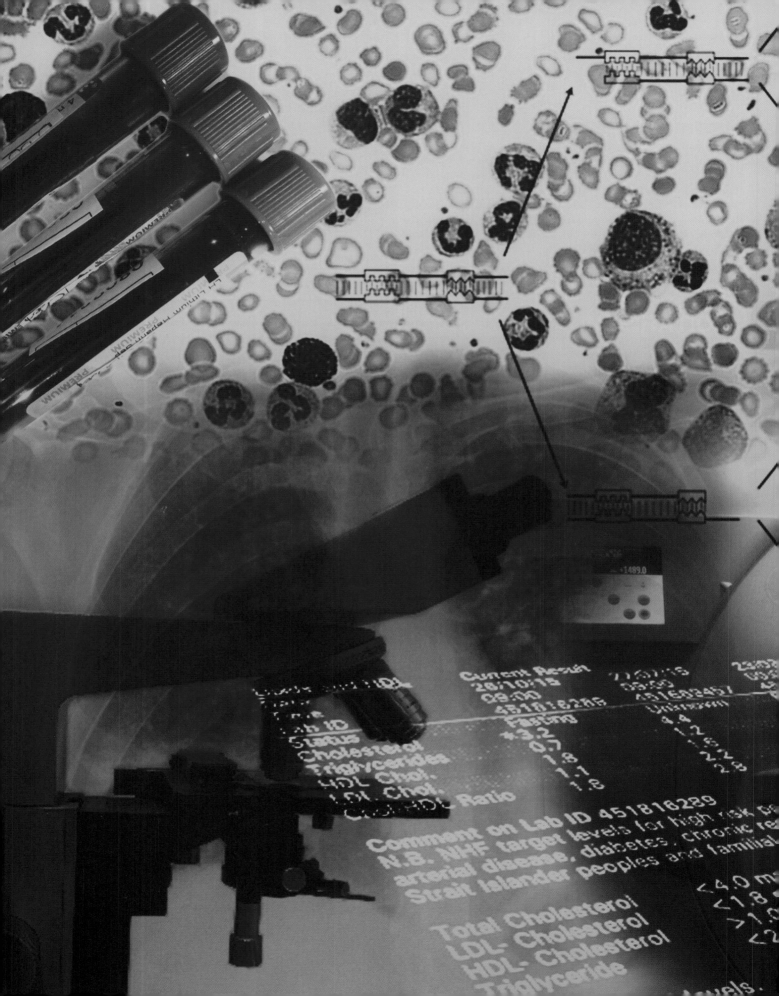

Common presentations

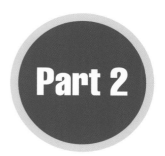

Part 2

Chapters

13 Chest pain

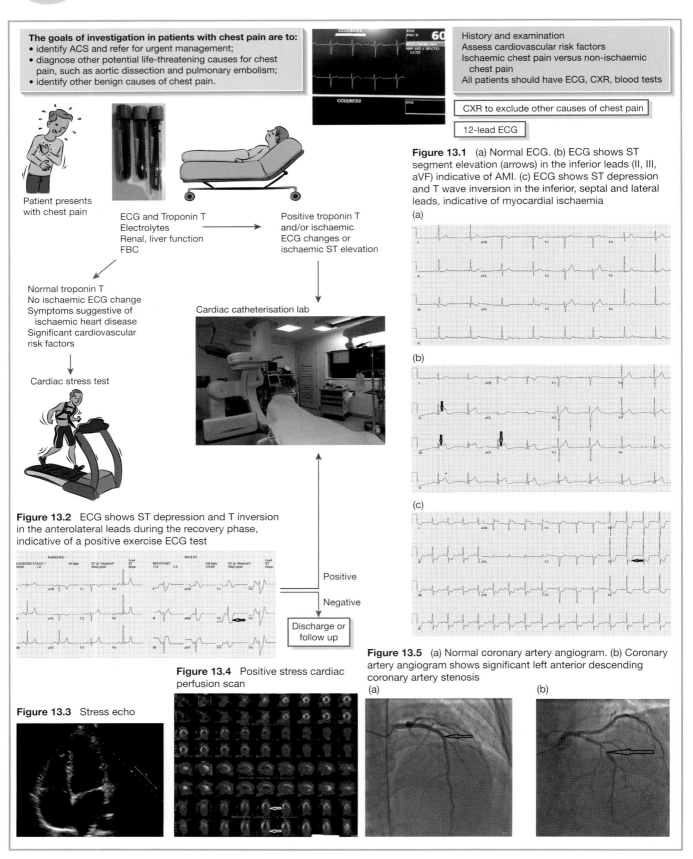

The goals of investigation in patients with chest pain are to:
- identify ACS and refer for urgent management;
- diagnose other potential life-threatening causes for chest pain, such as aortic dissection and pulmonary embolism;
- identify other benign causes of chest pain.

History and examination
Assess cardiovascular risk factors
Ischaemic chest pain versus non-ischaemic chest pain
All patients should have ECG, CXR, blood tests

CXR to exclude other causes of chest pain

12-lead ECG

Patient presents with chest pain

ECG and Troponin T
Electrolytes
Renal, liver function
FBC

Positive troponin T and/or ischaemic ECG changes or ischaemic ST elevation

Normal troponin T
No ischaemic ECG change
Symptoms suggestive of ischaemic heart disease
Significant cardiovascular risk factors

Cardiac stress test

Cardiac catheterisation lab

Figure 13.1 (a) Normal ECG. (b) ECG shows ST segment elevation (arrows) in the inferior leads (II, III, aVF) indicative of AMI. (c) ECG shows ST depression and T wave inversion in the inferior, septal and lateral leads, indicative of myocardial ischaemia

(a)

(b)

(c)

Figure 13.2 ECG shows ST depression and T inversion in the anterolateral leads during the recovery phase, indicative of a positive exercise ECG test

Positive

Negative

Discharge or follow up

Figure 13.4 Positive stress cardiac perfusion scan

Figure 13.5 (a) Normal coronary artery angiogram. (b) Coronary artery angiogram shows significant left anterior descending coronary artery stenosis

(a)

(b)

Figure 13.3 Stress echo

Clinical Investigations at a Glance, First Edition. Jonathan Gleadle, Jordan Li and Tuck Yong. © 2017 John Wiley & Sons, Ltd. Published 2017 by John Wiley & Sons, Ltd.

Chest pain is one of the commonest presentations to emergency departments. The initial investigations should be focused on the possibility of acute coronary syndrome (ACS) or other serious conditions such as pulmonary embolism and aortic dissection, which cannot be excluded on clinical grounds alone. This chapter will focus on investigating patients with chest pain in whom the diagnosis of ACS/myocardial ischaemia requires exclusion. However, it is important to recognise that ACS does not always present with chest pain, but sometimes as exertional dyspnoea, sweating or discomfort in the arm, back or jaw. A third of patients with acute myocardial infarction (AMI) may not experience pain.

Initial investigations

ECG

All patients who present with chest pain should have an ECG done immediately. An ECG may reveal the following:
- ST elevation myocardial infarction (STEMI) (Figure 13.1b) or new left bundle branch block (LBBB). Patients with these findings require urgent cardiologist review and consideration of reperfusion therapy. However, there are other causes of ST segment elevation, such as pericarditis. For patients with ST elevation and symptoms of ACS, reperfusion therapy should be initiated without waiting for troponin levels.
- Acute ischaemic changes, such as ST-segment depression or T-wave inversion (Figure 13.1c), which warrant further investigations.
- Evidence of prior myocardial infarction (MI) – pathological Q-waves, LBBB or persistent T-wave abnormalities.
- Arrhythmia or arrhythmia with a rapid ventricular response resulting in rate-associated ischaemia.
- Significant conduction abnormalities.

It is important to realise that an ECG may be normal in some patients with ACS.

Cardiac biomarkers: troponin

Troponins are regulatory muscle proteins released into the circulation following myocardial injury. Troponin has three subunits: TnC, TnT and TnI. Troponin-C has no diagnostic value. Both troponin I and T are derived from heart.

Troponin levels are very low or undetectable in healthy individuals. Significant increase in troponins reflects myocardial injury. Troponin levels rise 2–3 hours after onset of myocardial injury and can persist for up to 10 days after MI. Assays that quantify cardiac troponin have greater specificity and sensitivity for the diagnosis of AMI than traditional cardiac enzymes do. Measurement of creatine kinase MB and myoglobin in patients with chest pain is no longer recommended. There are many other conditions associated with cardiac troponin elevations.

High-sensitivity cardiac troponin

High-sensitivity cardiac troponin assays can detect troponin in concentrations 10- to 100-fold lower than previous assays and can detect troponin in the circulation of healthy people. The advantages of using a high-sensitivity troponin assay include:
- increases the diagnosis of AMI by improving sensitivity from 73–91% with modest reductions in specificity from 94–90%;
- the negative predictive value at 3 hours is over 99%, providing a safe early method of excluding AMI.

Improvements in assay sensitivity have inevitably reduced specificity, as these assays do not define the cause of myocardial injury and troponin concentrations are elevated in other acute illnesses (Table 13.1). The specificity of high-sensitivity troponin assays is critically dependent on whether clinicians restrict the use of these assays to patients with suspected ACS. Furthermore, troponin concentrations may be permanently raised in patients with chronic heart diseases, including stable coronary artery disease (CAD), congestive cardiac failure and CKD. Demonstrating a dynamic change in troponin concentration is therefore very helpful in identifying patients with AMI.

CXR

In the evaluation of chest pain, the CXR can be useful in detecting:
- cardiomegaly, suggesting long-standing cardiac pathology;
- globular heart shadow due to a significant pericardial effusion;
- widened mediastinum due to acute aortic dissection;
- upper lobe redistribution of blood vessels, pulmonary oedema or pleural effusion due to left ventricular failure;
- pneumonia, pneumothorax.

Further investigations

Cardiac stress tests

Coronary ischaemia is caused by a mismatch between supply (coronary blood flow) and demand (myocardial oxygen consumption) as workload increases. This is commonly caused by coronary artery stenosis. Cardiac stress tests work by demonstrating inducible ischaemia as workload increases (either through exercise or pharmacological stress). Cardiac stress tests stratify the risk of known or possible CAD as the underlying cause of chest pain.

Stress testing is most valuable in patients of intermediate pre-test probability of ACS (10% < pre-test probability < 90%), as it is in this group of patients that a change in risk stratification is most likely (i.e. from low to high risk). In patients with high pre-test probability of ACS (e.g. typical angina) coronary angiography can be the initial diagnostic test.

Absolute contraindications to cardiac stress testing include AMI; unstable angina; severe aortic stenosis; uncontrolled arrhythmia; decompensated heart failure; acute pulmonary embolus; aortic dissection.

Relative contraindications include left main coronary artery stenosis; uncontrolled hypertension; electrolyte abnormalities; hypertrophic obstructive cardiomyopathy; uncontrolled arrhythmia.

It is important to ensure that the appropriate stress modality is requested: if patients cannot walk at a reasonable workload, request a pharmacological stress test (e.g. dobutamine stress echocardiogram). Although the test is generally safe, there is a small risk of AMI (~1:5000 tests) and death (~1:10,000 tests).

Withholding rate-controlling medications such as beta-blockers is standard before stress testing (withhold the night before and morning of the test for twice-daily beta-blocker, and the morning of the test for once-daily beta-blocker); 85% of maximal predicted heart rate (MPHR = 220 bpm − age) must be achieved for the test to be diagnostically accurate.

An exercise stress ECG identifies ischaemia if horizontal or down-sloping ST depression of >1 mm at 80 m/s after the J-point is induced with exercise (Figure 13.2). Stress echocardiography assesses the ECG response to stress as well as obtaining an immediate post-stress echocardiogram to assess for inducible wall motion abnormalities as a marker of ischaemia. It may show the effect of exercise on valvular function (e.g. degree of stenosis or regurgitation), pulmonary pressure, inducibility of outflow tract gradients (obstruction) and cardiac shunting.

Depending on the clinical scenario, a positive exercise stress test (EST) or stress echocardiography may be an indication for

Table 13.1 Conditions commonly associated with cardiac troponin elevations

Congestive heart failure
Myocarditis
Pericarditis
Arrhythmias
Aortic dissection
Pulmonary embolism
Malignant hypertension
Chronic kidney disease
Sepsis
Systemic inflammatory diseases
Trauma
Severe neurological diseases such as stroke
Critically ill patients, multi-organ failure

Table 13.2 Summary of different investigations for the evaluation of myocardial ischaemia

Test	Sensitivity	Specificity	Advantages	Limitations
Exercise stress test	68%	70–77%	Assessment of exercise capacity First-line test in absence of contraindications	Lowest sensitivity of all stress tests Risk of false-negative test Lowest diagnostic accuracy in women
Stress Echocardiogram	80–85%	78–86%	Assessment of exercise capacity, cardiac structure/function No radiation High specificity	False negatives in single vessel or circumflex territory ischaemia
Myocardial perfusion study	85–90%	70–75%	Assessment of exercise capacity High sensitivity	Radiation False positives due to higher sensitivity or diaphragmatic attenuation
CT coronary angiography	85–99%	64–90%	High negative predictive value (especially in low to intermediate-risk group)	Radiation Functional effect of stenoses not routinely assessed
Coronary angiography	100%	100%	Gold standard	Invasive and radiation Functional effect of stenoses not routinely assessed

Key points in investigating chest pain

- All patients who present with chest pain should have an immediate ECG and a CXR.
- Troponin levels begin to rise 2 h after myocardial injury and can persist for up to 10 days after AMI.
- Cardiac stress tests have good but not perfect predictive value in determining flow-limiting coronary disease.
- Invasive coronary angiography is considered the gold standard for diagnosing CAD.

coronary angiography (Figure 13.3). A negative test may be reassuring but it cannot exclude myocardial ischaemia as no stress test has 100% sensitivity. If the clinical presentation does not correlate with the negative stress test, a repeat test, alternative test modality or coronary angiogram may be indicated. An inconclusive test is most commonly due to submaximal heart rate achieved (e.g. due to beta-blockade) or intermediate ECG changes (e.g. T-wave changes without ST segment depression).

Myocardial perfusion scan

In patients with flow-limiting CAD, an intravenous vasodilator such as adenosine or dipyridamole increases the difference between perfusion of normal myocardium and that supplied by a stenosed artery. This can be visualised with myocardial perfusion scintigraphy (sensitivity 91%, specificity 78%). Images acquired during vasodilator stress and at rest are compared to assess whether perfusion is impaired within a coronary artery territory (Figure 13.4). Adenosine is contraindicated in severe asthma and in patients with second- or third-degree heart block. Patients should not ingest caffeine in the 24 hours before the test due to competitive inhibition of adenosine.

CT coronary artery calcium score

CT coronary artery calcium scoring is a screening test for CAD that also has prognostic value for future cardiac events. Calcium scoring has a negative predictive value of 99% for obstructive CAD in low-risk populations, and a normal study result predicts a <2% cardiac event rate over the next 5 years. If the calcium score is zero then non-coronary causes of chest pain should be considered. However, obstructive CAD may go undetected in younger patients in whom atherosclerotic plaque has not advanced to the stage of calcification.

CT coronary angiography

CT coronary angiography is used to determine whether patients with a CT calcium score of 1–400 have obstructive CAD (sensitivity 98%, specificity 92%). Three-dimensional images of the angiogram are reconstructed to visualise coronary stenoses caused by calcified or non-calcified plaque. The positive predictive value for detecting a coronary stenosis of 50% or more is 91%, and the negative predictive value is 83%.

Coronary artery angiography

Invasive coronary angiography is considered the gold standard for diagnosing CAD (Figures 13.5a and b) and should be considered in the following situations:
- high pre-test probability (70–90%) of CAD;
- functional or anatomical coronary imaging is non-diagnostic;
- functional or anatomical coronary imaging is positive and the patient is a candidate for revascularisation.

As well as diagnosing CAD, patients may proceed to coronary stenting if a suitable stenosis is identified. It may be difficult to define the importance of an intermediate stenosis on an angiogram, so the flow-limiting effect can be assessed by using a pressure-recording catheter. The overall complication rate for coronary angiogram is 7.4 per 1000, with a mortality rate of 0.7 per 1000. The most common complications are arrhythmias, vascular injury and myocardial ischaemia.

Cardiac MRI

Cardiac MRI, where first-pass contrast-enhanced imaging of the heart is performed during a vasodilator infusion, can be used to assess myocardial perfusion (sensitivity 90%, specificity 79%). This test has a higher negative predictive value than myocardial perfusion scintigraphy (91% versus 79%). Cardiac MRI is not suitable for patients with an incompatible pacemaker or claustrophobia.

14 Acute abdominal pain

Acute abdominal pains

Suggests serious pathology and requires urgent investigations

- Systemically unwell/septic-looking
- Associated with severe vomiting, fever
- Patient lying very still
- Hypotension/shock
- Impaired consciousness
- Peritonism (guarding, rigid abdomen, rebound pain)
- Absent or altered bowel sounds
- Evidence of gastrointestinal bleeding
- Suspicion of a medical cause for abdominal pain

Arterial blood gas
Acidosis may develop and lactate level may be elevated in ischaemic bowel, severe necrotising pancreatitis and perforation

Blood tests
FBC
CRP
Electrolyte, serum creatinine
Blood glucose level
Liver function tests
Serum lipase or amylase
Troponin will need to be performed if a cardiac cause is suspected

Pregnancy test

Urine tests
Urine analysis may reveal urinary infection, haematuria due to renal calculi
Mid-stream urine for microscopy and culture
Urine pregnancy test

Stool tests
Harmful bacteria, intestinal parasites and *Clostridium difficile* toxin
Excessive fats may suggest chronic pancreatitis, malabsorption

Other investigations:
- ERCP
- Tissue biopsy
- Examination under anaesthesia
- Laparoscopy and exploratory laparotomy

AXR

Figure 14.1 (a) Normal AXR. AXR shows (b) small bowel obstruction. (c) Gas under right hemidiaphragm due to a perforated duodenal ulcer

(a)
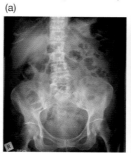

(b)
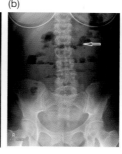

(c)
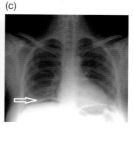

Abdominal USS

Figure 14.2 Abdominal USS shows (a) thickened gallbladder wall consistent with cholecystitis. (b) Obstructed right kidney with proximal stone in the right ureter. (c) Ectopic pregnancy

(a)

(b)
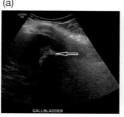

(c)
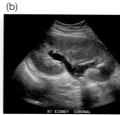

Abdominal CT

Figure 14.3 (a) CT abdomen shows normal appendix. (b) Acute appendicitis. (c) CT abdomen shows intra-abdominal free air due to ischaemic small bowel perforation

(a)
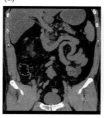

(b)
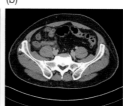

(c)
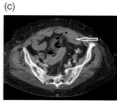

Endoscopy indications
- Signs of GI bleeding or anaemia
- Weight loss
- Vomiting
- Progression of symptoms
- Dysphagia
- Previous gastric surgery
- Family history of GI carcinoma
- Over 55 years of age

Colonoscopy indications
- Signs of GI bleeding or anaemia
- Weight loss
- Altered bowel habit
- Family history of GI carcinoma

Figure 14.4 (a) Colonoscopy shows diverticular disease. (b) Endoscopy shows gastric ulcer

(a)
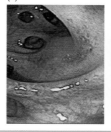

(b)
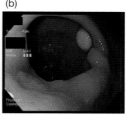

Key points in investigating acute abdominal pain

- Plain AXR has little role in the diagnosis of most causes of abdominal pain except suspected bowel obstruction or perforated viscus.
- If a patient is suspected to have a leaking aortic aneurysm, a CT scan is the first-choice investigation, provided the patient is stable.
- CT abdomen can improve the accuracy of diagnosis in patients with appendicitis.
- Always consider pregnancy, including ectopic ones, in any woman of childbearing age who presents with abdominal pain, and a pregnancy test must be performed.

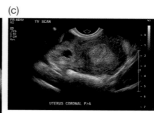

Abdominal pain is one of the commonest reasons for presentation to hospital or general practice. Abdominal pain can be caused by a wide range of surgical and non-surgical conditions. It can be classified as acute (acute abdomen) or chronic abdominal pain, which is defined as pain of more than 2 weeks' duration. Acute abdomen may require immediate surgical or medical intervention and is usually accompanied by signs of peritoneal irritation.

The investigations for acute abdominal pain can be considered according to the location of the pain: whether it is upper or lower abdominal pain. However, patients may present with generalised abdominal pain.

A history that includes a complete description of the abdominal pain and associated symptoms is essential for accurate diagnosis. The choice of investigations is dependent on the likely differential diagnosis of the cause of abdominal pain.

Laboratory investigations

Blood tests

• The basic blood tests should be performed. A normal WBC count or CRP should never be used alone as the decision trigger to discharge a patient who continues to remain clinically unwell. Both investigations are not sensitive or specific enough to be used in such a manner.
• CRP: raised CRP is suggestive of sepsis, inflammatory, or malignant causes.
• Electrolytes: all patients with abdominal pain should have a baseline electrolyte and renal function done.
• Blood glucose: to exclude diabetic ketoacidosis.
• Liver function test: elevated markers in liver function tests can suggest cholecystitis, cholangitis, choledocholithiasis, hepatitis and pancreatitis.
• Serum lipase or amylase: may be increased in pancreatitis but also in peritonitis, cholecystitis, strangulated or infarcted bowel and pancreatic cyst.
• Arterial blood gas: acidosis may develop and lactate level may be elevated in ischaemic bowel, severe pancreatitis and perforation.
• Troponin levels will need to be performed if a cardiac cause is suspected.

Urine tests

• Urine analysis: may reveal urinary tract infection, haematuria due to renal calculi or Henoch–Schönlein purpura.
• Mid-stream urine for microscopy and culture: should be performed in patients presenting with lower abdominal pain.
• Urine pregnancy test or blood quantitative β-hCG test: is essential in females of reproductive age to exclude ectopic pregnancy and assess safety of investigations involving radiation.

Stool tests

• This may reveal harmful bacteria, intestinal parasites and *Clostridium difficile* toxin.

ECG

Inferior AMI may present with epigastric or upper abdominal pain. ECG should be performed in patients with severe abdominal pain and/or suspected coronary artery disease.

Radiological investigations

Plain X-rays

A plain AXR has little role in the diagnosis of most causes of abdominal pain and should not be performed routinely. AXRs are only useful when bowel obstruction (Figures 14.1a and b), perforated viscus (pneumoperitoneum Figure 14.1c), urinary calculus, ischaemic bowel or megacolon complicating inflammatory bowel disease (IBD) is suspected. For other pathologies, an ultrasound scan (USS) and CT of the abdomen should be considered. A normal AXR does not exclude other pathologies and may falsely reassure. CXR can identify areas of consolidation, effusion or pneumothorax.

Ultrasound

An USS is useful to image the hepatobiliary (Figure 14.2a), pancreatic, pelvic organs and urinary systems. However, obesity and bowel gas can prevent adequate visualisation of pancreases. Hydronephrosis is a relatively late development of acute ureteric obstruction (Figure 14.2b). USS also aids diagnosis of any condition that result in free abdominal fluid or intra-abdominal collections, as well as for guiding drainage. An USS can assess abdominal aortic aneurysm (AAA) if it is not thought to have ruptured, and it is useful to exclude ectopic pregnancy (Figure 14.2c).

CT

CT is better than USS for the demonstration of small gallstones, renal calculi, changes in solid abdominal organs (Figure 14.3a), tumours in the abdominal cavity and intra-abdominal collections, especially in the retroperitoneum or between bowel loops. CT may also detect unsuspected bowel pathology such as a tumour or IBD and associated complications.

If a patient is suspected of having a leaking AAA, a CT scan is the first choice of investigation, provided the patient is stable. Angiography or CT angiography is useful for establishing a diagnosis of ischaemic abdominal organs and for providing intervention.

Endoscopic investigations

The indications for upper GI endoscopy or sigmoidoscopy/colonoscopy (Figures 14.4a and b) are listed opposite.

Endoscopic retrograde cholangiopancreatography (ERCP) has both a diagnostic and therapeutic role. ERCP is useful to assess the site and cause of biliary obstruction, prior to surgical, endoscopic or radiological intervention. It also allows sphincterotomy to be performed to facilitate the passage of stones lodged in the common bile duct.

Body fluid

There is no role for diagnostic lavage in evaluation of acute or chronic abdominal pain.

Laparoscopy and exploratory laparotomy

Laparoscopy is used in gynaecology and general surgery as a diagnostic and therapeutic tool. Laparotomy is now required only when less invasive procedures have failed to provide a clear diagnosis or when treatment to relieve symptoms such as bowel obstruction is required urgently.

Investigations for specific conditions

Acute appendicitis

Acute appendicitis is a common condition and is usually diagnosed by typical history and physical signs. However, the finding of a normal appendix at surgical exploration varies between 10 and 30% if diagnosis is made on clinical grounds only. Delayed diagnosis/surgery is associated with an increased rate of perforation and post-operative complications. This must be balanced against the negative appendectomy rate. Preoperative imaging of suspected appendicitis is associated with a significantly lower rate of negative appendectomies, without delaying time-to-surgery, or the perioperative complication rate. CT abdomen has significantly improved the accuracy of diagnosis in patients with appendicitis. The finding of an appendiceal diameter greater than 6 mm has a positive predictive value of 98%. Other CT signs of acute appendicitis include periappendiceal fat inflammation, fluid in the right lower quadrant and failure of contrast to fill the appendix (Figure 14.3b). An USS has a sensitivity and specificity of 80% and 90% respectively for the diagnosis of acute appendicitis. Features of appendicitis on ultrasound include:

- an outer appendix diameter of 6 mm or larger;
- positive sonographic McBurney sign;
- non-compressibility of the appendix;
- echogenic periappendiceal inflammatory fat change.

Biliary disease/cholecystitis

An USS is the investigation of choice for patients suspected to have biliary disease. The finding of gallstones, gallbladder wall thickening (Figure 14.2a), pericholecystic fluid and pain on compression of the gallbladder with ultrasound probe (sonographic Murphy's sign) is diagnostic for cholecystitis. ERCP may be required if the clinical features are suggestive of ascending cholangitis (right upper quadrant pain, fever, jaundice).

Cholescintigraphy scan (^{99}Tc-hepatobiliary iminodiacetic acid scan) is a nuclear imaging used to evaluate the function of the gallbladder. ^{99}Tc-iminodiacetic acid chelate complex is given intravenously, excreted into the biliary system and stored by the gallbladder and biliary system. In the absence of disease, the gallbladder is visualised within 1 hour of the injection of the radioactive tracer. If the gallbladder is not visualised within 4 hours after the injection or 30 min post-morphine, cholescintigraphy for acute cholecystitis has sensitivity of 97%, specificity of 94% and is superior compared with an USS.

Diverticulitis

CT is the first choice of investigation in patients with suspected diverticulitis. It can confirm the diagnosis of diverticulitis (>97% sensitivity), but a negative CT scan does not completely exclude the diagnosis. The CT features of diverticulitis include presence of diverticula with pericolic infiltration of fatty tissue, thickening of colonic wall and abscess formation. Although an USS has 85% sensitivity for diagnosing acute diverticulitis it usually requires CT for further delineation.

Pancreatitis

See Chapter 78 on acute pancreatitis.

Ischaemic bowel

CT is the best initial diagnostic test (Figure 14.3b). Mesenteric angiography is useful for determining the cause of intestinal ischaemia and defining the extent of disease.

Abdominal aortic aneurysm

See Chapter 54 on peripheral arterial disease.

Renal colic

Plain AXR has a sensitivity of 45–59% and specificity of 64–77% for detecting ureteric calculi. Uric acid stones are usually radiolucent and unlikely to be detected. AXR in combination with USS has a sensitivity of 80% and specificity of 90% for calculus detection. Stones missed on USS are typically small (<5 mm) and pass spontaneously. Non-contrast CT has a sensitivity of 97% and specificity of 92%. It can also detect alternative pathology. Intravenous pyelography is no longer used because of lower sensitivity and specificity and being time consuming.

Ectopic pregnancy and gynaecological disorders

Clinicians should always consider ectopic pregnancy in any woman of childbearing age who presents with abdominal pain. In patients with elevated β-hCG, USS identification of an intrauterine pregnancy rules out ectopic pregnancy.

A transabdominal USS is the first imaging modality of choice for evaluation of ectopic pregnancy and gynaecological disorders in females in the reproductive age group. It provides information regarding the uterus, adnexa and ovaries. A transvaginal USS (Figure 14.2c) can provide a more detailed examination for gynaecological disease.

15 Headache

Key points in investigating headache

- CRP should be done if patients have visual symptoms, jaw claudication or other findings suggesting giant cell arteritis.
- Urgent neuroimaging (CT and/or MRI) is mandatory for patients with altered mental status, seizures, papilledema, focal neurologic deficits or thunderclap headache.
- LP and CSF analysis should be done if headache is progressive or clinical findings suggest idiopathic intracranial hypertension, and there are no signs of increased intracranial pressure.
- Patients with thunderclap headache require CSF analysis even if CT and examination findings are normal.

Table 15.1 Classification and common causes of headache

Primary headache
- Tension headache
- Tension–vascular headache
- Migraine
- Cluster headache

Secondary headache
- Intracranial causes:
  - Haemorrhagic
  - Tumour
  - Infection
- Extracranial causes:
  - Arteries – temporal arteritis
  - Skull – tumour
  - Dentition – temporomandibular joint dysfunction, dental caries, apical tooth abscess
  - Scalp – bacterial infection, herpes zoster
  - Sinuses – sinusitis, tumours
  - Eyes – glaucoma, conjunctivitis
  - Ears – otitis externa, otitis media

Table 15.2 Common causes of cerebral ring-enhancing lesion

M	Metastasis
A	Abscess
G	Glioblastoma multiforme
I	Infarct (subacute phase)
C	Contusion
D	Demyelinating disease
R	Radiation necrosis

Symptoms and signs in headache investigation

New-onset headache in patient:	Clinical possibilities
Having seizures but who has no epilepsy	Space-occupying lesion (Figure 15.1)
Who is pregnant or post-partum	Cerebral venous thrombosis (Figure 15.2)
Who is taking an anticoagulant	Intracranial haemorrhage, subdural haematoma (Figure 15.3)
Who has taken amphetamine or cocaine	Intracranial haemorrhage (Figure 15.4)
Who has a history of cancer or immunodeficiency	Opportunistic infections, lymphoma, metastases
Who is >50 years	Malignancy, temporal arteritis
Who is young and morbidly obese	Cerebral venous thrombosis or benign intracranial hypertension

Headache associated with:	
Head injury especially with loss of consciousness	Intracranial haemorrhage, subdural or extradural haemorrhage (Figure 15.5)
Waking the person from sleep	Space-occupying lesion
Confusion, drowsiness or vomiting	Encephalitis, intracranial abscess, hypertensive encephalopathy and other space-occupying lesion
Fever or neck stiffness	Meningitis, subarachnoid haemorrhage
Focal neurological deficit	Space occupying lesion
Symptoms worsened by coughing or physical activity	Increased intracranial pressure (Figure 15.6)
Stroke-like symptoms or signs	Subdural haematoma and other space-occupying lesion
Abrupt onset and intense ('thunderclap')	Subarachnoid haemorrhage (Figure 15.7)
Progressive worsening	Brain tumour or other space-occupying lesion
Jaw claudication, or visual disturbance	Temporal arteritis

Figure 15.1 T1-weighted MRI of the head shows a space-occupying lesion – glioblastoma multiforme

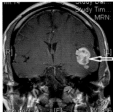

Figure 15.2 MR venography shows a left-sided cerebral venous thrombosis

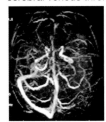

Figure 15.3 CT head shows a right-sided large subdural haematoma

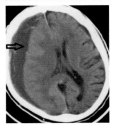

Figure 15.4 CT head shows left-sided intracranial haemorrhage

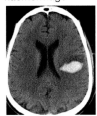

Figure 15.5 CT head shows a right-sided epidural haematoma

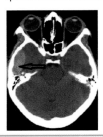

Figure 15.6 CT head shows severe cerebral oedema

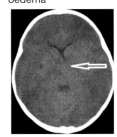

Figure 15.7 CT head shows subarachnoid haemorrhage

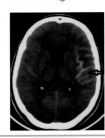

Figure 15.8 CT head shows a left hemispheric ring-enhancing space-occupying lesion, confirmed to be an abscess

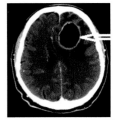

Clinical Investigations at a Glance, First Edition. Jonathan Gleadle, Jordan Li and Tuck Yong. © 2017 John Wiley & Sons, Ltd. Published 2017 by John Wiley & Sons, Ltd.

eadache is very common. Headache can be classified as primary and secondary (Table 15.1). Most patients with headache who present to primary care have primary headache (>90%), which is benign and self-limiting, but some primary headaches can be recurrent or persistent and disabling. In primary headache, findings on neurological examination are usually normal and investigations are not helpful for diagnosis. Identifying a serious cause of secondary headache is an essential part of the initial investigation. This requires a detailed history and physical examination. The presence of 'red flags' symptoms or signs in patient with headache indicate the need for investigations.

Neuroimaging

A CT of the head is the first choice of imaging when 'red flag' features (red flag box) are present or intracranial pathology is suspected. If a haemorrhage is small or below the foramen magnum, the CT head can be normal and a lumbar puncture (LP) may be required to make the definitive diagnosis of a subarachnoid haemorrhage (Figure 15.7) (Chapter 136). If a ring-enhancing space-occupying lesion is found on CT head (Figure 15.8), the differential diagnoses to consider are shown in Table 15.2.

An MRI is more sensitive than CT, but in primary headache is more likely to pick up incidental findings and not more likely to reveal clinically relevant findings. CT is therefore adequate in most patients, with MRI reserved for selected patients where the clinical history suggests MRI may be more useful (e.g. in patients with brainstem symptoms).

In patients with suspected raised intracranial pressure, CT head also remains the initial imaging modality. MRI should be considered if the CT is normal or may be required to give further information on the lesion found on CT. In patients with headache precipitated by valsalva (coughing, sneezing, straining, stooping, exertion) MRI is required to exclude an Arnold Chiari malformation or a posterior fossa lesion. Venous sinus thrombosis must be excluded either by CT venography or MR venography (Figure 15.2). Other secondary causes to consider include medications (most commonly tetracyclines), infective or inflammatory meningitis, malignant meningitis (carcinoma, lymphoma or leukaemia) and carbon dioxide retention.

Neuroimaging has costs and risks, such as incidental findings and false positives or negatives. CT scans can detect incidental findings in over 20% of cases compared with only 2% of findings potentially related to headache. Neuroimaging used incorrectly can also be falsely reassuring. There is therefore good evidence that neuroimaging is not required in stable migraine, and should be restricted to patients with 'red flags'. There is insufficient evidence to make recommendations in tension headache or trigeminal autonomic cephalalgias (cluster headache).

Should patients be imaged for reassurance? Patients increasingly expect a scan when they attend for assessment, particularly in secondary care. Explanation may suffice, but neuroimaging is required for reassurance with some patients. This has to be balanced against the risk of incidental findings, and patients should be counselled about the risk of finding an incidental abnormality. In a prospective randomised controlled trial of 150 patients with chronic daily headache and no 'red flag' features, patients were randomised to receive no imaging or an MRI scan. Those randomised to a scan had significantly lower anxiety levels at 3 months, but this was not maintained and anxiety levels returned to baseline at 1 year. There was a significant reduction in health-care costs in patients with psychiatric co-morbidity who were scanned compared with those who were not, presumably by altering the referral patterns of their primary care physicians.

Plain X-ray and/or coronal CT scans of the paranasal sinuses may be useful in patients whose headaches are localised to the supraorbital or infraorbital regions. Both migraine and cluster headache may mimic the pain of sinusitis, in that all three conditions have a similar distribution. A skull X-ray has a negligible diagnostic yield and should be done only in cases where bony pathology is suspected.

Lumbar puncture

Acute severe headache with stiff neck and fever suggests meningitis or encephalitis and a LP is mandatory unless there is a contraindication and should be carried out without delay. It can confirm the diagnosis and identify the causative organism, allowing determination of antibiotic sensitivities and rationalisation of treatment. If a focal neurological symptom or sign is present, a LP can be potentially dangerous and lead to brainstem herniation and a CT head should be performed before performing a LP. However, if there are no focal neurological symptoms and signs, LP can be performed without imaging. See Chapter 136 regarding the indication for LP in a patient with suspected subarachnoid haemorrhage.

Laboratory investigations

In an elderly patient presenting with recent onset of headache, a FBC and CRP should be obtained, to evaluate for the possibility of temporal arteritis. A normal CRP does not exclude temporal arteritis. If the clinical suspicion is high, a temporal artery biopsy should be organised (Chapter 152).

Angle closure glaucoma should be considered in a patient with headache associated with a red eye, halos or unilateral visual symptoms.

16 Nausea and vomiting

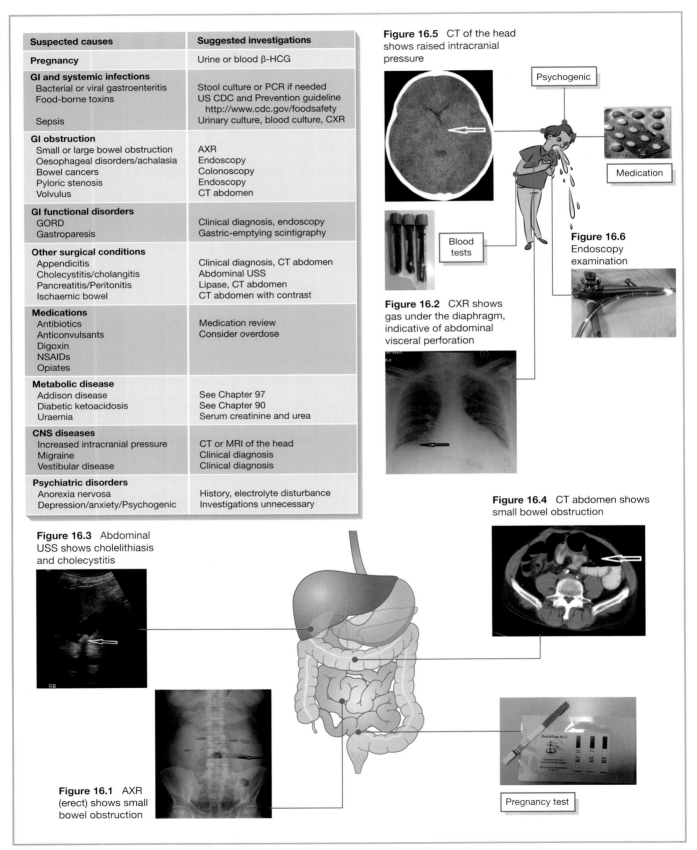

Suspected causes	Suggested investigations
Pregnancy	Urine or blood β-HCG
GI and systemic infections Bacterial or viral gastroenteritis Food-borne toxins Sepsis	Stool culture or PCR if needed US CDC and Prevention guideline http://www.cdc.gov/foodsafety Urinary culture, blood culture, CXR
GI obstruction Small or large bowel obstruction Oesophageal disorders/achalasia Bowel cancers Pyloric stenosis Volvulus	AXR Endoscopy Colonoscopy Endoscopy CT abdomen
GI functional disorders GORD Gastroparesis	Clinical diagnosis, endoscopy Gastric-emptying scintigraphy
Other surgical conditions Appendicitis Cholecystitis/cholangitis Pancreatitis/Peritonitis Ischaemic bowel	Clinical diagnosis, CT abdomen Abdominal USS Lipase, CT abdomen CT abdomen with contrast
Medications Antibiotics Anticonvulsants Digoxin NSAIDs Opiates	Medication review Consider overdose
Metabolic disease Addison disease Diabetic ketoacidosis Uraemia	See Chapter 97 See Chapter 90 Serum creatinine and urea
CNS diseases Increased intracranial pressure Migraine Vestibular disease	CT or MRI of the head Clinical diagnosis Clinical diagnosis
Psychiatric disorders Anorexia nervosa Depression/anxiety/Psychogenic	History, electrolyte disturbance Investigations unnecessary

Figure 16.5 CT of the head shows raised intracranial pressure

Psychogenic

Medication

Figure 16.6 Endoscopy examination

Blood tests

Figure 16.2 CXR shows gas under the diaphragm, indicative of abdominal visceral perforation

Figure 16.4 CT abdomen shows small bowel obstruction

Figure 16.3 Abdominal USS shows cholelithiasis and cholecystitis

GB

Figure 16.1 AXR (erect) shows small bowel obstruction

Pregnancy test

Clinical Investigations at a Glance, First Edition. Jonathan Gleadle, Jordan Li and Tuck Yong. © 2017 John Wiley & Sons, Ltd. Published 2017 by John Wiley & Sons, Ltd.

Nausea is the subjective, unpleasant sensation that one may experience immediately preceding vomiting. Vomiting is a highly organised physical event that results in the rapid, forceful evacuation of gastric contents in retrograde fashion from the stomach and out of the mouth. Vomiting must be distinguished from regurgitation, which is the retrograde flow of oesophageal contents into the mouth passively.

The causes of nausea and vomiting are extensive and include a broad range of physiological and pathological conditions affecting the gastrointestinal tract, the peritoneal cavity and the CNS as well as endocrine and metabolic functions. Given the vast number and diversity of potential causes of nausea and vomiting, a carefully considered and orderly approach to the investigation of patients with nausea and vomiting is needed to maintain cost-effective investigations and avoid misdiagnosis. The most common cause of acute nausea/vomiting is viral gastroenteritis or bacterial food poisoning. This illness is commonly self-limiting and does not required extensive investigations.

The plan for investigation of nausea and vomiting can be divided into whether the symptoms are acute or chronic. Chronic symptoms are defined as those lasting more than 1 month. A comprehensive history and physical examination are helpful in revealing the cause of nausea and vomiting and guiding the selection of laboratory studies and diagnostic tests.

> **The goals of investigating nausea and vomiting are:**
> - To a detect surgical or medical emergency that requires urgent intervention or hospitalisation
> - To identify the underlying cause
> - To evaluate for consequences of nausea and vomiting, such as dehydration

Laboratory investigations

Basic laboratory tests in patients with nausea and vomiting are listed below. These laboratory tests may also provide the first clues to detection of other systemic disorders; for example, suspicion of Addison's disease will be aroused by the detection of hyponatraemia.

> **Basic laboratory tests for nausea and vomiting**
> - **Pregnancy test.** For any female of childbearing age, a urine pregnancy test should be performed first not only to define whether pregnancy might be the cause of symptoms, but also as a prerequisite to performing any radiologic studies and treatment.
> - **FBC.** Leukocytosis indicates an inflammatory process; microcytic anaemia requires further investigation.
> - **Electrolytes and glucose level.** This can reveal the consequences of nausea and vomiting (e.g. acidosis, alkalosis, AKI, hypokalaemia).
> - **Liver function tests and lipase.** These tests are useful for patients with upper abdominal pain or jaundice.
> - **Serum drug levels.** These tests may indicate toxicity among patients who are taking digoxin, theophylline or salicylates.
> - **Urine analysis and culture.** These tests help to exclude urinary tract infection.

Radiological imaging

Plain erect and supine AXR is useful for assessment of acute episodes of vomiting suggestive of bowel obstruction (Figure 16.1). False-negative results occur in up to 22% of patients with a partial obstruction. CXR can help identify gas under the diaphragm, which is indicative of abdominal visceral perforation (Figure 16.2).

Upper GI and small bowel radiography with barium contrast media follow through can identify mucosal lesions and higher grade obstructions and evaluate small bowel to the terminal ileum.

CT and USS of the abdomen may provide valuable information if gallbladder, pancreatic or hepatobiliary pathology (Figure 16.3) is suspected. CT abdomen with oral contrast is the study of choice for detecting intestinal obstructions (Figure 16.4) and also allows evaluation of the surrounding abdominal structures.

CT or MRI of the head is indicated if raised intracranial pressure might be responsible for nausea and vomiting (Figure 16.5).

Upper GI endoscopy

Proximal mucosal lesions and obstructions may be detected by endoscopy (Figure 16.6). A duodenal biopsy should be taken to assess for coeliac disease, infection or eosinophilic enteritis. Gastroparesis is suggested by retained food at the time of the endoscopy.

Investigating gut motility disorder

If no diagnosis is determined after initial evaluation, gastric and intestinal motility studies may be considered. However, a trial of antiemetic or prokinetic medications may be an alternative.

Gastric-emptying scintigraphy

Scintigraphy is the gold-standard test for measurement of gastric emptying. Gastric emptying can be tested using liquid, solid or mixed meals labelled with the radioactive isotopes ^{99m}Tc and ^{113}In. Concurrent uses of both isotopes makes it possible to study emptying of the liquid and solid components of a mixed meal. Gastric emptying is dependent on the contents of the meal, and therefore normal values differ between meals. Important parameters are the time interval between completion of the meal and the start of emptying (lag phase), gastric emptying speed (percentage per hour) and retention after 1 hour and 2 hours.

^{13}C breath test of gastric emptying

After consumption of a meal with ^{13}C, ^{13}C-containing breakdown products produced in the small bowel will be absorbed and ^{13}CO$_2$ will be exhaled through the lungs. The time–^{13}CO$_2$ concentration curve provides information about gastric emptying, as this is the rate-limiting step. The ^{13}C breath test is widely used as it is a simple and inexpensive test for gastric emptying and the results correlate well with those obtained with a scintigraphy study.

For problematic cases of recurrent vomiting, wireless motility capsules or antroduodenal manometry may be informative. Finally, if all organic, gastrointestinal and central causes of chronic nausea and vomiting have been explored, psychogenic vomiting or functional nausea and vomiting should be considered.

> **Key points**
>
> - When investigating the cause of nausea and vomiting, always consider non-gastrointestinal disorders.
> - Pregnancy test should be performed in any woman of childbearing age presenting with nausea and vomiting.
> - CT abdomen should be considered in patients with unexplained nausea. It helps to identify abdominal masses, pancreatic, hepatobiliary or retroperitoneal pathology.

17 Diarrhoea

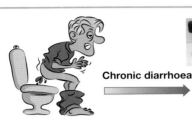

Chronic diarrhoea

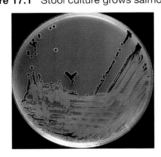

Acute diarrhoea

Stool study
- Inspection of the stool sample
- *C. difficile* toxin test and faecal leucocytes, ova and parasites
- Enzyme-linked immunosorbent assay for giardia antigen if initial investigations are unrevealing.
- Stool pH <5.3 is diagnostic of carbohydrate intolerance
- If laxative abuse is suspected, test faecal electrolytes and osmolality, and alkalinisation assay for phenolphthalein may be useful

Blood tests
- FBC – provides clues for an infective cause and identify anaemia.
- CRP – indicates severity of inflammatory disease.
- Electrolytes, urea, creatinine, LFTs – determine any biochemical complications.
- Thyroid function test.
- Iron studies, folate, vitamin B12 and 25-hydroxy-vitamin D if malabsorption is suspected.
- Coeliac disease serology – coeliac disease is the most common small bowel enteropathy in the western world (up to 1% of asymptomatic adults).
- If diarrhoea is >1 L/day and especially if there is hypokalaemia, vasoactive intestinal polypeptide, substance P, calcitonin, histamine should be measured. If there is flushing, urine 5-hydroxyindoleacetic acid should be measured.

Breath test
Breath tests for fat malabsorption include ^{14}C-triolein or a ^{13}C-labelled mixed triglyceride as substrates

Symptoms and indications for further investigation in acute diarrhoea
- Bloody diarrhoea
- Pus in the stool
- Recent hospital treatment or antibiotic treatment
- Persistent vomiting
- Severe dehydration, watery, high-volume diarrhoea
- Significant weight loss
- Patient is involved in handling food
- History of recent foreign travel

Radiological investigations
- AXR
- SBBFT

Figure 17.1 Stool culture grows salmonella

Figure 17.2 AXR shows pancreatic calcification indicative of chronic pancreatitis

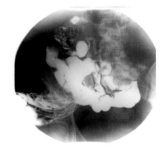

Figure 17.3 SBBFT shows normal small bowel mucosa

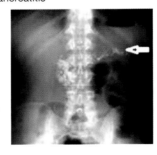

Key points in investigating diarrhoea
- Acute diarrhoea is most likely to be infectious.
- Infective diarrhoea is usually self-limiting. Microbiologic investigation is usually unnecessary unless there are red flag symptoms and indications.
- Investigations for chronic diarrhoea should focus on the identification of likely causes, the severity of the illness and any nutritional deficiency.

Endoscopic investigations

Figure 17.4 Colonoscopy shows (a) melanosis, characteristic in laxative abuse; (b) colon cancer; (c) a normal appearance in a patient with microscopic colitis

(a)

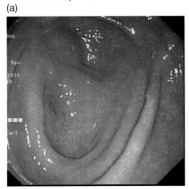

(b)

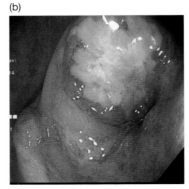

(c)

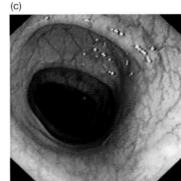

Clinical Investigations at a Glance, First Edition. Jonathan Gleadle, Jordan Li and Tuck Yong. © 2017 John Wiley & Sons, Ltd. Published 2017 by John Wiley & Sons, Ltd.

D iarrhoea is defined as an increased frequency of stools (more than three times per day being abnormal) or a change in stool consistency (becoming loose or watery). An objective measurement of diarrhoea is stool weight: a stool weight of greater than 200 g per day in a western population is regarded as abnormal. Faecal incontinence is commonly misinterpreted as diarrhoea. Acute diarrhoea is defined as terminating within 4 weeks and may be accompanied by nausea, vomiting, abdominal cramps and systemic symptoms. Symptoms persisting for >4 weeks are regarded as chronic diarrhoea and require further investigation.

Acute diarrhoea

Acute diarrhoea is more likely to have an infectious cause (bacteria, viruses, parasites). Other causes may include lactose intolerance and medications. Antibiotic-associated diarrhoea is otherwise unexplained diarrhoea in association with the administration of antibiotics. Infection with *Clostridium difficile* accounts for 10–20% of antibiotic-associated diarrhoea. Clindamycin, cephalosporins and penicillins are most frequently associated with *C. difficile* diarrhoea, but they also cause diarrhoea that is unrelated to superinfection with this organism. Clinical investigation of the patient with acute diarrhoea is usually unnecessary unless the patient has 'red flag symptoms' (red flag box). The investigation should focus on the assessment of the severity of the illness, the need for rehydration and the identification of likely causes on the basis of the history and clinical findings.

Laboratory investigations

FBC may reveal leucocytosis and neutrophilia in patients with an infective cause of diarrhoea. The haemoglobin and platelet counts are important in patients with diarrhoea complicated by haemolytic–uraemic syndrome caused by enterohaemorrhagic *Escherichia coli*.

For acute enteritis and colitis, maintaining adequate intravascular volume and correcting fluid and electrolyte disturbances take priority over the identification of the causative agent. Therefore, electrolytes, urea and creatinine should be measured in patients, especially the elderly, with moderate or severe dehydration.

Infective diarrhoea is usually self-limiting. Microbiologic investigation is usually unnecessary for patients who present within 24 hours after the onset of diarrhoea. However, systemic illness, fever or bloody stools should prompt routine stool testing for salmonella (Figure 17.1), shigella, campylobacter and Shiga toxin-producing *E. coli*. If the patient is involved in handling food or has a history of foreign travel, three stool specimens for microscopy, culture and sensitivity should be performed.

C. difficile infection (CDI) cannot be distinguished clinically from other causes of acute diarrhoea without laboratory testing. However, asymptomatic carriage of toxigenic *C. difficile* is not infrequent. Patients hospitalised >72 hours with unformed stool or patients with clinical suspicion should be tested for CDI.

The current recommendation in many centres is a two-step process. Step 1: perform an initial screen on stool samples using a test for a *C. difficile* antigen called glutamate dehydrogenase, which is produced by both toxin- and non-toxin-producing strains. It is very sensitive, but not specific for toxin-producing *C. difficile*. Step 2: follow up positive screening results with PCR assay, which is rapid and very sensitive to confirm the presence of *C. difficile* toxin.

Other investigations

An AXR or CT of the abdomen is non-specific and insensitive for identifying the cause of acute diarrhoea. Endoscopic investigations are not required for acute diarrhoea except for patients who are immunocompromised.

Chronic diarrhoea

A detailed history is essential in the assessment of patients with chronic diarrhoea. It can help distinguish organic as opposed to functional diarrhoea or distinguish malabsorption from colonic/inflammatory forms of diarrhoea. Symptoms suggestive of an organic cause of diarrhoea include: <3 months' duration, predominately nocturnal or continuous diarrhoea and significant weight loss. In patients <45 years old who have no symptoms and risk factors suggestive of organic diarrhoea and negative initial investigations, then a diagnosis of irritable bowel syndrome may be made without further investigations. In patients over 45 years with diarrhoea, functional symptoms are less reliably differentiated from symptoms of organic disease and, given the higher prevalence of colonic neoplasia in this age group, further investigation is recommended.

Laboratory investigations

An initial clinical evaluation and limited laboratory investigations often point to the cause of diarrhoea. The passage of bulky malodorous stools is suggestive of malabsorption. Colonic inflammatory or secretory forms of diarrhoea typically present with liquid or loose stools with the passage of blood or mucus. In steatorrhoea, stools are fatty, pale coloured, extremely smelly, float and are difficult to flush away. The common stool and blood tests are listed opposite. Breath tests for fat malabsorption include ^{14}C-triolein or a ^{13}C-labelled mixed triglyceride as substrates. Breath tests have a low sensitivity for mild or moderate fat malabsorption and are inappropriate in patients with diabetes, liver disease or obesity.

Radiological investigations

AXR may reveal pancreatic calcification (Figure 17.2). The small bowel barium follow through (SBBFT) or barium enteroclysis remains the standard means of assessing small bowel mucosa (Figure 17.3), although sensitivity and specificity are low. However, a negative result offers reasonably reliable exclusion of macroscopic small bowel disease. Small bowel enteroscopy has been regarded as a complementary investigation to SBBFT, to distinguish small bowel abnormalities or to assess further the small bowel after a negative radiological investigation.

Endoscopic investigations

In most patients with chronic diarrhoea, some form of endoscopic investigation will be necessary. Sigmoidoscopy and biopsy can be performed before a barium study and without hyperosmotic preparation. This is an appropriate examination in younger patients who on clinical grounds are believed to have a functional bowel disorder. Melanosis coli can be found with laxative abuse (Figure 17.4a).

Colonoscopy yields a prevalence of colonic neoplasms (Figure 17.4b) of 27% in those patients undergoing colonoscopy for a change in bowel habit including diarrhoea. In addition to neoplasia, colonoscopy also has a diagnostic yield for other conditions (ranging from 7% to 31%), with inflammatory bowel disease and microscopic colitis (Figure 17.4c) being most commonly found.

18 Constipation

Constipation is common, and the majority of constipation does not need investigation, especially in young patients without any of the following red flag alarm features.

Indications for investigation in patients presenting with constipation

- Age >50 years
- An acute or recent onset of constipation
- Progressive worsening constipation
- Unintentional weight loss
- Associated with rectal bleeding, melaena or mucus
- Change in stool calibre
- Associated with nausea, vomiting
- Family history of inflammatory bowel disease or colorectal cancer

Physiological testing

Physiological testing is required only infrequently, in those with symptoms not responding to treatment and who do not have a secondary cause or in whom a trial of a high-fibre diet and laxatives was not effective. Tests include:
- colonic-transit measurement
- anorectal manometry
- balloon expulsion
- defecography

Laboratory investigations
- FBC
- Thyroid function
- Electrolytes, including serum calcium, glucose levels

Radiological investigations
AXR should not be performed routinely to evaluate constipation. Radiological investigations are performed if intestinal obstruction or secondary causes of constipation, such as colorectal cancer, are suspected.

Endoscopic investigations
In patients with 'alarm' symptoms as listed in red flag box, the colon should be examined endoscopically

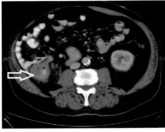

Figure 18.1 CT abdomen shows significant circumferential caecal colonic wall thickening and mass indicative of caecal malignancy

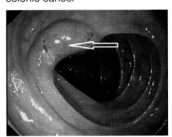

Figure 18.2 Colonoscopy shows colonic cancer

Figure 18.3 Nuclear small and large bowel transit study shows left-sided colonic delay

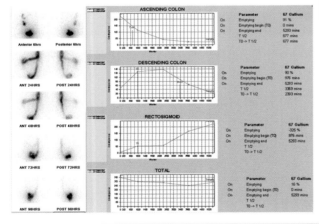

Key points in investigating constipation

- Laboratory investigations that may be useful in patients with constipation include thyroid function tests, electrolytes (including serum calcium and glucose level), and FBC.
- Radiological investigations do not add much value to the diagnosis of constipation when it can be achieved with clinical information.
- Physiological testing is required only infrequently, in those with symptoms not responding to treatment.

Clinical Investigations at a Glance, First Edition. Jonathan Gleadle, Jordan Li and Tuck Yong. © 2017 John Wiley & Sons, Ltd. Published 2017 by John Wiley & Sons, Ltd.

Constipation is a common symptom affecting 15% of the population worldwide. Predisposing factors include female sex, increasing age, low socioeconomic status and depression. There is no single definition of constipation. Most patients define constipation by one or more symptoms: infrequent stools (usually fewer than three per week), hard and dry stools, difficult stool passage with straining or discomfort, a sense of incomplete bowel evacuation and excessive time spent on the toilet or unsuccessful defecation. Though symptoms associated with constipation are often intermittent and mild, they can also be chronic (symptoms >6 months), challenging to treat and debilitating to the patient. Constipation can be a presenting symptom of colorectal cancer. Constipation is frequently multifactorial and can result from systemic and neurological disorders or medications.

Clinical evaluation

The majority of constipation does not need investigation, especially in young patients without any red flag alarm features (red flag box). History and physical examination can help identify secondary causes of constipation. A digital rectal examination should be performed in every patient with constipation because it often yields important clinical information, such as whether faecal impaction, anal stricture or rectal masses are present.

Laboratory investigations

Laboratory investigations that may be useful in patients with constipation include thyroid function tests, electrolytes (including serum calcium and glucose level), and FBC.

Radiological investigations

Radiological investigations usually do not add value to the diagnosis of constipation which can be achieved with clinical information. An AXR should not just be performed to confirm constipation. Radiological investigations are performed if intestinal obstruction or secondary causes of constipation such as colorectal cancer is suspected (Figure 18.1).

Endoscopic investigations

In patients with 'alarm' symptoms (red flag box), the colon should be examined endoscopically to exclude the possibility of structural diseases such as colorectal cancer (Figure 18.2). In patients without 'alarm' symptoms who are <50 years, sigmoidoscopy may be the first choice of investigation.

Physiological testing

Physiological testing is required very infrequently in those with symptoms not responding to treatment and who do not have a secondary cause or in whom a trial of a high-fibre diet and laxatives was not effective. In patients with clinical features suggestive of a defecatory disorder (commonly due to pelvic floor or anal sphincter dysfunction), the initial physiological investigations to consider are anorectal manometry and balloon expulsion. Defecography may be considered if the results of these tests are equivocal or if there is a clinical suspicion of a structural abnormality in the rectum that impedes defecation, such as rectal prolapse. A defecatory disorder can be associated with delayed colonic transit, and measurement of the colonic transit time should be considered after the underlying pelvic floor dysfunction has been corrected.

In patients without clinical features of defecatory disorders, the initial physiological test to consider is colonic transit testing, to differentiate slow-transit constipation from normal-transit constipation. Then anorectal manometry and balloon-expulsion tests should be considered for patients who do not have a response to treatment with fibre and laxatives.

Colonic-transit measurement

Colonic transit time is measured by performing abdominal radiography 120 hours after the patient has ingested radiopaque markers in a gelatine capsule. Before the study, the patient should be on a high-fibre diet and not taking laxatives or medications that can affect bowel function. Normal colonic transit time is <72 hours. Retention of >20% of the markers indicates prolonged transit. If the markers are retained exclusively in the lower left colon and rectum, the patient may have a defecatory disorder. A nuclear small and large bowel transit study is an alternative method (Figure 18.3).

Anorectal manometry

Anorectal manometry can measure the pressure of the anal sphincter at rest (predominantly the internal anal sphincter) and the maximal voluntary contraction of the external sphincter, the presence or absence of relaxation of the internal anal sphincter during balloon distention (the anorectal inhibitory reflex), rectal sensation and the ability of the anal sphincters to relax during straining. Inappropriate contraction of the anal sphincter at rest and bearing down is commonly observed in patients with defecatory disorder.

Balloon expulsion

Balloon expulsion is a simple office-based screening test for defecatory disorders. After insertion of the latex balloon into the rectum, 50 mL of water or air is instilled into the balloon and the patient is expected to expel the balloon within 2 min. Inability to expel the balloon within that time suggests a defecatory disorder.

19 Haematemesis and melaena

Goals of investigation
- Ascertain if a patient has had a UGIB if the history is inadequate to clarify
- Determine the extent of blood loss
- Identify the cause of bleeding
- Identify patients with a low or high probability of re-bleeding

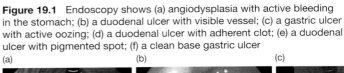

Blood tests
- FBC
- Group and cross-match blood
- Coagulation studies
- Electrolytes, urea, creatinine
- Liver function tests

Endoscopy is the primary diagnostic investigation in patients with acute UGIB

Timing of endoscopy
- Endoscopy should be undertaken immediately after resuscitation for unstable patients and patients with suspected liver disease or with continued bleeding
- Endoscopy should be undertaken within 24 h of admission for all other patients with UGIB

Figure 19.1 Endoscopy shows (a) angiodysplasia with active bleeding in the stomach; (b) a duodenal ulcer with visible vessel; (c) a gastric ulcer with active oozing; (d) a duodenal ulcer with adherent clot; (e) a duodenal ulcer with pigmented spot; (f) a clean base gastric ulcer

Assess the risk of re-bleeding
- Active spurting (Figure 19.1a)
- Non-bleeding visible vessel (Figure 19.1b)
- Active oozing (Figure 19.1c)
- Adherent clot (Figure 19.1d)
- Flat pigmented spot (Figure 19.1e)
- Clean base ulcer (Figure 19.1f)

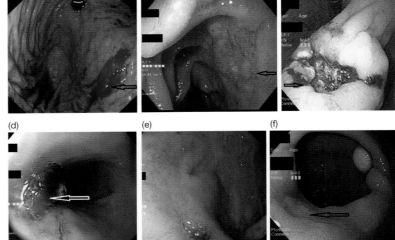

Repeat endoscopy
- Repeat endoscopy within 24 hours after initial endoscopic haemostatic therapy is not recommended
- Repeat endoscopy only to be performed in patients with evidence of recurrent bleeding
- Recurrent bleeding after a second endoscopic therapeutic session, consider surgery or interventional radiology

Further investigations
If the endoscopy finding is normal and there is clinical evidence of bleeding or recurrent bleeding:
- Abdominal CT with intravenous contrast (Figure 19.2)
- Ultrasound
- Radionuclide RBC scans (Figure 19.3)
- Angiography

Investigate *H. pylori* status (Chapter 21)

Figure 19.2 CT abdomen with intravenous contrast shows no evidence of active gastrointestinal bleeding

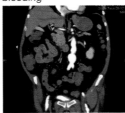

Figure 19.3 Radionuclide-labelled RBC gastrointestinal bleeding study shows active bleeding

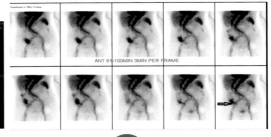

Key points in investigating UGIB

- Haemoglobin level is a poor indicator of the amount of recent blood loss as anaemia does not become apparent until haemodilution has occurred.
- Endoscopy is the primary diagnostic investigation in patients with acute UGIB and can identify the cause of haemorrhage in the majority of patients.
- At endoscopy, examine for stigmata of recent haemorrhage and indicators of likely re-bleeding.
- Repeat endoscopy should only be performed in patients with clinical evidence of recurrent bleeding.

Clinical Investigations at a Glance, First Edition. Jonathan Gleadle, Jordan Li and Tuck Yong. © 2017 John Wiley & Sons, Ltd. Published 2017 by John Wiley & Sons, Ltd.

Haematemesis, the vomiting of blood, indicates active haemorrhage from the upper gastrointestinal (UGI) tract, which requires rapid clinical assessment, investigation and management. Haematemesis must be distinguished from haemoptysis. Coffee-ground vomit refers to the vomiting of black material that is assumed to be altered blood; it often implies that bleeding has been relatively modest or has ceased. Melaena is the consequence of a significant haemorrhage into the UGI tract. A varying degree of digestive alteration of blood makes the stools black and tarry. Haematochezia is the passage of fresh or altered blood per rectum, usually due to colonic bleeding but can rarely be due to rapid and profuse UGI bleeding (UGIB). Acute UGIB is a medical emergency with a hospital mortality of 6–13%.

Laboratory investigations

Full blood examination

A FBC will provide an estimation of haemoglobin and platelet count. A fall in haemoglobin is expected with blood loss. However, anaemia does not develop immediately because haemodilution has not taken place. Therefore, haemoglobin level is a poor indicator of the need to transfuse. The mean corpuscular volume is usually normal in acute blood loss but can be reduced in chronic blood loss if there is iron deficiency. Haemoglobin (or haematocrit) can be measured serially (4–6 hourly in the first day) to help assess whether there is ongoing blood loss.

Group and cross-match blood

Usually between two and six units of RBCs should be cross-matched according to rate of active bleeding. Indications for blood transfusion are patients who are in shock and/or show signs of ongoing bleed. Blood transfusions should target haemoglobin ≥70 g/L, with higher haemoglobins targeted in patients with comorbidities such as coronary artery disease or clinical evidence of intravascular volume depletion.

Coagulation studies

INR and activated partial thromboplastin time (APTT) should be checked in patients with suspected chronic liver disease and those taking anticoagulant therapy.

Biochemistry and liver function tests

A raised urea/creatinine ratio is useful for the diagnosis of bleeding from the UGI tract in patients who do not present with overt vomiting of blood. Elevated creatinine may point towards AKI complicating hypovolaemic shock. Deranged liver function may suggest liver disease, potentially with bleeding from varices.

Upper GI endoscopy

Endoscopy is the primary diagnostic investigation in patients with acute UGIB. Endoscopy can identify the cause of haemorrhage in 80% of patients (Figures 19.1a–f), but in 20% no definite cause is found. Depending on the cause of the bleed, therapeutic interventions can also be performed endoscopically.

Assess the risk of re-bleeding

Stigmata of recent haemorrhage should be recorded as they predict risk of further bleeding and guide management decisions. The stigmata, in descending risk of further bleeding, are listed opposite.

Repeat endoscopy

Routine second-look endoscopy, in which repeat endoscopy is performed 24 hours after initial endoscopic haemostatic therapy, is not recommended. Repeat endoscopy should only be performed in patients with clinical evidence of recurrent bleeding. If further bleeding occurs after a second endoscopic therapeutic session, surgery or interventional radiology with transcatheter arterial embolisation should be considered.

Investigate *H. pylori* status

Biopsy-based *H. pylori* testing is recommended in patients presenting with a bleeding ulcer. Some studies suggest sensitivity may be decreased with acute UGIB; confirmation of a negative test with a subsequent non-endoscopic test such as urea breath test is needed. However, if histological examination of the biopsy specimens shows no mucosal mononuclear cell infiltrate, the predictive value for absence of *H. pylori* approaches 100%, while a neutrophilic infiltrate has >95% positive predictive value for *H. pylori* infection.

Imaging

CXR

CXR may identify aspiration pneumonia, pleural effusion, perforated oesophagus.

Abdominal CT with contrast and ultrasound

These can identify liver disease, potential haemorrhagic sites and aortoenteric fistulae.

Nuclear medicine scans

This scan uses technetium-labelled RBCs. It can identify areas of active haemorrhage with a bleeding rate >0.5 mL/min.

Angiography

Angiography may be useful if there is evidence of ongoing bleeding and endoscopy fails to identify site of bleeding or unstable patients who re-bleed after endoscopic treatment. It can determine the site of bleeding but not the cause and can lead to therapeutic intra-arterial injection of vasopressin or arterial embolisation.

20 Rectal bleeding

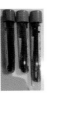

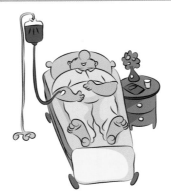

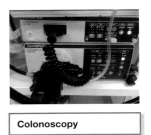

Colonoscopy

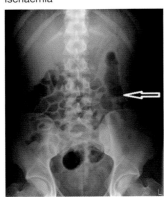

Figure 20.1 AXR (erect) shows thumbprinting in descending colon compatible with mucosal thickening and segmental bowel ischaemia

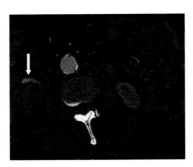

Figure 20.2 CT abdominal angiogram shows contrast in the large bowel due to bleeding

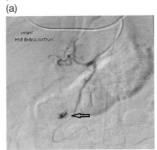

Figure 20.3 Angiogram shows (a) a focal bleeding point from rectum prior to embolisation; (b) cessation of bleeding post-embolisation

(a) (b)

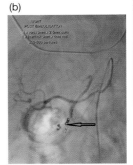

Figure 20.4 Radionuclide-labelled red blood cells study shows active bleeding in the caecum area

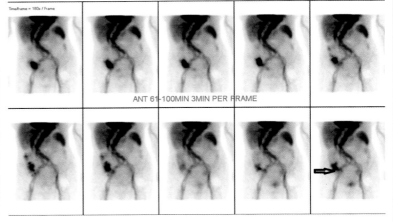

ANT 61-100MIN 3MIN PER FRAME

Key points in investigating per rectum bleeding

- Undertake proctoscopy, sigmoidoscopy or colonoscopy if bleeding is persistent or recurrent.
- Consider mesenteric angiography if there has been significant bleeding and/or colonoscopy has failed to identify a bleeding site.
- Technetium-labelled red blood cell scintigraphy may help localise the bleeding source.
- If rectal bleeding continues, consider laparotomy.

The passage of blood through the rectum is a common symptom, and any lesion of the small or large bowel may be implicated. Although haemorrhoids is the most common cause of rectal bleeding, there are many other aetiologies to consider that can be classified according to the location of pathology in the gastrointestinal tract. However, in as many as 20% of patients no aetiology can be identified even when there has been considerable blood loss and thorough investigation.

Rectal bleeding always warrants further investigation. The investigations chosen will depend on the presenting symptoms, age and likely diagnosis. A digital rectal examination should always be performed first to confirm blood in the rectum and to exclude any rectal or pelvic masses before other investigations. Proctoscopy enables lesions felt digitally to be seen and biopsied and is particularly useful in the assessment of haemorrhoids. The purpose of investigations is to determine the cause of the bleeding and consequences arising from the bleed.

Laboratory investigations

FBC is performed to provide information about the haemoglobin level. Electrolytes, urea and creatinine and liver function tests are indicated in patients with significant rectal bleeding. Coagulation studies should also be performed, especially in patients with bleeding disorders or taking anticoagulants.

Blood group and cross-match should be performed for anaemic patients, major haemorrhage or when major surgery is being considered. Ferritin and iron studies are indicated if iron-deficiency anaemia is suspected.

Radiological investigations

Plain X-rays and barium enema

An AXR may reveal gross thickening of the bowel wall and/or gas within the bowel wall in late stages of acute intestinal ischaemia (Figure 20.1). Barium enema has a significant miss rate for colorectal cancer and other pathologies, and does not have a role in investigation of rectal bleeding.

CT of abdomen

A CT scan can be used to diagnose diverticulitis or advanced colorectal cancer that may be the cause of rectal bleeding. CT has been found to be highly accurate in the diagnosis of ischaemic colitis. Typically, CT scans show irregular thickening of the bowel wall, but other inflammatory or infectious conditions can have the similar features. Vascular extravasation of the contrast medium points out the location of the bleeding (Figure 20.2). The sensitivity of CT angiography in the detection of colonic angiodysplasia is 70% and specificity is 100%.

Angiography

Mesenteric angiography is the best option in haemodynamically unstable patients with massive bleeding. Angiography is also performed if colonoscopy has failed to identify a bleeding site. The advantage of angiography over colonoscopy or scintigraphy is that no special preparation is needed and it can be performed in a relatively short period; angiography also provides a means for immediate treatment (Figures 20.3a and b). On angiography, haemorrhage is identified as the extravasation of contrast into the lumen of the bowel.

Angiography can reveal the site of acute arterial occlusion of a diseased bowel segment. Images may show attenuation, vasoconstriction or complete arterial occlusion of the vessel involved. Angiographic findings are highly sensitive for vascular narrowing or stenosis when the ischaemia is arterial in origin. However, in established colonic ischaemia, no angiographic changes may be observed, or the angiographic changes may be indistinguishable from those of inflammatory bowel disease.

Radionuclide study

Technetium-labelled red blood cell scintigraphy (Figure 20.4) may help localise the source of active gastrointestinal haemorrhage when other techniques such as endoscopy have failed. It is more sensitive and less invasive than angiography for intermittent bleeding, and repeat imaging can be performed on several occasions within 24 hours. Whilst the site of bleeding may be identified, it cannot determine the underlying cause.

Endoscopic investigations

Sigmoidoscopy

Flexible sigmoidoscopy enables the rectum and distal portion of the colon to be visualised and lesions to be biopsied. It is the investigation of choice for patients under the age of 45 years with rectal bleeding not explained by haemorrhoids or who have received treatment for haemorrhoids and still have bleeding.

Colonoscopy

Patients over the age of 45 years with persistent rectal bleeding should be offered a colonoscopy. Colonoscopy after rapid oral purging is the procedure of choice for patients with acute lower gastrointestinal bleeding and who are haemodynamically stable, and it also provides a potential route to therapy. In elderly, frail or unfit patients, virtual colonoscopy may be preferable as it is minimally invasive and better tolerated for patients and may also provide additional extra colonic information.

Laparotomy

Infrequently, all investigations may be unrevealing. If rectal bleeding continues, laparotomy may be indicated.

21 Dyspepsia

Indications for endoscopy in patients presented with dyspepsia

- Age 50 years with new-onset dyspepsia
- Anorexia or unintentional weight loss
- Dysphagia or odynophagia
- Protracted vomiting
- Persisting upper abdominal pain radiating to the back
- Unexplained iron-deficiency anaemia
- Haematemesis or melaena
- Epigastric mass
- Failure of two courses of empirical treatments
- Strong history of familial cancer
- Previous gastric surgery or ulcer

Key points in investigating dyspepsia, GORD and PUD

- The response of symptoms to PPI for 14 days is about as specific and sensitive for the diagnosis of GORD as the results of 24-hour pH monitoring.
- Ambulatory pH monitoring is generally considered the diagnostic gold standard for GORD, but the test is time consuming and inconvenient, requiring good technical placement of the probe and experienced interpretation of the results.
- Endoscopic biopsy is the only test that can detect the columnar mucosal changes of Barrett oesophagus.

Table 21.1 Summary of tests used in *H. pylori* infection

Test	Advantages	Disadvantages	Use	Sensitivity	Specificity
Serology test	Inexpensive Quick Easy to perform Non-invasive	Need local validation: accuracy dependent on purification of strains and suitability of strain types for group being tested	Pre-eradication	92%	70%
Urea breath tests	High sensitivity and specificity Can confirm efficacy of eradication using ^{13}C testing	^{13}C urea and isotope ratio mass spectrometry are expensive	Pre- and post-eradication	95%	96%
Endoscopy/urease test	High specificity Rapid and inexpensive	Invasive, sampling error Cannot determine antibiotic resistance	Pre- and post-eradication	92–100%	79–100%
Endoscopy/histopathology	High specificity	Invasive, sampling error Observer dependent Cannot determine antibiotic resistance	Pre- and post-eradication	97%	100%
Endoscopy /H. pylori culture	High specificity Allows determination of antibiotic resistance	Invasive, sampling error Time consuming	Antibiotic sensitivity	65%	100%

Clinical Investigations at a Glance, First Edition. Jonathan Gleadle, Jordan Li and Tuck Yong. © 2017 John Wiley & Sons, Ltd. Published 2017 by John Wiley & Sons, Ltd.

Dyspepsia is pain or discomfort in the epigastric region, anorexia, nausea, bloating, fullness, early satiety and heartburn. It is a common complaint. An organic cause is found in 60% of patients, and 40% of dyspepsia is considered to be functional or idiopathic. Dyspepsia is more common in patients who take non-steroidal anti-inflammatory drugs (NSAIDs) and drugs such as corticosteroids and bisphosphonates and in patients infected with *Helicobacter pylori*.

Functional dyspepsia is defined as no macroscopic mucosal abnormality. Non-erosive reflux, hiatus hernia, non-erosive duodenitis and gastritis are reported at endoscopy in patients with dyspepsia. The cause of symptoms in these patients is usually unclear. It is likely that multiple factors are involved, including acid, defective motility, *H. pylori* infection and depression.

A firm clinical diagnosis can be difficult to make when patients present with dyspepsia as few symptoms are discriminatory and symptoms show little correlation with endoscopic findings. As dyspepsia is common and investigations can be costly and invasive, it is acceptable to institute treatment with an anti-secretory agent, such as proton pump inhibitor (PPI), in patients under 50 with dyspepsia but without red flags (see red flag box). While this treatment is attempted it is recommended that *H. pylori* testing is undertaken.

Diagnostic tests for *H. pylori* infection

H. pylori infection can be diagnosed by showing urease activity in the stomach using breath tests or by examination of gastric biopsies (Table 21.1).

Serological test

Serological testing can demonstrate antibodies to *H. pylori* in serum. The test is inexpensive, non-invasive and widely available but not useful in demonstrating successful eradication. Serological testing performs less well than breath testing. The resultant lower positive predictive value (64% versus 88%) leads to concerns about the unnecessary use of antibiotics when serology testing is used only.

Breath tests

Carbon-tagged breath tests, which depend on *H. pylori* urease degradation of urea to produce tagged carbon dioxide that appears in exhaled breath, are of intermediate cost, but are non-invasive and accurate. Two methods have been used with urea labelled either with ^{14}C (a small radioactive dose, but cheap) or ^{13}C (a stable, non-radioactive dose but more expensive). ^{13}C urea breath tests are available as kits on prescription. These tests are the only tests that can confirm successful eradication, but they must be performed when patients are not taking PPIs or bismuth, nor within 4 weeks of antibiotic use.

Upper GI endoscopy and biopsy

Methods of identifying *H. pylori* in endoscopy include biopsy urease tests, histology and culture of the organism, which involves significant cost. Routine use of endoscopy for diagnosis of *H. pylori* is not recommended.

If the *H. pylori* test is positive, eradication therapy is recommended. The value of confirming the success of eradication therapy has been questioned because of the high efficacy of *H. pylori* eradication therapies and the cost involved to detect <5% who would be expected to remain *H. pylori* positive. A pragmatic approach is to confirm eradication for patients who have had complicated ulcer disease. Once eradicated, the risk of *H. pylori* re-infection is small (0.5–1.0% per annum).

Endoscopy

Endoscopy is the procedure of choice for the evaluation of dyspepsia. Routine endoscopic investigation of patients <50 years with dyspepsia and without red flag symptoms, is not necessary. Endoscopy is indicated if there are signs or symptoms suggesting an important underlying cause (see red flag box).

Radiology investigation

A double contrast barium upper GI study may be an acceptable alternative to endoscopy, but does not allow biopsies to be taken and is thus considered second choice. However, it provides valuable complementary information in diagnosis of minor strictures that may be missed endoscopically, motility disorders, extrinsic and possibly intra-mural abnormalities as well as the diagnosis of malrotations, herniations and other structural abnormalities.

Gastric scintigraphy may help confirm delayed gastric emptying, particularly in patients with postprandial distress-type symptoms, to direct treatment, but the correlation between gastric emptying rates and symptoms is poor.

Gastro-oesophageal reflux disease (GORD)

GORD is defined as reflux that causes symptoms and mucosal injury in the oesophagus. The two most typical symptoms of GORD are heartburn and regurgitation. Extra-oesophageal symptoms such as cough, hoarseness and exacerbation of asthma can occur.

When symptoms of GORD are characteristic and the patient responds to PPI therapy, no diagnostic tests are necessary. This is known as a PPI test. This test may also be positive in other acid-related disorders, such as peptic ulcer disease and functional dyspepsia. It only has a specificity of 24–65%. In primary care, a short trial of a PPI is useful because the combination of a favourable response and absence of alarm symptoms makes additional diagnostic testing unnecessary.

However, further diagnostic testing may be required to evaluate treatment non-responsiveness and identify GORD-related complications such as esophagitis, Barrett's metaplasia and adenocarcinoma.

Ambulatory reflux monitoring

Oesophageal pH monitoring records the overall oesophageal acid exposure (pH <4). More importantly it shows whether there is a temporal relation between symptoms and reflux events (Figure 21.1). This is done by a transnasally inserted catheter with pH sensor, which is connected to a portable data logger enabling measurements over a 24-hour period. This investigation should be performed after acid-suppressive drugs have been discontinued for >5 days.

However, two-thirds of all reflux episodes are non-acidic but still trigger reflux symptoms. In this situation, oesophageal impedance measurement can be used to detect reflux independent of the pH of the refluxate. Impedance and pH monitoring are usually done in combination.

Figure 21.1 Oesophageal pH monitoring showing GORD (left) and normal (right)

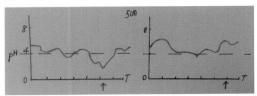

Figure 21.2 Endoscopy showing (a) normal gastroesophageal junction and (b) reflux oesophagitis

(a)

(b)

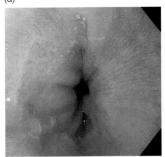

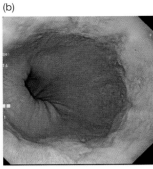

Figure 21.3 Endoscopy showing oesophageal candidiasis

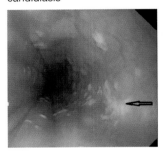

Figure 21.4 Endoscopy showing Barrett's oesophagus

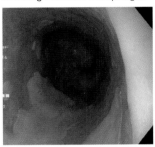

Figure 21.5 Endoscopy showing oesophageal carcinoma

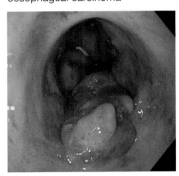

Figure 21.6 Endoscopy showing gastric carcinoma

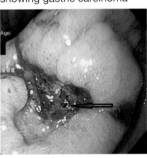

Figure 21.7 Endoscopy showing gastric ulcer with visible vessel

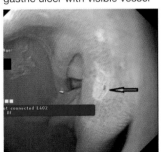

Upper GI endoscopy

Patients who present with alarm symptoms (red flag box) warrant upper GI endoscopy because they might have complications of GORD or other pathologies. An observation of typical reflux oesophagitis (Figure 21.2) confirms the diagnosis of GORD. This investigation also serves to exclude alternative diagnoses such as eosinophilic oesophagitis or infection (Figure 21.3). The overall diagnostic yield of upper GI endoscopy in GORD is low because most patients with GORD do not have visible erosions in the oesophagus. It is a test with high specificity but low sensitivity for GORD.

Barrett's oesophagus (Figure 21.4) is a complication of GORD in which potentially precancerous metaplastic columnar cells replace the normal squamous mucosa. There is still controversy surrounding the appropriate role of endoscopy in screening patients for Barrett's oesophagus and in surveillance of those known to have the condition. The risk of oesophageal adenocarcinoma in patients with Barrett's oesophagus is 0.50–0.75% per year. Therefore, screening patients for Barrett's oesophagus, followed by surveillance of affected patients for the development of dysplasia and adenocarcinoma, can potentially enable early diagnosis of oesophageal carcinoma (Figure 21.5) or even prevention of cancer by ablation of dysplastic lesions. However, despite widespread screening for Barrett's oesophagus with endoscopy, evidence that this strategy reduces the rate of death from oesophageal adenocarcinoma is lacking.

Manometry

Oesophageal manometry is not required for the diagnosis of GORD because motor dysfunction associated with reflux is non-specific. The main reasons for manometry are to determine the correct placement of the pH monitor and to rule out severe oesophageal motility disorder such as achalasia and absent peristalsis prior to anti-reflux surgery. Manometry is also potentially useful in patients with predominant regurgitation because it can help to distinguish the rumination syndrome from GORD.

Peptic ulcer disease (PUD)

PUD is characterised by mucosal inflammation and damage of the mucosal barrier in the lower oesophagus, stomach or duodenum. The use of NSAIDs and presence of *H. pylori* infection are the most common causes. Patients with PUD can be asymptomatic or present as chronic, epigastric pain related to eating a meal. Asymptomatic PUD should be suspected if there is no obvious cause of anaemia, especially iron-deficiency anaemia. Some patients present with complications of PUD, such as haematemesis, melaena, and perforated ulcer.

Upper GI endoscopy

Endoscopy is not indicated in patients <55 years with typical symptoms of PUD and absence of alarming symptoms (red flag box). Treatment with PPIs usually leads to healing within 6 weeks. *H. pylori* testing (Table 21.1) is recommended. If *H. pylori* infection is diagnosed, the infection should be eradicated.

Endoscopy is essential for accurate diagnosis and differential diagnosis of PUD and ulcer complications:
- Gastric ulcer can be biopsied to exclude malignancy (Figure 21.6).
- PUD can be biopsied for an *H. pylori* diagnostic test (Figure 21.7).
- Bleeding due to PUD can treated by endoscopy. Endoscopic healing is the gold standard used to evaluate ulcer healing, which is necessary in gastric ulcer but not in duodenal ulcer.

Diagnostic tests for *H. pylori* infection

H. pylori infection can be diagnosed by non-invasive methods or by endoscopic biopsy of the gastric mucosa (Table 21.1).

Investigating complications of PUD

In addition to haemorrhage (Chapter 20), PUD can be complicated by perforation and pyloric stenosis. About 90% of perforations are on the anterior wall of the first part of the duodenum. A plain erect CXR is the first investigation for a patient with suspected perforation. It will often reveal gas under the diaphragm, which confirms the perforation but not its origin. CT of the abdomen may be able to reveal the site of the perforation. Diagnostic upper GI endoscopy is **contraindicated** if perforation is present or suspected because the stomach must be inflated during the examination and air and gastric contents would spill into the peritoneal cavity.

In patients with suspected pyloric stenosis, plain AXR may reveal a grossly dilated stomach filled with mottled food material. Barium meal generally shows gastric dilatation, sometimes with increased peristalsis, a narrowed pyloro-duodenal area and delayed gastric emptying. Upper GI endoscopy can show the narrowed and oedematous pyloric canal. Several gastric washouts using a large-bore tube are necessary to clear the gastric content before barium meal or endoscopy is attempted.

22 Dysphagia

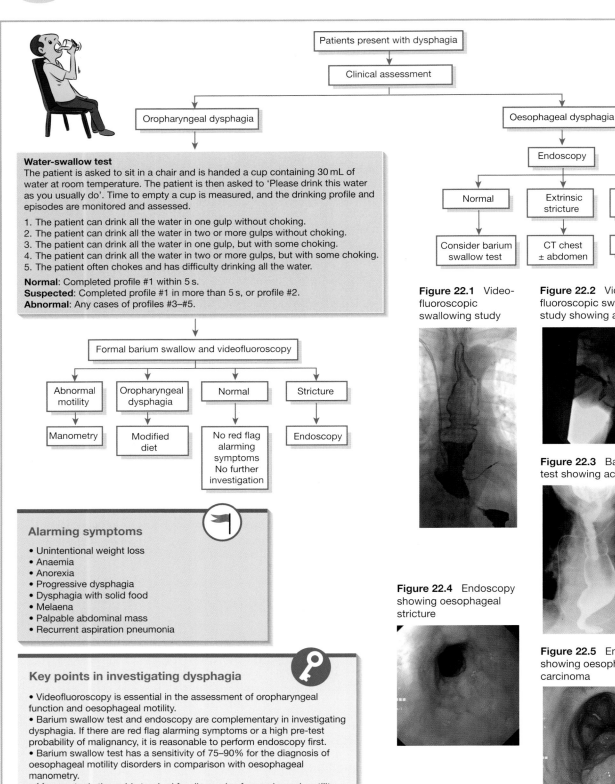

Patients present with dysphagia

↓

Clinical assessment

Oropharyngeal dysphagia | Oesophageal dysphagia

Water-swallow test
The patient is asked to sit in a chair and is handed a cup containing 30 mL of water at room temperature. The patient is then asked to 'Please drink this water as you usually do'. Time to empty a cup is measured, and the drinking profile and episodes are monitored and assessed.

1. The patient can drink all the water in one gulp without choking.
2. The patient can drink all the water in two or more gulps without choking.
3. The patient can drink all the water in one gulp, but with some choking.
4. The patient can drink all the water in two or more gulps, but with some choking.
5. The patient often chokes and has difficulty drinking all the water.

Normal: Completed profile #1 within 5 s.
Suspected: Completed profile #1 in more than 5 s, or profile #2.
Abnormal: Any cases of profiles #3–#5.

Oesophageal dysphagia → Endoscopy → Normal / Extrinsic stricture / Intrinsic stricture

Normal → Consider barium swallow test
Extrinsic stricture → CT chest ± abdomen
Intrinsic stricture → Biopsy

Formal barium swallow and videofluoroscopy

Abnormal motility → Manometry
Oropharyngeal dysphagia → Modified diet
Normal → No red flag alarming symptoms No further investigation
Stricture → Endoscopy

Alarming symptoms

- Unintentional weight loss
- Anaemia
- Anorexia
- Progressive dysphagia
- Dysphagia with solid food
- Melaena
- Palpable abdominal mass
- Recurrent aspiration pneumonia

Key points in investigating dysphagia

- Videofluoroscopy is essential in the assessment of oropharyngeal function and oesophageal motility.
- Barium swallow test and endoscopy are complementary in investigating dysphagia. If there are red flag alarming symptoms or a high pre-test probability of malignancy, it is reasonable to perform endoscopy first.
- Barium swallow test has a sensitivity of 75–90% for the diagnosis of oesophageal motility disorders in comparison with oesophageal manometry.
- Manometry is the gold standard for diagnosis of oesophageal motility disorders, especially achalasia.

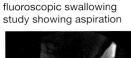

Figure 22.1 Video-fluoroscopic swallowing study

Figure 22.2 Video-fluoroscopic swallowing study showing aspiration

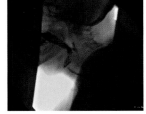

Figure 22.3 Barium swallow test showing achalasia

Figure 22.4 Endoscopy showing oesophageal stricture

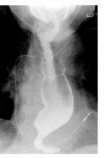

Figure 22.5 Endoscopy showing oesophageal carcinoma

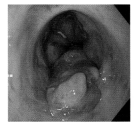

Clinical Investigations at a Glance, First Edition. Jonathan Gleadle, Jordan Li and Tuck Yong. © 2017 John Wiley & Sons, Ltd. Published 2017 by John Wiley & Sons, Ltd.

Dysphagia is difficulty with swallowing or a perception that there is an impediment to the normal passage of swallowed food.

Initial clinical evaluation

Determine whether the dysphagia is oropharyngeal or oesophageal. If the patient reports of 'lump in the throat' or difficulty initiating swallowing or complains of fluid regurgitating into the nose or choking on trying to swallow, these findings are suggestive of oropharyngeal dysphagia with an accuracy of 85%. If the patient reports food sticking in the oesophagus, it is likely oesophageal dysphagia. The history should concentrate on location, dysphagia for solid foods or liquids or both, whether progressive or intermittent and duration. The next step is to identify the cause of the dysphagia and consequences such as nutritional deficiency or aspiration.

Investigations for suspected oropharyngeal dysphagia

Oropharyngeal dysphagia is common in elderly patients. Post-stroke dysphagia occurs in about 50% of cases. Up to 50% of Parkinson patients have some symptoms suggestive of oropharyngeal dysphagia and up to 95% show abnormalities on barium swallow.

The water-swallow test is an inexpensive and useful screening test to complement clinical history and physical examination. This test has a predictive sensitivity of >85% for identifying the presence of dysphagia. This test may be complemented by a 'food test'. However, water-swallow test fails to identify aspiration in 20–40% of cases when followed up by videofluoroscopy. A videofluoroscopic swallowing study (also known as the 'modified barium swallow') is the gold standard for diagnosing oropharyngeal dysphagia (Figure 22.1) and may predict the risk of aspiration pneumonia (Figure 22.2), and endoscopy is the best test for the evaluation of structural causes of dysphagia.

Investigations for suspected oesophageal dysphagia

The main goal in investigating oesophageal dysphagia is to exclude malignancy. The following symptoms would suggest possibility of malignancy: duration <3 months, progressive dysphagia, dysphagia more for solids than for liquids and weight loss.

Laboratory investigations

- FBC: anaemia may relate to iron deficiency or chronic disease.
- Serum electrolytes: low albumin may indicate chronic malnutrition.
- Liver function tests: deranged liver functions may indicate metastatic disease involving the liver.

Radiological imaging

CXR

A CXR can help to identify changes suggestive of aspiration pneumonia, mediastinal masses and goitre.

Barium swallow

Barium swallow is a fluoroscopic study of swallowing that allows a structural and functional assessment of the oesophagus and hypopharynx. The examination should include all phases of swallowing, including an assessment of motility. Videofluorography provides an assessment of the tongue, pharynx and epiglottis, as well as information on oesophageal motility. To assess emptying of the oesophagus, a timed barium swallow can be done, in which the height of the barium column 5 min after ingestion of diluted barium is a measure of emptying. The results correlate well with manometry.

Barium swallow in patients with achalasia often shows a typical bird-beak appearance at the junction (Figure 22.3), with a dilated oesophageal body, sometimes with an air–fluid level and absence of an intragastric air bubble. In more advanced achalasia, severe dilatation with stasis of food and a sigmoid-like appearance can occur. Although radiology is not as sensitive as manometry, this investigation remains important to rule out structural abnormalities and estimate the diameter of the oesophagus.

CT

CT can be used to assess extrinsic lesions and tumour staging prior to surgery.

Manometry

Manometry is most helpful in the detection of early achalasia. Absence of peristalsis, sometimes with increased intraoesophageal pressure owing to stasis of food and saliva, and incomplete relaxation of the lower oesophageal sphincter are the hallmarks of achalasia. High-resolution manometry (HRM) is increasingly being used to provide more detailed information on oesophageal motility. By means of catheters incorporating 36 or more pressure sensors, HRM allows detailed pressure recording from the pharynx to the stomach.

Upper gastrointestinal endoscopy

Upper GI endoscopy is indicated for patients with dysphagia, especially with any symptoms suggesting malignancy. It helps to identify oesophageal stricture (Figure 22.4), oesophageal carcinoma (Figure 22.5) and pharyngeal pouch. If oesophageal carcinoma is suspected, endoscopy will enable tissue biopsy to be performed, and endoscopic ultrasound can also be undertaken. The overall rate of oesophageal perforation after flexible endoscopy involving oesophageal instrumentation, biopsy or dilatation is 1.5–2.6%. In the early stage of achalasia, both endoscopy and radiology are less sensitive than manometry and only identify about half (or even less) of patients with early-stage achalasia. In advanced cases, endoscopy might reveal a dilated oesophagus with retained food and increased resistance at the gastro-oesophageal junction.

23 Weight loss

Is there a clinically significant unintentional weight loss? That is, 5 kg or more than 5% of usual body weight lost over 6–12 months. What is the body mass index?

Weigh the patient

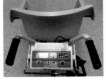

- Any documented weight change?
- How much weight loss over how much time?
- Any clothing or belt size changes?
- Any associated symptoms such as GI and/or constitutional symptoms?
- Any dietary history and food chart available?
- Any psychiatric symptoms?
- Has the patient been screened for depression and cognitive impairment?
- Any abnormal findings on physical examination?

Food chart

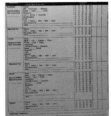

First-line investigation
- FBC
- Serum electrolytes, urea, creatinine
- LFTs
- Thyroid function tests
- CRP
- Serum glucose and HbA1c
- LDH
- Urinalysis
- FOBT
- CXR

Abnormal findings →

3 months of 'watchful waiting'

No abnormal findings

Persistent weight loss →

Table 23.1 Common causes of unintentional weight loss

Organic causes

- Common organic causes:
  - malignancy (16-36%)
  - GI disorders (10–20%) – dentition, diarrhoea, dysphagia, IBD
  - endocrine disorders (5–12%) – diabetes, thyroid disease
- Less common organic causes:
  - cardiovascular disease – heart failure
  - respiratory disease – chronic obstructive pulmonary disease
  - chronic infection
  - renal disease – advanced CKD
  - medication side effect
  - neurological disease – stroke

Psychosocial causes
- Depression - Eating disorders - Dementia - Poor nutritional intake – poverty or inadequate access to food

Idiopathic

Second-line investigation

Endoscopy and/or colonoscopy
- GI disorders (malignant and non-malignant) account for a third of all causes of unexplained weight loss in studies of adults of all ages, so upper GI endoscopy and/or colonoscopy is a reasonable second-line investigation.

Other investigations
- Other investigations should be considered in the appropriate clinical context:
  - HIV screen test
  - mammogram
  - coeliac disease serology test
  - malabsorption test (Chapter 71).

Tests not recommended to be routinely performed in investigating weight loss
- Tumour markers: not useful diagnostic tests in weight loss.
- Abdominal ultrasound
- CT scan

Figure 23.1 CXR shows right upper lobe lung cancer

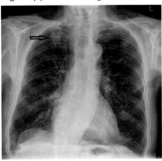

Figure 23.2 FOBT test kit

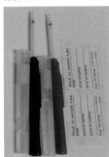

Figure 23.3 Endoscopy shows oesophageal cancer

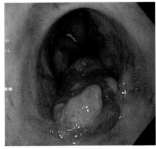

Key points in investigating weight loss

- Unintentional weight loss is common in elderly people and is associated with increased morbidity and mortality.
- All patients should be assessed by a dietitian and screened for depression and cognitive impairment.
- If initial history, examination, and investigations are normal, three months of "watchful waiting" is preferable to further blind investigations.

Clinical Investigations at a Glance, First Edition. Jonathan Gleadle, Jordan Li and Tuck Yong. © 2017 John Wiley & Sons, Ltd. Published 2017 by John Wiley & Sons, Ltd.

Clinically significant unintentional weight loss is defined as a loss of 5 kg or >5% of usual body weight lost over 6–12 months. It may reflect underlying disease severity or a yet undiagnosed disease and is associated with increased morbidity and mortality.

Unintentional weight loss may be the presenting problem or be identified during a consultation for other problems. Unintentional weight loss has a diverse cause but can be classified into three groups: organic (malignant and non-malignant), psychosocial and idiopathic (Table 23.1). Among organic causes, malignancy is the most common cause. The cause of unintentional weight loss is evident without extensive evaluation in most patients. Observational studies have shown that in as many as 25% of cases no identifiable cause is found despite extensive investigation.

Unintentional weight loss should not be dismissed as natural age-related change and should be investigated. A complete history, physical examination and selected basic investigations are the first step. One should objectively quantify food intake and assess cognitive function and mood.

First-line investigations

FBC
Anaemia is suggestive of an organic cause of weight loss and it should prompt further investigations, which will depend on the type of anaemia (e.g. microcytic, macrocytic). A raised white cell count may also suggest organic disease, such as malignant, infection or inflammatory diseases.

Serum electrolytes and creatinine
Although this is not a particularly helpful test in predicting an organic versus non-organic cause for weight loss, it is a reasonable investigation to perform because abnormal results may point towards an organic cause.

Liver function tests, including albumin
Normal LFTs and albumin level make serious organic causes for weight loss less likely, particularly cancer, which is usually advanced by the time weight loss occurs.

Thyroid function tests
Hyperthyroidism is a common cause of weight loss.

CRP
A raised CRP may suggest a possible organic cause for the weight loss. A normal CRP makes a serious organic cause for the weight loss less likely.

Blood glucose and HbA$_1$C
Uncontrolled diabetes is a cause of weight loss.

LDH
LDH >500 IU/L is associated with an increased likelihood of a malignant cause of involuntary weight loss.

CXR
CXR should be performed in all patients to identify respiratory disease, including malignant and non-malignant causes (Figure 23.1).

Urinalysis
Urinalysis should be part of the initial investigation and is non-invasive and inexpensive; however, its diagnostic benefit in elderly patients with unintentional weight loss is uncertain.

Faecal occult blood test (FOBT)
Because GI disorders (malignant and non-malignant) account for a third of all causes of unexplained weight loss, a FOBT is a reasonable first-line investigation (Figure 23.2). It is non-invasive and, although it is not particularly sensitive or specific, a positive result would prompt further investigation with colonoscopy and/or endoscopy.

Second-line investigations
If initial history, examination and investigations are all normal, 3 months of 'watchful waiting' is preferable to further blind investigations because organic disease is found only rarely in patients with normal results from physical examination and initial investigations. This waiting period is unlikely to have an adverse outcome. Abnormal findings on initial evaluation should be used to guide further investigations into the cause of the weight loss.

Tumour markers
They are not useful diagnostic tests; they should not be used as part of the initial investigation and may be misleading. Their role is in monitoring response to treatment in patients with cancer or detecting tumour recurrence early after treatment.

CT scan
There is currently no evidence that whole-body CT scanning ('globalgram') is helpful in investigating patients with unintentional weight loss. The yield of whole-body CT scanning is low and the likelihood of finding an 'incidentaloma' is high.

Abdominal ultrasound
Several studies have used abdominal ultrasound as part of their initial routine evaluation, but its usefulness in this setting is not clear. Abnormal findings on examination (or abnormal LFTs) would usually have prompted further investigation.

Endoscopy and/or colonoscopy
Upper GI endoscopy and/or colonoscopy is a reasonable second-line investigation (Figure 23.3) given GI disorders are common in patients with unexplained weight loss in adults of all ages. However, they are invasive and not without risk; they should be reserved for patients in whom it is indicated on the basis of history, examination or baseline investigations, such as a history of GI bleeding or evidence of iron-deficiency anaemia.

Other investigations
These investigations should be considered in the appropriate clinical context:
- HIV screen test
- mammogram
- coeliac disease serology test.

24 Obesity

The purposes of the investigations are to:
- Assess the severity of obesity
- Identify any underlying specific cause of weight gain
- Assess the presence and severity of coexisting and obesity-related conditions

Table 24.1 WHO classification of weight and the risk of morbidities according to BMI values

WHO classification	BMI (kg/m^2)	Risk for morbidities
Normal weight	18.5–24.9	—
Overweight	25.0–29.9	Mildly increased
Obese	30.0	—
Class I	>30.0–34.9	Moderate
Class II	35.0–39.9	Severe
Class III	40.0	Very severe

Key points in investigation of obesity

- Investigate secondary causes of obesity if clinical features are suggestive.
- Features of monogenic forms of obesity should prompt genetic testing.
- Patients who are overweight or obese should be screened and assessed for absolute cardiovascular risk factors, which include hyperlipidaemia, hypertension and type II diabetes.

Table 24.2 Diseases commonly associated with overweight and obesity

Cardiovascular diseases
- Premature coronary artery disease
- Hypertension
- Stroke

Metabolic diseases
- Type II diabetes
- Polycystic ovarian syndrome

Gastrointestinal diseases
- Non-alcoholic fatty liver disease
- Gastro-oesophageal reflux disease
- Gallbladder disease

Musculoskeletal diseases
- Osteoarthritis
- Lower back pain

Cancers
- Breast cancer
- Colon cancer
- Ovarian cancer

Other diseases
- Chronic kidney disease
- Obstructive sleep apnoea
- Stress urinary incontinence
- Depression

Obesity is a state of excess adipose tissue mass. The body mass index (BMI) is the most widely used method of measuring obesity. It is calculated as body weight in kilograms divided by the square of the height in metres [BMI (kg/m^2) = weight/height^2]. The World Health Organisation (WHO) classification of weight in adults is useful in identifying individuals at increased risk of morbidity and mortality from obesity (Table 24.1). An alternative measure of obesity is the waist-to-hip ratio (WHR). This indicates abdominal fat, and the upper limit is 0.90 in men and 0.85 in women. WHR is a more accurate predictor for cardiovascular risk than BMI is.

The prevalence of obesity in many countries has increased dramatically in recent years and is predicted to increase further. Overweight and obesity are associated with increased risk of many diseases (Table 24.2). Obesity significantly increases the risk of mortality at any given age.

Combinations of genetic, developmental and environmental determinants alter the body's normal system for weight regulation, which leads to obesity. Obesity can be secondary to specific conditions such as Cushing's syndrome, hypothyroidism, insulinoma and other disorders involving the hypothalamus. Mutations in specific genes can cause severe obesity such as Prader–Willi syndrome.

Clinical evaluation

The evaluation of obese patients should include the history of weight gain, the maximum body weight, the patterns of food intake and physical activity. A detailed family history is also important and often suggests a genetic predisposition. Drug history should be taken to identify possible drugs that may be contributing to weight gain, such as steroid hormones, antidepressants (tricyclics), antipsychotics (olanzapine), anticonvulsants (sodium valproate), insulin and other hypoglycaemics (sulfonylurea, thiazolidinediones). The psychological aspects of eating behaviour should be explored.

Laboratory investigations

Standard laboratory studies in the evaluation of obesity should include the following:
- biochemical profile
- fasting lipid panel
- liver function tests
- thyroid function tests
- fasting glucose and HbA1c
- serum uric acid
- microalbuminuria screen.

Other tests are performed as indicated by clinical findings. For example, the 24-h urinary free-cortisol test is needed if Cushing's syndrome or other hypercortisolaemic states are clinically suspected. The measurement of plasma leptin is not routinely indicated but may be useful in suspected cases of leptin deficiency (morbid obesity, increased appetite and hyperphagia, and hypogonadotropic hypogonadism) or in severe lipodystrophy. Consider performing screening investigations for polycystic ovarian syndrome if clinically indicated (Chapter 107).

Genetic testing

In young patients with features of monogenic forms of obesity, genetic testing is required to identify obesity-related monogenic syndromes.

Investigations for fat mass and distribution

BMI, waist circumference and WHR are the common measures of the degree of body fat mass and distribution in routine clinical practice. Other measures include:
- caliper-derived measurements of skin-fold thickness;
- dual-energy X-ray absorptiometry;
- bioelectrical impedance analysis;
- ultrasound to determine fat thickness;
- MRI and CT scanning for direct measurement of visceral fat.

Investigations for obesity-related complications

The following investigations may be required to evaluate obesity-related complications:
- ECG and exercise stress test should be performed for suspected coronary artery disease;
- formal sleep study for suspected obstructive sleep apnoea;
- Screening mammography and faecal occult blood test for breast and colon cancers.

25 Fatigue

Table 25.1 Common causes for secondary fatigue

Cardiopulmonary
Congestive cardiac failure (CCF), COPD, peripheral vascular disease, atypical angina
Disturbed sleep
Sleep apnoea, gastro-oesophageal reflux disease
Endocrine/metabolic
Diabetes mellitus, hypothyroidism, pituitary insufficiency, CKD, chronic liver disease, hypercalcaemia, adrenal insufficiency
Infection
Infective endocarditis, tuberculosis, infectious mononucleosis, hepatitis, HIV, CMV infection
Inflammatory
Rheumatoid arthritis, SLE
Medications
Sedative-hypnotics, analgesics, antihypertensive medications, antidepressants, or substance abuse
Psychiatric
Depression, anxiety, somatisation disorder

Symptoms and signs for fatigue

- New onset of fatigue in a previously well, elderly patient
- Unintentional weight gain or loss
- Abnormal bleeding
- Dyspnoea
- Fever or night sweats
- Patient at risk for HIV, hepatitis or tuberculosis
- Lymphadenopathy
- Cardiac murmurs, signs of CCF
- Symptoms suggestive of malignancy – haemoptysis, dysphagia, postmenopausal bleeding
- Goitre
- Peripheral oedema
- Focal neurological signs

Table 25.2 Diagnostic criteria for chronic fatigue syndrome

Fatigue
Clinically evaluated, unexplained, or relapsing fatigue persistent for 6 months or more, that:
- is of new or definite onset
- is not the result of ongoing exertion
- is not substantially alleviated by rest
- results in substantial reduction in previous levels of occupational, educational, social or personal activities

and

Other symptoms
Four or more of the following symptoms that are concurrent, persistent for 6 months or more and which did not predate the fatigue:
- impaired short-term memory or concentration
- sore throat
- tender cervical or axillary lymph nodes
- muscle pain
- multi-joint pain without arthritis
- headaches of a new type, pattern or severity
- unrefreshing sleep
- post-exertional malaise lasting >24 h

The goals of investigation in fatigue are:
- To identify an underlying cause, if present
- To reassure the patient of negative investigation results

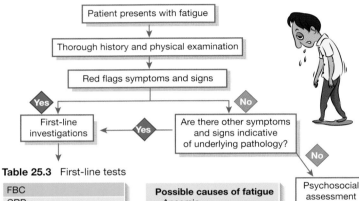

Table 25.3 First-line tests

FBC
CRP
Biochemistry panel
Blood glucose level
Liver function tests
Thyroid function tests
Iron study
Urinalysis, pregnancy test if indicated

Possible causes of fatigue
Anaemia
Inflammatory diseases
CKD, hyponatraemia
Protein malnutrition
Diabetes
Hepatitis, liver disease
Hypothyroidism
Iron deficiency
Urinary tract infection

Table 25.4 Selected second-line investigations for fatigue

Test	Possible causes of fatigue
Serology for EBV, CMV	Infectious mononucleosis, CMV infection
HIV serology	HIV infection
Hepatitis serology	Hepatitis B,C
Coeliac serology	Coeliac disease
Toxicology screen	Substance abuse
CXR	Adenopathy, cancer, tuberculosis
ECG	Arrhythmia
Echocardiography	Valvular heart disease, CCF
Pulmonary function tests	COPD
Sleep polysomnography	Obstructive sleep apnoea
MRI of the brain and spine	Multiple sclerosis

Key points in investigating fatigue

- There is no single test that can diagnose a cause for fatigue.
- In patients presenting with fatigue but no red flags, watchful waiting is a reasonable approach instead of performing unnecessary investigations.
- Over half of patients presenting with fatigue will have laboratory tests requested for fatigue but only 3% of these tests will result in a significant clinical diagnosis.
- Minor laboratory test abnormalities are common and they may not indicate the cause of fatigue.

Clinical Investigations at a Glance, First Edition. Jonathan Gleadle, Jordan Li and Tuck Yong. © 2017 John Wiley & Sons, Ltd. Published 2017 by John Wiley & Sons, Ltd.

Fatigue is a very common presenting symptom and negatively impacts work performance, family life and social relationships. Chronic fatigue is defined as fatigue that lasts longer than 6 months and is not relieved by rest. Patients with fatigue report a lack of energy, mental exhaustion, poor muscle endurance, delayed recovery after physical exertion and non-restorative sleep. Fatigue can be classified as:

• **Secondary fatigue** – caused by an underlying medical condition and may last 1 month or longer, but generally lasts <6 months. Medical conditions that may cause or contribute to chronic fatigue are listed in Table 25.1.

• **Physiological fatigue** – an imbalance in the routines of exercise, sleep, diet or other activity that is not caused by an underlying medical condition and is relieved with rest. Overexertion, deconditioning, post-viral illness, anaemia, lung disease, medications and depression are common causes.

• **Chronic fatigue syndrome** – no aetiology can be identified after clinical evaluation.

Clinical evaluation

Fatigue is a subjective symptom. The importance of the history cannot be overemphasised, because in most cases a fairly clear cause will be apparent from the history and physical examination. The subsequent investigations are carried out to confirm the initial impression. Clinicians should begin the evaluation by seeking common causes. The red flag box lists the symptoms and signs for fatigue that require further investigation. However, there is no organic cause for at least half of the cases of fatigue, and extensive laboratory and radiological investigation may not be necessary. The diagnostic criteria for chronic fatigue syndrome are listed in Table 25.2.

First-line investigations

The first-line laboratory investigations are listed in Table 25.3. These tests may identify a potentially reversible medical disorder in about 5% of patients presented with chronic fatigue. Women of childbearing age should have a pregnancy test. No specific test has been shown to be diagnostic of the cause of fatigue unless the history or physical examination suggests a specific medical condition.

Second-line investigations

The second-line investigations should only be performed if specific alternative diagnoses are suggested by clinical history, physical examination and first-line investigation results (Table 25.4). The diagnostic yield of investigations beyond the aforementioned first-line investigations is very low.

26 Coma and impaired consciousness

The goals of investigation are to:
- Assess the severity of altered state of consciousness, is the patient comatose?
- Investigate for reversible causes of coma
- Prognostic evaluation

Key points in investigating coma

- Capillary glucose levels must be measured at bedside to exclude hypoglycaemia, which is reversible.
- Blood tests should include a comprehensive metabolic panel (serum electrolytes, urea, creatinine). ABGs are measured, and carboxyhaemoglobin level if carbon monoxide toxicity is suspected.
- Toxicology screening and additional toxicology tests are done based on clinical suspicion.
- Non-contrast head CT should be done as soon as possible to check for masses, haemorrhage, oedema, evidence of bone trauma.

Table 26.1 Common causes of coma

Structural brain disease	Diffuse neuronal dysfunction	Toxins
• Brain tumour • Hypoxic brain injury after cardiac arrest • Raised intracranial pressure • Subdural, intracerebral haemorrhage • Acute ischaemic stroke • Hydrocephalus • Cerebral or cerebellar oedema secondary to stroke • Cerebral venous sinus thrombosis • Sepsis • Central nervous system (CNS) infections • Non-convulsive status epilepticus	• Hypoglycaemia • Hyperglycaemia, diabetic ketoacidosis (DKA) • Hyponatraemia • Hypercalcaemia • Hyperammonaemia • Acute kidney injury (AKI) or advanced CKD • Hepatic encephalopathy • Hypothyroidism myxoedema coma • Pituitary apoplexy • Wernicke's encephalopathy • Addison's disease	• Sedative hypnotic agents • Opioids • Dissociative agents (e.g. ketamine) • Alcohols • Histotoxic agents (e.g. cyanide) • Carbon monoxide • Methaemoglobinaemia • Psychiatric medications • Antiepileptic drugs • Salicylate overdose • Neuroleptic malignant syndrome • Serotonin syndrome

Table 26.2 Initial stabilisation protocol

- Confirm airway patency
- Intubate when necessary to ensure adequate oxygenation and protection from aspiration
- Assess circulation, establish intravenous access, administer saline if the patient is hypotensive, measure blood glucose level (BGL) and treat hypoglycaemia if present
- Until trauma of the cervical spine has been excluded (by history or imaging), it should be immobilised
- The history and clinical examination can give important diagnostic clues

Table 26.3 Initial investigations for patients with altered consciousness

Test	Results	Possible causes
Blood glucose	Hypoglycaemia	Insulin, sulfonylureas, β blockers
	Hyperglycaemia	DKA, non-ketotic hyperosmolar coma
Electrolytes	Hyponatraemia	MDMA (Ecstasy), carbamazepine
	Hypernatraemia	Severe dehydration
	Hypercalcaemia	Metastatic bone disease, multiple myeloma
Renal function	Markedly raised serum creatinine and urea	Advanced CKD or AKI
LFTs	Abnormal LFTs, coagulopathy	Liver failure
	Raised ammonia	Hepatic encephalopathy, valproate, urea cycle disorder
FBC	Neutrophilia	Sepsis
Troponin T	Raised troponin	AMI
Arterial blood gas (ABG)	Metabolic acidosis	Methanol, ethylene glycol, or salicylate poisoning, lactic acidosis of any cause (cyanide poisoning, Wernicke's encephalopathy), DKA, uraemia
	Respiratory acidosis	CNS depressant (opioid, benzodiazepine), hypercarbic respiratory failure
	Respiratory alkalosis	Central hyperventilation, salicylates
	Bradycardia	Increased intracranial pressure, sick sinus syndrome
ECG	Tachycardia	Ventricular tachycardia, supraventricular tachycardia
	ST–T change	Acute myocardial infarction
	Prolonged QTc interval	Tricyclic antidepressant or antipsychotic intoxication, various forms of acute structural brain injury
Thyroid function tests	Hypothyroidism	Myxoedemic coma
	Hyperthyroidism	Thyroid storm with agitated delirium, which can progress to coma, may have bulbar paralysis
Toxins	Alcohol level	Alcohol intoxication
Urine toxins	Urine drug screen	Drug overdose
CXR	Consolidation	Pneumonia

Figure 26.1 CT head showing: (a) moderate acute subdural haemorrhage extending around the left hemisphere; (b) extensive acute multicompartment intracranial haemorrhage

(a)   (b)

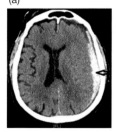
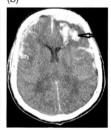

Figure 26.2 (a) EEG showing continuous, bilateral synchronous, high-voltage spike-and-wave activity consistent with non-convulsive status epilepticus. (b) Post-treatment with intravenous clonazepam, EEC showing no spike-and-wave activity consistent with termination of non-convulsive status epilepticus

(a)   (b)

Many patients present to hospitals with an altered state of consciousness. The Glasgow coma scale is used to indicate the degree of impairment of consciousness and monitor for changes. It loses discriminative value in intubated patients and those with very low scores, and it assesses brainstem function poorly. The aetiology of coma can be classified into three groups: structural brain disease, diffuse neuronal dysfunction and toxins (Table 26.1).

Initial stabilisation

As with any unstable patient, the patient should be resuscitated according to basic life support ABCD protocol (Table 26.2).

Initial investigation

The components of the initial assessment are the history, physical examination and simple laboratory tests. The history and physical examination aim to distinguish a structural cause from diffuse neuronal dysfunction or psychiatric cause. The initial investigations are listed in Table 26.3.

Blood test for toxin or keep blood for future toxin test if clinically indicated. Poisoning remains a clinical diagnosis. Routine toxicological testing rarely changes acute management. Co-oximetry should be included if carbon monoxide poisoning or methaemoglobinaemia is suspected. Reliance on serum ammonia to diagnose hepatic encephalopathy is controversial because a single value is neither sensitive nor specific. High ammonia concentrations can also occur with valproate-induced encephalopathy and rare deficiencies of urea cycle enzymes. Blood culture should be taken if there is suspicion of sepsis. A CXR should be performed in all comatose patients.

In patients with metabolic acidosis, a widened anion gap suggests one of four mechanisms (ketones, uraemia, lactate, toxins). Ketosis can occur in diabetes, alcohol misuse or starvation. Uraemia generally produces acidosis only in later stages. Elevated lactate can occur in sepsis, hypoperfusion or Wernicke's encephalopathy, with toxins such as cyanide or metformin usage.

CT of the brain

Neurological examination is essential before performing CT of the brain. The first step is to decide whether the lesion is in one hemisphere causing a mass effect, or in both hemispheres, or in the brainstem. Imaging results cannot be properly interpreted without knowing whether brainstem signs are present. Fundoscopy can reveal subhyaloid haemorrhages (in subarachnoid haemorrhage or asphyxia) or papilloedema, which indicates increased intracranial pressure.

CT head should be done without delay in comatose patients with unclear diagnoses, those with suspected structural injury and those with preceding head trauma. CT brain can be truly positive (intracranial haemorrhage), truly negative (normal scan in a poisoned patient), falsely positive (a unilateral frontal lobe mass without shift or mass effect) or falsely negative (normal scan in a patient with basilar artery occlusion). CT head of comatose patients should be checked for tissue shift, hydrocephalus, intracranial haemorrhage (Figure 26.1) (including bilateral isodense subdural haematoma), obliteration of the basal cisterns, subtle thalamic abnormalities and a hyperdense basilar artery. CT head that shows diffuse brain oedema should prompt consideration of inserting a device to monitor intracranial pressure.

Not every comatose patient needs a brain CT. Hypoglycaemic patients who respond to dextrose, those with DKA and patients admitted from nursing homes with fever and urosepsis do not usually need CT brain. However, continuous monitoring of comatose patients is crucial; failure to improve as expected should trigger diagnostic reassessment and CT.

When the CT result is negative, a timely re-evaluation to avoid missing any reversible causes of coma should be considered:
- Does the patient need MRI or vascular imaging?
- Does the patient need a lumbar puncture (LP)?
- Does the patient need an emergency EEG?
- Does the patient need treatment for poisoning?
- Dose the patient need empirical intravenous antimicrobials?

MRI and vascular imaging

CT can miss treatable cerebrovascular causes of coma, including basilar artery occlusion, posterior reversible encephalopathy syndrome, early thalamic and brainstem ischaemic stroke, cerebral venous sinus thrombosis, locked-in syndrome from pontine damage, an embolic shower with several small cortical infarctions, and hypertensive encephalopathy. Therefore, clinicians must consider whether a patient needs MRI, MR angiography and magnetic resonance venography (MRV). CT angiography is useful to expeditiously exclude basilar occlusion. MRI can be falsely negative within the first 48 hours of brainstem strokes. Patients who have seizures with headache, especially with neurological deficits not localising to an arterial territory, should undergo MRV to exclude cerebral venous sinus thrombosis.

Lumbar puncture

If meningitis or encephalitis is suspected, LP should be performed. For patients with decreased conscious level, CT head should be done before LP. If LP is delayed, blood cultures should be obtained and appropriate intravenous antimicrobials given immediately, as delays in antibiotic administration of as little as a few hours substantially increase mortality. In cases of suspected brain abscess or other mass lesion, LP should be avoided because it can worsen tissue shifts and the CSF rarely yields diagnostic information. MRI is needed for diagnosing limbic or brainstem encephalitis.

Septic patients can develop encephalopathy in the absence of hypotension, hypoxia or CNS infection. Renal or hepatic failure can causes diffuse neuronal dysfunction and lead to altered conscious level.

EEG

An EEG can confirm psychogenic unresponsiveness. Patients who remain comatose after several generalised seizures can benefit from an EEG to exclude non-convulsive status epilepticus (Figure 26.2), defined as prolonged seizure activity in the absence of major motor signs. Clinical clues to the presence of this disorder include nystagmus-like eye movements, myoclonic jerks and staring into space. Patients whose eyes are open but who are otherwise unresponsive can have non-convulsive status epilepticus.

An EEG should be performed in comatose patients with no clear cause, and in patients intubated for convulsive status epilepticus because electrical seizures can persist even though paralytic or sedative drugs obscure their motor manifestations.

27 Preoperative investigations for elective surgery

Table 27.1 The American Society of Anesthesiologists' (ASA) grades for patients

ASA grade	Advantages	Examples	Mortality (%)
Grade 1	Normal healthy patient	No clinically important comorbidity, no clinically significant past/present medical history	0.1
Grade 2	A patient with mild systemic disease	Stable angina, not limiting activity, well-controlled hypertension, diabetes, COPD/asthma, stable CKD with creatinine <200 µmol/L	0.2
Grade 3	A patient with severe systemic disease	Unstable angina, limited activity, not well controlled hypertension, diabetes, COPD/asthma, CKD with creatinine of >200 µmol/L or on renal replacement therapy	1.8
Grade 4	A patient with severe systemic disease that is a constant threat to life	Immediate post-myocardial infarction, decompensated congestive cardiac failure, type II respiratory failure	7.8
Grade 5	A moribund patient unlikely to survive 24 hours with or without surgery		9.4

Figure 27.1 Preoperative ECG showing sinus arrhythmia

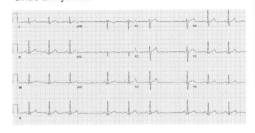

Table 27.2 Grading of surgical procedures

Classification	Operations
Minor, grade 1	Excision of lesion of skin; drainage of breast or skin abscess, tooth extraction, release of carpal tunnel syndrome
Intermediate, grade 2	Primary repair of inguinal hernia; excision of varicose vein(s) of leg; tonsillectomy; knee arthroscopy; partial excision of breast
Major, grade 3	Total abdominal hysterectomy; endoscopic resection of prostate; lumbar discectomy; thyroidectomy
Major plus, grade 4	Total joint replacement; lung operations; colonic resection; radical neck dissection
Cardiovascular surgery, grade 5	CABG; AAA repair

Table 27.4 Indication for echo

- Suspected aortic stenosis and mitral stenosis
- To establish LV function in patients with suspected heart failure who are breathless climbing a flight of stairs
- Suspected pulmonary hypertension
- Not indicated for patients with stable IHD or those with Mild regurgitant lesions with normal LV and no change in symptoms and last echo is within 18 months

Table 27.3 Suggested investigations for patients with conditions posing a risk of intra- or postoperative complications

Conditions	Suggested investigations
Risk of perioperative hypotension	FBC, creatinine, electrolytes, LFTs
Significant risk of major blood loss (e.g. major vascular procedures)	FBC, coagulation study, group and save, creatinine, electrolytes, LFTs
Cardiovascular disease	FBC, creatinine, electrolytes (potassium within 1 week if on digoxin or diuretics), ECG, CXR
Hepatic disease	LFTs, coagulation study and hepatitis B and C as appropriate
Renal disease	Urea, creatinine, electrolytes, FBC
Diuretics	Serum potassium, magnesium levels
COPD	FBC, CXR, pulmonary function tests (PFTs)
Bleeding history	Coagulation studies (aspirin is not an indication for coagulation tests)
Anticoagulants	Coagulation studies
Diabetes mellitus	Urea, creatinine, electrolytes, regular blood glucose on day of surgery
Thyroid disease	Thyroid function tests

Key points in preoperative investigations

- Haemoglobin measurement is useful in detecting unsuspected anaemia and providing a baseline level for surgeries with anticipated blood loss and potential haemorrhagic complications.
- Coagulation studies should be reserved for patients with a history of bleeding disorders or medical conditions that predispose them to bleeding, and for those taking anticoagulants.
- Preoperative biochemistry and creatinine testing should be performed in patients at risk of electrolyte abnormalities or renal impairment only.
- Patients in whom cardiac stress testing was normal within the past 2 years or who have had CABG within the past 5 years, and are asymptomatic, require no further investigations.

Clinical Investigations at a Glance, First Edition. Jonathan Gleadle, Jordan Li and Tuck Yong. © 2017 John Wiley & Sons, Ltd. Published 2017 by John Wiley & Sons, Ltd.

The goal of preoperative assessments is to identify factors associated with increased risks of specific complications and to recommend further investigations and a management plan that minimises operative risks. The risk of postoperative complications is influenced by patient-related factors (Table 27.1) and surgery-related factors (Table 27.2). The need for preoperative clinical investigations should be directed by:

- the patient's known medical conditions;
- the findings of a thorough history and physical examination;
- the grading of surgical procedures (Table 27.2);
- the potential intra- and postoperative complications of the proposed surgery and the anaesthesia.

Investigations should be individualised to the patient for specific clinical indications, balancing the patient's clinical status with the potential risks of anaesthesia and surgery. Investigations of healthy patients for low-risk surgery are generally not indicated. For grade 1–3 surgery, unless there has been a change in clinical status, many previously normal tests need not be repeated within 3 months; exceptions include potassium in those taking diuretics and blood glucose in patients with diabetes.

Full blood count (FBC)

FBC should be performed preoperatively if:

- history is suggestive of underlying anaemia;
- a significant blood loss is anticipated during the operation;
- all patients aged ≥65 years;
- previous history of haematological disorders.

Even mild degrees of preoperative anaemia or polycythaemia can be associated with an increased risk of 30-day postoperative mortality and cardiac events in older patients undergoing major non-cardiac surgery.

Electrolytes

Unanticipated electrolyte abnormalities (sodium, potassium, bicarbonate) are found in only 0.2–5.0% of surgical patients. Routine electrolyte measurement is not recommended for elective surgery in healthy individuals.

Blood glucose

The frequency of abnormal glucose results in asymptomatic patients is 1.8–5.5%. This frequency increases with age, so that nearly 25% of patients >60 years have a fasting blood glucose level (BGL) >6.7 mmol/L. However, mild asymptomatic hyperglycaemia (<10 mmol/L) is unlikely to contribute to postoperative complications, and routine measurement of BGL is not recommended in all cases. However, diabetes is associated with higher perioperative risks in vascular surgery and coronary artery bypass grafting (CABG); routine BGL determination is recommended in such cases.

Renal function

The prevalence of undiagnosed CKD in asymptomatic patients ranges from 0.2% to 2.4% and increases with age (9.8% of patients aged 46–60 years). Patients with stage 2 to 3 CKD are usually asymptomatic but have an increased risk of perioperative morbidity and mortality. Accordingly, measuring serum creatinine level is recommended for all patients aged >50 years, especially if hypotension or the use of nephrotoxic medications is anticipated. Some medications may need dose adjustment based on creatinine clearance.

Liver function test

The frequency of hepatic aminotransferase enzyme abnormalities is estimated to be approximately 0.3–0.5%. Routine preoperative testing is not recommended for healthy individuals.

Coagulation studies

In the absence of a history of bleeding diathesis in elective surgery patients, abnormal INR and activated partial thromboplastin time (APTT) results are estimated to be <1%. Bleeding time is not a useful predictor of bleeding risk, and a normal bleeding time does not exclude the possibility of excessive bleeding. Accordingly, INR, APTT and bleeding time are not recommended for routine preoperative testing (preoperative screening).

Urinalysis

The primary rationale for doing a urinalysis preoperatively is to detect either asymptomatic renal disease or an underlying urinary tract infection (UTI). There is no correlation between asymptomatic UTI and surgical wound infection. Urinalysis should not be routinely done for asymptomatic patients.

Group and save or cross-match

Anticipating that there may be a requirement for blood transfusion, but not routinely for this operation, the patient's blood type is identified and held, pending a possible (later) request for units of blood or blood products. If the blood transfusion is likely to be needed the blood should be cross-matched and the blood or blood products held in the blood bank for 24 hours.

Pregnancy testing

Pregnancy has an important bearing in the perioperative care of a woman of childbearing age. History alone may not be completely reliable to exclude pregnancy. Therefore, a pregnancy test is recommended for a woman of reproductive age.

ECG

The prevalence of abnormal ECG findings among healthy elective surgery patients is about 14–53% and increases with age in a continuous fashion. The rationale for obtaining an ECG preoperatively is to identify high-risk patients with previous myocardial infarction or arrhythmia. Detecting a silent myocardial infarction is the main clinical benefit, because numerous investigations have shown an association between preoperative myocardial infarction and surgical mortality. In addition, any rhythm other than sinus, including frequent premature ventricular contractions, is associated with increased surgical risk. Routine ECG is recommended for all patients >50 years undergoing elective intermediate surgery.

An ECG is not routinely recommended in asymptomatic patients <50 years without any clinical risk factors who are to undergo low-risk surgery. However, an ECG is recommended for all patients undergoing vascular or cardiac surgery.

CXR

A CXR adds little to clinical evaluation in healthy patients. A CXR should not be performed routinely for preoperative evaluation in patients without risk factors. Routine CXR is recommended only for patients older than 60–70 years unless underlying heart or lung disease is a possibility.

Echocardiogram

This indications for echocardiogram are listed in Table 27.4.

28 Syncope

Table 28.1 Serious causes of syncope

- Cardiac arrhythmias
- Low cardiac output
- Valvular heart disease
- Pulmonary embolism
- Aortic dissection
- Leaking aneurysm
- Gastrointestinal bleeding

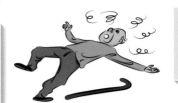

The initial assessment
- Careful history-taking and physical examination
- Postural blood pressure measurement
- ECG

High-risk syncope patients

- History of severe structural heart or coronary artery disease (heart failure, low left ventricular ejection fraction, previous myocardial infarction)
- Family history of sudden cardiac death
- Syncope during exertion or supine
- Preceded by palpitations or associated with chest pain or dyspnoea
- Systolic blood pressure <90 mmHg
- Haematocrit <30% or presence of AKI
- Significant electrolyte disturbance
- ECG features suggesting arrhythmic syncope (Table 28.3)

Table 28.2 ECG features suggesting arrhythmic syncope

- Bifascicular block
- Intraventricular conduction abnormalities with QRS duration of 0.12 s
- Sinus bradycardia (<50 beats/min) (Figure 28.1a), sinoatrial block
- Pre-excited QRS complexes, suggesting Wolff–Parkinson–White (WPW) syndrome (Figure 28.1b)
- Prolonged QT interval (Figure 28.1c)
- Q wave suggesting myocardial infarction
- Right bundle branch block pattern with ST-elevation in leads V1 to V3 (Brugada syndrome)

Figure 28.1 ECG showing (a) significant bradycardia, (b) WPW syndrome and (c) prolonged QT interval

(a)

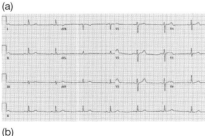

(b)

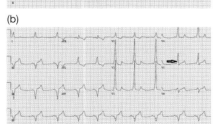

(c)

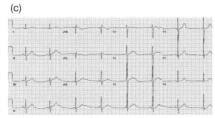

Figure 28.2 Tilt table testing

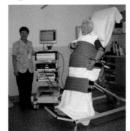

Diagnostic of postural hypotension or neurally mediated syncope → No further investigation

Unexplained syncope, red flag high-risk patients → Echocardiography; consider exercise test or evaluation of myocardial ischaemia

Abnormal → Treat structural heart disease or ischaemia; consider electrophysiology study

Normal → Single, benign episode → No further investigation

Normal → Recurrent syncope → Holter monitor or implantable loop recorder

Sinus rhythm with symptoms → Consider tilt-table test or no further investigation

Arrhythmia with symptoms → Treat as appropriate

Key points in investigating syncope

- Syncope in a person with no cardiac history and normal ECG is less likely to have a cardiac-related cause.
- In-hospital ECG monitoring is only recommended in syncopal patients with structural heart disease who are at high risk for life-threatening arrhythmias.
- Holter monitor is indicated in patients with a significant ECG abnormality, with known heart disease, syncope preceded by palpitation or during exertion or a family history of sudden death.

Clinical Investigations at a Glance, First Edition. Jonathan Gleadle, Jordan Li and Tuck Yong. © 2017 John Wiley & Sons, Ltd. Published 2017 by John Wiley & Sons, Ltd.

Syncope is a transient loss of consciousness caused by cerebral hypoperfusion and usually associated with spontaneous, rapid and complete recovery. There are many causes, ranging from benign vasogenic syncope to sinister cardiac causes such as ventricular tachycardia (Table 28.1). Investigating the cause of the syncope can be difficult, and in 45% of patients a cause is not found even after admission and extensive investigations. Patients with a cardiac cause for syncope have a mortality of 33% within a year.

Initial investigation

The initial assessment for **all patients** presenting with syncope should include:
- a detailed history-taking and physical examination;
- a postural blood pressure measurement;
- an ECG.

About 45% of patients will have their cause of syncope identified after this assessment.

ECG

90% of patients with cardiac syncope will have an abnormal ECG, while 6% of patients with reflex-mediated syncope have an abnormal ECG (Figure 28.1). A patient with a negative cardiac history and normal ECG is much less likely to have a cardiac cause.

Laboratory studies

Glucose, electrolyte testing, renal function and haemoglobin/ haematocrit should be checked.

Risk stratification

If the diagnosis is uncertain following the initial evaluation, further investigation should be undertaken in high-risk patients (Table 28.2). In-hospital ECG monitoring is recommended in patients with structural heart disease who are at high risk for life-threatening arrhythmias. Although the diagnostic yield of in-hospital monitoring is only 16%, it is justified by the risk of a life-threatening event. If there has been a single syncope with low-risk clinical features and normal blood pressure and ECG, no further evaluation is usually indicated. If there are recurrent episodes, further investigations should include tests for cardiac or reflex-mediated causes.

Suspected cardiac syncope

Echocardiogram

Echocardiography is useful in providing detailed evaluation of cardiac structure. Indications include recurrent syncope, abnormal ECG, abnormal cardiovascular examination, chest pain, exercise-induced symptoms and palpitations preceding the syncope.

The finding of structural heart disease does not definitely establish the aetiology of syncope; echocardiography may establish a causative diagnosis in 5% of patients with suspected cardiac syncope with the following uncommon but important findings: severe aortic stenosis, obstructive tumour or thrombus (e.g. atrial myxoma), cardiac tamponade, aortic dissection and congenital anomaly of the coronary artery.

Holter monitor

The most helpful diagnostic test is an ECG recording during an attack. Some patients have transient arrhythmias that lead to syncope but resolve before presentation. In this group, non-invasive ambulatory ECG monitoring can be performed for 24 hours (Holter monitor). However, if the patient does not have any symptoms during monitoring, serious cardiac arrhythmias are not excluded. It should be considered in patients with a significant ECG abnormality (Table 28.3) known heart disease, syncope preceded by palpitation or during exertion or a family history of sudden death. The diagnostic yield is 1–2% in unselected patients with syncope.

External loop recorder

An external loop recorder can be used to investigate patients with unexplained recurrent syncopal episodes. However, the diagnostic yield is variable and influenced by the ability to activate the recorder. The diagnostic yield is 25–35% in selected patients with suspected cardiac syncope (2- to 3-week records).

Implantable loop recorder

An implantable loop recorder is a subcutaneous monitoring device implanted in the left parasternal or pectoral region. It is programmed to save any abnormal heart rates or runs of arrhythmia or be patient activated. The indications include:
- patients with recurrent syncope;
- patients with high-risk features in whom a thorough evaluation did not demonstrate a cause of syncope;
- to assess the contribution of bradycardia before embarking on cardiac pacing in patients with suspected or certain reflex syncope.

Diagnostic yield is 60% in selected patients with suspected cardiac syncope.

Electrophysiology studies

Electrophysiology studies directly assess intracardiac conduction and ascertain if there is inducible supraventricular and ventricular arrhythmias by intracardiac stimulation. They are performed in patients with underlying heart disease and unexplained syncope or with conduction disease. The diagnostic yield is 11% in patients without structural heart disease and 49% in patients with structure heart disease.

Suspected reflex-mediated syncope: tilt-table testing

Tilt-table testing involves a patient lying supine for 15 min and then the bed is tilted at an angle of 60° for a further 45 min (Figure 28.2). The patient is monitored with ECG and blood pressure measurements every 5 min. It can be useful to confirm the diagnosis in patients who have suspected reflex-mediated vasovagal syncope, but it has limited specificity, sensitivity and reproducibility. It is undertaken for unexplained syncope, especially in patients with a structurally normal heart, to confirm that recurrent syncope is reflex mediated. The diagnostic yield is 25–62% in unexplained syncope.

Suspected cerebrovascular syncope

Cerebrovascular causes of syncope are very rare. Head CT, MRI, EEG and carotid ultrasound should be requested only when the initial assessment is suggestive for cerebrovascular syncope. The yield of such tests in unselected patients with syncope is <1%.

29 Back pain

Clinical features of back pain

- Age >50 years
- History of malignancy
- Recent unintentional weight loss
- History of trauma, including minor trauma in the elderly, osteoporotic or those on corticosteroids
- Symptoms or signs of infection such as fever, raised CRP
- High-risk patients for infection; e.g. with immunosuppression, steroid use or history of intravenous drug use
- Neurological signs or cauda equina syndrome

Table 29.1 Common causes of low back pain

Mechanical causes (97%)	Non-mechanical spinal condition (~1%)	Visceral disease (2%)
• Lumbar muscular strain/sprain (70%)	• Malignancy (0.7%) 　Multiple myeloma 　Metastatic carcinoma 　Spinal cord tumours 　Retroperitoneal tumours	• Diseases of pelvic organs 　Endometriosis 　Chronic pelvic inflammatory disease
• Age-related degenerative disorder (10%)		
• Herniated disc (4%)	• Infection (0.01%) 　Osteomyelitis 　Septic discitis 　Paraspinous abscess 　Epidural abscess	• Renal disease 　Nephrolithiasis 　Pyelonephritis 　Perinephric abscess
• Spinal canal stenosis (3%)		
• Osteoporotic crush fractures (4%)		
• Spondylolisthesis (2%)		• Aortic abdominal aneurysm
• Traumatic fracture (<1%)	• Inflammatory arthritis (0.3%) 　Ankylosing spondylitis 　Paget's disease	• Pancreatitis
• Congenital disease (<1%)		
• Severe kyphosis		

Figure 29.1 X-ray of thoracolumbar spine shows T9, T12, L3 vertebral body anterior wedge crush fracture

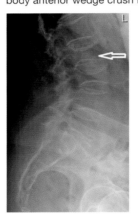

Figure 29.2 MRI of lumbar spine shows disc herniation in L5 and S1

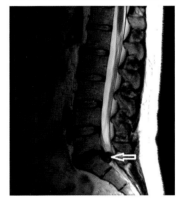

Figure 29.3 MRI without gadolinium enhancement of the thoracolumbar region shows endplate erosion, marrow oedema and high T2 signal within T11–12, indicative of discitis–osteomyelitis

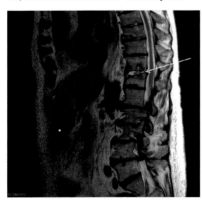

Figure 29.4 Whole-body bone scan shows multifocal bony metastatic disease from a prostate cancer

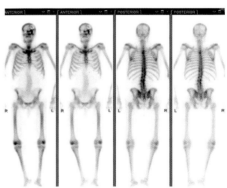

ack pain, especially low back pain (LBP), is a very common complaint. The annual incidence is 10–15% with a point prevalence of approximately 30% in developed countries. Approximately 90% of patients recover without sequelae, but relapse can occur. A subset of patients may be incapacitated from chronic LBP, defined as symptoms persistent for >6 months and often associated with depression, job dissatisfaction and medico-legal issues involving financial compensation.

LBP has many causes (Table 29.1) and the most common ones are musculoligamentous strain/sprains and age-related degenerative processes in the intervertebral discs and facet joints. The other common causes include spinal canal stenosis and disc herniation. The L5 and S1 nerve roots are involved in about 95% of lumbar disc herniations. However, a precise pathoanatomical diagnosis cannot be given in about 80% of patients with isolated back pain.

Careful history taking and physical examination can be helpful, and imaging in patients without 'red flag' clinical features (see red flag box) is usually unnecessary. In contrast, a presumed diagnosis of cauda equina syndrome in a patient presenting with new bowel or bladder dysfunction, bilateral sciatica and saddle anaesthesia necessitates urgent investigations. Furthermore, the prevalence of serious disorders in patient with back pain is low and the sensitivity and specificity of most 'red flag' clinical features is modest.

Radiological investigations

Patients presenting with back pain without 'red flags' do not require radiological imaging at initial presentation. CT or MRI is indicated to exclude infection, tumour, and bone- or disc-related disease with nerve root or spinal cord compression.

High-risk patients – such as those on immunosuppression, those taking corticosteroids and those with a history of intravenous drug use – presenting with back pain should be considered for blood culture and radiological studies. Patients with unrelenting pain despite recumbency, systemic features such as fevers, chills, history of malignancy, unintentional weight loss and neurological deficits warrant urgent MRI or CT. Imaging is indicated in patients with trauma, especially minor trauma in the elderly, those with osteoporosis and those on long-term corticosteroid treatment.

Plain X-ray

Plain X-rays are used to assess the entire lumbar spine, sacroiliac joints and the sagittal dimension of the bony canal. Evidence of compression vertebral fractures, malignancy, and ankylosis may be demonstrated (Figure 29.1). Plain X-rays are good at demonstrating skeletal detail but inadequate for the evaluation of soft-tissue abnormalities. Plain X-rays are not sensitive for early cancer or infection; MRI and other laboratory investigations are needed to evaluate the possibility of these conditions. Radiation exposure is a concern for plain X-ray and CT as both modalities result in substantial irradiation of the gonads.

CT

CT is useful if there are localising neurological features. CT offers direct visualisation of the disc margin, theca, nerve roots, facet joints and pars interarticularis. In cases of spinal canal stenosis, CT clearly demonstrates the cause, level and severity of stenosis. CT-guided biopsy is used to confirm the diagnosis of vertebral discitis–osteomyelitis, paraspinous or epidural abscess. CT can also be used to assess aortic aneurysm, which may be the source of referred pain.

MRI

MRI is the preferred investigation for back pain with neurological features. Its ability to scan the entire spine in both the sagittal and axial planes and the myelographic effect of cerebrospinal fluid enables MRI to provide an assessment of the extent, level and severity of disease. MRI is useful in detecting metastases in the marrow cavity and is the most sensitive method for evaluating degenerative disc disease, disc herniation and infection (Figures 29.2 and 29.3). However, MRI is limited in the assessment of bony detail, and correlation with plain X-rays or CT may be required.

Radionuclide studies

Radionuclide studies are indicated to further evaluate patients with persistent back pain and features suggestive of malignancy or Paget's disease of the bone. These studies can detect tumour infiltration, infection, disc degeneration, facet joint disease and stress fracture (Figure 29.4).

Laboratory investigations

Routine laboratory studies are not necessary in the evaluation of back pain unless there are 'red flag' clinical features. However, in patients with back pain with a possible inflammatory disorder, malignancy or infection, a FBC and biochemistry including calcium, urate, LDH, CRP and blood cultures are typically obtained. Although non-specific in nature, these values should not be elevated in the setting of mechanical back pain. Urinalysis and urine culture should also be ordered when considering the possibility of pyelonephritis or renal colic.

Key points in investigating back pain

- Do not offer radiological imaging at the initial presentation with LBP but no 'red flag' features.
- Patients with unrelenting pain despite recumbency, systemic features such as fevers, chills, history of malignancy, unintentional weight loss and neurological deficits warrant urgent MRI or CT.
- MRI is the preferred investigation for back pain with neurological deficits.
- Plain X-ray has limited value in investigating back pain.

30 Peripheral oedema

The **goal of investigation of peripheral oedema** is to determine the underlying cause and identify any serious illness, such as DVT, heart, liver or kidney failure.

Key points in investigating peripheral oedema

- Duplex ultrasound is used to assess for DVT or chronic venous insufficiency.
- CT abdomen and pelvis should be considered in patients aged >40 years without an apparent cause for oedema or in younger patients with suspicious findings such as unilateral oedema, pelvic symptoms/signs, or weight loss.
- Lymphoscintigraphy can be helpful to distinguish lymphoedema from other causes of oedema and to determine the cause of lymphoedema.

Table 30.1 Causes of lower limb oedema

Unilateral		Bilateral	
Acute (<72 h)	Chronic	Acute (<72 h)	Chronic

DVT
Cellulitis
Ruptured Baker's cyst
Compartment syndrome
	Venous insufficiency
	Secondary lymphoedema:
	  tumour, radiation, surgery,
	  infection
	Primary lymphoedema
	Pelvic mass causing
	  external compression
	Reflex sympathetic
	  dystrophy
	Congenital venous
	  malformations
		Bilateral
		DVT
			Venous insufficiency
			Congestive heart failure
			Pulmonary hypertension
			Lymphoedema
			Drugs
			Pregnancy
			Nephrotic syndrome
			Cirrhosis
			Idiopathic oedema
			Malnutrition
			Pelvic mass causing
			  external compression
			Myxoedema
			Obesity

Table 30.2 Drugs that may cause peripheral oedema

Calcium channel blockers
Hydralazine
Methyldopa
Corticosteroids
Oestrogen and/or progesterone
Non-steroidal anti-inflammatory drugs
Pioglitazone

Figure 30.1 Echo shows severe pulmonary hypertension

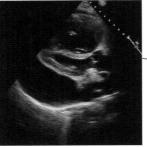

Figure 30.2 CXR shows decompensated congestive heart failure

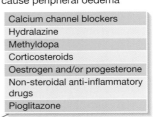

Figure 30.3 Duplex ultrasound shows left DVT

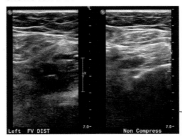

Figure 30.4 CT abdomen shows a large soft tissue mass arising from ovary causing bilateral leg and periperal oedema

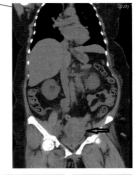

Figure 30.5 Normal lymphoscintigram

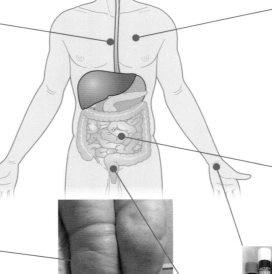

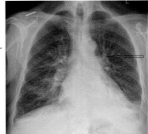

Urine protein : creatinine ratio

FBC
Electrolyte
Creatinine
Albumin
LFTs
TFTs

? BNP

? D-dimer

Oedema is a palpable swelling caused by an increase in interstitial fluid volume. Causes of peripheral oedema range from the benign to the potentially life threatening. The most likely cause of leg oedema in patients >50 years of age is venous insufficiency. The distribution of oedema is an important clue to the underlying cause. Unilateral leg swelling usually suggests a local disease process, whereas bilateral peripheral oedema is often due to a systemic disorder. The causes of lower limb oedema are shown in Table 30.1.

The initial evaluation should identify any risks for deep vein thrombosis (DVT), any systemic diseases (heart, liver or kidney), history of pelvic/abdominal neoplasm or radiation, history of surgery, distribution of the oedema (unilateral or bilateral), whether there is pitting (myxoedema and advanced fibrotic form of lymphoedema typically do not pit), associated tenderness and skin changes. Drug-induced oedema is relatively common (Table 30.2).

Laboratory investigations

If the cause of the oedema is unclear, the basic laboratory tests, including FBC electrolytes, creatinine, albumin, LFTs and TFTs, should be performed. This will usually guide further investigation.

A normal B-type natriuretic peptide (BNP) can be used to rule out heart failure as the cause of oedema. A normal D-dimer will help to rule out DVT in patients with acute oedema. However, an elevated D-dimer should be followed up with a Doppler examination because false-positive D-dimers are common. A spot urine protein : creatinine ratio >350 mg/mmol indicates the cause of oedema is likely the nephrotic syndrome, whilst a normal albumin excludes nephrotic syndrome as the cause and makes liver disease or malnutrition unlikely. Patients with suspected nephrotic syndrome should have serum lipids measured.

ECG and echocardiography should be performed if heart failure and/or pulmonary hypertension (Figure 30.1) is suspected as the cause of oedema. Sleep polysomnography is indicated if a patient is suspected to have pulmonary hypertension secondary to obstructive sleep-breathing disorder.

Radiological investigations

A CXR is indicated if a cardiopulmonary cause of the peripheral oedema is suspected (Figure 30.2).

Duplex ultrasound is used to assess DVT or chronic venous insufficiency (Figure 30.3). It may also show other conditions that may mimic DVT, including Baker's cyst and muscle haematoma. Ultrasound of the liver or kidney is indicated if underlying liver or kidney disease is suspected.

A CT of the abdomen and pelvis should be considered in patients aged >40 years without an apparent cause for oedema or in younger patients with suspicious findings, such as unilateral oedema, pelvic symptoms/signs or weight loss. Patients aged >35 years with undiagnosed lymphoedema should have a CT scan. Tumours commonly associated with leg oedema include prostate cancer, ovarian cancer and lymphoma (Figure 30.4).

Lymphoscintigraphy (Figure 30.5) can be helpful to distinguish lymphoedema from other causes of oedema and to determine the cause of lymphoedema. Lymphoscintigraphy is performed by injecting a radioactive tracer into the first web space and monitoring lymphatic flow with a gamma camera. It has a sensitivity >90% and specificity of 100%. Normal lymphoscintigraphy excludes a diagnosis of lymphoedema.

Other investigations

Diagnosis of idiopathic oedema is usually made clinically after excluding systemic disease by history, examination and other related investigations. Confirmatory tests (e.g. morning and evening weights with a gain of >0.7 kg) may be helpful if there is significant doubt about the diagnosis.

31 Jaundice

Patient presents with jaundice or serum bilirubin level >40 mmol/L

Does the jaundice have a
• prehepatic
• hepatic or
• posthepatic cause?

First line of imaging investigation is abdominal USS

Blood tests
FBC
Bilirubin levels
LFTs: AST, ALT, ALP, GGT
Hepatitis serology
Autoimmune markers
Amylase

Prehepatic causes?

Hepatic causes?

Posthepatic causes?

Urine tests
Bilirubin positive:
  conjugated bilirubinaemia
  is due to obstructive or
  hepatic causes
Absent urobilinogen:
  obstruction to the CBD
Excess urobilinogen:
  liver damage and
  haemolytic jaundice

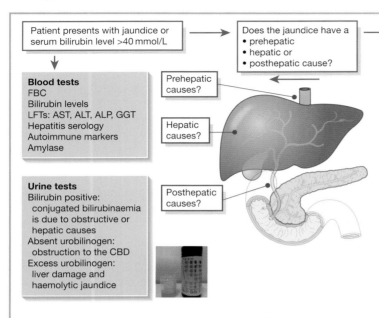

Figure 31.1 USS shows (a) normal CBD and (b) dilated CBD due to tumour compression
(a)   (b)

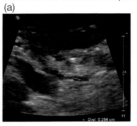
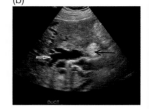

Figure 31.2 USS shows a gallbladder stone

Figure 31.3 USS shows a metastatic liver cancer

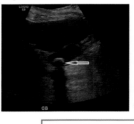
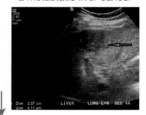

Consider CT abdomen if USS is indeterminate

Figure 31.4 CT abdomen (coronal) shows gallbladder wall thickening, gallstones within gallbladder, dilated intra and extra-hepatic biliary trees
*dilated CBD; # gallstones

Figure 31.5 CT abdomen (post-contrast) shows a hypo-enhancing ill-defined lesion in pancreatic head (arrow) causing ductal dilatation (*)

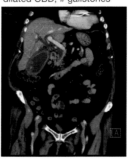
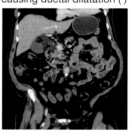

Key points 🔑

• A urinalysis positive for bilirubin indicates the presence of conjugated bilirubinaemia, which is likely due to obstructive or hepatic causes.
• Ultrasound can be used to determine the presence of bile duct obstruction by detecting ductal dilatation.
• Ultrasound is less effective than CT and MRCP/ERCP in determining the cause and site of obstruction.

Figure 31.7 ERCP shows extraction of stone in the biliary duct

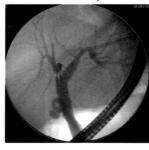

Consider ERCP, which has both a diagnostic and, more importantly, a therapeutic role but has risks

A percutaneous liver biopsy should be considered in patients with unexplained jaundice after initial investigations

Figure 31.8 Liver biopsy of alcoholic hepatitis

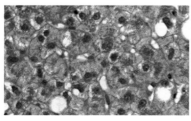

Consider MRCP in patients with obstructive LFTs, suspected gallstones, a dilated bile duct on USS and abnormal LFTs following cholecystectomy.

Figure 31.6 MRCP coronal image shows (a) normal MRCP appearances and (b) dilatation of the intrahepatic biliary tree
(a)   (b)

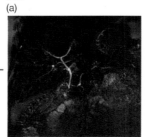
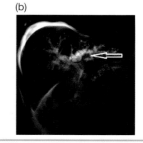

Jaundice is yellow staining of the body tissues produced by an excess of circulating bilirubin. Jaundice is detectable clinically when the bilirubin level rises above 40 mmol/L. Jaundice is classified into three groups: (1) prehepatic, resulting from excessive red cell destruction (Chapter 122); (2) hepatic due to liver injury; and (3) posthepatic due to obstruction of the biliary tree. However, this classification has limitations. Jaundice may be related to mixed mechanisms in diseases such as intrahepatic cholestasis.

Unconjugated hyperbilirubinaemia can be caused by disorders of enzyme metabolism affecting conjugation. Gilbert syndrome is a common, benign, hereditary disease due to a decrease in the activity of enzyme glucuronosyltransferase, causing unconjugated hyperbilirubinaemia, which is usually an incidental finding with normal liver function. Jaundice or worsening of hyperbilirubinaemia may occur during stress, fasting and acute illness. However, these changes are transient and there is **no** need for further investigation.

Clinical investigation

Is the jaundice caused by prehepatic, intrahepatic or extrahepatic causes? This distinction can be made in the majority of patients by a thorough history and examination. Clinically important clues to extrahepatic obstructions include abdominal pain, a palpable gallbladder or upper abdominal mass, evidence of cholangitis, and a history of previous biliary surgery. In patients with clinical and biochemical evidence suggestive of cholestasis, the major role of imaging is to determine the site and cause of obstruction.

Laboratory investigations

Urine test

The initial investigation in jaundice is to determine whether the hyperbilirubinaemia is conjugated or unconjugated. A urinalysis that is positive for bilirubin indicates the presence of conjugated bilirubinaemia, which is likely due to obstructive or hepatic causes. Conjugated bilirubinaemia is absent in prehepatic causes such as haemolytic anaemia. Absent urobilinogen indicates obstruction to the common bile duct (CBD). On the other hand, excess urobilinogen occurs sometimes in liver damage and haemolytic jaundice.

FBC

This is useful to exclude haemolysis.

Bilirubin levels

A raised bilirubin will confirm the presence of jaundice and give some indication of its severity.

Liver function tests

• Aspartate transaminase (AST) and alanine transaminase (ALT) are markers of hepatocellular injury.
• Alkaline phosphatase (ALP) and gamma-glutamyltransferase (GGT) are markers of cholestasis.

Other laboratory investigations

• Hepatitis A, B, C serology.
• Autoimmune markers: ANA, anti-smooth muscle, antimitochondrial, anti-liver–kidney, antimicrosomal, antineutrophil cytoplasmic antibodies.
• Lipase or amylase.

Imaging

Ultrasound is a non-invasive, low-cost and quick imaging modality to evaluate jaundice. It can determine the presence of bile duct obstruction by detecting ductal dilatation with sensitivity of 70% and specificity 90% (Figure 31.1). The false negative is usually due to inability to see the extrahepatic biliary tree because of bowel gas, obesity or the absence of biliary dilatation in the presence of obstruction. It can assess cholelithiasis (Figure 31.2), choledocholithiasis and acute cholecystitis. Ultrasound has a sensitivity and specificity of 95% for the diagnosis of cholelithiasis. Its sensitivity is much less for choledocholithiasis (missed in up to 60% of patients). Overall, ultrasound is less effective than CT and magnetic resonance cholangiopancreatography (MRCP)/endoscopic retrograde cholangiopancreatography (ERCP) in determining the cause and site of obstruction. Ultrasound is also useful for the detection of liver metastases (Figure 31.3) and other diffuse liver diseases, such as cirrhosis.

CT of abdomen is indicated if ultrasound is indeterminate. It is more sensitive (90%) and specific (94%) than ultrasound in detection of biliary obstruction, especially for imaging extramural causes of obstruction (Figure 31.4). CT is also superior to ultrasound in displaying the entire pancreas and detecting pancreatic tumours (Figure 31.5).

MRCP is the most sensitive of the non-invasive techniques that can provide the three-dimensional anatomy of the biliary and pancreatic duct. It is usually performed in patients presenting with obstructive LFTs and with suspected gallstones and/or a dilated bile duct on ultrasound and in patients who have persistent symptoms and abnormal liver function following cholecystectomy. When compared with ERCP, MRCP has a sensitivity, specificity, positive predictive value and negative predictive value of 85%, 93%, 87% and 82% respectively. Stones (as small as 2 mm) appear as dependent low-signal-filling defects within the CBD, surrounded by high-signal-intensity bile (Figure 31.6).

Pancreatic adenocarcinoma usually appears as a focal mass, most often in the head of the pancreas, leading to encasement and obstruction of the pancreatic duct and/or CBD. Dilatation of both ducts is seen in 75% of cases appearing as the 'double duct' sign on MRCP. Peri-ampullary carcinoma can lead to high-grade obstruction of the CBD with abrupt termination on MRCP. There is usually only mild dilatation of the pancreatic duct.

ERCP has a diagnostic and therapeutic role but has risks (9% pancreatitis, 0.4% mortality). ERCP is useful to assess the site and cause of obstruction prior to surgical, endoscopic or radiological intervention. In general, ERCP is more reliable for detecting low obstruction (Figure 31.7). It is of value in the demonstration of ampullary lesions and to delineate the level of biliary tree obstruction. It allows sphincterotomy to be performed to facilitate the passage of stones lodged in the CBD.

Percutaneous transhepatic cholangiography (PTC) is both diagnostic for assessing the level of obstruction and therapeutic for biliary obstruction by being used as a precursor to a biliary drainage procedure or prior to stent insertion. In general, PTC is more reliable for high obstructions. It is contraindicated if bleeding disorder or ascites is present.

Liver biopsy

A percutaneous liver biopsy should be considered in patients with unexplained jaundice after initial investigations (Figure 31.8). Major complications, such as clinically significant intra-abdominal bleeding, are uncommon, and mortality is 0.01%. Percutaneous liver biopsy is contraindicated in patients with a significant coagulopathy or substantial ascites; in these instances, transjugular liver biopsy can be an alternative. Liver biopsy may be of value in differentiating hepatocellular cholestasis from obstructive jaundice.

32 Meningitis

Patients with suspected meningitis: headache, fever, neck stiffness and altered mental status

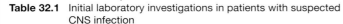

Table 32.1 Initial laboratory investigations in patients with suspected CNS infection

FBC with differential may demonstrate neutrophilia with a left shift in bacterial meningitis

Serum electrolytes can help to determine dehydration or SIADH

Serum glucose and protein are used to compare with the CSF results

Urea, creatinine and LFTs are needed to assess organ function and adjust antibiotic dose

Coagulation profile and platelet count are indicated before LP and in cases of suspected disseminated intravascular coagulopathy. Patients with coagulopathies may require platelets or fresh frozen plasma before LP

CRP is raised in patients with bacterial meningitis; in patients where the CSF Gram stain is negative and the differential diagnosis is between bacterial and viral meningitis, a normal CRP excludes bacterial meningitis with 99% certainty.

Key points

- Confirming the diagnosis of meningitis requires CSF analysis.
- Identification of the causative bacteria involves Gram staining, culture and PCR when available.
- CT of the head should be considered before LP in the presence of focal neurological deficit, new-onset seizures, papilloedema, altered mental state, or immunocompromise to exclude generalised cerebral oedema, brain tissue shift and brain abscess.

Figure 32.1 A typical skin rash (petechiae and purpura) due to meningococcaemia

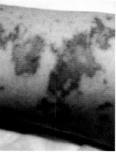

Any contraindications for LP:
- Altered mental status
- History of CNS disease
- Severely immunocompromised
- Focal neurological signs
- New-onset seizures
- Papilloedema

Figure 32.2 CT head shows increased intracranial pressure

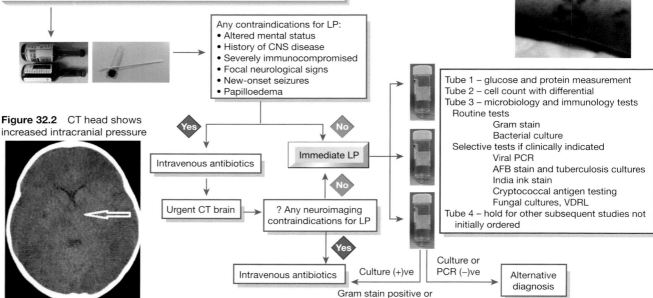

Yes → Intravenous antibiotics → Urgent CT brain → ? Any neuroimaging contraindications for LP

No → Immediate LP

No → ? Any neuroimaging contraindications for LP

Yes → Intravenous antibiotics

Gram stain positive or cell count suggestive of bacterial or viral meningitis

Culture (+)ve

Tube 1 – glucose and protein measurement
Tube 2 – cell count with differential
Tube 3 – microbiology and immunology tests
　Routine tests
　　　Gram stain
　　　Bacterial culture
　Selective tests if clinically indicated
　　　Viral PCR
　　　AFB stain and tuberculosis cultures
　　　India ink stain
　　　Cryptococcal antigen testing
　　　Fungal cultures, VDRL
Tube 4 – hold for other subsequent studies not initially ordered

Culture or PCR (–)ve → Alternative diagnosis

Table 32.2 Typical findings in the CSF with different conditions

Condition	Glucose	Protein	Cells/mm³	Comments
Bacterial meningitis	↓	↑	Often >300	Polymorphs
Viral meningitis	N	N/↑	<300 mononuclear	Viral PCR
Fungal meningitis	↓	↑	<300 mononuclear	Culture and antigen detection
Tuberculous meningitis	↓	↑	Mixed pleocytosis <300	Acid-fast bacillus (AFB) stain, culture and PCR
Herpes simplex encephalitis	N	Mildly ↑	5–500 lymphocytes	PCR
HIV meningitis	N	N/↑	Mononuclear pleocytosis	Culture, antigen detection, antiviral antibodies
Neurosyphilis – early	N/↓	↑	<300 lymphocytes	Venereal Disease Research Laboratory (VDRL) test
Neurosyphilis – late	N	↑	<300 lymphocytes	Treponema pallidum immobilisation test
Malignant meningitis	↓	↑	Mononuclear	Rapid cytospin and look for malignant cells

Meningitis is a syndrome characterised by inflammation of the meninges. Meningitis is usually caused by bacterial, viral, parasites or fungal infection, but may rarely result from injury, cancer or drugs such as non-steroidal anti-inflammatory drugs. *Streptococcus pneumonia*, *Haemophilus influenzae type b* (Hib) and *Neisseria meningitidis* are responsible for 90% of all cases of bacterial meningitis.

Clinical evaluation

Bacterial meningitis has a high fatality rate, and 30% of survivors have long-term sequelae, including hearing loss and focal neurologic deficits. Therefore, a high index of suspicion and prompt investigation are imperative. Classic symptoms of meningitis include headache, fever, neck stiffness, nausea or vomiting, and altered mental status. In adults with community-acquired bacterial meningitis, the sensitivity of the classic triad of fever, neck stiffness and altered mental status is low (44%), but almost all such patients present with at least two of these symptoms.

Bacterial meningitis may prove fatal within hours. All patients with suspected acute bacterial meningitis should be rapidly admitted to hospital and isolated droplet precautions taken. Patients should be assessed for whether LP is clinically safe. If LP cannot be performed or is delayed because a CT of the head is needed, broad-spectrum antibiotics that encompass coverage of *Streptococcus pneumoniae* and *Staphylococcus aureus* should be started before the CT scan and after blood cultures have been taken. This may reduce the diagnostic yield of LP, but administration of antibiotics should not be delayed.

Initial laboratory investigations

In patients with suspected meningitis, the initial investigations are listed in Table 32.1.

Blood culture: All patients with suspected meningitis should have blood samples obtained for culture immediately and before instituting antibiotics. The result may be influenced by previous antimicrobial therapy. Positive blood cultures occur in 40–70% of cases of *H. influenzae*, *S. pneumoniae* or *N. meningitidis* meningitis.

Other cultures: Nasopharynx aspirate, respiratory secretions, urine and skin lesions (Figure 32.1) should be sent for culture.

LP and cerebrospinal fluid (CSF) analysis

LP is mandatory in any patient in whom meningitis is suspected, although the procedure has potential risks. Reports have emphasised the risk of brain herniation as a complication of diagnostic LP in patients with meningitis. However, if the patient has
- no history of being immunocompromised
- no focal neurological signs and symptoms and
- no decrease in consciousness level

then it is **not** necessary to perform CT/MRI of the brain prior to LP to look for evidence of raised intracranial pressure. The CSF analysis is listed in Table 32.2.

The opening pressure of the CSF is elevated in most patients with bacterial meningitis. Gram staining of CSF permits the rapid identification of the causative organism (sensitivity: 60–90%; specificity: ≥97%). Bacterial antigen tests have a limited sensitivity, but may be helpful in patients with negative Gram staining and cultures. *N. meningitidis* capsular polysaccharide antigen can be detected by latex agglutination in 40–95% of patients with meningococcal meningitis.

In viral meningitis, the WBC count is 10–300/µL; the glucose concentration is typically normal but can be low in meningitis from herpes simplex and mumps viruses. The use of PCR assay has revolutionised the diagnosis of viral meningitis, especially herpes viruses meningitis. PCR for herpes viruses has sensitivity and specificity of >95% for all herpes CNS infections. The PCR assay for enteroviruses is more sensitive than viral culture and is 94–100% specific.

The most important differential diagnoses for viral meningitis are encephalitis and bacterial meningitis. Reduced Glasgow coma scale score suggests encephalitis and should prompt empirical treatment with acyclovir and further investigations to establish the diagnosis (see Chapter 138). Distinguishing viral meningitis from bacterial meningitis may be difficult clinically. If the patient is very ill or immunocompromised, empirical antibiotics should be instituted. A LP may confirm a diagnosis of viral meningitis and allow cessation of antibiotics and earlier hospital discharge.

In patients with tuberculous meningitis, the CSF is characterised by a predominantly lymphocytic pleocytosis; an elevated protein level and a low glucose level. PCR testing can provide a rapid diagnosis, though false-negative results may occur in samples containing very few organisms (less than two colony-forming units per millilitre). The demonstration of acid-fast bacillus (AFB) by Ziehl–Neelsen stain in the CSF is difficult and usually requires a large volume of CSF.

Progressive, life-threatening, subacute meningitis can be caused by *Cryptococcus* species. Risk factors include immunosuppression, HIV infection, neutropenia and neurosurgery. *Cryptococcus neoformans* may be cultured from the CSF or identified with India ink preparation or detection of CSF cryptococcal antigen.

The analysis of the CSF should be repeated only in patients whose condition has not responded clinically after 48 hours of appropriate antimicrobial therapy.

Neuroimaging

CT or MRI of the head should be considered before LP in the presence of focal neurological deficit, new-onset seizures, papilloedema, altered mental state, or immunocompromise to exclude generalised cerebral oedema, brain tissue shift and brain abscess. It may identify underlying conditions and meningitis-associated complications such as brain infarction, cerebral oedema and hydrocephalus. When these criteria are met, indications for neuroimaging before LP are present in about 45% of patients with bacterial meningitis confirmed by CSF culture.

For patients with a decline in consciousness, or those whose condition fails to improve after the initiation of appropriate antimicrobial therapy, brain imaging is indicated. On neuroimaging, early signs of brain oedema are the disappearance of sylvian fissures and a narrowing of ventricular size. In patients with an advanced stage of brain oedema and raised intracranial pressure, basal cisterns and sulci may become obliterated (Figure 32.2).

33 Anaemia

Table 33.1 Morphological classification of anaemia

Diagnosis	Microcytic hypochromic)	Normocytic, normochromic	Macrocytic
Mean cell volume (MCV, fl)	<80	80–95	>95
Mean cell Hb (MCH, pg)	<27	27–33	>33
Possible causes	Iron deficiency Thalassaemia Anaemia of chronic disease (some cases) Lead poisoning Sideroblastic anaemia	Haemolytic anaemia Anaemia of chronic disease Acute blood loss Mixed deficiencies Bone marrow failure CKD	Alcoholism Folate or vitamin B12 deficiency Liver disease Myelodysplastic syndromes Hypothyroidism

Table 33.2 Diagnostic blood film abnormalities

Abnormality	Appearance	Possible causes
Oval macrocytes (Figure 33.1)	A red cell that is larger than normal	B12 or folate deficiency
Hypersegmented neutrophils (Figure 33.2)	A neutrophil with an increased number of nuclear lobes (six or more)	B12 or folate deficiency
Poikilocytosis	Increased variation in red cell shape	Vitamin deficiencies, hereditary abnormalities such as sickle cell disease
Polychromasia	A blue tinge to red cell, characteristic of reticulocytes	Haemolytic anaemia
Spherocytes	A red cell that has lost its central pallor and biconcave shape and is spherical	Haemolytic anaemia, hereditary spherocytosis
Target cells (Figure 33.3)	A red cell with a strongly staining area within the area of central pallor	Liver disease, thalassaemia
Hypogranular or hyposegmented neutrophils	A neutrophil with reduced cytoplasmic granulation or reduced nuclear lobes (two lobes or none)	Myelodysplastic syndrome, severe infection
Monocytosis (Figure 33.4)	Increased circulating monocytes	Chronic inflammation (e.g. tuberculosis)
Circulating blasts (Figure 33.5)	Circulation of primitive blast cells	Acute leukaemia

Table 33.3 Iron status in different conditions

Diagnosis	Hb	MCV (fL) MCH (pg)	Serum ferritin (µg/L)	Transferrin (g/L)	Transferrin saturation (%)	Serum iron (µmol/L)
Normal iron store	See Table 33.1	80–95 27–33	20–300	1.7–3.4	>20	10–30
Iron deficiency without anaemia	N	N/↓	<20	N/↑	N/↓	↓
Iron deficiency anaemia (IDA)	↓	↓	<15–30	↑	↓	↓
Anaemia of chronic disease or inflammation	↓	N (or mildly ↓)	N/↑	N	↓	↓
IDA with coexistent chronic disease or inflammation	↓	↓	N/↓ (usually <60–100)	N/↑	↓	↓
Thalassaemia	↓/N	↓/N	N/↑	N	N/↑	N

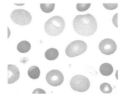

Figure 33.1 Macrocytosis

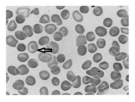

Figure 33.2 Hyper-segmented neutrophils

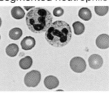

Figure 33.3 Target cells

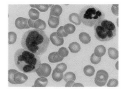

Figure 33.4 Monocytosis

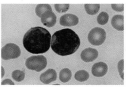

Figure 33.5 Circulating blast cells

Key points

- Confirm anaemia, assess severity and classify into microcytic, normocytic or macrocytic.
- Measurement of serum ferritin is the most accurate test to diagnose IDA.
- Macrocytic anaemia should prompt investigation for vitamin B12 or folate deficiency.
- Bone marrow examination is indicated in unexplained anaemia, macrocytosis, pancytopenia; suspected malignancy (lymphoma, leukaemia, multiple myeloma).

Anaemia is a haemoglobin (Hb) concentration below the reference range for the age and sex of an individual. Anaemia is a common problem often discovered on routine laboratory tests and a major cause of morbidity and mortality worldwide.

Anaemia may result from reduced formation or increased destruction of RBCs or their loss from the circulation by bleeding. When adaptive changes are unable to maintain tissue oxygenation in anaemia, symptoms including fatigue, dyspnoea on exertion, palpitation and angina can occur.

Initial investigation

The initial investigation is to confirm the anaemia, assess its severity and classify the anaemia into microcytic, normocytic or macrocytic anaemia (Table 33.1). The initial investigations should include:

- FBC, blood film;
- red cell indices, including mean corpuscular volume (MCV);
- reticulocyte count.

Pancytopenia (reduced Hb, WBC and platelet count) may suggest a bone marrow defect or general 'destruction' of haemopoietic cells (e.g. hypersplenism). Neutrophil and platelet count can be raised with haemolysis or haemorrhage. If reticulocyte count is not raised in a patient with anaemia, this may suggest impaired marrow function or lack of erythropoietin stimulus. It is essential to examine the blood film in all cases of anaemia (Table 33.2).

Underlying cause of anaemia

The underlying cause of anaemia should always be investigated as anaemia is a syndrome only. Anaemia is a manifestation of many diseases. Depending on the FBC results and red cell indices, the following investigations can be undertaken:

- biochemistry, including serum creatinine, urea, LFTs and LDH;
- iron studies;
- folate and vitamin B12 levels;
- thyroid function tests;
- protein electrophoresis (see Chapter 125);
- Hb electrophoresis and red cell enzymes – used in diagnosing α- or β-thalassaemia and haemoglobinopathy;
- haptoglobin and other tests for the evaluation of haemolysis (see Chapter 122);
- radiological investigations if lymphoproliferative disorders or malignancy with bone marrow involvement are suspected;
- bone marrow examination, indicated in unexplained anaemia, macrocytosis, pancytopenia; suspected malignancy (lymphoma, leukaemia, multiple myeloma);
- cytogenetic and molecular analyses, which can be done on aspirate material in hematopoietic or other tumours.

Microcytic anaemia

Microcytic anaemia is most commonly due to iron deficiency. Confirmation with iron study is required. The important differential diagnoses are thalassaemic conditions. Table 33.3 provides guidance for interpretation of results of laboratory tests of iron status. Serum ferritin is the most useful index of iron deficiency. In an adult patient with anaemia, a ferritin level <15 μg/L is diagnostic of iron deficiency, while levels of 15–30 μg/L are highly suggestive. However, ferritin is an acute-phase protein elevated in infection, inflammation and malignancy. A serum ferritin in the normal range does not exclude iron deficiency in the presence of concurrent illness. Serum iron levels have significant diurnal variation, are low in both iron deficiency and inflammation, and should not be used alone to diagnose iron deficiency. Serum iron is reduced in iron deficiency, with an increase in total iron binding capacity (TIBC), so that iron saturation is <10%. Iron is also low in anaemia of chronic disease, with reduced TIBC, giving normal iron saturation. Bone marrow aspirate with Perls' Prussian blue stain is the gold-standard test for iron deficiency anaemia (IDA).

The cause of IDA needs to be investigated. Menstrual blood loss is the commonest cause of IDA in premenopausal women, while gastrointestinal blood loss is the commonest cause in postmenopausal women and men. Patients without a clear physiological explanation for iron deficiency should be evaluated by upper gastrointestinal endoscopy and/or colonoscopy to exclude a source of gastrointestinal bleeding, particularly a malignant lesion. Patients with IDA should be assessed for coeliac disease and malabsorption. Functional iron deficiency exists when, despite adequate stores, iron cannot be mobilised for erythropoiesis. It is commonly seen in patients with end-stage kidney disease.

Microcytic anaemia can be caused by other conditions. If thalassaemia is suspected, Hb electrophoresis with an estimation of HbA$_2$ and F is carried out. β-thalassaemia minor is diagnosed by HbA$_2$ >3.5%, but the Hb electrophoresis is usually normal in adults with α-thalassaemia trait. DNA analysis of both α- and β-globin genes can be performed.

Macrocytic anaemia

The commonest causes of macrocytosis are vitamin B12 or folate deficiency, liver disease, alcoholism and reticulocytosis and can usually be differentiated on the basis of red cell indices and morphologic findings. Bone marrow studies are not usually indicated. In liver disease and alcoholism, macrocytosis is mild and uniform. Megaloblastic anaemia is a group of disorders in which the erythroblasts in the bone marrow show a characteristic abnormality, maturation of the nucleus being delayed relative to that of the cytoplasm. The underlying cause is usually due to deficiency of vitamin B12 or folate. Other causes include abnormalities in vitamin B12 or folate metabolism, anti-folate drugs and defects of DNA synthesis.

Following the identification of folate or B12 deficiency, a cause must be sought. The common tests used to determine the cause of vitamin B12 deficiency leading to pernicious anaemia are anti-intrinsic factor antibodies and anti-parietal-cell antibodies and endoscopy. Tests for determining the cause of folate deficiency depend on the clinical picture and may include upper gastrointestinal endoscopy, jejunal biopsy, and tests for intestinal malabsorption.

Normocytic anaemia

Bleeding is an important cause of normochromic, normocytic anaemia where symptoms of anaemia are of recent onset. Anaemia of chronic disease (ACD) is usually mild to moderate (Hb 80–95 g/L) normochromic, normocytic anaemia. Patients with ACD have a low reticulocyte count. In investigating ACD CKD, congestive cardiac failure and malignancy should be considered.

34 Lymphadenopathy

Table 34.1 Common causes of localised and generalised lymphadenopathy

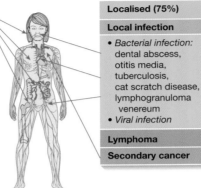

Generalised (25%)

Infections

- *Viral infection*: EBV, CMV, HIV, Dengue fever
- *Bacterial infection*: septicaemia, brucellosis, tuberculosis, syphilis
- *Fungal infection*: histoplasmosis
- *Protozoal*: toxoplasmosis

Non-infectious inflammatory disease

- Sarcoidosis, SLE, connective tissue disease

Malignancy

- Leukaemia, especially CLL, ALL
- Lymphoma
- Secondary cancer

Localised (75%)

Local infection

- *Bacterial infection:* dental abscess, otitis media, tuberculosis, cat scratch disease, lymphogranuloma venereum
- *Viral infection*

Lymphoma

Secondary cancer

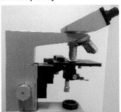

Figure 34.1 Blood film examination is useful in initial investigation of lymphadenopathy

Table 34.2 Evaluation of some suspected causes of lymphadenopathy

Disorder	Associated findings	Investigations
EBV infection	Splenomegaly in 50% of patients	Monospot, IgM, EA or VCA
Toxoplasmosis	Majority (80–90%) of patients are asymptomatic	IgM toxoplasma antibody
CMV infection	Often mild symptoms, patients may have hepatitis	IgM CMV antibody, blood viral polymerase chain reaction
Initial stages of HIV infection	"Flu-like" illness, rash	HIV antibody
Acute hepatitis B infection	Fever, nausea, vomiting, jaundice	LFTs, hepatitis B serology
Pharyngitis due to group A streptococcus, gonococcus	Fever, pharyngeal exudates, cervical nodes	Culture of throat swab on appropriate medium
Cat-scratch disease	Fever in one-third of patients; cervical or axillary nodes	Usually clinical criteria, biopsy if necessary
Tuberculosis lymphadenitis	Painless, matted cervical nodes	TST or IGRA, biopsy
Secondary syphilis	Rash	RPR
Lymphogranuloma venereum	Tender, matted inguinal nodes	Serology
Chancroid	Painful ulcer, painful inguinal nodes	Clinical criteria, culture
Sarcoidosis	Hilar nodes, skin lesions, dyspnoea	Biopsy
SLE	Arthritis, rash, serositis, renal, neurological, haematological disorders	Clinical criteria, Ds-DNA, complement levels
Serum sickness	Fever, malaise, arthralgia, urticaria; exposure to antisera or medications	Clinical criteria, complement assays
Lymphoma	Fever, night sweats, weight loss in 20–30% of patients	Biopsy
Leukaemia	Blood dyscrasias, bruising	Blood smear, bone marrow

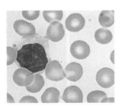

Figure 34.2 Blood film shows atypical lymphocyte in a patient with EBV infection

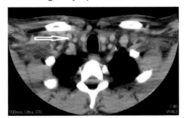

Figure 34.3 CT of the neck shows cervical lymphadenopathy due to non-Hodgkin lymphoma

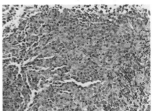

Figure 34.4 Lymph node biopsy shows non-Hodgkin lymphoma

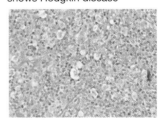

Figure 34.5 Lymph node biopsy shows Hodgkin disease

Key points

- Initial investigations should include FBC, biochemistry, CRP and viral serology (as clinically indicated).
- Radiological imaging may include CXR, ultrasound and CT scan to determine distribution of lymphadenopathy and guide the site of biopsy if indicated.
- Excisional biopsy of the most abnormal node is the best investigation to achieve a diagnosis.

Lymphadenopathy refers to lymph nodes that are abnormal in size, consistency or number. The extent of lymphadenopathy can be classified as localised (only one area is involved) or generalised (lymph nodes enlarged in two or more non-contiguous areas). About 75% of all lymphadenopathies are localised and often caused by a specific pathology in the area of drainage; 25% of lymphadenopathies are generalised and are often a sign of a significant underlying disease, such as lymphoma or malignancy. However, generalised lymphadenopathy can be caused by benign self-limiting disease, such as viral or bacterial infection. Distinguishing between localised and generalised lymphadenopathy is important in formulating a differential diagnosis and guiding investigation (Table 34.1).

Basic laboratory investigations

In the majority of patients, a careful history and physical examination will identify a cause of the lymphadenopathy such as viral or bacterial infection and no further investigation is necessary. In other cases, a definitive diagnosis cannot be made on the basis of the history and physical examination alone; further investigations should be performed in order to correctly identify the underlying illness.

The initial investigation of lymphadenopathy should be directed by the history and physical examination and the likely cause of lymphadenopathy. The following basic investigations should be performed:

- FBC, including peripheral blood smear (Figures 34.1 and 34.2);
- CRP;
- LFTs;
- electrolyte, creatinine, urea, LDH and uric acid;
- blood cultures if suspected septicaemia;
- tuberculosis interferon-gamma release assay;
- CXR.

When evaluating specific regional lymphadenopathy, lymph node aspirate for culture may be important if lymphadenitis is clinically suspected. Serological tests for specific microorganisms may be indicated, particularly if generalised adenopathy is present. These may include EBV, CMV, toxoplasma species, syphilis, hepatitis and HIV. If non-infectious inflammatory disease is suspected, autoantibody screen for SLE, rheumatoid arthritis and Sjögren's syndrome is indicated (Table 34.2).

Radiological investigations

Ultrasound

Ultrasonography is helpful in assessing the extent of lymph node involvement in patients with lymphadenopathy and any changes in the lymph nodes. Abdominal ultrasound can assess the liver and spleen size.

CT

Supraclavicular lymphadenopathy, with its high associated rate of serious underlying disease, is an indication for a CT scan of the chest and abdomen (Figure 34.3).

Positron-emission tomography (PET)

PET scan is not a first-line investigation modality, as benign and malignant conditions may cause intense uptake. However, PET scanning is helpful in the staging of lymphomas once a diagnosis is made.

Lymph node biopsy

Indications for lymph node biopsy and histological examination include:

- patients with generalised lymphadenopathy in whom the initial studies are non-diagnostic;
- patients with localised persistent lymphadenopathy, non-diagnostic initial studies and a high risk for malignancy;
- if the size, location or character of the lymphadenopathy is suggestive of malignancy.

In general, excisional biopsy is preferred, particularly if lymphoma is suspected (Figures 34.4 and 34.5). It allows an assessment of the architecture of the lymph node as well as histological, immunohistochemical, cytogenetic and molecular investigations. Fine-needle aspiration or core needle biopsy of a lymph node has limited ability to undertake flow cytometry and chromosomal analysis; it is occasionally useful for the diagnosis of underlying carcinomas or recurrent malignancy. Excisional biopsy also has limitations and may yield a definitive diagnosis in only 40–60% of patients because of inadequate specimen size, improper handling or node-sampling error.

Biopsies should be obtained at the most abnormal or largest lymph node site, even if it is technically difficult. Sampling more accessible nodes may miss the underlying malignancy. Inguinal node biopsy should be avoided, since the diagnostic yield at this site is often low. Empiric therapy with corticosteroids or antibiotics should be avoided before the biopsy as they may confound the results of a lymph node biopsy due to their lympholytic effect. Even in a patient with superior vena cava syndrome, which is not a medical emergency unless neurological symptoms are present, a biopsy should be obtained prior to the initiation of therapy. Endobronchial ultrasound-guided transbronchial needle aspiration can be used for tissue sampling from hilar and mediastinal lymph nodes.

Biopsies that reveal atypical lymphoid hyperplasia should be considered non-diagnostic rather than negative for a malignancy, and these patients should be carefully followed and a second biopsy should be strongly considered. Specific infections can be diagnosed if tissues are appropriately stained. For patients with high suspicion of underlying malignancy, an unrevealing lymph node biopsy should be considered non-diagnostic rather than negative for malignancy, and further investigations should be pursued.

35 Cough

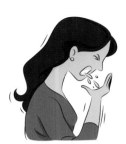

Table 35.1 Clinical approach

- History and examination will often suggest the most likely diagnoses
- A period of observation for 4 weeks in a patient with a history indicative of an upper respiratory tract infection is reasonable prior to further investigations
- Patient with 'red flag' symptoms (see box 35.1) should undergo investigation immediately
- Initial investigations may be limited to a CXR, if there is a high suspicion of a tumour, especially in patients with a smoking history, and pulmonary function tests if asthma is suspected
- Post-nasal drip, asthma and GORD are three of the most common conditions associated with chronic cough in non-smokers
- A cause for chronic cough can be found in 90% of cases after investigations

Figure 35.1 Portable spirometer

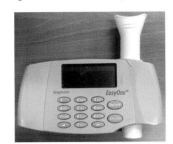

Symptoms in chronic persistent cough

- Copious sputum production
- Associated with fever, night sweats
- Haemoptysis
- Exertional or resting dyspnoea
- Unintentional weight loss

Figure 35.2 (a) Normal CXR (b) CXR shows pulmonary fibrosis

(a)

(b)

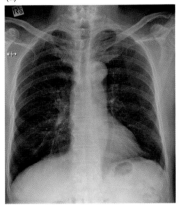
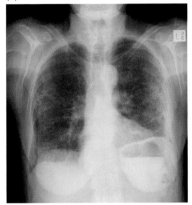

Figure 35.3 CT chest shows pulmonary fibrosis

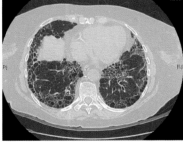
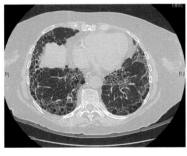

Figure 35.4 Bronchoscopy shows an endobronchial foreign body

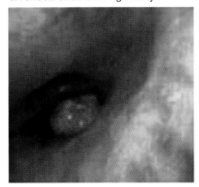

Key points

- The most important initial investigation of chronic cough is a CXR.
- Asthma is the commonest cause of chronic cough in adults.
- Spirometry is required to diagnose asthma and can be reliably used to demonstrate airflow obstruction and assess reversibility.
- Chest CT and bronchoscopy should be done in patients in whom lung cancer or another bronchial tumour is suspected.

Cough is a common symptom of most respiratory disorders and a frequent reason for medical consultations. Cough is a useful protective reflex to clear excessive secretions from the respiratory tract. Persistent cough also occurs in the absence of excessive mucus production and can be triggered by a tumour or foreign body. Cough can be divided into acute self-limiting cough, lasting less than 3 weeks, or chronic persistent cough, which usually lasts for more than 8 weeks with an overlap period of 3–8 weeks. Persistent chronic cough has been estimated to occur in 10–23% of adults. Chronic cough is a debilitating symptom that can significantly interfere with quality of life. The differential diagnosis of chronic cough is extensive and includes infections, inflammatory and neoplastic conditions, and many other pulmonary conditions. A clinical approach is listed in Table 35.1.

Laboratory investigations

In patients with chronic infections, suspected neoplasm and red flag symptoms (see red flag box), laboratory investigations are indicated. This includes FBC, urea, creatinine and electrolytes, LFTs and CRP. Sputum should also be collected for microscopy, Gram stain, acid-fast bacillus smear, culture and cytology if clinically indicated.

When a patient has paroxysms of cough, posttussive vomiting, and/or an inspiratory whooping sound, *Bordetella pertussis* infection is the likely culprit. A definitive diagnosis can be confirmed with a PCR test from a nasopharyngeal aspirate swab.

Pulmonary function tests

In patients with suspected asthma, pulmonary function tests should be undertaken (Chapter 61). Spirometric values of forced expiratory volume in 1 second/forced vital capacity of <70% and a positive bronchodilator response (≥12%) are consistent with an asthma diagnosis (Figure 35.1). The methacholine challenge test can demonstrate bronchial hyperresponsiveness.

CXR

A CXR should be done to rule out more ominous causes of chronic cough. Other abnormalities may suggest alternative diagnosis and avoid unnecessary investigation. For example, CXR findings of cardiomegaly and increased pulmonary vascular distribution are suggestive of congestive heart failure as a possible cause of chronic cough. Other findings could include pneumonia, pulmonary fibrosis (Figure 35.2) and lung cancer.

CT

A CT chest is warranted if mass lesions are discovered in the lung parenchyma, mediastinal mass or cavitary lesions on CXR. HRCT chest is indicated in patients suspected to have interstitial lung disease (Figure 35.3) or bronchiectasis. However, there is no role for thoracic CT scanning in the routine evaluation of chronic cough.

There is no gold-standard diagnostic test to confirm or rule out postnasal drip as the cause of cough. Direct inspection of the nasal passages and throat, together with a CT scan of the sinuses, may be indicated, However, CT scan of sinuses has a poor positive predictive value and is not recommended for initial work-up, but may be useful for patients whose symptoms persist longer than 3 weeks.

Bronchoscopy

The diagnostic yield from bronchoscopy in the routine evaluation of chronic cough is only about 5%. In spite of this, bronchoscopy has significant diagnostic potential in selected patients who have risk factors for malignancy, such as male sex, older than 40 years, a smoking history of more than 40 pack-years, and duration of haemoptysis for more than 1 week. Other potential bronchoscopic diagnoses include broncholithiasis, laryngeal dyskinesia and unrecognised aspirated foreign bodies (Figure 35.4).

Gastro-oesophageal investigations

GORD has been reported in 10–40% of patients with chronic cough. In patients with severe GORD, in addition to a trial of proton pump inhibitors, ambulatory pH monitoring and possible upper GI endoscopy may be warranted (Chapter 21). Patients suspected to have aspiration may require a barium swallow to evaluate further.

36 Haemoptysis

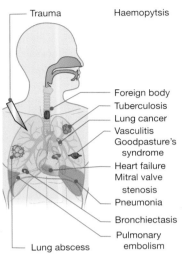

Trauma Haemopytsis

- Foreign body
- Tuberculosis
- Lung cancer
- Vasculitis
  Goodpasture's
  syndrome
- Heart failure
  Mitral valve
    stenosis
- Pneumonia
- Bronchiectasis
- Pulmonary
  embolism
- Lung abscess

Table 36.1 Laboratory tests to evaluate patients with haemoptysis

Tests	Findings
WBC count	Elevated WBC may indicate respiratory tract infections
Haemoglobin	Decreased in massive haemoptysis, inflammatory conditions, advanced lung cancer
Platelet count	Decreased in thrombocytopenia resulting in coagulopathy
Coagulation study	INR and activated partial thromboplastin time increased in anticoagulant use or disorders of coagulation
Electrolytes, urea and creatinine	Renal impairment may occur in Goodpasture's syndrome and granulomatosis with polyangiitis
CRP	Elevated in infections, inflammatory disorders and neoplasia
Arterial blood gases	Assess ventilation, hypoxia and/or hypercapnea
Sputum Gram stain, acid-fast bacillus smear and culture	Pneumonia, lung abscess, tuberculosis, mycobacterial infections
Sputum cytology (low diagnostic yield)	Neoplasm
Immunological tests	ANA, ANCA, anti-glomerular basement membrane antibody are indicated if vasculitis or Goodpasture's syndrome are suspected

Figure 36.1 CXR shows right middle lobe pneumonia

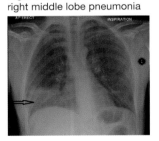

Figure 36.2 CXR lateral view shows a cavitary lesion

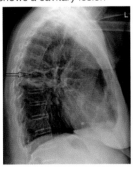

Figure 36.3 CXR shows pulmonary oedema

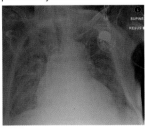

Figure 36.4 CXR shows patchy alveolar infiltrate due to vasculitis

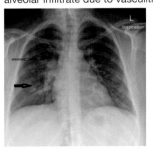

Figure 36.5 CXR shows bilateral hilar lymphadenopathy due to sarcoidosis

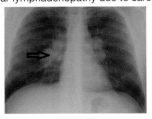

Figure 36.6 CXR shows right upper lobe lesion due to lung cancer

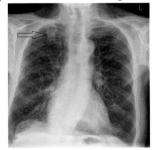

Figure 36.7 CT chest shows pulmonary haemorrhage

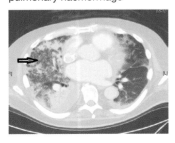

Figure 36.8 CTPA shows extensive bilateral pulmonary emboli

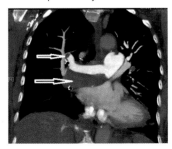

Figure 36.9 Bronchoscopy showing endobronchial cancer

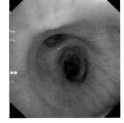
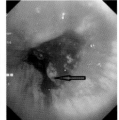

Clinical Investigations at a Glance, First Edition. Jonathan Gleadle, Jordan Li and Tuck Yong. © 2017 John Wiley & Sons, Ltd. Published 2017 by John Wiley & Sons, Ltd.

Haemoptysis is the coughing up of blood from the respiratory tract below the level of the larynx. Haemoptysis is a common and alarming symptom. Haemoptysis should be differentiated from haematemesis and pseudohaemoptysis, where a cough reflex is stimulated by blood from the oral cavity or nasopharynx, such as epistaxis. Haemoptysis is classified as non-massive or massive based on the volume of blood loss. Massive haemoptysis is arbitrarily defined as a blood loss of more than 200 mL over 24 hours, which can be potentially life threatening.

The common causes of haemoptysis are acute and chronic bronchitis, pneumonia, tuberculosis, and lung cancer. Infection remains the most common cause of haemoptysis, accounting for 60–70% of cases. The underlying aetiologies are:

- **Tracheobronchial source**
  - Bronchitis (acute or chronic)
  - Bronchiectasis
  - Bronchogenic carcinoma
  - Airway trauma
  - Foreign body
- **Pulmonary parenchymal source**
  - Pneumonia
  - Tuberculosis
  - Lung abscess
  - Fungal infection mycetoma ('fungus ball')
  - Goodpasture's syndrome
  - Granulomatosis with polyangiitis
  - Lung contusion
- **Primary vascular source**
  - Pulmonary embolism
  - Arteriovenous malformation
  - Elevated pulmonary
  - Venous pressure (especially mitral stenosis)
- **Miscellaneous and rare causes**
  - Systemic coagulopathy
  - Use of anticoagulants or thrombolytic agents
  - Pulmonary endometriosis.

Laboratory investigations

The laboratory tests that should be used in the evaluation of patients presenting with haemoptysis are summarised in Table 35.1.

CXR

A CXR should be obtained in every patient presenting with haemoptysis. Haemoptysis is an important diagnostic clue to potentially resectable lung cancer or other significant lung pathology. More frequently haemoptysis is due to benign pulmonary pathology such as bronchitis. CXR may be normal in up to 40% of patients presenting with haemoptysis. If a diagnosis remains unclear and patient has no risk factors for malignancy, patient can be followed by observation. However, a patient with smoking history or older than 50 years needs to be further investigated with chest CT and bronchoscopy. The rate of malignancy is 9.6% in smokers who present with haemoptysis regardless of the amount and frequency, even when initial CXR is normal.

CT

Conventional or high-resolution CT is the next investigation in patients with normal CXR or abnormal CXR which will further characterise the nature and extent of a lesion shown by CXR or bronchoscopy (Figure 36.7). It is the most sensitive diagnostic test with a positive yield of 67% in patients presenting with haemoptysis. It should be performed before bronchoscopy as it will improve the diagnostic yield or eliminate the need of bronchoscopy in some cases. CTPA is indicated in patients with features suggestive of pulmonary embolism (Figure 36.8).

Bronchoscopy

In high-risk patients with a normal CXR and/or chest CT, bronchoscopy should be considered to rule out malignancy. Risk factors that increase the likelihood of finding lung cancer on bronchoscopy include: older than 50 years, a smoking history of more than 40 pack-years and duration of haemoptysis for more than 1 week.

Bronchoscopy is needed if neoplasia is suspected clinically; it is diagnostic for central endobronchial disease (Figure 36.9) and allows for direct visualisation of the bleeding site. It also allows for tissue biopsies, bronchial lavage, or brushings for cytology and microbiology diagnosis. Fibre-optic bronchoscopy also can provide direct therapy in cases of continued bleeding. Rigid bronchoscopy is the preferred tool for cases of massive bleeding because of its greater suctioning and airway maintenance capabilities. The limitation of bronchoscopy is failure to visualise peripheral lesions and is associated with a risk of complications.

Bronchial angiography

Bronchial angiography is indicated when bronchial embolisation is intended, particularly if the bleeding is massive. Angiographic signs of pulmonary haemorrhage include extravasation of contrast media, hypervascularisation, and abnormal arborisation of bronchial arteries, systemic-pulmonary shunts and bronchial artery aneurysms.

Key points

- Sputum should be collected when patient presents with haemoptysis to check for the presence of acid-fast bacilli or malignant cells, but the diagnostic yield may be modest.
- CXR is the initial diagnostic test for haemodynamically stable patients with haemoptysis.
- CT chest with or without bronchoscopy is recommended in patients with massive haemoptysis (>200 mL/24 hours), those with abnormal CXR findings and those with risk factors for malignancy despite a normal CXR.
- Urine analysis for haematuria and proteinuria should be performed in patients with haemoptysis to consider the possibility of vasculitis.

37 Palpitations and cardiac arrhythmias

Table 37.1 Indications for further investigations of palpitations

- Recurrent tachyarrhythmia
- Palpitations associated with dyspnoea or syncope
- Structural heart disease or high risk factors for structural heart disease
- Palpitations during exercise
- Family history of inheritable heart disease or sudden cardiac death
- Abnormal ECG

Blood test: thyroid function test, anaemia
Holter monitor
Implanted loop event recording
Echocardiography
Electrophysiological studies

Key points

- A 12-lead ECG with a rhythm strip must be performed in all patient reporting palpitations; even if asymptomatic, the ECG may show changes that suggest a diagnosis.
- A 12-lead ECG may be normal between paroxysmal episodes of palpitations.
- A 24-hour Holter monitor or implantable loop recorder should be considered if symptoms are recurrent and the cause is unclear.
- In a patient with arrhythmias as the cause of palpitations, investigate whether there is associated structural heart disease or a non-cardiac precipitant such as electrolyte disorders.

Figure 37.1 ECG shows atrial flutter

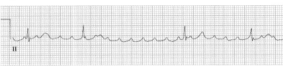

Figure 37.2 ECG shows atrial fibrillation

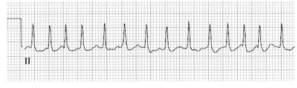

Figure 37.3 ECG shows sinus arrhythmia

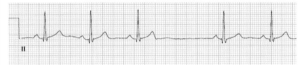

Figure 37.4 ECG shows sinus rhythm with premature ectopics

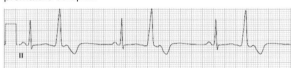

Figure 37.5 ECG shows junctional tachycardia.

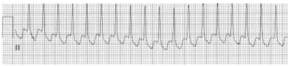

Figure 37.6 ECG shows WPW syndrome

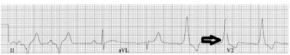

Figure 37.7 ECG shows ventricular tachycardia

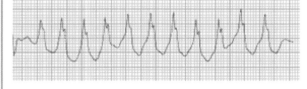

Figure 37.9 Holter monitor shows significant bradycardia with pause >3 seconds

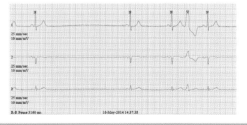

Figure 37.8 ECG shows complete heart block

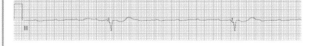

Clinical Investigations at a Glance, First Edition. Jonathan Gleadle, Jordan Li and Tuck Yong. © 2017 John Wiley & Sons, Ltd. Published 2017 by John Wiley & Sons, Ltd.

Palpitations are an inappropriate awareness of the heart beating. This symptom often causes considerable distress, but palpitations are often benign, with less than half of patients with palpitations suffering from an arrhythmia. Not every identified arrhythmia is of clinical or prognostic significance. Palpitations may be due to a primary cardiac disorder or to an extra-cardiac condition that is having a secondary effect on the heart.

Initial clinical investigation

The cause of palpitations can often be determined through a careful history and physical examination. The first question should clarify what the patient actually means by palpitations. Then ask about the speed, regularity (regular or irregular), onset and offset (instantaneous or gradual), frequency, duration of episode, precipitating or relieving factors and associated symptoms. A detailed family history is important to alert the clinician to a potentially inheritable cardiac condition that will require further investigation.

If the palpitations are present at the time of review, the radial pulse should be assessed and an ECG performed. If no symptom is present, a cardiovascular and general examination should be performed. Blood tests should exclude anaemia, thyroid dysfunction and electrolyte disturbance as potential causes of palpitations.

In patients who have no cardiovascular risk factors, no palpitation-associated symptoms such as dizziness, no abnormal findings on physical examination and normal ECG, further evaluation may not be required.

Further investigation

The purpose of further investigations is to:
• identify any arrhythmia causing the palpitation;
• to identify the patients who are more likely to have a significant arrhythmia and need to be investigated carefully (Table 37.1);
• identify any associated structural heart disease or non-cardiac precipitant of the arrhythmia
• guide the treatment of the arrhythmia.

ECG

The 12-lead ECG with a rhythm strip must be recorded at once for any patient reporting of palpitations whose symptoms are present. Even if asymptomatic, the ECG may show changes that suggest a diagnosis. The following are common arrhythmias that are associated with palpitations:
• atrial flutter (Figure 37.1)
• atrial fibrillation with rapid ventricular response (Figure 37.2)
• sinus tachycardia or arrhythmia (Figure 37.3)
• sinus rhythm with frequent premature supraventricular or ventricular extra-systoles (Figure 37.4)
• supraventricular tachycardia (Figure 37.5)
• Wolff–Parkinson–White (WPW) syndrome (Figure 37.6)
• ventricular tachycardia (VT) (Figure 37.7)
• bradycardia–tachycardia syndrome (sick sinus syndrome) (Figure 37.8)
• bradycardia caused by advanced arteriovenous block or sinus node dysfunction (Figure 37.9).

Many other ECG findings warrant further cardiac investigation. These findings include evidence of previous myocardial infarction, left or right ventricular hypertrophy, atrial enlargement, short PR interval and prolonged QT interval.

Investigating patients with infrequent symptoms can be more challenging. If episodes are prolonged when they occur, an ECG recording during the episode is probably the best approach. The patient can be given a letter to present to the closest emergency department and asked for an ECG to be performed without delay.

Ambulatory (Holter) monitoring and continuous-loop event monitors

The resting ECG can often be normal between episodes of palpitations. If symptoms are occurring on most days, a 24-hour Holter monitor should be arranged (Figure 37.9). The aim is to correlate the patient's symptoms with an ECG trace. The patient is given a diary to record the times of any symptoms. If the recording shows normal sinus rhythm during a typical episode of palpitation, this reassures that the symptom is due to awareness of heart beats only.

Twenty-four-hour recordings are often not long enough to capture patient's symptoms; therefore, the diagnostic yield is very low. As a rule of thumb, patients need to experience symptoms at least three or four times per week to make 24-hour monitoring a sensible choice. A recording of a symptom-free period is of limited value and can easily lead to false reassurance. For infrequent symptoms, a continuous implanted loop event recording system is a better choice as it allows longer recording periods and can be patient activated. The diagnostic yield has been reported as high as 66% and is more cost-effective.

If the symptoms suggest a potentially life-threatening arrhythmia, such as palpitations associated with syncope in patient with known ischaemic heart disease, further and more urgent investigations may be required including monitoring in a coronary care unit until the problem is identified and treated.

Echocardiography

Transthoracic echocardiography (TTE) is performed to evaluate left and right ventricular structure and function, including left ventricular ejection fraction. Any regional wall motion abnormalities in a coronary artery distribution may suggest coronary artery disease, which is the most common aetiology of VT. Echo can also confirm or exclude mitral valve prolapse, pericarditis and dilated or restrictive cardiomyopathy.

Electrophysiological studies

Electrophysiology studies directly assess intracardiac conduction and ascertain if there is inducible supraventricular and ventricular arrhythmias by intracardiac stimulation and are indicated for:
• palpitations associated with syncope or near syncope but normal other tests;
• palpitations with family history of sudden cardiac death;
• palpitations with suspected sinoatrial or atrioventricular node disease;
• self-limiting or sustained VT;
• WPW who have symptoms or those with WPW found on routine ECG and have a high-risk occupation.

Cardiac MRI

Cardiac MRI can provide detailed structural and functional information that is particularly useful in the diagnosis of arrhythmogenic right ventricular cardiomyopathy and infiltrative cardiomyopathies and has been shown to be beneficial in planning mapping and radiofrequency catheter ablation strategies.

38 Red eye

Table 38.1 Common causes of a red eye

Conjunctival

Allergic conjunctivitis
Bacterial or viral conjunctivitis
Chlamydial conjunctivitis
Spontaneous subconjunctival haemorrhage

Corneal

Corneal ulcer (bacterial, viral or fungal)
Contact-lens-related red eye
Corneal foreign body
Corneal abrasion
Keratitis

Inflammatory

Episcleritis
Scleritis
Anterior uveitis
Endophthalmitis

Traumatic

Penetrating ocular trauma
Chemical trauma

Other

Angle-closure glaucoma
Contact lens problems

The purpose of investigation in red eye is to:
- Differentiate between benign conditions and sight-threatening diseases
- Determine the underlying cause
- Guide the need for urgent referral to an ophthalmologist

Initial evaluation of red eye:
- Unilateral or bilateral eye involvement
- Evidence of visual impairments
- Onset and duration of symptoms
- Type and amount of discharge
- The presence of pain and/or photophobia
- The presence of allergies or systemic disease
- The use of contact lenses

Figure 38.2 Cyclitis as part of uveitis

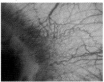

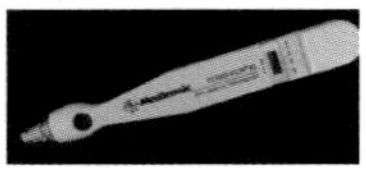

Figure 38.3 Tonometer

Patient presented with red eye with any of these alarming symptoms or signs needs urgent referral to ophthalmologist for further investigation

- Using contact lens
- Previous eye surgery
- Decreased vision
- Severe pain
- Nausea and vomiting
- Cloudy or opaque cornea
- Dendritic ulcer
- Hypopyon (pus in the anterior chamber)
- Non-reactive pupils
- Ocular trauma
- Persisting or worsening symptoms

Figure 38.1 Slit-lamp examination

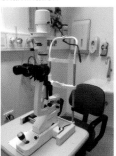

Table 38.2 Laboratory investigations for patients with episcleritis, scleritis and anterior uveitis

Tests	Interpretations
FBC	Normocytic normochromic anaemia may be seen with underlying autoimmune disorders
Electrolytes, calcium, urea, creatinine	Abnormal biochemistry results may occur with sarcoidosis, SLE and vasculitis
CRP	Elevated in inflammatory diseases
RF and anti-CCP antibodies	Positive in patients with rheumatoid arthritis
ANA	Positive in most patients with autoimmune diseases
Ds-DNA	Positive in patients with SLE
ANCA	c-ANCA is positive in granulomatosis with polyangiitis
Syphilis serology	If syphilis is suspected to cause anterior uveitis
HLA B-27	Uveitis can be associated with HLA B-27

Figure 38.4 CXR shows pulmonary fibrosis

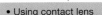

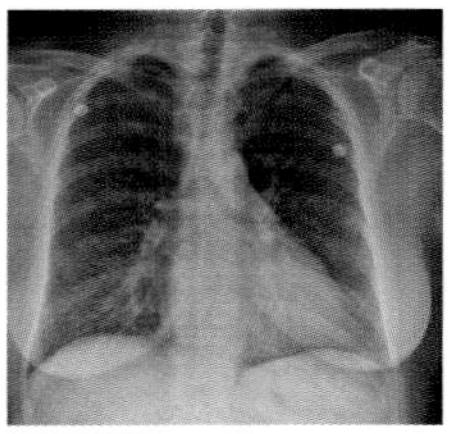

Figure 38.5 CT bony windows axial image shows bilateral sacroiliac joint sclerosis and fusion consistent with advanced sacroiliitis

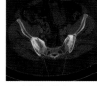

Figure 38.6 CT chest shows pulmonary fibrosis

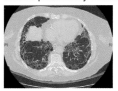

Figure 38.7 Colonoscopy shows ulcerative colitis

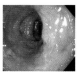

Table 38.3 Other investigations of patients with conditions associated with anterior uveitis

Images	Interpretations
CXR	May reveal pulmonary fibrosis in association with ankylosing spondylitis or hilar lymphadenopathy in sarcoidosis (Figure 38.4)
X-ray or CT of spine and sacroiliac joints	May reveal bilateral symmetric sacroiliitis and ossification of the annulus fibrosus in the lumbar spine in ankylosing spondylitis (Figure 38.5)
HRCT	May reveal interstitial lung diseases or pulmonary fibrosis in association with ankylosing spondylitis (Figure 38.6)
Colonoscopy	May reveal IBD (Figure 38.7)

Key points in investigating red eye

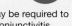

- Conjunctival swab for culture and viral PCR may be required to distinguish between bacterial, viral and allergic conjunctivitis.
- The diagnosis of scleritis and uveitis requires further work-up for associated systemic disease.
- In subconjunctival haemorrhage due to trauma, CT scan is needed to rule out a ruptured globe or retrobulbar haemorrhage.
- FBC and coagulation study should only performed if there is severe recurrent subconjunctival haemorrhage.

Clinical Investigations at a Glance, First Edition. Jonathan Gleadle, Jordan Li and Tuck Yong. © 2017 John Wiley & Sons, Ltd. Published 2017 by John Wiley & Sons, Ltd.

A red eye, a sign of ocular inflammation, is one of the commonest ophthalmological presentations. The common causes of red eye include benign conditions such as allergic conjunctivitis, subconjunctival haemorrhage and causes that can threaten vision, such as angle-closure glaucoma and uveitis (Table 38.1).

A thorough history and eye examination is the first step in the clinical evaluation of red eye. Examination should include testing visual acuity, pupillary reaction and performing fluorescein staining of the cornea. The focus is to answer the questions listed opposite to provide the clues for the underlying causes and guide further investigations and referral. Steroid eye drops should never be initiated in a patient with red eye unless in consultation with an ophthalmologist.

Conjunctivitis

The most common cause of red eye is conjunctivitis. Swabs for bacterial, viral and chlamydial culture and/or PCR should be taken in suspected cases of infectious conjunctivitis. Viral conjunctivitis usually presents with one or two red eyes, and is often associated with recent upper respiratory tract infection. If there is suspicion of herpes simplex virus involving the cornea or eyelid, corneal staining and slit lamp examination should be performed. Herpes zoster virus ophthalmicus occurs when the varicella-zoster virus is reactivated in the ophthalmic division of the trigeminal nerve. An ophthalmologist should be consulted regarding investigations and systemic or topical antiviral agents and topical steroids. Wood's lamp or slit-lamp examination (Figure 38.1) after fluorescein staining should be performed.

Bacterial conjunctivitis is usually caused by *Streptococcus pneumonia*, *Staphylococcus aureus* and *Haemophilus influenzae*. Antibiotic drops or ointment should be initiated after swab for culture. Hyperacute conjunctivitis is caused by *Neisseria gonorrhoeae* or *Chlamydia trachomatis*. Ocular chlamydial infection leads to two forms of conjunctivitis: trachoma and inclusion conjunctivitis. Inclusion conjunctivitis is a sexually transmitted disease (STD). It should be suspected if unilateral viral conjunctivitis-like symptoms last >4 weeks. A work-up for other STDs, such as syphilis and gonorrhoea, should also be performed (Chapter 116) because co-infection rate is high.

The contact lens user who has pain or red eye should remove the lens immediately. If one suspects an infectious complication, smears and cultures should be performed with urgent ophthalmology consultation. Allergic conjunctivitis is a clinical diagnosis, and further investigation is usually not required.

Subconjunctival haemorrhage is a clinical diagnosis. If there is a history of trauma, CT of the orbits should be performed to rule out a ruptured globe or retrobulbar haemorrhage. If subconjunctival haemorrhage is recurrent or there is a history of bleeding problems, such as easy bruising, a FBC and coagulation study should be performed.

Inflammatory eye disorders

Making a diagnosis of inflammatory eye disorder early in patients presenting with red eye is important because it can cause serious complications, such as impaired vision and glaucoma. Investigation into the underlying systemic causes should be performed after a definite ophthalmic diagnosis of inflammatory eye disorder has been confirmed.

Scleritis

The diagnosis of scleritis requires further investigations (Table 38.2) for associated systemic diseases, such as rheumatoid arthritis, SLE, inflammatory bowel disease (IBD), sarcoidosis and granulomatosis with polyangiitis, as 50% of the cases are associated with a systemic disorder. Approximately 10% of anterior scleritis is infectious. If suspected, serological and conjunctival scrapings for smears and cultures are required. If these tests are negative after 48 hours and the scleritis continues to progress, scleral or corneoscleral biopsy is essential. Posterior scleritis can be detected by orbital magnetic resonance imaging.

Uveitis

Uveitis is the inflammation of the iris (iritis), ciliary body (cyclitis) (Figure 38.2) and choroid (choroiditis). It can be classified as anterior uveitis, posterior uveitis and panuveitis. The diagnosis of uveitis is often confirmed by the presence of inflammatory cells and a proteinaceous flare in the anterior or posterior chambers of the eye on slit-lamp examination.

The causes of uveitis can be inflammatory, traumatic or infectious. About half of these patients have an associated systemic disease, such as ankylosing spondylitis, psoriatic arthritis, reactive arthritis or IBD. Many other systemic diseases may present with uveitis, including sarcoidosis and granulomatosis with polyangiitis. Although infection is an uncommon cause of uveitis, it is important to rule it out by specific serology testing before instituting immunosuppressive therapy. Other investigations are listed in Tables 38.2 and 38.3.

Glaucoma and other local causes of red eye

Patients with acute angle-closure glaucoma usually present with severe ocular pain, redness, a decrease in vision and nausea or vomiting. A slit-lamp examination and measurement of intraocular pressure by tonometer (Figure 38.3) are required for diagnosis. If angle-closure glaucoma is suspected, the definitive investigation involves gonioscopy, which can view the internal junction of the base of the iris with the trabecular network. A fundoscopic examination that reveals optic nerve cupping indicates the need for urgent referral and treatment. Laboratory studies are not required for most patients.

Other local causes of red eye, including ectropion, entropion, corneal ulcer, contact-lens-related red eye, corneal abrasion, corneal foreign body, penetrating and chemical trauma, scleritis and angle-closure glaucoma, should be evaluated further by an ophthalmologist.

Foreign body, trauma and others

If a foreign body is suspected, examine the surface of the eye and under lids using a slit lamp; stain with fluorescein to assess corneal and epithelial injury. Refer embedded or metallic foreign bodies to ophthalmologist.

Corneal ulceration may be caused by trauma (including foreign body), bacterial infection (often in a contact lens wearer) or herpes simplex infection and be visible after fluorescein staining.

In chemical burns, assess damage with fluorescein staining and slit-lamp examination. In trauma, consider penetrating injury, which may need a CT scan.

39 Vertigo

Table 39.1 Common causes of vertigo

Peripheral causes	Central causes	Central causes
Benign positional paroxysmal vertigo (BPPV)	Brainstem stroke or transient ischaemic attack	Cervical vertigo
Acute vestibular neuronitis (vestibular neuritis)	Multiple sclerosis	Drug-induced vertigo
Ménière's disease (endolymphatic hydrops)	Brain tumour (cerebellopontine angle tumour)	Psychological
Acute labyrinthitis	Basilar migraine	Physiologic (motion sickness)
Herpes zoster oticus (Ramsay Hunt syndrome)	Cerebellar haemorrhage	
Otosclerosis	Arnold–Chiari deformity	

Table 39.2 Distinguishing characteristics of peripheral and central vertigo

Feature	Peripheral vertigo	Central vertigo
Onset	Sudden	Subacute
Nystagmus	Combined horizontal and torsional; inhibited by fixation of eyes onto object; fades after a few days; does not change direction with gaze to either side	Purely vertical, horizontal or torsional; not inhibited by fixation of eyes onto object; may last weeks to months; may change direction with gaze towards fast phase of nystagmus
Imbalance	Mild to moderate; able to walk	Severe; unable to stand still or walk
Nausea, vomiting	Usually present	Usually absent
Hearing loss, tinnitus	Common	Rare
Brainstem or cranial nerve signs	Absent	Common
Latency following provocative diagnostic manoeuvre	Longer (up to 20 seconds)	Shorter (up to 5 seconds)

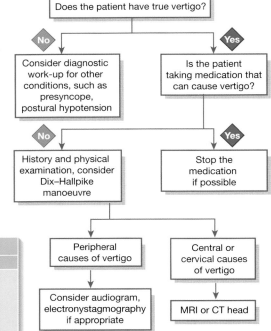

Patient presents with dizziness

↓

Does the patient have true vertigo?

No → Consider diagnostic work-up for other conditions, such as presyncope, postural hypotension

Yes → Is the patient taking medication that can cause vertigo?

No → History and physical examination, consider Dix–Hallpike manoeuvre

Yes → Stop the medication if possible

Peripheral causes of vertigo → Consider audiogram, electronystagmography if appropriate

Central or cervical causes of vertigo → MRI or CT head

Figure 39.1 Audiogram

Key points
- Laboratory tests identify the aetiology of vertigo in less than 1% of patients with dizziness.
- Radiological studies should be performed in patients with neurologic signs and symptoms, risk factors for cerebrovascular disease or progressive unilateral hearing loss.
- Audio-vestibular investigations are useful for confirming and characterising suspected vestibular dysfunction.
- An audiogram may be helpful in suggesting a labyrinthine cause of the vertigo. Low-frequency sensorineural hearing loss is seen in Ménière's syndrome.

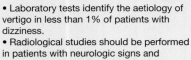
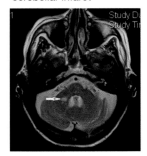

Figure 39.2 MRI shows small cerebellar infarct

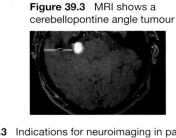
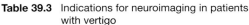

Figure 39.3 MRI shows a cerebellopontine angle tumour

Table 39.3 Indications for neuroimaging in patients with vertigo

Very sudden onset (seconds) of vertigo that persists and not provoked by position
Association with new onset of (occipital) headache
Association with hearing loss but no previous Ménière history
Associated with central neurological signs
Risk factors for cerebrovascular disease

Vertigo is a false sense of motion, either of self or of the environment, and is often of vestibular origin. It should be distinguished from dizziness, light-headedness and presyncope. The causes of vertigo include central vestibular causes (originating in the central nervous system) and peripheral vestibular causes (originating in the peripheral nervous system) (Table 39.1). Central vertigo is commonly associated with other signs of brainstem dysfunction, such as double vision, dysarthria or dysphagia. Peripheral vertigo can be associated with tinnitus or hearing loss.

Initial evaluation

The initial evaluation is to determine whether the patient has a peripheral or central cause of vertigo. Key information from the history that can be used to make this distinction includes the timing and duration of the vertigo; what provokes or aggravates it; and whether any associated symptoms exist, especially neurologic symptoms and hearing loss. Characteristics distinguishing peripheral and central vertigo are listed in Table 39.2. The Dix–Hallpike manoeuvre may be the most helpful test to perform on patients with vertigo. It has a positive predictive value of 83% and a negative predictive value of 52% for the diagnosis of benign positional paroxysmal vertigo (BPPV).

Audiogram (Figure 39.1) helps to establish the diagnosis of Ménière's disease by demonstrating a sensorineural hearing loss, usually unilateral and initially worse in the low frequencies. Vestibular function can be examined by electronystagmography, calorimetry and brainstem-evoked responses.

Laboratory tests, including electrolytes, glucose, FBC and thyroid function tests, can be performed in patients with vertigo who exhibit signs or symptoms that suggest the presence of other causative conditions. It identifies the causes in <1% of patients with vertigo.

Radiological investigations

Radiological investigations should only be considered in patients with vertigo who have neurologic signs and symptoms, risk factors for cerebrovascular disease or progressive unilateral hearing loss (Table 39.3). In general, MRI is more appropriate than CT for investigating the causes of vertigo because of its superiority in visualising the posterior fossa, where most central nervous system disease that causes vertigo is found (Figure 39.2). MRI is also useful if lesion of the cerebellopontine angle (Figure 39.3) or multiple sclerosis is suspected as a cause of vertigo. MR angiography or CT angiography of the posterior fossa vasculature may be useful in diagnosing vascular causes of vertigo, such as vertebrobasilar insufficiency, thrombosis of the labyrinthine artery, anterior or posterior inferior cerebellar artery insufficiency and subclavian steal syndrome.

Radiological investigations can be used to rule out tumours or developmental abnormalities. However, they are not indicated in patients who have BPPV or vestibular neuronitis. Radiological imaging may aid in the diagnosis of cervical vertigo (i.e. vertigo triggered by somatosensory input from head and neck movements) in patients with a history suggestive of this diagnosis; however, other conditions should be excluded before considering this diagnosis.

41 Haematuria

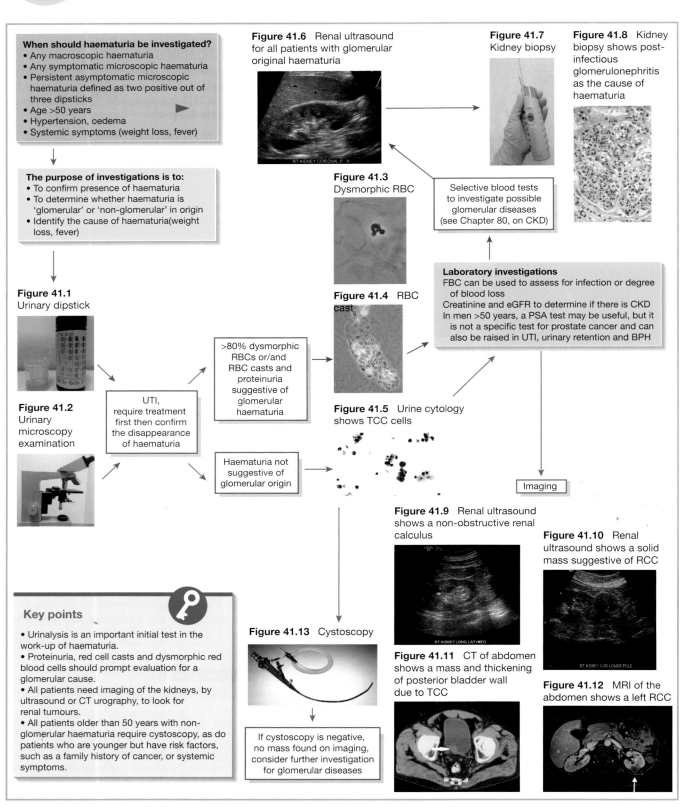

When should haematuria be investigated?
- Any macroscopic haematuria
- Any symptomatic microscopic haematuria
- Persistent asymptomatic microscopic haematuria defined as two positive out of three dipsticks
- Age >50 years
- Hypertension, oedema
- Systemic symptoms (weight loss, fever)

The purpose of investigations is to:
- To confirm presence of haematuria
- To determine whether haematuria is 'glomerular' or 'non-glomerular' in origin
- Identify the cause of haematuria(weight loss, fever)

Figure 41.1 Urinary dipstick

Figure 41.2 Urinary microscopy examination

UTI, require treatment first then confirm the disappearance of haematuria

>80% dysmorphic RBCs or/and RBC casts and proteinuria suggestive of glomerular haematuria

Haematuria not suggestive of glomerular origin

Figure 41.6 Renal ultrasound for all patients with glomerular original haematuria

Figure 41.3 Dysmorphic RBC

Figure 41.4 RBC cast

Figure 41.5 Urine cytology shows TCC cells

Selective blood tests to investigate possible glomerular diseases (see Chapter 80, on CKD)

Laboratory investigations
FBC can be used to assess for infection or degree of blood loss
Creatinine and eGFR to determine if there is CKD
In men >50 years, a PSA test may be useful, but it is not a specific test for prostate cancer and can also be raised in UTI, urinary retention and BPH

Figure 41.7 Kidney biopsy

Figure 41.8 Kidney biopsy shows post-infectious glomerulonephritis as the cause of haematuria

Imaging

Figure 41.9 Renal ultrasound shows a non-obstructive renal calculus

Figure 41.10 Renal ultrasound shows a solid mass suggestive of RCC

Figure 41.11 CT of abdomen shows a mass and thickening of posterior bladder wall due to TCC

Figure 41.12 MRI of the abdomen shows a left RCC

Figure 41.13 Cystoscopy

If cystoscopy is negative, no mass found on imaging, consider further investigation for glomerular diseases

Key points
- Urinalysis is an important initial test in the work-up of haematuria.
- Proteinuria, red cell casts and dysmorphic red blood cells should prompt evaluation for a glomerular cause.
- All patients need imaging of the kidneys, by ultrasound or CT urography, to look for renal tumours.
- All patients older than 50 years with non-glomerular haematuria require cystoscopy, as do patients who are younger but have risk factors, such as a family history of cancer, or systemic symptoms.

Haematuria is the presence of an abnormally high number of red blood cells (RBCs) in the urine and can be classified as macroscopic haematuria ('gross or visible haematuria') and microscopic haematuria, which can only be detected by urine dipstick or under microscopy. Haematuria can be symptomatic or asymptomatic. Macroscopic haematuria has a high diagnostic yield for urological malignancy. About 79–90% of patients with bladder tumours present with haematuria, and 30% of patients with painless haematuria are found to have a malignancy. The common causes of haematuria can be divided into nephrological and urological causes.

If there is current menstruation, a repeat sample at a later date is appropriate. Painful haematuria indicates the presence of UTI, stones, ureteric blood clot or renal infarction. Painless haematuria usually indicates urinary tract malignancy or glomerular diseases.

Urinalysis

Urine dipstick of a fresh voided urine sample has a sensitivity of 90–100% and specificity of 85–90% in detecting haematuria (Figure 41.1). Significant haematuria is considered to be 1+ or greater. Trace haematuria should be considered negative. The dipstick is sensitive to 1–2 RBCs/high-power field (hpf) and may therefore overdiagnose haematuria. If a urine dipstick is positive for blood, the urine specimen should be sent for formal microscopic evaluation. Symptom-free patients with dipstick haematuria without microscopic haematuria do not need urologic evaluation.

The dipstick relies on haemoglobin to catalyse the oxidation of a chromagen by organic hydrogen peroxide. However, myoglobin, bacterial peroxidase, povidone and hypochlorite can also catalyse this reaction, leading to false positives. Urine dipstick checking blood and protein is often part of routine life insurance and employment medical examinations. The presence of haematuria should not be attributed to anticoagulant or antiplatelet therapy, and patients should be evaluated regardless of these medications. Exercise-induced haematuria or rarely myoglobinuria should be excluded.

Urine microscopy and culture

UTI is one of the most common causes of haematuria and should be excluded by urine culture before further investigations of haematuria. A dipstick should be repeated 6 weeks post-treatment to confirm the post-treatment absence of haematuria.

Microscopic haematuria is defined as ≥3 RBCs/hpf in the sediment of a spun specimen. It is very prevalent, occurring in up to 5% of adults on a single test. Red cell morphology and casts (Figures 41.2 to 41.4) can be useful in determining if the haematuria is glomerular in origin. The specimen must be examined within 3 hours by phase-contrast microscopy. If microscopic haematuria is predominantly glomerular in origin (>80% of RBCs appear dysmorphic or/and presence of RBC casts or/and presence of proteinuria), the source of the haematuria is highly likely to be in the renal parenchyma and the risk of urinary tract cancer is minimal. In this situation there is generally no need for detailed imaging except renal ultrasound and urological investigation unless the risk profile of the patient is high for urinary tract cancer. If the haematuria is non-glomerular in origin, not associated with proteinuria or normal kidney function, it is essential to investigate for a structural lesion with imaging and cystoscopy as urothelial cancer is the main consideration.

Urine protein measurement

Measuring proteinuria by protein:creatinine ratio or albumin:creatinine ratio is helpful to determine whether the haematuria has a glomerular or non-glomerular cause.

Urine cytology

The yield from urine cytology varies with grade of tumour, number of samples examined and experience of the cytopathologist. The sensitivity of urine cytology in high-grade transitional cell carcinoma (TCC) varies from 40% to 76%, and for low-grade TCC is as low as 15–25% (Figure 41.5). A negative result from three consecutive, daily, early morning urine specimens can be used for patients at low risk of TCC, as an alternative to cystoscopy. Any positive cytological finding indicates the need to proceed to cystoscopy.

Ultrasound

All patients with persistent microscopic haematuria or macroscopic haematuria should have an ultrasound to exclude kidney and bladder pathology (Figure 41.6). Ultrasound is used to characterise renal mass/tumours, cystic lesions and the pelvicalyceal system. It can detect hydronephrosis, renal calculi and moderately large bladder lesions. It also allows for an assessment of the prostate gland and the effects of bladder emptying. Compared with CT, ultrasound has a lower diagnostic yield and is less sensitive for ureteric and bladder tumours.

CT urogram

CT urogram is the preferred modality of imaging for detecting genitourinary malignancy, stones and other disease (Figure 41.11). It has a sensitivity of 94–100% and specificity of 97% for detecting pathology in patients with haematuria. Spiral CT (with or without contrast), particularly with thin slices, has superseded both intravenous pyelography and ultrasonography in detecting urothelial cancer especially small tumours (<3 cm). If stone disease is suspected, spiral CT should initially be performed without contrast. If negative, a CT with contrast should follow to provide full information about lesions and cysts. In patients allergic to contrast, ultrasound followed by cystoscopy and retrograde pyelogram can provide equivalent diagnostic information gained from a CT with contrast.

MRI

MRI urography is as accurate as CT for diagnosing many urologic conditions, so it can be performed in lieu of a CT urogram in patients with iodine allergy, or any reason to avoid ionising radiation (Figure 41.12).

Cystoscopy

If diagnostic imaging is negative, cystoscopy is recommended for patients aged over 50, in whom the risk of bladder cancer is increased. Under 50 the diagnostic yield from cystoscopy is very low. Cystoscopy should be performed at any age if there are risk factors for TCC. Cystoscopy visualises the entire bladder and is an effective way to diagnose urethral and bladder pathology (Figure 41.13). Flexible cystoscopy can be performed under local anaesthetic and tissue can be biopsied.

42 Attempted suicide and self-poisoning

Table 42.2

Compounds commonly causing poisoning

• Carbon monoxide	• Ethylene glycol	• Mushrooms:
• Organophosphates	• Methanol	*Amanita*
• Cyanide	• Metals	*phalloides*
• Digoxin	Lithium	• Paracetamol
• Carbamazepine	Iron	• Paraquat
• Sodium valproate	Lead	• Salicylates
• Antidepressants	Mercury	• Benzodiazepine
		• NSAIDs

Table 42.3

Examples of drugs that can be measured quantitatively in the blood

- Paracetamol
- Salicylates
- Anticonvulsants
- Digoxin
- Carbon monoxide
- Toxic alcohols
- Methaemoglobin

Key points

- An ECG should be obtained in patients who have ingested cardiotoxic medications (e.g. antidepressants, digoxin, calcium channel blockers, beta blockers, antiarrhythmics). Cardiac monitoring should be continued if any abnormalities are seen.
- Drug screening has limited value because in most cases of toxic ingestion care is supportive and not affected by identification of the drug.
- Urine drug screens typically test for substance abuse (e.g. amphetamines, cocaine, marijuana, opioids, phencyclidine, and benzodiazepine).

Figure 42.1 History from family or witnesses including the nature of the poisonous substance, the degree of exposure and the time since exposure is essential

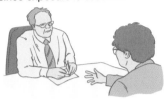

Figure 42.2 Records of prescribed medications are helpful

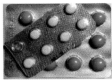

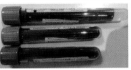

Figure 42.3 ECG showing prolonged QT interval

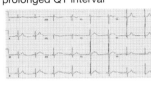

Figure 42.4 Urine analysis

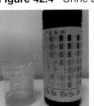

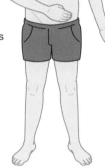

Electrolytes, FBC
Creatinine
LFTs
Glucose
Coagulation study
Urine β-HCG
CK
ABG
Serum osmolarity
Paracetamol level
Specific drug levels
  (e.g. salicylates,
  iron, digoxin,
  anticonvulsants,
  alcohol)
Urine drug screen
Urinalysis

Figure 42.5 Urine microscopy showing calcium oxalate crystals which may indicate ethylene glycol poisoning

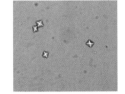

Figure 42.6 Rumack–Matthew nomogram is used for predicting hepatotoxicity and guiding the need for antidote treatment of paracetamol overdose

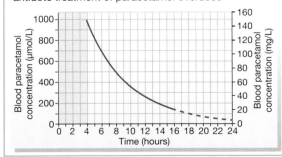

Attempted suicide

Self-harm refers to episodes of self-inflicted harm regardless of lethal intent. Attempted suicide is an episode where there was at least some suicidal intent. The major risk factors for attempted suicide are summarised in Table 42.1. However, demographic risk factors are poor predictors of an individual's suicide risk. It is important to carefully enquire about each individual's current suicidality.

In evaluating a suicidal patient, a thorough examination of past psychiatric history is important. Assessment of suicide risk is paramount for all patients presenting with possible suicide attempts, self-harm or depressive symptoms, regardless of overt suicidal statements. (For a detailed guide to assessment of suicide risk, see Gleadle, 2012: chapter 60.) Although patients will often detail the specific ingestion, at times a patient will be unwilling or unable to acknowledge ingestion of toxic substances. A high index of suspicion should remain for potential co-ingestion of multiple substances. Poisoning remains the most common method of suicide, especially among women.

It is recommended that basic laboratory tests should be performed in a patient presenting with attempted suicide, including:

- FBC;
- urinalysis and pregnancy test (if indicated);
- electrolytes, creatinine, glucose, LFTs;
- drug (paracetamol, aspirin) and alcohol levels;
- urine toxicology screen for drugs of abuse;
- ECG;
- pulse oximetry and arterial blood gases (ABGs) if any alteration in conscious level or respiratory signs or symptoms.

Acute poisoning

Poisoning is a common cause of morbidity and mortality, and acute medication poisonings account for nearly one-half of all poisonings in developed countries. The types of poisoning include:

- intentional – self-harm, attempted suicide, substance abuse;
- accidental – medication error, dosage error, recreational use;
- environmental – plants, food, venomous stings, occupational exposures.

Clinical evaluation

Acute poisoning requires urgent investigation, accurate diagnosis and prompt treatment. All patients must be initially stabilised using the ABCD Adult Basic Life Support guideline. History from patients or witnesses, including the nature of the poisonous substance, the degree of exposure and the time since exposure, is essential. Attempts should be made to identify the specific poison (Table 42.2) as soon as possible, but this should not delay life-saving supportive care. Any patient with suspected poisoning should be admitted for observation. Patients with intentional self-poisoning should undergo a full psychiatric evaluation and risk assessment for further attempted suicide before discharge.

Blood or urine toxicology

Blood or urine toxicological analysis is used to confirm the diagnosis of poisoning, to determine and monitor treatment, to establish the time to restart chronic drug therapy or for medico-legal purposes.

The majority of toxicology-related diagnoses and therapeutic decisions are made from the history or clinical examination. Toxicology analytical tests are limited by a prolonged turnaround time and high cost. Furthermore, the cut-off levels of toxicity have not been determined for many toxins, making the interpretation of tests difficult. The timing of specimen collection is also important. If collected too early or too late the results may have little clinical correlation. If doubt exists about the need for a toxicology test, a sample of blood and urine should be taken and stored for subsequent analysis. The use of quantitative blood tests should be limited to those drugs and toxins where the specific blood level will either predict toxicity or guide specific therapy (Table 42.3).

A serum paracetamol level is recommended for ingestions of an unknown drug because paracetamol is a common drug ingested in self-poisoning, is often compounded with other drugs, has delayed signs and symptoms of toxicity, and levels guide specific treatment. The presence of calcium oxalate crystals in the urine microscopy examination may indicate ethylene glycol poisoning. Qualitative urine toxicology screening tests are available for 'drugs of abuse', and the range of drugs tested for depends on individual laboratories. A negative screening test does not imply that poisoning has not occurred, but only that the compounds tested for are not implicated in the poisoning.

Other laboratory investigations

Basic laboratory investigations, including glucose, serum electrolytes, creatinine, LFTs and ABGs are often helpful for diagnostic purposes. An ECG should be performed if the patient is hypotensive, has an arrhythmia or underlying heart disease or is suspected of taking a proarrhythmic agent. A CXR is needed if aspiration is suspected. Serious poisonings are often characterised by hypoglycaemia, acid–base and electrolyte disturbances, liver and renal impairment, and respiratory failure.

Paracetamol overdose

Paracetamol is one of the most common medicinal poisonings. The key factors to consider are the dose and concentration (early), clinical and laboratory features suggesting liver injury (late) and any history suggesting increased susceptibility to toxicity. Serum paracetamol levels can guide the need for N-acetylcysteine administration in all patients with deliberate paracetamol poisoning, regardless of the stated dose of ingestion.

The best surrogate marker for injury is a timed serum paracetamol level plotted on a nomogram (e.g. Rumack–Matthew, Figure 42.6). However the nomogram cannot be applied to repeated or staggered doses, or if the time of ingestion cannot be determined with confidence. The nomogram can be used for predicting hepatotoxicity and serves as a guide to whether antidote is necessary. Interpretation of the nomogram is meaningless in chronic ingestions or for blood levels drawn <4 h or >24 h post-ingestion. Patients that are malnourished or have induced cytochrome P450 enzymes (e.g. alcoholics or those taking enzyme-inducing drugs concurrently) are at higher risk for hepatotoxicity and the lower 'high-risk' treatment line should be used as the guide to the necessity for antidote.

Serum creatinine, LFTs and coagulation study should be performed regularly to monitor for evidence of liver and renal failure, which may not be apparent for up to 24 h after acute paracetamol ingestion.

43 Immunosuppressed patients

Table 43.1 Suggested tests for monitoring immunosuppressive drugs treatment

Immunosuppressive drugs	Full blood count	Electrolytes, creatinine, fasting blood sugar level	Liver function tests	Lipid profile	Other tests
Corticosteroids	3-monthly	3-monthly	3-monthly	6-monthly	Eye review if symptomatic, bone density 2-yearly
Azathioprine	Monthly for first 3 months, then 3-monthly	3-monthly	Monthly for first 3 months, then 3-monthly	6-monthly	Consider thiopurine methyltransferase test before commencement
Mycophenolate	Monthly for first 3 months, then 3-monthly	Monthly for first 3 months then 3-monthly	Monthly for first 3 months, then 3-monthly	Not required	Annual skin check
Cyclosporin/tacrolimus	Monthly for first 3 months, then 3-monthly	Weekly for 4 weeks, then monthly for 3 months, then 3-monthly	Monthly for first 3 months, then 3-monthly	6-monthly	Annual skin check
Sirolimus	Initially weekly for 4 weeks, then monthly for 3 months, then 3-monthly	Monthly for first 3 months, then 3-monthly	Monthly for first 3 months, then 3-monthly	6-monthly	Urine protein ACR (albumin : creatinine ratio) monthly for 3 months, then 3-monthly
Methotrexate	Monthly initially, then 3 monthly	Monthly initially, then 3-monthly	3-monthly	12-monthly	Calculate cumulated dose
Cyclophosphamide	Weekly initially for 4 weeks, then monthly	Monthly	Monthly	12-monthly	Urinalysis 6-monthly

Table 43.2 Tests to be considered in suspected infection in the immunocompromised patient

Organisms	Test
Cryptococcus	Cryptococcal antigen test
CMV, EBV, HSV, VZV	Quantitative PCR for DNA
HIV	Reverse transcriptase PCR for RNA
Histoplasma capsulatum	Mycelial phase antigen
Legionella pneumophilia	Urinary antigen test
Pneumocystis jirovecii	Sputum, bronchoalveolar lavage silver-based stains or PCR; transbronchial biopsy may detect the organism
Tuberculosis	See Chapter 117
Clostridium difficile	*C. difficile* toxin

Table 43.4 Common qualitative markers of immunosuppression

Absolute neutrophil count
Total lymphocyte count
B-lymphocyte quantity and subsets
T helper cell or CD4 and CD8 cell count
Serum immunoglobulins – total and subgroups
Quantification of individual complement components
Functional assays of the classical and alternative complement pathway
Delayed hypersensitivity skin test

Table 43.3 Time line for infection in solid organ transplantation

Time line	Common infection	Examples
First 2 months post-transplant	Common infections post-surgery	Wound infections Pneumonias Urinary tract infections Catheter related infections Infected drainage tubes Infection from the donor organ (rare)
2–12 months post-transplant	Opportunistic infections as a consequence of immunosuppressive therapy	CMV *P. jirovecii* *Aspergillus* spp. *Nocardia* *Mycobacterium tuberculosis* Other viral infections: BK virus, EBV, hepatitis B and C, human herpes virus 6 and 7
12 months post-transplant	Majority are free from infection; those with rejection and on higher levels of immuno-suppression continue to be at high risk of infection	PTLD related to EBV Reinfecting hepatitis B in liver graft, a combination of pooled human hepatitis B immunoglobulin and the antiviral agent lamivudine is used to prevent reinfection. Lifelong monitoring and therapy are required

The purposes of investigation in immunocompromised patients:
- Recognise the immunocompromised patient
- To monitor during treatment with immunosuppressive drugs
- To diagnose infection and identify the pathogens as early as possible
- To diagnose malignancy as early as possible

Key points

- Blood cultures from peripheral sites and from an access device (if present) are mandatory in immunocompromised patients with suspected infection.
- Radiological investigations can assist in identification of infection site. Culture and biopsy of affected body fluid or tissue should be obtained.
- Annual examination of the skin and lip by a dermatologist (more frequently in high-risk patients, such as patients with a history of skin cancer) is recommended.
- Screen for cervical cancer given the high risk and aggressive nature of this disease in immunocompromised patients.

Clinical Investigations at a Glance, First Edition. Jonathan Gleadle, Jordan Li and Tuck Yong. © 2017 John Wiley & Sons, Ltd. Published 2017 by John Wiley & Sons, Ltd.

An immunosuppressed patient has an alteration in phagocytic, cellular or humoral immunity that increases the risk of infection, lymphoproliferative disorder or cancer. This chapter will focus on patients who are immunocompromised because of cancer or its treatment, transplantation of bone marrow or solid organs, taking immunosuppressants for autoimmune diseases and patients who have had a splenectomy.

Monitoring during treatment with immunosuppressive drugs

The number of patients taking immunosuppressive drugs for treatment of autoimmune disease and prevention of rejection in solid organ transplant (SOT) is increasing. Drugs that suppress the immune system are inevitably associated with increased risk of infection and malignancy. Table 43.1 shows a suggested frequency of monitoring for stable patients who are on immunosuppressive drugs. Patients with WBCs $<3.5 \times 10^9$ cells/L, or neutrophils $<2 \times 10^9$ cells/L or platelets $<150 \times 10^9$ cells/L should have repeat testing within 7 days. Immunosuppressive drugs may need to be suspended if there is significant neutropenia ($<1.5 \times 10^9$ cells/L).

In cancer chemotherapy, cytotoxic drug regimens cause cytopenia as a result of marrow toxicity. Neutropenia is the main predictor of infection (see Chapter 111).

Humanised monoclonal antibodies are increasingly used in SOT. These drugs are often used at the initiation of immunosuppression or as rescue treatment for acute rejection. They have the potential to induce profound T cell depletion, and the risks of subsequent infection are high. Monoclonal antibodies are also widely used in autoimmune disease, such as rheumatoid arthritis, ankylosing spondylitis, inflammatory bowel disease and haematological malignancy. Anti-tumour necrosis factor drugs have shown an increase in opportunistic infections, especially reactivation of tuberculosis and in the incidence of haematological malignancy.

Infections in immunosuppressed patients

Infection is the major cause of morbidity and mortality in immunosuppressed patients. Patients may be infected by common community-acquired and/or opportunistic organisms. The risk of infection increases with the degree of immunosuppression.

Laboratory investigations

A FBC is mandatory in the initial investigation, and attention should be given to the WBC and neutrophil count. Coagulation studies, biochemistry, creatinine and LFTs should be examined. Deranged liver markers may be present with disseminated viral infections. CRP is a non-specific marker of inflammation/infection.

Microbiology investigations

The spectrum of organisms responsible for infection in immunosuppressed patients is wide because virtually any organism can become invasive and multiple organisms may emerge during a single febrile episode, especially when immunosuppression is severe and prolonged (Table 43.2). Attention should be directed to the most common sites of infection, including the respiratory tract, lungs, urinary tract, oral cavity, gastrointestinal tract (including the perianal area), skin and soft tissues.

Sending adequate and appropriate samples to the microbiology laboratory is the cornerstone of investigation in suspected infection in the immunocompromised patient. Common microbiological specimens include blood, urine, sputum, and CSF, which can be immediately examined using Gram staining. More importantly, samples should be cultured and antimicrobial sensitivity checked using a range of growth media.

In transplant recipients, cytomegalovirus (CMV), herpes simplex virus (HSV) and varicella zoster virus (VZV) PCR assays are indicated as part of the work-up for a patient presenting with fever with no clear site of infection (Table 43.3). Serostatus mismatch, where the donor is sero-positive for CMV but the recipient is serologically negative, confers a higher risk of CMV disease. CSF analysis is indicated in patients with symptoms of meningism or suspected of CNS infection, especially for those who are asplenic or had a previous splenectomy.

Radiological investigations

Imaging may identify a source of infection; it does not contribute to the identification of the pathogen but can direct further microbiological sampling.

CXR may reveal atypical pneumonia, tuberculosis or bronchiectasis that is associated with ongoing immunosuppression.

Ultrasound may be useful for identifying and draining fluid-filled lesions.

CT of the chest can help in the diagnosis of suspected invasive fungal infection. CT of other areas (e.g. nasal sinuses, abdomen) should be considered.

MRI is indicated to evaluate suspected sinusitis, hepatosplenic candidiasis, liver abscess and infections in the brain, such as toxoplasmosis and viral encephalitis.

Infections following splenectomy

Patients following splenectomy have a life-long increased susceptibility to certain infections, particularly those caused by encapsulated bacteria (*Neisseria meningitidis*, *Streptococcus pneumoniae* and *Haemophilus influenzae*). Patients who undergo elective splenectomy should be immunised against these organisms prior to operation. Patients may need life-long prophylaxis with penicillin.

Malignancy in immunosuppressed patients

The incidence and risk of malignancy, especially cutaneous and haematological malignancies, is increased in immunosuppressed patients compared with the general population. The length of exposure to immunosuppressive therapy and the intensity of therapy (Table 43.4) are clearly related to the risk of malignancy; and once malignancy has developed, taking immunosuppression can translate into more aggressive tumour progression, metastasis and lower patient survival. The most common malignancies encountered in the post-SOT are non-melanoma skin cancers, post-transplant lymphoproliferative disorders (PTLDs) and Kaposi's sarcoma. The pathogenesis of these tumours is likely related to immunosuppressive drugs and subsequent viral infection.

Patients taking immunosuppressive drugs should have yearly skin checks and be up to date with the normal recommended cancer screening programs, such as faecal occult blood test over 50 years of age, cervical smears, PSA and mammography. Currently, there is no evidence to support increased frequency of screening.

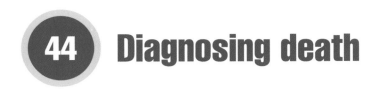

44 Diagnosing death

Box 44.1 Essential components for diagnosing brain death

History or physical examination findings provide a clear aetiology of an irreversible loss of consciousness combined with the irreversible loss of the capacity to breathe.

Exclusion of reversible conditions causing a state of apnoeic coma or capable of mimicking or confounding the diagnosis of brain death:
- shock/hypotension;
- hypothermia – temperature <32 °C;
- drugs known to alter neurologic, neuromuscular function and electroencephalographic testing, like anaesthetic agents, neuroparalytic drugs, benzodiazepines and alcohols;
- brainstem encephalitis;
- encephalopathy associated with hepatic failure, uraemia and hyperosmolar coma.

Full clinical examination of the patient, which demonstrates profound coma, apnoea and absent brainstem reflexes (Table 44.1).

Table 44.1 Full clinical examination for diagnosing brain death

Absence of spontaneous movement, decerebrate or decorticate posturing, seizures, and response to noxious stimuli administered through a cranial nerve pathway
Absent pupillary reflex to direct and consensual light
Absent corneal, oculocephalic, cough and gag reflexes
Absent oculovestibular reflex
Absent pharyngeal and tracheal reflexes
Absent of respiratory efforts in the presence of hypercarbia
Conduct the apnoea test; a positive test supports the diagnosis of brain death

Key points

The diagnosis of brain death requires:
- Unresponsive coma
- Absence of brainstem reflexes
- Absence of respiratory centre function
- The clinical setting in which these findings are irreversible.

Table 44.2 Confirmatory investigations sometimes used in assisting in the diagnosis of brain death

Confirmatory test	Description	Advantages	Disadvantages
Loss of electrical activity			
EEG	16-channel EEG recordings over 30 minutes	Portable	Artefacts from other sources Limited use in setting of sedation Cortical activity rather than deep cerebral activity
Evoked potentials	Visual, auditory, somatosensory and multimodal	Portable Less resistant to sedation compared with EEG	Restricted availability Complex interpretation Testing of isolated neural tracts
Cessation of cerebral circulation			
Four-vessel intra-arterial catheter angiography	Direct injection of contrast into both carotid arteries and both vertebral arteries	Direct visualisation of cerebral blood flow Current gold standard	Invasive Not portable Risk of complications
CT angiography	CT indicators include: absent enhancement bilaterally of the middle cerebral artery cortical branches, P2 segment of the posterior cerebral arteries, and internal cerebral veins; in the presence of contrast enhancement of external carotid arteries	Readily available Rapid acquisition Growing literature base Can be combined with perfusion studies	Not portable
MR angiography	MRI with contrast enhanced angiography	Can be combined with perfusion studies	Not practical because of magnet incompatibility with lines, ventilator tubing and other hardware
Single-photon emission CT	Imaging of brain tissue perfusion using a tracer isotope (e.g. 99mTc-HMPAO)	Images brain perfusion Quantitative	Restricted availability
PET scan	Imaging of brain with biologically active positron-emitting nuclides (e.g. 18F-fluorodeoxyglucose)	Can assess brain metabolism	Not portable Restricted availability

Clinical Investigations at a Glance, First Edition. Jonathan Gleadle, Jordan Li and Tuck Yong. © 2017 John Wiley & Sons, Ltd. Published 2017 by John Wiley & Sons, Ltd.

The diagnosis, confirmation and certification of death are usually the legal responsibility of medical practitioners. The diagnosis of death is often obvious. The body is cool, motionless and pale. In establishing the diagnosis of death an understanding of the recent history is important. For example, patients who are profoundly hypothermic may appear dead but in fact may be capable of resuscitation. It is vital to **establish with certainty the identity of the body**. Death is defined as the irreversible loss of those essential characteristics necessary to the existence of a living person and include the irreversible loss of the capacity for consciousness, combined with irreversible loss of the capacity to breathe. These two essential capacities are found in the brain, particularly the brainstem. Dying is a process, which affects different functions and cells of the body at different rates. Medical practitioners must decide at what moment along this process there is permanence and death can be appropriately declared. Death can be diagnosed using three different sets of criteria: circulatory, somatic and neurological.

Diagnosis and confirmation of death using somatic criteria

Somatic criteria for death are those that can be applied by simple external inspection of a body without a requirement to examine for signs of life or evidence of internal organ function. The criteria include signs such as rigor mortis, decapitation and decomposition. Somatic criteria unequivocally indicate irreversible loss of consciousness and irreversible apnoea.

Diagnosis and confirmation of death using circulatory criteria

For people suffering cardiorespiratory arrest (including failed resuscitation), death can be diagnosed when a registered medical practitioner or other appropriately trained and qualified individual confirms the irreversible cessation of neurological (pupillary), cardiac and respiratory activity. Diagnosing death in this situation requires confirmation that there has been irreversible damage to the vital centres in the brainstem, due to the length of time in which the circulation to the brain has been absent.

The simultaneous onset of circulatory arrest, unconsciousness and apnoea (cardiorespiratory arrest) has long been used as a basis for diagnosing death, both in the hospital and in the community. Within 15 seconds of cessation of cerebral circulation, consciousness is lost and the brain suffers irreversible anoxic structural damage; the EEG becomes iso-electric and apnoea rapidly ensues, if not already present. Circulatory criteria to diagnose death predict the permanent and irreversible loss of the capacity for consciousness and the capacity to breathe.

The observation period begins at the time of loss of the circulation, in association with coma and apnoea; the minimum acceptable duration of observation depends on the criterion used for diagnosing death. It is important to note that palpation of the pulse may be insufficient to ensure circulatory arrest as low output circulatory states can persist even when the pulse is impalpable. If it is in doubt or where the technology is readily available, intra-arterial pressure monitoring or electrocardiogram can be used to confirm circulatory arrest.

Diagnosis and confirmation of death using neurological criteria

Death by neurological criteria or brain death is defined as the irreversible loss of all functions of the brain, including the brainstem, whether induced by intra-cranial events or the result of extra-cranial events such as hypoxia while the cardio-respiratory activity is being maintained by continued mechanical ventilation. The three essential findings in brain death are coma, absence of brainstem reflexes, and apnoea. An evaluation for brain death should be considered in patients who have suffered a massive, irreversible brain injury of identifiable cause. A patient determined to be brain dead is legally and clinically dead.

The diagnosis of brain death is primarily clinical. Different countries may have different legal definitions of what constitutes brain death and how the tests should be undertaken. There are three essential components for diagnosing brain death (Box 44.1).

Clinical tests for diagnosing brain death should be carried out by two fully registered doctors who are competent with the procedures; one of these should be a senior doctor. The tests must be carried out on two occasions, separated by a period of time. No other tests are required if the full clinical examination of the patient, which demonstrates profound coma, apnoea and absent brainstem reflexes, including each of two assessments of brainstem reflexes and a single apnoea test, are conclusive.

Confirmatory investigations (Table 44.2) are not routinely required for the diagnosis of brain death. They should be performed when it is not possible to fully satisfy the stated three essential components for the diagnosis of brain death:
- a primary metabolic or pharmacological cause cannot be ruled out;
- in cases of high cervical cord injury preventing the formal assessment of the irreversible loss of the capacity to breathe secondary to functional and structural damage to the brainstem;
- a full neurological examination of the brainstem reflexes is impossible due to extensive facial injuries.

Any investigation should always be considered as additional to a full clinical assessment of the patient. The potential for error and misinterpretation with confirmatory investigations should be considered and local availability and familiarity with the tests used to guide request.

Brain death confirmed by documenting the absence of electrical activity during at least 30 minutes of EEG recording that adheres to the minimal technical criteria for EEG recording in suspected brain death has been adopted by the American Electroencephalographic Society. The intensive care unit setting may result in false readings due to electronic background noise creating innumerable artefacts. Furthermore, EEG cannot rule out a metabolic or pharmacological factor as potential causes.

No clinical or imaging tests can establish that every brain cell has died. If clinical testing cannot be relied upon because the above conditions are not all met, absence of intracranial blood flow is diagnostic. Four-vessel angiography and radionuclide imaging are the preferred imaging techniques for assessing intracranial blood flow.

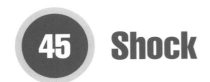

Shock

Table 45.1 Type of shock

Type of shock	Physiology	CVP	PAOP	CO
Hypovolaemic	Decreased circulatory volume	↓	↓	↓
Cardiogenic	Impaired cardiac pump function			
Left ventricular		↔	↑	↓
Right ventricular		↑	↔/↓	↓
Distributive	Pathologic peripheral blood vessel vasodilation			
Septic		↔	↔	↑
Anaphylactic		↓	↓	↔/↑
Neurogenic		↓	↓	↔
Obstructive	Non-cardiac obstruction to blood flow	↑	↑	↓
Pulmonary embolus		↑	↓	↓
Tension pneumothorax		↑	↑	↓
Tamponade		↑	↑	↓

Table 45.2 Basic investigation for shock

Tests	Purpose of the tests
FBC	Determine anaemia/blood loss, leucocytosis or leukopenia in infection, thrombocytopenia in infection or DIC
Coagulation study or extended coagulation study	Assess coagulopathy, recognise early DIC
Serum electrolyte	Determine electrolyte disturbance
Serum creatinine, urea	Assess renal function
LFTs	Assess liver failure
Lactate	Gauge the degree of hypoperfusion
Urine analysis	Exclude urosepsis
Urine pregnancy test	Exclude pregnancy
ABG	Assess oxygenation, acidosis, consider ARDS
ECG	Exclude cardiac arrhythmia/ischaemia
CXR	Exclude chest infection, CCF, ARDS

Table 45.3 Causes of hypovolaemic shock and tests

Haemorrhagic	
Bleeding from wounds	Physical examination
Bleeding from blunt traumatic injuries (haemothorax, lacerated liver, spleen or kidney, fracture)	Abdominal and/or chest CT, USS for haematoma
Bleeding from GI tract	Endoscopy, see Chapter 20
Bleeding from rupture AAA, retroperitoneal, ectopic pregnancy	CT abdominal/chest, pelvic USS

Non-haemorrhagic	
Severe diarrhoea	Faecal MCS and CD toxin
Severe, protracted vomiting	AXR, abdominal CT
Fluid loss to third space, pancreatitis, bowel obstruction, peritonitis	See Chapters 14, 70 and 78
Severe burn	Clinical assessment
Excessive nasogastric, fistula or enterostomy losses	Electrolyte, renal function Clinical assessment
Renal loss, diabetes mellitus or insipidus, Addison disease	Blood glucose level, serum cortisol levels

The purpose of investigations in patients with shock is to:
- Recognise shock early
- Assess the severity of shock
- Identify the cause of shock
- Assess end organ damage caused by shock
- Guide immediate management to stabilise the patient

Table 45.4 Causes of cardiogenic shock

Acute myocardial infarction (AMI)
Cardiomyopathy
Ventricular outflow obstruction (aortic stenosis or dissection)
Ventricular filling anomalies (atrial myxoma, mitral stenosis)
Acute valvular failure (aortic or mitral regurgitation), ventriculoseptal defects
Cardiac dysrhythmias
Cardiac bypass surgery
Cardiac trauma
Myocarditis

Table 45.5 Clinical features of SIRS

1. Body temperature >38 °C or <36 °C
2. Heart rate >90 beats/min
3. Respiratory rate >20 breaths/min or $PaCO_2$ of <32 mmHg
4. WBC count >12.0 ×10⁹/L or <4.0 ×10⁹/L or the presence of >10% immature neutrophils

Key points

- Arterial blood gases and lactate are measured to assess the severity of shock. Laboratory findings that support the diagnosis of shock include lactate >3 mmol/L, base deficit less than −4 mmol/L, and $PaCO_2$ <32 mmHg. However, none of these findings alone is diagnostic.
- In patient with suspected septic shock, the key is to do urine, blood culture and culture other suspect body fluids such as CSF, joint, pleural, and peritoneal fluids. In patients with a suspected surgical or occult cause of sepsis, ultrasonography, CT, or MRI may be required.
- If DIC is suspected, fibrin degradation products, D-dimer and fibrinogen levels should be measured.
- Echocardiography should be performed immediately to establish the cause of cardiogenic shock.

Clinical Investigations at a Glance, First Edition. Jonathan Gleadle, Jordan Li and Tuck Yong. © 2017 John Wiley & Sons, Ltd. Published 2017 by John Wiley & Sons, Ltd.

Shock is a clinical syndrome resulting in inadequate tissue perfusion and cellular oxygenation affecting multiple organ systems. Perfusion may be decreased systemically (as in hypotension) or limited to regional maldistribution (as in septic shock, where global perfusion is normal or even elevated). Decreased organ perfusion leads to tissue hypoxia, anaerobic metabolism, activation of an inflammatory cascade and eventual vital organ dysfunction. Clinically, it is characterised by hypotension (systolic blood pressure <90 mmHg or a mean arterial pressure <60 mmHg or reduced by >30%, for at least 30 minutes), and poor peripheral perfusion (cool and clammy skin demonstrating poor capillary refill) and often altered conscious state. Shock is classified as hypovolaemic, cardiogenic, distributive or obstructive (Table 45.1).

Basic investigations for all patients presenting with shock

All patients presenting with shock or suspected shock should have the basic investigations outlined in Table 45.2 performed during the resuscitation.

Further investigations for specific type of shock

If a particular type of shock is suspected from history and physical examination, further investigations may be directed accordingly.

Hypovolaemic shock

Hypovolaemic shock is caused by a loss of intravascular fluid (whole blood or plasma). The common causes of hypovolaemic shock and investigations are listed in Table 45.3.

Cardiogenic shock

Cardiogenic shock may occur with any disease that causes direct myocardial damage or otherwise inhibits cardiac contraction. The common causes of cardiogenic shock are shown in Table 45.4. In invasive monitoring, right-heart catheterisation will reveal a high central venous pressure (CVP), pulmonary artery occlusion pressure (PAOP) (>18 mmHg), and peripheral resistance; low cardiac output (cardiac index <2.2 L/(min m^2)) and mixed venous oxygen content. Further investigations include:
- ECG and troponin level for AMI;
- coronary artery angiogram for AMI;
- CXR for acute pulmonary oedema, CCF;
- echocardiography to demonstrate the defect and assess the regional and global ventricular function, and presence of a mechanical defect, including ventricular septal defect, papillary muscle or free wall rupture and tamponade.

Septic shock

Distributive shock can be caused by the systemic inflammatory response syndrome (SIRS), or shock provoked by the inhibition, or absence, of sympathetic tone (neurogenic shock) or vasoactive compounds such as anaphylactic shock (see Chapter 158).

The clinical features of septic shock include features that are characteristic of the underlying disorder (e.g. peritonitis, pyelonephritis, pneumonia) as well as the features of SIRS (Table 45.5).

The focus of investigation in septic shock is to identify the source of sepsis:
- blood and urine culture;
- culture various fluids – sputum, ascites, CSF, synovial fluid, drained collection fluid;
- wound swab;
- CXR for pneumonia, lung abscess;
- abdominal ultrasound for cholecystitis or cholangitis;
- CT abdomen for intra-abdominal collections, peritonitis;
- transoesophageal echocardiography for endocarditis;
- lumbar puncture for meningitis.

Obstructive shock

Obstructive shock is caused by a mechanical obstruction to normal cardiac output and a subsequent reduction in systemic perfusion. Clinical features include hypotension, tachycardia, respiratory distress, cyanosis and jugular veins distension. Invasive monitoring, such as CVP and pulmonary artery pressure (PAP), can help to establish diagnosis. Further investigation should include:
- CXR for tension pneumothorax;
- CT PA for pulmonary embolism;
- echocardiography for pericardial tamponade;
- CT abdomen for abdominal compartment syndrome.

Physiological monitoring

Physiologic monitoring is essential to the accurate diagnosis and appropriate management of the patient presenting with shock. Non-invasive monitoring includes heart rate, BP, temperature, urinary output and pulse oximetry.

Invasive monitoring includes indwelling arterial, central venous, intracranial and intravesicular pressure catheters; end-tidal carbon dioxide monitors; respiratory function monitors; and pulmonary artery catheters.

Pulmonary artery catheterisation is the 'gold standard' for bedside haemodynamic monitoring of a patient in shock. It provides three different types of variables: pressure, volume and flow. Combining these variables in various calculations provides pressures generated by either the left or right ventricle: an 'outgoing pressure' (mean arterial pressure or mean PAP) and an 'incoming pressure' or estimate of 'preload' (PAOP or CVP); cardiac output and systemic vascular resistance index. These physiologic data can be utilised to diagnose a patient's shock state (severity) and guide appropriate resuscitative treatment. The extent to which such pulmonary artery catheter monitoring improves clinical outcomes remains contentious, however.

46a Trauma

Table 46.1 Initial laboratory investigations in trauma patients

Tests	Indications
FBC	Routine
Biochemistry panel	Routine
Coagulation studies	Not indicated unless the patient is taking anticoagulants
Blood group and cross-match	Routine
Urine toxicology screen	Only if clinically suspected intoxication
Blood alcohol level	Only in patient with altered level of consciousness or local legal requirement
Creatine kinase	Only indicated to confirm rhabdomyolysis
Troponin	Suspected myocardial contusion
Liver function tests	Only if hepatic injury suspected
Arterial blood gas	Seriously injured patient with abnormal breathing or poor perfusion/hypovolaemia; elderly patient age >65 years
Serum lactate	Provides a useful monitor of perfusion

Table 46.2 Indications for imaging in suspected cervical spine injuries

Posterior midline tenderness
Reduction in conscious state/alertness
Intoxication
Presence of distracting injury
Long bone fracture
A visceral injury
A large laceration, degloving injury or crush injury
Large burns
Any other injury producing acute functional impairment
Focal neurological deficit

Table 46.3 Indications for CT as the first-line investigation rather than plain films

- Neurological deficits, irrespective of plain film findings
- Multi-trauma, major distracting injury
- High-speed traffic accidents (>60 km/h combined velocity)
- Pedestrian struck by motor vehicle, occupant ejected from motor vehicle
- Falls from height (>1 m or five stairs)

Table 46.4 Indications for head CT in head trauma

All patients with history of loss of consciousness
Vomiting, two episodes
Persistent Glasgow coma scale (GCS) <13
GCS <15 at 2 h after injury
Focal neurological deficit
Post-traumatic seizure
Amnesia
Persistent headache
Skull fractures
Fall from height
Intoxicated patients
Penetrating head injury
Patient taking anticoagulants, such as warfarin

Table 46.5 Primary and secondary surveys for thoracic trauma

Primary survey	Secondary survey
Tension pneumothorax	Contained rupture of the aorta
Flail chest	Perforation of the tracheobronchial tree
Open, blowing chest wound	Perforation of the oesophagus
Massive haemothorax	Rupture of the diaphragm
Cardiac tamponade	Myocardial contusion
	Pulmonary contusion

Figure 46.1 X-ray of the cervical spine shows a complete fracture of C7 spinous process with an inferior dislocation of the bone fragment

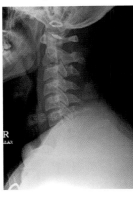

Figure 46.2 CT bony windows sagittal images of cervical spine show C-spine fracture dislocation with anterior displacement of C6 vertebra and disrupted facet articulation

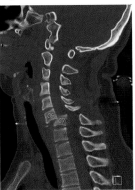

Figure 46.3 CT head shows (a) an acute subdural haematoma; (b) a lens-shaped epidural haematoma in the right temporal region; (c) a left frontal lobe intracranial haemorrhage post-fall; (d) a subarachnoid haemorrhage; (e) a post-head-trauma secondary hydrocephalus

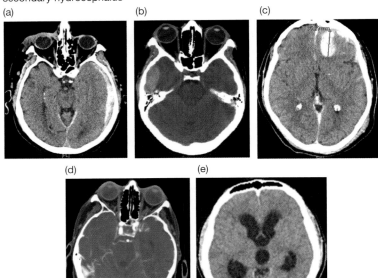

Box 46.1 Indications for monitoring intracranial pressure

- GCS = 8 with abnormal CT scan
- GCS = 8 with normal CT scan, if two or more of the following: (a) age >40, (b) BP <90, posturing
- GCS = 9–12 with abnormal CT scan if the patient will undergo a prolonged operation for other injuries

Figure 46.4 X-ray of the skull shows skull fracture

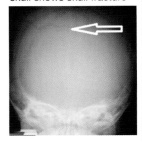

Clinical Investigations at a Glance, First Edition. Jonathan Gleadle, Jordan Li and Tuck Yong. © 2017 John Wiley & Sons, Ltd. Published 2017 by John Wiley & Sons, Ltd.

Trauma is a leading cause of hospitalisation or death worldwide. The common causes of trauma are motor vehicle accidents, falls, assaults, sports-related injuries and penetrating trauma.

Initial clinical evaluation

The initial evaluation of trauma patients involves resuscitation and assessment simultaneously according to the advanced trauma life support guidelines. The purpose of the initial evaluation is to diagnose and manage life-threatening conditions that can cause death or serious morbidity if not treated early. This is called 'primary survey', which includes the following five components:

A Airway maintenance with cervical spine protection
B Breathing and ventilation
C Circulation and haemorrhage control
D Disability/neurological status
E Exposure/environmental control.

The secondary survey is done after the primary survey is completed and the patient is stable from a cardiopulmonary standpoint. Complete examination from head to toe, including an appropriate neurological examination, is performed. The initial essential laboratory investigations are listed in Table 46.1.

Spinal trauma

Spinal fractures, dislocations and penetrating injuries are common in trauma patients. Some 90% of spinal injuries due to blunt trauma are located at C5–C6, T11–L1 and T4–T6. The diagnosis of the cervical spine injuries remains a challenge, especially in the presence of associated severe head injury or multiple injuries. When in doubt, protect the potentially injured spine; the indications for imaging are listed in Table 46.2.

Plain X-rays

Plain X-rays remain a useful initial investigation. Patients with suspected spinal injuries are investigated with a supine cross-table lateral film as part of a 'trauma' series. An adequate C-spine film should include C1 and T1. Soft tissue thickness of >5 mm in front of C3 or more than two-thirds of the thickness of the spinal body is suggestive of significant injury to the anterior structures. If a fracture or dislocation is found (Figure 46.1), further views are taken, with extreme care not to move the patient's neck but rather to position the X-ray tube and cassette appropriately for each view. Flexion and extension views are not useful.

CT

Patients at increased risk of cervical spine injury (Table 46.3) are imaged with CT as the first-line investigation rather than plain films. CT is more sensitive and specific than plain X-ray in detecting cervical injury. The difference in sensitivity is partly due to the technical difficulty of obtaining adequate plain films of the whole cervical spine in trauma patients. CT is indicated in patients with positive findings on plain X-rays or those with a strong suspicion of bony injury, to assess the relationship of bony fragments, dislocated facet joints, unsuspected fractures of posterior structures and disc herniation (Figure 46.2).

MRI

In the acute phase, MRI will demonstrate injuries involving the spinal cord, disc and ligaments. MRI can reveal chronic complications such as syringomyelia and arachnoid cyst formation.

Head trauma

Head trauma is divided into closed head injury and penetrating head injury. The main indications for head CT are summarised in Table 46.4.

CT

Potential findings on CT head as a result of trauma include subdural haemorrhage, epidural haematoma, intracerebral haemorrhage, subarachnoid haemorrhage, secondary hydrocephalus and skull fractures (Figure 46.3). Subsequent CT may be necessary if there is neurological deterioration.

Skull X-rays

Skull X-rays may show a fracture (Figure 46.4) in patients without significant intracranial injury. Conversely, they are often normal in patients with significant intracranial injury. Hence, they have little place in the investigation of head injuries. Do skull X-rays only if CT is not available (may show fractures, foreign bodies, air in the skull).

MRI

MRI has a limited role in the evaluation of acute head injury because of its long acquisition times and the difficulty in obtaining MRIs in a critically ill patient. MRI is used in the subacute setting to evaluate patients with unexplained neurologic deficits.

Monitoring intracranial pressure (ICP)

ICP monitoring is a diagnostic, monitoring, and therapeutic modality in severe head injuries. The insertion of intracranial catheters carries risks of haemorrhage and infection. International guidelines recommend the monitoring of ICP in all patients with survivable severe traumatic brain injury with specific indications (see Table 46.6) (Box 46.1).

Thoracic trauma

The extent and choice of imaging depends on clinical assessment, the severity of trauma and other associated injuries. During the primary and secondary surveys, the investigations are to identify the life-threatening conditions given in Table 46.5.

CXR

CXR may show findings of serious injuries, but often signs are subtle and may not be visible on plain X-rays. These may include flail chest (Figure 46.5), collapse and consolidation, mediastinal widening, pleural effusion, pneumothorax, pneumomediastinum (Figure 46.6), enlarged cardiac shadow (Figure 46.7), elevated hemidiaphragm and intrathoracic bowel gas. Additional skeletal projections are required to evaluate bony injuries, such as oblique rib, sternum, shoulder girdle and spine projections.

CT

CT is useful to confirm mediastinal haematoma, pericardial effusion (Figure 46.8) or haematoma, lung laceration (Figure 46.9) or haematoma and other associated upper abdominal injuries. It is also useful in assessing related spinal injury. CT angiogram may be able to demonstrate a traumatic aneurysm of the aorta.

Angiography

Angiography is the gold standard in the diagnosis of traumatic aortic rupture. An aortic arch angiogram should be considered in cases with non-diagnostic CT scan.

The aim of investigations in abdominal trauma is to assess the extent of injury and select patients who are most likely to benefit from non-operative management.

Table 46.6 Methods in investigation of blunt abdominal injuries

Type of shock	Serial physical examination	FAST	CT	DPL	Laparoscopy
Sensitivity (%)	90	50–80	92–97	80–95	50–100
Specificity (%)	90	50–95	98	50–90	75–90
Negative predictive value (%)	90	60–98	99	80–95	100 No
Patient cooperation	Yes	Yes	No		Yes
Invasive	No	No	No	No	No
Evaluates retroperitoneum	No	No	Yes	Yes No	Yes
Complication	No	No	Yes if CKD	Yes	

Table 46.7 Selected investigations in abdominal trauma

Organs	Special investigations
Kidney	Angiogram: indicated if a kidney does not take up contrast during CT scan, if evidence of false aneurysm or arteriovenous fistula on CT scan, if there is persistent gross haematuria
Bladder	Cystogram (the bladder should be filled and oblique X-rays should always be obtained). If an abdominal CT scan is performed, a CT cystogram may replace the standard cystogram
Urethral injuries	Urethrogram
Pancreatic injuries	Serum amylase (elevated in about 70% of blunt trauma and 30% of penetrating pancreatic trauma). MRCP for evaluation of the pancreatic duct
Colonic injuries	The diagnosis is made intraoperatively
Rectal injuries	Sigmoidoscopy or gastrografin enema

Table 46.8 Investigations for peripheral vascular injuries

- ABI in lower extremity injuries or brachio-brachial index for upper extremities <0.9 is suspicious of arterial injury and is an indication for further investigation. In minor injuries (small intimal tears or false aneurysm) the ABI may be normal
- Duplex ultrasound is the investigation of choice for all proximity injuries in the neck and the extremities
- Arteriogram: the indications for angiograms are a bruit or murmur in a stable patient, shotgun injuries, most vascular injuries due to blunt trauma and inconclusive duplex results

Table 46.9 Key points in investigating pregnant women with trauma

- X-ray or CT scans should not be deferred because of pregnancy; use abdominal shielding whenever possible
- Ultrasound examination of the uterus and fetus should be performed on all pregnant trauma patients
- Estimation of gestational age is critical to decision-making in pregnant trauma patients; if in doubt, confirm by ultrasound examination and fundal height
- The Rh-status should be checked and negative pregnant females should receive Rhogam to prevent isoimmunisation
- Fetal monitoring in advanced pregnancy with a viable fetus and immediate consultation with obstetricians

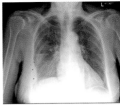

Figure 46.5 CXR shows flail chest

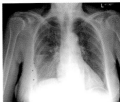

Figure 46.6 CXR shows pneumomediastinum

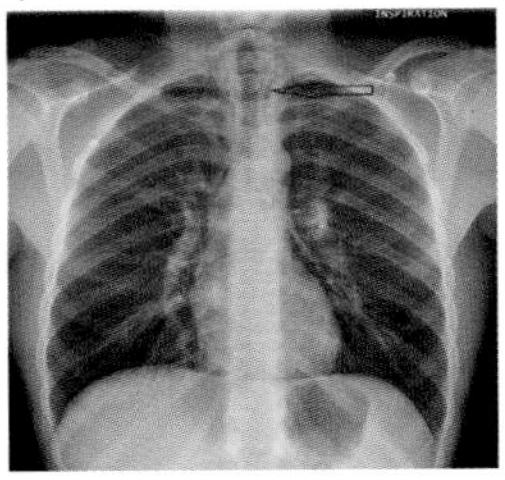

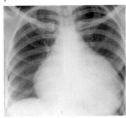

Figure 46.7 CXR shows enlarged cardiac shadow due to haemorrhagic pericardial effusion

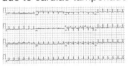

Figure 46.8 CT chest shows a large pericardial effusion

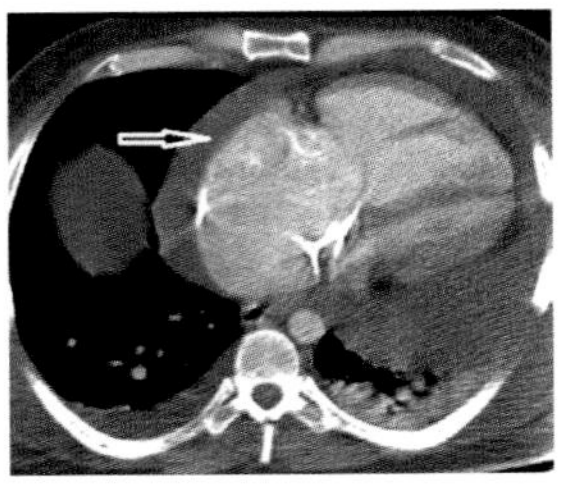

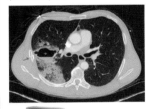

Figure 46.9 CT chest shows rib fracture with underlying lung pneumatocele (*) with surrounding ground glass change suggestive of a lung laceration and surrounding parenchymal haemorrhage

Figure 46.10 ECG showing low-voltage QRS complexes due to cardiac tamponade

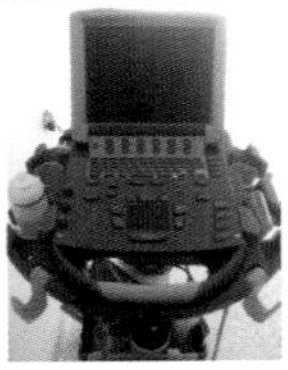

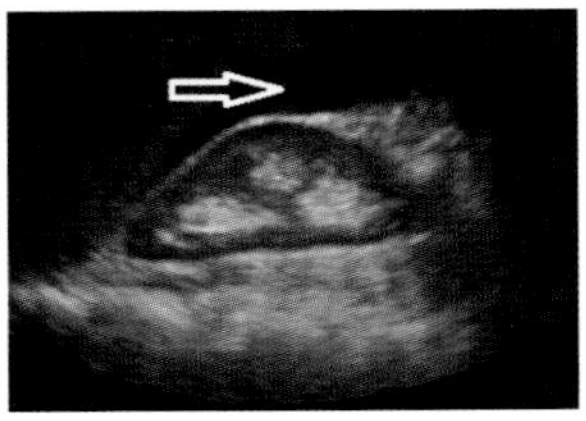

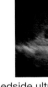

Figure 46.11 Bedside ultrasound machine for FAST scan

Figure 46.12 FAST scan shows right upper quadrant free fluid

Key points

- When imaging is indicated, cervical spine CT is superior to plain X-rays in cervical spine injury assessment and is preferred if available, feasible and safe.
- CT of the head may not be needed in patients with mild injury with no loss of consciousness, amnesia or disorientation and GCS 15.
- CXR and CT may be required to assess thoracic trauma.
- In a haemodynamically unstable patient, FAST ultrasound is useful to assess for intraperitoneal bleeding. In stable patients, CT is the investigation of choice.

Echocardiography

Echocardiography is used to confirm and follow up pericardial haematoma or effusion. Transoesophageal echocardiography can be used to assess aortic tear.

Cardiac trauma

Blunt cardiac trauma may vary from asymptomatic or symptomatic cardiac contusion to full cardiac rupture. Patients with cardiac ruptures or penetrating injury of the heart rarely reach the hospital alive. **Do not** waste valuable time on unnecessary investigations if the diagnosis is obvious. Investigations should be done only if the diagnosis is uncertain.

Routine ECG and troponins should be performed in all patients with a suspicious mechanism of injury. ECG may show signs of myocardial ischemia, arrhythmias or may be normal. In approximately one-third of the cases with tamponade, ECG shows low-voltage QRS complexes, elevated ST segments and inverted T waves (Figure 46.10). Normal ECG and troponins on admission reliably exclude any significant cardiac contusion. A focused abdominal sonography for trauma (FAST) or echocardiogram can diagnose tamponade due to cardiac rupture. Radiological signs on CXR suggestive of cardiac injury include:

- enlarged cardiac shadow
- pneumopericardium
- widened upper mediastinum.

Pericardiocentesis is rarely used and it is unreliable and falsely negative in up to 60% because of clot formation in the pericardial sac.

Abdominal trauma

Common blunt abdominal injuries are to the liver, spleen, kidney and mesentery. If the patient needs a laparotomy, undue delay for unnecessary investigations is unwarranted. The following different modalities of investigation are by no means equal. The decision on which modality or combination of methods, to choose will depend on patient conditions and hospital factors (Table 46.6).

CT

CT abdomen is the 'gold standard' in investigation of blunt abdominal trauma with sensitivity of 92–97% and specificity of 98%. Advantages include non-invasive nature, the ability to exclude retroperitoneal injuries and the ability to grade solid organ injury. The NPV of CT for diagnosis of intra-abdominal injuries is 99%; therefore, the majority of haemodynamically stable well patients with no findings on CT may be discharged after a period of observation and serial abdominal examination.

Hollow organ injury is rare (1–3% of blunt trauma admissions). CT is still the modality of choice for diagnosing small bowel perforation because of its high sensitivity for extraluminal air (87–100% sensitivity and specificity 99–100% when CT was obtained >8 h after injury).

When CT evaluation indicates hollow organ injury, exploratory laparotomy is required. Otherwise, patients are observed with serial abdominal examination. When hollow organ injury is suspected based on clinical signs without CT findings, exploratory laparotomy should be considered with a low threshold to reduce complications resulting from delayed treatment of hollow organ injuries.

Contrast extravasation found on CT is a sign of active bleeding and requires immediate surgical or angiographic intervention.

Plain X-rays

Plain CXR and AXR can demonstrate skeletal injuries, rupture of hollow viscus and large fluid collections. X-rays of the spine, pelvis, and ribs are obtained as indicated. Routine pelvis X-rays in an alert asymptomatic patient are not indicated. Important radiological findings include fractures, free intraperitoneal gas, retroperitoneal gas, an elevated diaphragm, a hollow viscus in the chest, soft tissue shadows, scoliosis and loss of the psoas shadow.

Focused abdominal sonography for trauma (FAST) scan

A FAST scan (Figure 46.11) is an abbreviated search for intraperitoneal fluid (Figure 46.12) that may indicate intraabdominal haemorrhage. The sensitivity and specificity of FAST in the detection of haemoperitoneum in haemodynamically unstable patients is 98%, with the presence of intraperitoneal fluid outside the pelvic cavity strongly associated with intra-abdominal injury. If FAST results are negative, other causes of haemodynamic instability must be searched for during the secondary survey.

Diagnostic peritoneal lavage (DPL)

The main indication for DPL is blunt or sometimes penetrating multi-trauma with unexplained hypotension, where the FAST exam is not diagnostic. DPL has a high sensitivity (95%) and specificity (99%) for intraperitoneal haemorrhage. However, DPL does not exclude retroperitoneal injury and is invasive with a 1% risk of complications.

Angiography

Angiography is necessary in suspected vascular trauma or ongoing blood loss from renal, splenic or pelvic injuries provided that immediate surgery is not indicated in unstable patients.

Other investigations

Microscopic urinalysis should be done on all patients with blunt abdominal trauma. Other selective investigations are summarised in Table 46.7.

Penetrating abdominal injuries

A distinction should be made between high-velocity and low-velocity injuries. High-velocity missiles cause extensive tissue damage and patients almost always require a laparotomy. Low-velocity injuries are usually due to 'civilian' violence (stab wounds, most handguns). The investigations, mainly plain X-ray and CT with contrast, should be performed only on stable patients. Many patients will need surgical intervention.

Peripheral vascular injuries

Penetrating injuries, fractures, dislocations and direct blunt trauma can cause peripheral vascular injuries. The presence of peripheral pulse does not exclude proximal arterial injury. The investigations are listed in Table 46.8.

Trauma in pregnancy

All female trauma patients of reproductive years should have a bedside urinary pregnancy test performed immediately. The important points in investigation of pregnant women with trauma are listed in Table 46.9.

46b Trauma

Indications for X-ray series of the ankle:
- Pain near either of the malleoli
- Unable to weight bear both immediately and in the emergency department
- Bone tenderness at the posterior edge or tip of either malleolus

Plain X-rays of the knee are indicated when any of the following factors are present:
- Tenderness at the head of the fibula
- Isolated tenderness of the patella
- Inability to flex knee to 90°
- Inability to walk four weight-bearing steps

The indications for imaging in thoraco-lumbar spine injury:
- Altered mental status
- Injury with evidence of intoxication with ethanol or drugs
- Neurologic deficits
- Spine pain or palpation tenderness
- Falls from significant height (>3 m)
- Motor vehicle/motorcycle/bicycle/all-terrain vehicle crash with or without ejection
- Pedestrians struck
- Assault, sport injury
- Concomitant cervical spine fracture

The indications for imaging in hip trauma:
- Severe pain in the hip or thigh after a fall
- Inability to move the hip
- Unable to weight bear
- Deformity, including shortening, adducted and internally rotated, or abducted and externally rotated
- Hip oedema and ecchymosis
- Severe hip pain in an osteoporotic patient without fall/injury

The indications for imaging in shoulder trauma:
- Severe pain
- Severe swelling and bruising of the should joint, clavicle area
- Impaired range of movement of the shoulder joint
- A grinding sensation when the shoulder joint is actively or passively moved
- Deformity
- A rotated arm

The indications for imaging in elbow trauma:
- Limited active range of motion
- Bruising
- Tenderness over the radial head, olecranon and medial epicondyle
- Or imaging studies may be unnecessary for the evaluation of elbow fractures and dislocations if the active range of motion (including extension, flexion, supination and pronation) remains normal

Indications for imaging in wrist and forearm injury:
- Severe pain and tenderness directly over the injury site
- Swelling of the wrist joint
- Limited range of motion in the wrist and hand
- Deformity
- Remember to always examine and image the elbow for associated injuries

Figure 46.13 (a, b) Plain X-ray shows bimalleolar fracture of the right ankle

(a)   (b)

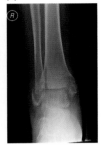

Figure 46.14 (a, b) Plain X-ray shows a left pertrochanteric fracture with significant displacement and avulsion of the left greater trochanter

(a)

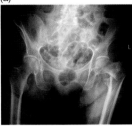

(b)

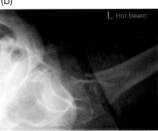

Figure 46.15 Plain X-ray shows a fracture involving the surgical neck of the humerus

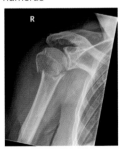

Figure 46.16 (a, b) Plain X-ray shows fracture of the olecranon with posterior dislocation of the fracture fragments

(a)

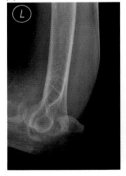

(b)

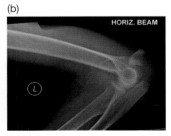

The following are additional indications for investigating possible scaphoid fractures:
- Provocative tests reproduce or exacerbate pain
- Snuffbox tenderness positive (sensitivity 90%, specificity 40%)
- Watson test (shift test, palpate scaphoid tubercle while wrist moved from ulnar to radial deviation) positive (sensitivity 85%, specificity 60%)

Ankle injury

Ankle injuries can occur at any age and are the most common sports injuries. Ankle injuries can be defined by the kind of tissue involved: bone, ligament or tendon. The most common ankle injuries are sprains and fractures. The indications for ankle X-ray series are listed opposite.

CT of the ankle is required for preoperative planning or if there is a high clinical suspicion of fracture despite normal plain X-ray or presence of an ankle effusion (correlated with an occult fracture in 40–80% of patients). MRI is useful in assessing ligamentous injuries (sensitivity 60%, specificity 100%), but routine MRI scan should be discouraged as most ligamentous injuries recover with conservative management. Ultrasound can detect lateral ankle ligament rupture with a sensitivity of 85% and specificity of 94%.

Knee injury

Most people who present with acute knee injuries have soft tissue rather than bony injuries, and where fracture is present there is often accompanying soft tissue injury. Imaging of injured knees is commonly ordered, even though fractures are found in only 6% of such patients. Ottawa Rules in acute knee injury in adults has sensitivity of 98.5% and specificity 48.6%. The indications for plain films of the knee are listed opposite.

MRI is useful for the detection of ongoing knee instability following trauma to the knee, as it can accurately delineate the soft tissues of the joint, especially meniscal tears, cruciate ligament tears, collateral ligamentous injuries, and osseous and chondral lesions. CT has a lesser role in the assessment of post-traumatic knee pain, though it is useful in demonstrating subtle bony injury and loose bodies within the knee joint and for preoperative planning. Ultrasound is useful in the rapid evaluation of meniscus, ligamental injury, tendon lesions, joint effusions, bursitis and cysts.

Hip injury

Plain X-ray is the initial investigation for suspected fracture and it will show a fracture in the majority of cases (Figure 46.14). It misses 5–14% of occult, non-displaced fractures. If clinical suspicion of occult hip fracture persists, CT of the hip is the next investigation of choice. It may still miss a small percentage of hip fractures, particularly in osteoporotic bone, small impacted fractures or undisplaced fractures that run parallel to the axial plane. Timely surgical management is important as delayed diagnosis increases the rate of secondary fracture displacement and morbidity; an MRI may be warranted when CT is negative but a high clinical suspicion remains. MRI is superior to other imaging modalities in detecting occult hip fractures with 100% sensitivity and specificity.

Thoraco-lumbar spine injury

The indications for imaging are listed opposite. Plain X-rays are adequate for the investigation of thoracolumbar spine if the patient does not require a CT scan for another reason. MRI is indicated for patients with neurologic deficits as well as when clinical suspicion is high despite a normal plain film or normal CT scans.

Shoulder injury

Plain X-ray is the initial modality for investigating suspected traumatic shoulder injury and can demonstrate most fractures and dislocations (Figure 46.15). If an impingement syndrome or rotator cuff tear is suspected, ultrasound is recommended in addition to plain X-ray. CT of the shoulder is useful in complex fracture–dislocation injuries of the shoulder. MRI (91% sensitivity, 97% specificity for full-thickness rotator cuff tears) is useful as an alternative in suspected rotator cuff injury.

Elbow injury

Plain X-ray is the initial choice for the investigation of acute elbow injuries and is best for showing fracture (sensitivity 70%, specificity 56%), soft tissue swelling and joint effusions (Figure 46.16). When no fracture is apparent, X-ray findings of a joint effusion or displacement of the fat pads can raise the suspicion of an occult fracture. Occult fractures are found in 80% of patients with isolated posterior fat pad displacement on initial or follow-up X-ray.

MRI is the preferred imaging modality for chronic elbow pain after injury. Whilst MRI scans detect more injuries than X-rays, the vast majority of these will make no difference to patient management or outcome. CT is used for fracture characterisation (sensitive 92%, specificity 79%) and preoperative planning of complex fractures.

Wrist injury

Fractures of the forearm are common injuries in adults. Initial assessment includes history, examination and standard plain X-rays. Small, occult, or intra-articular fractures may not be seen on initial X-ray. When suspicion of a fracture is high, the X-ray should be repeated in 2 weeks. If immediate confirmation or exclusion of fracture is required or if there is a question about the presence of joint instability or associated ligament injury, MRI should be performed.

The initial diagnostic modality for suspected scaphoid fracture is plain X-ray, but up to 30% of fractures are radiographically occult at the time of presentation. Early MRI is recommended as it is most accurate in detecting occult scaphoid fracture, and has the advantage of simultaneously evaluating bone marrow abnormalities and surrounding soft tissue injuries. Early imaging results in faster identification of fractures and other injuries and reduces unnecessary immobilisation and prevention of complications, such as avascular necrosis, non-union and osteoarthritis. If early MRI is unavailable or contraindicated, CT is an alternative. Depending on local resources, presumptive casting and repeat plain X-ray in 7–10 days is an alternative.

Facial and orbital injury

Maxillofacial injuries are common, and more than 50% of patients with these injuries have multisystem trauma. CT is the modality of choice in investigating facial trauma and suspected orbital fracture. Mandibular fractures are often imaged by conventional radiography and orthopantomogram (OPG), but CT has surpassed OPG as the current gold standard for the radiological evaluation and diagnosis of mandible fractures. MRI is a useful adjunct to CT, particularly in identifying soft tissue, optic nerve and globe injury. However, metallic fragments in the orbit should first be excluded on plain film or CT before undergoing MRI.

In summary, clinical judgment is important and imaging may additionally be needed if the patient is uncooperative, has impaired consciousness, marked swelling around a limb or joint, or impaired sensation.

47 Alcohol-use disorder

The purpose of investigation of alcohol-use disorders is to:
- Screen alcohol-use disorders
- Assess the severity of alcohol-use disorders especially alcohol dependence
- Identify alcohol-related medical complications
- Assess the need for assisted alcohol withdrawal

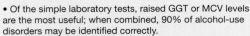

Key points
- Of the simple laboratory tests, raised GGT or MCV levels are the most useful; when combined, 90% of alcohol-use disorders may be identified correctly.
- Laboratory tests may be used to confirm the diagnosis of suspected alcohol-use disorders and help ascertain the extent of disease.
- Patients with alcohol-use disorders should be assessed for nutritional status.

Table 47.1 Investigations of patients with alcohol dependence

General	Specfic
• FBC • Electrolytes, urea, creatinine, calcium, magnesium, glucose and urate • LFTs • Blood alcohol levels • Fasting lipids • Coagulation study	• Lipase: if pancreatitis is suspected • CK: if myopathy is suspected • Serum folate: if anaemia, macrocytosis or poor nutrition is present • Transketolase (thiamine assay): if poor nutrition, neuropathy, cardiomyopathy or neurological changes • Hepatitis B and C and HIV testing: if liver pathology confirmed or other illicit drug use suspected

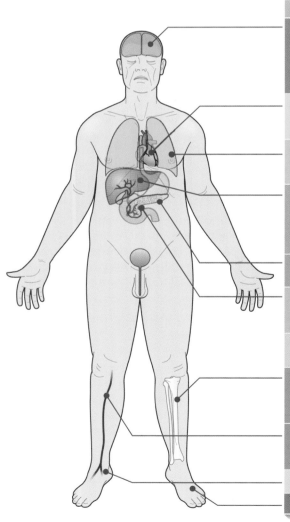

Table 47.2 Investigation of alcohol-related medical complications

Alcohol-related complication	Investigations
Alcohol-related brain damage (Wernicke encephalopathy, Korsakoff syndrome, cerebellar degeneration, subdural haematoma); peripheral neuropathy	CT or MRI of brain Nerve conduction test
Atrial fibrillation Cardiomyopathy Congestive heart failure	ECG, CXR, echocardiography, brain natriuretic peptide
Pulmonary infections – aspiration pneumonia, lung abscess	FBC, CXR, CT chest (for abscess)
Fatty liver, alcoholic hepatitis, cirrhosis Portal hypertension Hepatocellular carcinoma (HCC)	LFTs, coagulation study, hepatitis B and C serology, abdominal ultrasound, AFP (for HCC), upper GI endoscopy (for varices), liver biopsy if the hepatitis is severe enough to require corticosteroid treatment
Diabetes mellitus (related to chronic pancreatitis)	Fasting blood glucose level, oral glucose tolerance test, glycated haemoglobin
Pancreatitis Pancreatic exocrine insufficiency	Lipase, faecal elastase-1, serum trypsinogen, vitamin levels, CT abdomen
Nutritional deficiency (vitamin B, folic acid), hypoalbuminaemia	Thiamine, folic acid level, serum albumin level
Metabolic complications: ketoacidosis, hypo or hyper-glycaemia, hyponatraemia, osteoporosis	Serum electrolyte, blood glucose level, DEXA scan of bone
Haematological complications: anaemia, leukopenia, thrombocytopenia, coagulopathy	FBC, coagulation study
Peripheral vascular disease	Duplex ultrasound
Peripheral neuropathy	Nerve conduction test

Alcohol-use disorder is a chronic, relapsing disorder characterised by increased tolerance to the effects of alcohol, the presence of characteristic withdrawal signs and symptoms, and impaired control over the quantity and frequency of alcohol use. Alcohol-use disorders include hazardous and harmful drinking and alcohol dependence. Alcohol-use disorder can cause a variety of medical and psychiatric sequelae. Alcohol is one of the leading causes of preventable morbidity and mortality and exerts a heavy social cost. Early identification of problem patterns of use and complications can lead to timely intervention and lessen these adverse effects.

Excessive alcohol intake may occur in different forms, including regular daily drinking above recommended levels (more than two standard drinks on each occasion for both men and women) and episodic drinking to intoxication (binge-drinking). If no harm has yet been experienced, these consumption patterns are described as 'hazardous drinking'. If the drinking has caused physical or mental harm, it is called 'harmful drinking', and drinking that has resulted in becoming dependent on alcohol is 'alcohol dependence'.

Investigations for identifying problem drinking

Routine screening may help to identify and treat alcohol-use disorder early. Characteristic history and examination findings are often sufficient to diagnose problem alcohol use. The Alcohol Use Disorders Identification Test is considered to be the most accurate test for identifying problem drinking. Laboratory studies can be useful to provide confirmatory evidence.

Blood or breath alcohol concentration

Evidence of recent alcohol use can be detected by blood or breath alcohol levels, especially for legal purposes. Values in the range of 50 to 100 mg/dL are typically associated with some impairment in memory, coordination and judgement in non-dependent users. A high blood alcohol concentration (e.g. >200 mg/dL) with minimal signs of intoxication may indicate tolerance to alcohol effects, but does not itself diagnose dependence.

Clinical Institute Withdrawal Assessment for Alcohol (CIWA-Ar) scale

The revised CIWA-Ar is the standard assessment instrument used to quantify the severity of alcohol withdrawal symptoms. A score ≥8 to 10 indicates the presence of significant alcohol withdrawal symptoms.

Laboratory tests in suspected excessive alcohol intake

Simple and complex laboratory tests may be used. Of the simple laboratory tests, raised gamma-glutamyl-transpeptidase (GGT) or mean corpuscular volume (MCV) levels are the most useful; and when these values are combined, 90% of alcoholics may be identified correctly.

FBC: elevated MCV or macrocytosis can be associated with excessive alcohol use. Normal to low haemoglobin, mild thrombocytopenia (platelet $<100,000$ mm^3) is seen in about one-third of heavy alcohol users.

LFTs: aspartate aminotransferase (AST) is typically higher than alanine aminotransferase (ALT) when alcohol is the cause of liver disease. GGT is usually elevated in patients with excessive alcohol intake and is closely correlated with alcohol consumption. Other potential abnormalities in laboratory tests in excessive alcohol use include elevated urate and high-density lipoprotein. Biological markers are not as reliable as a good clinical history or brief screening questionnaire in detecting alcohol problems. The carbohydrate-deficient transferrin (CDT) test is the most sensitive test for heavy drinking. Serum CDT is reduced after regular high alcohol intake.

Investigation of patients with alcohol dependence

Table 47.1 summarises the general and specific investigations performed in the evaluation of patients with alcohol dependence.

Investigation of alcohol-related complications

Table 47.2 shows the major medical complications related to chronic excessive alcohol intake and investigations of these problems.

48 Eating disorders

The purpose of investigations is to:
- Exclude other medical conditions which can mimic anorexia nervosa (Table 48.1)
- Assess nutritional status
- Identify any metabolic complications related to low body weight
- Monitor for refeeding syndrome

Key points

- Eating disorders are diagnosed based on clinical findings and no diagnostic investigations are required.
- Starvation with anorexia nervosa may affect multiple organs, and investigations are required to determine these effects.
- Biochemistry should be monitored closely during refeeding.

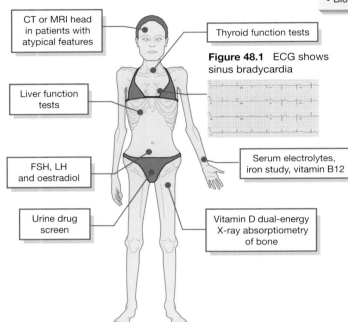

CT or MRI head in patients with atypical features

Thyroid function tests

Liver function tests

FSH, LH and oestradiol

Urine drug screen

Serum electrolytes, iron study, vitamin B12

Vitamin D dual-energy X-ray absorptiometry of bone

Figure 48.1 ECG shows sinus bradycardia

Table 48.1 Main differential diagnoses of eating disorders

Nephrological causes
Gastrointestinal disorders
• inflammatory bowel disease • coeliac disease • chronic liver disease
Endocrine
• diabetes mellitus • hyperthyroidism • Addison's disease
Malignancy
• solid organ tumours, such as pancreatic cancer • haematological malignancy: lymphoma, leukaemia

Eating disorders are serious illnesses with significant mortality and morbidity and comprise:

- anorexia nervosa
- bulimia nervosa
- eating disorders not otherwise specified.

Anorexia nervosa is characterised by determined dieting, often accompanied by compulsive exercise, and in a subgroup of patients, purging behaviour with or without binge eating, resulting in sustained low weight with body mass index <17.5 kg/m^2. Anorexia nervosa can be classified into two types:

- Food-restricting type – characterised by marked caloric reduction, typically to 300–700 kcal per day, often accompanied by compulsive exercise.
- Binge-eating and purging type – the binge may consist of food in a range from small amounts ('subjective' binge) to several thousands of calories. Purging usually begins after dieting commences, most commonly with the use of self-induced vomiting, or by abuse of laxatives, and occasionally with the use of diet pills or diuretics.

Eating disorders are more common in young people. The lifetime risk of the eating disorder is 0.3–1.0% among women and <0.1% among men. Standardised mortality ratios for anorexia nervosa (compared with the general population) are elevated for all causes of death (ratio 11.6), especially suicide (ratio 56.9).

The diagnosis of anorexia nervosa is made on the basis of history, including information from family members, friends and teachers. Other psychiatric disorders often coexist with anorexia nervosa, including major depression or dysthymia (50–75%), anxiety disorders (>60%), obsessive–compulsive disorder (40%) and alcohol or substance abuse (10–30%). There is no specific laboratory investigation that can confirm the diagnosis of anorexia nervosa. In most cases, patients with an eating disorder will have normal laboratory results and the biochemical markers may not be an accurate indicator of the severity of illness or medical instability.

Initial basic investigations

- FBC
- Serum electrolytes, including calcium, phosphate and magnesium, creatinine, urea, fasting glucose
- Liver function tests
- Thyroid function test
- Urinalysis, including pH (possibility of diuretic use).

Further investigations for selected patients

- Iron studies, serum vitamin B12, folate level in patients with anaemia.
- Follicle-stimulating hormone (FSH), luteinising hormone (LH) and oestradiol.

- Coeliac disease serology in patients with iron deficiency.
- Urine drug screen.
- An ECG may be helpful in detecting arrhythmias. The most common arrhythmia is sinus bradycardia (Figure 48.1). An ECG should be performed before initiation of atypical antipsychotic medications.
- Serum vitamin D level and dual-energy X-ray absorptiometry of bone, for patients who have been underweight for >6 months.
- CT or MRI of the brain for patients with atypical features, such as hallucinations, delusions, delirium and persistent cognitive impairment, despite weight restoration.

In anorexia nervosa, elevated amylase is primarily secreted by the salivary gland. Hypocalcaemia may result from chronic malnutrition or alkalosis and may be associated with changes on ECG. Magnesium deficiency may result from malnutrition, diarrhoea or misuse of diuretic agents and may be associated with hypokalaemia, hypophosphataemia and changes on ECG. Malnutrition may produce hepatomegaly, fatty liver and, rarely, cirrhosis. Elevated levels of liver enzymes may also reflect alcohol abuse or the use of medications with toxic effects on the liver. Patients may need regular follow-up in the clinic to monitor weight and laboratory indicators, such as electrolyte levels, and ECG may need to be repeated.

Refeeding syndrome

Refeeding syndrome is defined as the potentially fatal shifts in fluids and electrolytes that may occur in malnourished patients receiving artificial refeeding (whether enterally or parenterally). These shifts result from hormonal and metabolic changes and may cause serious clinical complications. The hallmark biochemical feature of refeeding syndrome is hypophosphataemia. However, the syndrome is complex and may also feature abnormal sodium and fluid balance; changes in glucose, protein and fat metabolism; thiamine deficiency; hypokalaemia; and hypomagnesaemia.

Phosphate, magnesium, electrolyte levels and kidney function should be followed closely. Clinical changes and laboratory results requiring immediate attention include altered consciousness, tachycardia, congestive heart failure, atypical abdominal pain, a prolonged QT interval or QT dispersion, which is a marker of abnormal ventricular repolarisation associated with an increased risk of arrhythmia, serum potassium levels <3 mmol/L and serum phosphate <0.3 mmol/L.

Refeeding syndrome is detected by considering the possibility of its existence and by using the simple biochemical investigations described. If the syndrome is detected, the rate of feeding should be slowed down and essential electrolytes should be replenished.

49 Seizure

The purpose of investigations in a patient presenting with suspected seizure is to:
- Establish if the episode of loss of consciousness is a seizure
- Classify the type of seizure and determine whether this is a first seizure
- Identify any underlying cause of the seizure
- Stratify the risk of seizure recurrence and the need of treatment

Table 49.2 Initial laboratory investigation in patient with seizure

Tests	Seizure-provoking factors
Glucose	Hypoglycaemia or hyperglycaemia
Electrolytes	Hyponatraemia or hypernatremia, hypocalcaemia
Creatinine and urea	Uraemia
Liver function tests	Liver failure
Alcohol level	Excessive alcohol intake or alcohol withdrawal
Urine drug screen	Drug intoxication
FBC, CRP	Infection, although mild leukocytosis can occur after a seizure, eosinophilia (a clue to parasitic infection)

Table 49.1 Common types of seizures
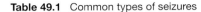

Seizure type	Clinical features	EEG features
Generalised		
Primarily generalised tonic-clonic seizures ('grand mal')	Loss of consciousness, tonic–clonic seizures, sometimes preceded by myoclonic jerks	Spike-wave complexes (3–5 Hz)
Absence seizures ('petit mal')	Brief episode of unresponsiveness (average, 10 seconds) and rapid recovery; increased or decreased muscle tone, automatism; triggered by hyperventilation	Spike-wave pattern (3 Hz)
Partial		
Simple partial (focal) seizures	May be motor, sensory, autonomic or psychic, depending on location of electrical discharge; consciousness is not impaired	Localised slowing or sharp wave activity, or both
Complex partial seizures (temporal lobe or psychomotor)	Begin with motor, sensory, autonomic or psychic features; consciousness is impaired; automatisms may occur	Focal slowing or sharp wave activity, or both
Secondarily generalised partial seizure	Focal seizures evolving to a bilateral convulsive seizure	Focal slowing or sharp wave activity, or both

Figure 49.1 MRI brain shows right-sided mesial temporal sclerosis with volume loss and enlargement of the temporal horn of the lateral ventricle

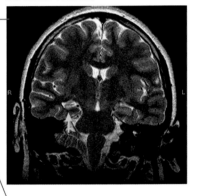

Figure 49.2 CT head non-contrast shows hyperdense mass lesion in left cerebral deep white matter due to lymphoma

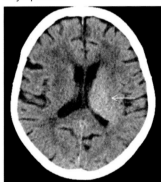

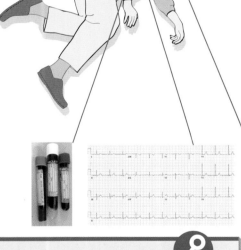

Figure 49.3 Normal EEG

Figure 49.4 Epileptiform EEG

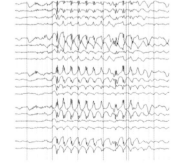

Key points in investigating seizures

- Patients with first seizure in the absence of a provoked cause require investigation with an MRI of the brain and an EEG.
- A single routine EEG consisting of half an hour recording during wakefulness, hyperventilation and intermittent photic stimulation provides diagnostic findings in approximately half of patients with epilepsy.
- A negative serial EEG study in a patient with continuing paroxysmal events should raise suspicion of non-epileptic episodes.

A seizure is a clinical manifestation of abnormal electrical activity in the brain. Epilepsy is defined as more than one seizure. There are different types of seizures (Table 49.1).

The cumulative lifetime risk of a single seizure is 8% and epilepsy is 3%. If a first seizure is unprovoked, 30–50% of patients will recur; after a second unprovoked seizure, 70–80% will recur, justifying the diagnosis of epilepsy (a tendency for recurrent seizures).

Worldwide, provoked seizures in adults are commonly caused by infections such as acute meningitis, encephalitis, malaria; intoxication and withdrawal from alcohol and other drugs. In later life, cerebral vascular disease becomes the most common cause. Brain tumours, including metastases, are responsible for about 4% of first seizures.

Clinical evaluation

Seizure is a clinical diagnosis; a detailed history from patient and witness is paramount. The differential diagnosis of seizure is wide, including syncope, transient ischaemic attack, metabolic encephalopathy (hypoglycaemia or electrolyte disturbance), cardiac arrhythmias and pseudoseizures.

If the first event is ambiguous, waiting for a recurrence is a good strategy. The diagnosis may become clearer and in the meantime a diagnosis of 'don't know' may be better than an incorrect diagnosis of epilepsy with its psychosocial consequences.

Laboratory investigations

The initial laboratory tests are performed to investigate whether the seizure is provoked (Table 49.2). Elevated serum prolactin usually two times baseline or three standard deviations above normal, when measured 10–20 minutes after a suspected seizure, is a useful adjunct for the differentiation of generalised tonic–clonic or complex partial seizure from psychogenic nonepileptic seizure. Serum prolactin level does not distinguish epileptic seizures from syncope.

ECG is mandatory in anyone with loss of consciousness, as syncope of cardiac cause may present as a secondary hypoxic seizure, and potentially fatal arrhythmias, particularly long QT syndromes, will otherwise be missed. Patients without a provoked cause of first seizure require further evaluation with imaging.

Brain imaging

The main purpose of brain imaging is to identify a cause of the patient's seizure that may need treatment. MRI is the modality of choice in all adults with first unprovoked seizure. However, relevant lesions on MRI are usually not found in patients with electroencephalogram (EEG)-proven idiopathic epilepsy. Overall, MRI has a yield of 10% in first seizures and is more sensitive than CT, especially in identifying subtle lesions, such as cortical dysplasia or mesial temporal sclerosis (Figure 49.1).

CT head is useful for first seizure patients with acute head injury or patients with reduced level of consciousness in the emergency setting. It is safer and faster than MRI for acutely unwell patients, and it may influence acute management in 15% of patients.

Neuroimaging is not a diagnostic test for epilepsy. However, if a patient has attacks of uncertain nature and their neuroimaging reveals an epileptogenic lesion such as a malignant glioma or lymphoma (Figure 49.2), then a diagnosis of epilepsy becomes highly probable.

Neurological deficits (prenatal injury, neurological deficit, intellectual disability) or relevant MRI or EEG abnormalities (spikes, slow waves, or both) are the strongest predictors of seizure recurrence. For patients with one or both of these factors, the risk of recurrence is 70% over 5 years. For patients without these factors, recurrence is 35%.

EEG

All patients who are suspected of having seizure or epilepsy should have an EEG (Figures 49.3 and 49.4). An EEG is useful in confirming the presence of abnormal electrical activity, providing information about the type of seizure (Table 49.1) and the location of seizure focus. Yield is highest in the first 24 hours after the seizure. Relevant abnormalities (spikes and/or slow waves occurring with an irregular frequency of about 3–5 Hz) are found in 10–50% of cases. The yield is increased by activation procedures (hyperventilation and photic stimulation) and after sleep deprivation (up to 80% yield, but also an increase to 4% in false positives).

False-negative interictal EEG results occur in 50% of patients with seizure in routine recordings. A normal EEG does not rule out seizure. Repeating the EEG in highly suspicious seizure reduces the false-negative rate to 30%, and a sleep-deprived recording reduces them to 20%. False-positive interictal EEGs occur in up to 0.5–2% of healthy young adults. Seizure/epilepsy cannot be diagnosed from an EEG alone. There must be a clinical description of episodes that are compatible with seizure/epilepsy.

Video–EEG monitoring

The indication for video–EEG monitoring is patients with probable epilepsy or patients with frequent attacks of uncertain nature. Ictal video–EEG monitoring is the most sensitive and specific test for epilepsy. It is also used to capture ictal and interictal focal discharges as part of the pre-surgical assessment of patients with mesial temporal sclerosis. Video recording may be crucial to diagnose cases when the EEG is normal.

50 Muscle weakness

Table 50.1 Common causes and investigations for muscle weakness

Cause	Weakness	Investigations
Medications		
Corticosteroids	Proximal	Medication history
Antiretroviral drugs	Generalised	Medication history
Infections		
EBV infection	Generalised	EBV immunoglobulin M and G antibodies
Alcohol		
	Proximal	Raised ALP, GGT, anaemia
Endocrine disorders		
Addison disease	Generalised	Hyponatraemia, adrenocorticotropic hormone stimulation test
Cushing syndrome	Proximal	Elevated urine free cortisol level
Hyperthyroidism	Proximal	Raised T4, suppressed TSH
Hypothyroidism	Proximal	Raised TSH, reduced T4
Electrolyte disturbance		
Hyperkalaemia/ hypokalaemia	Variable	Serum electrolytes
Hypomagnesemia	Variable	Serum electrolytes
Inflammatory disorders		
Polymyositis	Proximal	Elevated myoglobin; ANA (+); myositis autoantibodies may be present (see Table 50.2)
Dermatomyositis	Proximal	Elevated myoglobin; ANA (+); myositis autoantibodies (see Table 50.2)
Inclusion body myositis	Distal, forearm and hands	Elevated myoglobin; ANA (+); myositis autoantibodies (see Table 50.2)
Rheumatologic disorders		
Rheumatoid arthritis	Local	Elevated rheumatoid factor, anti-CCP antibodies (+)
SLE	Proximal	ANA, anti-dsDNA antibodies, depressed C3 and C4
Genetic disorders		
Becker muscular dystrophy	Hip; proximal leg and arm	EMG, muscle biopsy
Limb–girdle muscular dystrophy	Variable, proximal limb, pelvic and shoulder girdle	EMG, muscle biopsy
Myotonic dystrophy	Distal greater than proximal, temporal and masseter wasting	EMG, muscle biopsy
Metabolic disorders		
Mitochondrial disease	Proximal	EMG, muscle biopsy
Glycogen and lipid storage	Proximal	EMG, muscle biopsy
Neurological disorders		
Cerebrovascular accident	Focal neurological signs	CT head
Motor neurone disease	Neurological signs	EMG
Demyelinating disorders	Variable	MRI, nerve conduction test
Guillain–Barré syndrome		
Multiple sclerosis		See Table 50.2
Botulism	Variable	
Lambert–Eaton		
Myasthenia gravis		

Figure 50.1 EMG report

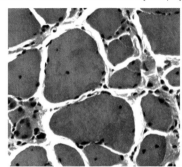

Figure 50.2 Muscle biopsy shows histological features of Duchenne muscular dystrophy

Key points

- If muscle weakness, or neuromuscular junction disorders are suspected, the key tests that help differentiate these mechanisms of weakness are neurophysiological studies.
- Elevated muscle enzymes (CK, lactate dehydrogenase) are consistent with myopathy but can also be high in neuropathies (reflecting muscle atrophy) and rhabdomyolysis.
- Muscle biopsy is the gold standard to diagnose myopathy or myositis.

Muscle weakness is a common presentation. It is important to distinguish muscle weakness from fatigue or exhaustion. Fatigue is the inability to continue performing a task after multiple repetitions; in contrast, a patient with muscle weakness is unable to perform the first repetition of the task. The causes of muscle weakness are listed in Table 50.1.

The first step in the investigation of muscle weakness is to determine the level of the neuromuscular pathway that is compromised. History and examination can usually differentiate between peripheral neuropathy, neuromuscular junction disorders and myopathy. Muscle weakness can occur with systemic disorders such as endocrine disorders or electrolyte disturbance.

Clinical Investigations at a Glance, First Edition. Jonathan Gleadle, Jordan Li and Tuck Yong. © 2017 John Wiley & Sons, Ltd. Published 2017 by John Wiley & Sons, Ltd.

Investigations for muscle disorders

Initial investigations aim to identify any reversible causes of myopathy. Basic laboratory tests include serum electrolytes, including calcium, phosphate and magnesium; glucose and thyroid function tests should be routinely performed.

Creatine kinase (CK) level should be checked. A persistently elevated CK level usually indicates myositis, a muscular dystrophy or recurrent rhabdomyolysis. However, it is not specific for myopathy because it can be influenced by muscle mass, or recent physical exercise. Furthermore, CK can be elevated in some neuropathies and systemic diseases, such as hypothyroidism and hypokalaemia. Slightly elevated CK levels can be found in some families without an obvious underlying cause, often referred to as familial hyperCKaemia, which has a benign prognosis. CK can be normal in some myopathies; a normal CK does not exclude muscle disease.

In patients with suspected immune-mediated myopathies, CRP, rheumatoid factor, anti-CCP antibodies, ANA and myositis-specific antibodies (Table 50.2) should be tested.

Electromyography (EMG)

EMG can distinguish myopathies from motor neuropathies, anterior horn cell and neuromuscular junction disorders (Figure 50.1). EMG assesses different aspects of muscle activity: the spontaneous activity of the muscle, its response to the insertion of a probe, the character of the individual motor unit action potentials and the rapidity with which additional motor units are recruited in response to an electrical signal. In inflammatory myopathy, there is increased spontaneous activity with the presence of fibrillations, complex repetitive discharges and positive sharp waves. EMG can also identify myotonic disorders when the insertion of the electrode may trigger an extended series of repetitive discharges lasting up to 30 seconds.

Muscle imaging

Muscle MRI is a non-invasive tool in the assessment of skeletal muscle disorders, especially for deep muscles not readily accessible to EMG. MRI can identify the pattern of muscles involved and subclinical muscle involvement.

Muscle biopsy

Muscle biopsy is the gold-standard investigation for muscle weakness (Figure 50.2). A muscle biopsy is undertaken when diagnosis remains inconclusive after non-invasive investigations have been completed. The best muscles to biopsy are those moderately affected by the disease process but not diseased to the point of severe atrophy or necrosis. Common biopsy sites are the deltoid, biceps and quadriceps for proximal myopathies and the gastrocnemius for distal myopathies. The pathologic examination should focus on the histologic, histochemical, electron microscopic, genetic and biochemical changes in the affected muscle. Histology may show atrophic, degenerating and regenerating muscle fibres, or it may confirm the specific diagnosis such as ragged red fibres in mitochondrial myopathies.

Investigations for neuromuscular junction disorders

Myasthenia gravis (MG) is an autoimmune disorder of neuromuscular junctions characterised by fatigable weakness. It is caused by antibodies against the postsynaptic acetylcholine receptor. Any muscle group can be affected in MG, but typically patients present with ocular symptoms, namely diplopia and ptosis. Fatigability can be elicited by watching for ptosis during sustained up gaze.

Lambert–Eaton myasthenic syndrome is an autoimmune disease in which autoantibodies are directed against the presynaptic voltage-gated calcium channels. It can occur sporadically or as a paraneoplastic syndrome, usually due to small cell lung cancer.

Ice cooling test

In patients with ptosis, the ice test is a simple first-line test. This distinguishes MG from other causes of ptosis. It involves application of crushed ice in a latex glove to the eye for 3 minutes. In MG this leads to improvement of ptosis and has a sensitivity and specificity of >90%.

Laboratory investigations

MG is a clinical diagnosis supported by serological and electrophysiological tests. The presence of antibodies to the acetylcholine receptor (AchR) or to muscle-specific tyrosine kinase (MuSK) is highly specific (99%) for MG. About 85% of patients with generalised MG have antibodies to the AchR and up to 50% of patients with ocular MG. If the result is negative or equivocal, test for MuSK antibodies and up to 70% of AchR seronegative generalised MG will be positive. CK levels are usually normal in MG. Serological testing for voltage-gated calcium channel antibodies is positive in 85% of patients with Lambert–Eaton syndrome.

Neurophysiological studies

Electrophysiology tests are generally normal in MG and the diagnosis may be missed if repetitive nerve stimulation (RNS) and single-fibre electromyography (SFEMG) tests are not requested. RNS is specific for MG, but the sensitivity is only 70%, and lower in disease that is purely ocular. SFEMG is a selective recording technique that allows identification of action potentials from individual muscle fibres. It is more sensitive (92–100%) than RNS for MG but is not specific. In Lambert–Eaton syndrome, electrophysiological studies show decreased amplitude of motor nerve. RNS is normal at low frequency (1–3 Hz). At high frequency (20, 30 and 50 Hz), an incremental increase in amplitude is seen after exercise.

Imaging

About 10% of patients with MG have a thymoma. CT of the chest is required in all patients with a diagnosis of MG. Some 50–70% of patients with Lambert–Eaton syndrome have associated cancers, most commonly small cell lung cancer. Therefore, CT chest is required.

Table 50.2 Common auto-antibodies in myositis

Myositis-specific antibodies	Disease association
Anti-tRNA synthetases: Anti-Jo-1, Anti-PL-7, Anti-PL-12, Anti-OJ, Anti-EJ	Antisynthetase syndrome (in polymyositis or dermatomyositis)
Anti-signal recognition particle	Necrotising autoimmune myositis
Anti-Mi-2	Dermatomyositis
Anti-MDAS	Dermatomyositis
Anti-TIF1 (Anti-155/140)	Dermatomyositis with higher risk of malignancy
Anti-NXP-2	Juvenile dermatomyositis
Anti-HMG-CoA reductase	Statin-induced necrotising autoimmune myositis
Anti-cytosolic 5'-nucleotidase 1A (NT5C1A)	Sporadic inclusion body myositis
Anti-PM/SCL	Polymyositis, dermatomyositis, scleroderma
Anti-U1RNP	Overlap syndrome (SLE, systemic sclerosis and mixed connective tissue disease)
Anti-RNA polymerase	Overlap syndrome
Anti-TH/TO	Overlap syndrome (systemic sclerosis)

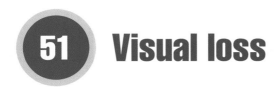

51 Visual loss

The purpose of investigations in vision loss is to:
- Determine the pattern and severity of vision loss
- Determine the cause of the vision loss
- Identify risk factors contributing the aetiology of the vision loss

Table 51.2 The common causes of gradual vision loss

Cataract
Age-related macular degeneration
Glaucoma
Diabetic retinopathy
Hypertension
Optic atrophy
Slow retinal detachment
Choroidal melanoma

Table 51.1 The common causes of acute vision loss and suggested investigations

Cause	Investigations
Common causes and investigations for acute loss of vision without eye pain	
Central retinal artery or vein occlusion	Risk factors, clinical assessment
Ischaemic optic neuropathy due to temporal arteritis	CRP, ESR, temporal artery biopsy
Amaurosis fugax (transient ischaemic attack)	CT or MRI of brain, carotid ultrasound
Retinal detachment	Clinical assessment
Macular haemorrhage due to macular degeneration	Clinical assessment
Vitreous haemorrhage due to diabetic retinopathy or trauma	Clinical assessment and possible ultrasound
Functional vision loss	
Common causes and investigations for acute loss of vision with eye pain	
Acute angle-closure glaucoma	Ophthalmologic assessment
Optic neuritis	MRI of the brain
Endophthalmitis	Ophthalmologic assessment, cultures of anterior chamber and vitreous fluids
Corneal ulcer	Ophthalmologic assessment
Anterior uveitis	Ophthalmologic assessment

Symptoms and signs in patients with chronic vision loss that requires urgent ophthalmologist referral:

- Sudden deterioration of vision
- Painful eye, especially with eye movement
- Visual field defect
- Abnormality of the retina or optic disk
- Systemic diseases that can cause progressive retinopathy, such as diabetes, malignant hypertension
- Patients with HIV/AIDS or receiving immunosuppressants

Key points

- Acute visual loss should be investigated with FBC, biochemistry, coagulation profile, ESR or CRP, lipid profile, ECG, echocardiography and carotid Doppler ultrasound according to the clinical context.
- Fluorescein angiography is helpful for detecting embolic retinal vascular occlusion.
- Radiological imaging is useful to determine the underlying cause of gradual visual loss.

Clinical Investigations at a Glance, First Edition. Jonathan Gleadle, Jordan Li and Tuck Yong. © 2017 John Wiley & Sons, Ltd. Published 2017 by John Wiley & Sons, Ltd.

Loss of vision is an alarming symptom and may be unilateral or bilateral. Unilateral visual loss is either due to a lesion of the eye itself or between the eye and the optic chiasm. Loss of vision can be sudden or gradual. Loss of vision is usually considered acute if it develops within a few minutes to a couple of days. Visual loss can be defined into two categories of severity:

1 Legal blindness is defined as a visual acuity (VA) worse than 6/60 and/or a visual field of <10° in the better eye.

2 Visual impairment is defined as a VA worse than 6/12 and/or a visual field of <20° in the better eye or a homonymous hemianopia.

Acute visual loss

Acute loss of vision has three general causes: (1) opacification of normally transparent structures through which light rays pass to reach the retina (e.g. cornea, vitreous); (2) retinal abnormalities; (3) abnormalities affecting the optic nerve or visual pathways. The common causes of acute visual loss and suggested investigations are listed in Table 51.1. History and general examination are vital, and a detailed ophthalmological examination, including assessment of VA, visual fields and fundoscopy, is required.

Laboratory investigations

These should include FBC and coagulation studies. Lipid profile should be assessed in patients with an ischaemic aetiology. If giant cell arteritis is suspected, patients should have ESR or CRP measured (see Chapter 152), and be referred urgently for ophthalmology review and initiation of steroids.

Radiological investigations

Patients with transient monocular blindness (amaurosis fugax) are at increased risk of stroke. Prompt evaluation of the carotid artery and heart (e.g. echocardiography, carotid Doppler) for embolic source is necessary. Carotid duplex ultrasound provides information on the degree of stenosis. Echocardiography can detect abnormal valves and dyskinetic wall segments that predispose to the formation of emboli. Ulceration is more difficult to detect noninvasively than invasively, so angiography remains the diagnostic gold standard for detecting carotid atherosclerotic disease.

Fluorescein angiography is helpful for detecting embolic retinal vascular occlusion. The most common embolic particles are cholesterol crystals, which are often small; they disappear rapidly but not without damaging the vessel wall. Fluorescein angiography may show hyperfluorescent crystals or areas of fluorescein leakage that are caused by crystal-related endothelial damage. Other causes of vascular occlusion include small vessel vasculitis or retinal infection (e.g. toxoplasmosis, fungal infection) and require systemic workup.

Cardiac investigations

An ECG is performed to assess the cardiac rhythm. Holter monitoring is the preferred method to screen for intermittent cardiac arrhythmias.

Other investigations

Temporal artery biopsy can be performed to rule out giant cell arteritis. The risk of missing the diagnosis of giant cell arteritis often outweighs the minor inconvenience of this slightly invasive procedure.

Gradual visual loss

Common causes of gradual loss of vision are listed in Table 51.2. Patients should be routinely screened for visual impairment. Routine eye examinations with dilated fundus should be performed in persons with diabetes every 2 years to identify and prevent progression of retinopathy. Many patients with diabetes will have additional risk factors, necessitating yearly screening.

Colour vision is more decreased in patients with optic nerve disorders than in those with retinal disorders. Colour vision is profoundly decreased compared with VA in patients with compressive and ischaemic optic neuropathy.

Evaluation of the optic disc during retinal examination may yield useful information. Optic disc changes can present with temporal pallor (as seen in toxic neuropathy and nutritional deficiency), focal pallor or bow-tie pallor (as seen in compression of the optic chiasma) and cupping (as seen in glaucoma). Visual field testing is also important in determining the site of a lesion involving the optic nerve head or visual pathways.

Laboratory investigations

Patients with diabetic and/or hypertensive retinopathy should have their FBC, HbA$_{1C}$ and lipid profile evaluated.

Radiological investigations

Different types of radiological studies can be performed to evaluate the different suspected disease processes:
- Ultrasound is recommended for neoplasms located in the orbit.
- B-scan ultrasound is recommended to look for optic sheath dilatation in papilloedema.
- CT or MRI is recommended to identify a cystic or solid lesion. For solid lesions, MRI (with contrast or fat suppression) is preferred in areas in close proximity to the bony wall.
- A non-contrast CT scan is preferred for peri-orbital fractures associated with trauma.
- A gadolinium-enhanced MRI with fluid-attenuated inversion recovery sequence is useful to detect multiple sclerosis lesions.

Retinal imaging

Traditionally fundus fluorescein angiography is performed to assess age-related macular degeneration, but it is an invasive investigation. Optical coherence tomography (OCT) is a non-invasive optical imaging method using near-infrared light and interferometric analysis, allowing visualisation of the retinal microarchitecture. It is used for early diagnosis of wet age-related macular degeneration and to guide management, particularly the need for retreatment.

Structural change of the optic disc with glaucoma can be detected with OCT or scanning laser polarimetry. For the diagnosis of angle-closure glaucoma, the anterior chamber angle is assessed with gonioscopy.

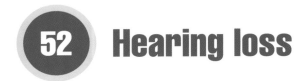

52 Hearing loss

The goals of investigation in hearing loss are:
- To determine objectively whether there is a hearing loss
- To determine whether the hearing loss is unilateral versus bilateral; sudden versus progressive; complete versus partial; fluctuating versus constant
- To define whether the hearing loss is conductive or sensorineural
- To determine the underlying causes of hearing loss, which may be reversible

Table 52.1 Common causes of CHL and SNHL

CHL	SNHL
Outer ear	**Inner ear**
• Wax	• Idiopathic
• Foreign body	• Presbycusis – deafness of old age
• Otitis externa	• Noise-induced – prolonged exposure to high noise level
Middle ear	• Congenital
• Acute or chronic otitis media	• Ménière's disease
• Otitis media with effusion	• Late otosclerosis
• Barotrauma	• Drug-induced – aminoglycosides, quinine
• Otosclerosis	• Infections – CMV, mumps, herpes zoster, meningitis
• Tympanic membrane perforation	• Acoustic neuroma
• Agenesis of the middle ear	• Head injury
• Tumours of the middle ear	• Paget's disease of the bone
	• Psychogenic

Figure 52.1 Otoscope examination

Figure 52.2 Otoscope examination shows otitis media with perforation and pus discharge

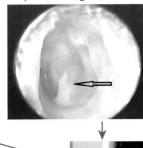

Figure 52.3 Tuning fork test

Routine laboratory testing is not recommended. Laboratory studies should be directed by clinical findings

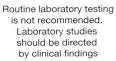

Figure 52.5 Audiogram

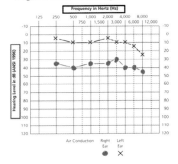

Figure 52.4 Audiometer

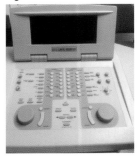

Figure 52.6 MRI of the head shows a cerebellopontine angle tumour

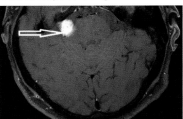

Key points

- Screen persons older than 65 years for hearing loss during periodic health examinations.
- Older patients who report hearing loss should have a formal audiometry test.
- A pure tone audiogram is the initial test and it will determine whether there is any hearing loss, the degree and the type of loss (conductive loss versus sensorineural loss). Tympanometry assesses tympanic membrane mobility and middle ear function.
- MRI with gadolinium is recommended for patients presenting with idiopathic sudden SNHL to identify those with serious underlying conditions.

Hearing loss is a common presenting symptom. Approximately 25% of people aged 65–74 years are estimated to have impaired hearing. For people over 75 years, this incidence rises to 40–50%. Hearing loss can be classified as conductive, sensorineural or mixed hearing loss.

• Conductive hearing loss (CHL) occurs in the external and middle ear due to interference with transmission of sound to the inner ear. Many causes (Table 52.1) can be treated successfully with surgery.

• Sensorineural hearing loss (SNHL) occurs in the inner ear (sensory) or auditory nerve/auditory pathway (neural). Many SNHLs are permanent because the human inner ear and hair cells have limited ability to regenerate.

Sudden onset of hearing loss (SOHL) is defined when there is a 30 dB or greater hearing loss over less than 72 hours. The vast majority of cases of SOHL loss are unilateral and the prognosis for some recovery of hearing is good; bilateral involvement is rare, and simultaneous bilateral involvement is very rare. Presbycusis refers to sensorineural hearing impairment in older adults. Typically, presbycusis involves bilateral high-frequency hearing loss associated with difficulty in speech discrimination and central auditory processing of information.

Clinical investigation

A thorough history and physical examination are essential prior to the investigation. Several systemic illnesses, such as granulomatosis with polyangiitis, can feature hearing loss as a complication.

Otoscope examination

An otoscope (Figure 52.1) can identify or rule out disorders of the outer ear and middle ear disorders (Figure 52.2) involving the tympanic membrane, such as such as otitis media or a foreign body. A microbiological swab of discharge in otitis externa is useful to direct antibiotic therapy.

Tuning fork tests

These tests help to differentiate the type of hearing loss. A 512 Hz tuning fork provides the most reliable response (Figure 52.3). The Rinne test is normal (positive) if air conduction persists twice as long as bone conduction. If bone conduction is better than air conduction, this suggests CHL and referred to as a 'negative test'. In the Weber test, sound should radiate to both ears equally. If sound lateralises to one ear, it indicates ipsilateral CHL or contralateral SNHL.

Audiometry

Audiometric testing is important and can assess the degree of hearing loss and whether hearing loss is conductive, sensorineural or mixed (Figures 52.4 and 52.5).

Pure tone audiometry: while the patient is wearing headphones, various tones of different frequencies varying from 250 to 8000 Hz are played at different volumes, and the threshold is determined at the lowest level at which tones can be detected 50% of the time. Normal hearing has a threshold of 0–20 dB.

Speech audiometry: the speech threshold is the lowest level at which the patient can repeat 50% of words. A recorded word list is supplied to the patient through the audiometer at increasing loudness levels, and the score is plotted on a graph. The word discrimination score can be helpful to decide whether a hearing aid would be useful. It is usually tested at a level 40 dB above the speech threshold.

Oto-acoustic emissions (OAEs) are faint sounds produced by hair cells in the cochlea, and a microphone sealed in the external ear canal can detect them. Their absence can confirm SNHL. They are used to screen neonates and infants. OAEs may also be a useful test to monitor recovery from damage due to ototoxic drugs. OAE testing can provide information about cochlear function, and the auditory brainstem response can be used to assess auditory nerve function.

Diagnostic testing for presbycusis: audiometric testing with pure-tone average and speech discrimination forms the basis of diagnostic testing for presbycusis. The need for additional testing can usually be determined from the audiometric test results. For example, individuals with asymmetric hearing loss (i.e. more than 10 dB difference at any two consecutive frequencies) and individuals with a conductive component require further evaluation.

Laboratory investigations

Routine laboratory testing is not recommended. Laboratory studies should be directed by clinical findings, and one or some of the following tests can be considered:

• FBC and differential, CRP for infection;

• fluorescent treponemal antibody-absorption for syphilis;

• ANA, anti-neutrophil cytoplasmic antibody, and rheumatoid factor for autoimmune diseases and/or vasculitis;

• viral (HIV, CMV, HSV mumps, rubella) serology and/or PCR;

• thyroid function test;

• fasting glucose for diabetes mellitus and lipid studies for hyperlipidaemia.

Radiological investigations

MRI with gadolinium enhancement of the internal acoustic meatus and brain is essential for investigating unilateral or asymmetrical SNHLs. Approximately 1–2% of patients with SOHL have internal auditory canal or cerebellopontine angle tumours (Figure 52.6). Conversely, 3–12% of patients with vestibular schwannomas present with SOHL. It may also identify other diagnoses relevant to the SNHL, such as demyelination, typically seen in multiple sclerosis, and small vessel ischaemic changes.

CT scans are not recommended in patients with presumptive SNHL. CT of the temporal bones and head can be used in patients with contraindications to MRI. A CT can exclude large acoustic neuromas in SNHL, and can evaluate the middle ear/ossicular chain in CHL.

Vestibular testing (video nystagmography, rotary chair) should be considered when hearing loss is associated with vertigo.

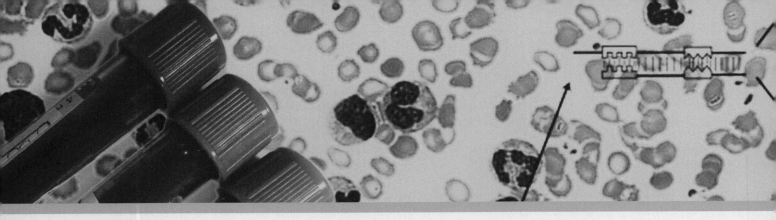

Chapters

Conditions

53 Heart failure

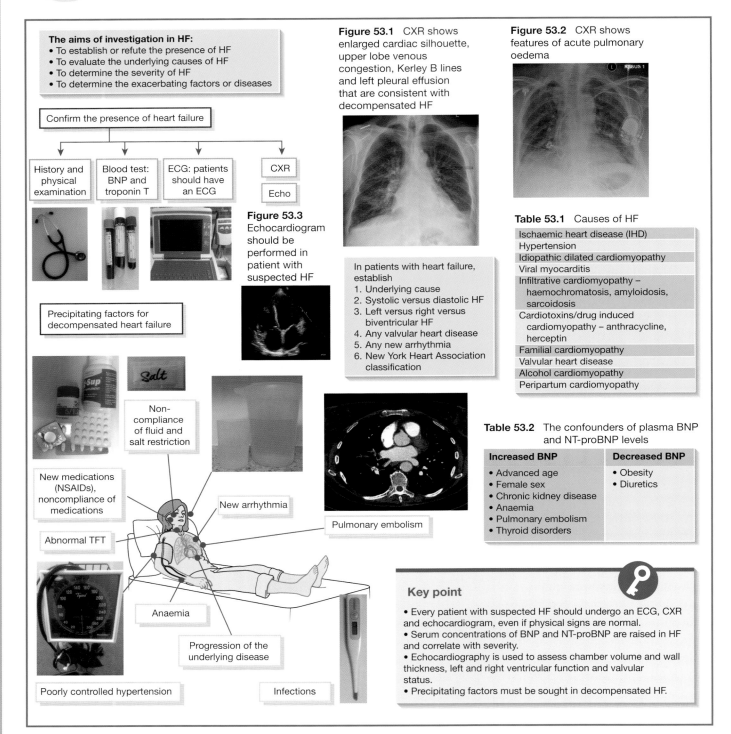

The aims of investigation in HF:
- To establish or refute the presence of HF
- To evaluate the underlying causes of HF
- To determine the severity of HF
- To determine the exacerbating factors or diseases

Confirm the presence of heart failure

History and physical examination

Blood test: BNP and troponin T

ECG: patients should have an ECG

CXR

Echo

Figure 53.3 Echocardiogram should be performed in patient with suspected HF

Precipitating factors for decompensated heart failure

Non-compliance of fluid and salt restriction

New medications (NSAIDs), noncompliance of medications

Abnormal TFT

New arrhythmia

Anaemia

Progression of the underlying disease

Poorly controlled hypertension

Infections

Pulmonary embolism

Figure 53.1 CXR shows enlarged cardiac silhouette, upper lobe venous congestion, Kerley B lines and left pleural effusion that are consistent with decompensated HF

In patients with heart failure, establish
1. Underlying cause
2. Systolic versus diastolic HF
3. Left versus right versus biventricular HF
4. Any valvular heart disease
5. Any new arrhythmia
6. New York Heart Association classification

Figure 53.2 CXR shows features of acute pulmonary oedema

Table 53.1 Causes of HF

Ischaemic heart disease (IHD)
Hypertension
Idiopathic dilated cardiomyopathy
Viral myocarditis
Infiltrative cardiomyopathy – haemochromatosis, amyloidosis, sarcoidosis
Cardiotoxins/drug induced cardiomyopathy – anthracycline, herceptin
Familial cardiomyopathy
Valvular heart disease
Alcohol cardiomyopathy
Peripartum cardiomyopathy

Table 53.2 The confounders of plasma BNP and NT-proBNP levels

Increased BNP	Decreased BNP
• Advanced age	• Obesity
• Female sex	• Diuretics
• Chronic kidney disease	
• Anaemia	
• Pulmonary embolism	
• Thyroid disorders	

Key point
- Every patient with suspected HF should undergo an ECG, CXR and echocardiogram, even if physical signs are normal.
- Serum concentrations of BNP and NT-proBNP are raised in HF and correlate with severity.
- Echocardiography is used to assess chamber volume and wall thickness, left and right ventricular function and valvular status.
- Precipitating factors must be sought in decompensated HF.

Clinical Investigations at a Glance, First Edition. Jonathan Gleadle, Jordan Li and Tuck Yong. © 2017 John Wiley & Sons, Ltd. Published 2017 by John Wiley & Sons, Ltd.

Heart failure (HF) is an abnormality of cardiac function leading to failure of the heart to pump blood at a rate required to perfuse the tissues of the body. HF can be classified as acute pulmonary oedema, decompensated HF and stable HF. In a least half of patients with HF it is associated with evidence of left ventricular systolic dysfunction (ejection fraction EF ≤40%). HF with preserved EF (HF-PEF) is also called diastolic HF.

The cardinal symptoms of HF (e.g. breathlessness and fatigue) and signs (e.g. peripheral oedema) are non-specific. Other symptoms, such as orthopnoea and paroxysmal nocturnal dyspnoea and signs such as jugular venous distension, cardiac enlargement and a third heart sound, have 70–90% specificity for diagnosis but only 11–55% sensitivity.

HF is a clinical syndrome and it should never be the final diagnosis. A cause of HF must be sought in all cases (Table 53.1). IHD is the cause in two-thirds of patients with systolic HF.

Laboratory investigations

FBC: Anaemia may precipitate HF or provide an alternative reason for dyspnoea. Neutrophilia may suggest an infective precipitant for decompensated HF.

Serum electrolytes and creatinine: Advanced renal impairment may cause or be associated with decompensated HF, a syndrome called cardio-renal syndrome. Patients with hyponatraemia and renal dysfunction in the setting of HF have a worse prognosis. Baseline kidney function is essential in monitoring diuretic therapy. Check blood glucose and hyperlipidaemia.

Iron study: Iron deficiency is common in patients with chronic HF, relates to disease severity, and is a strong and independent predictor of outcome regardless of anaemia.

LFTs: Abnormal tests with an obstructive pattern may indicate hepatic congestion resulting from right ventricular failure.

TFTs: Thyrotoxicosis can cause HF and is frequently associated with rapid atrial fibrillation. Hypothyroidism may also present as HF.

Cardiac markers: Troponins T and I are markers of myocyte injury and have improved the diagnosis and risk stratification with acute coronary syndromes. Modest elevation of cardiac troponin levels is often found in patients with HF without ischaemia. Troponin measurements (especially high-sensitivity assay) are a predictor of outcome in hospitalised patients with acute decompensated HF.

Serum natriuretic peptides: Serum concentration of B-type natriuretic peptide (BNP) and N-terminal pro-BNP (NT-proBNP) are raised in HF and correlate with severity. BNP >100 pg/mL and NT-proBNP >900 pg/mL each have a 90% sensitivity for the diagnosis of HF. Both are prognostic predictors of mortality and adverse cardiovascular events. The confounders of plasma BNP and NT-proBNP are summarised in Table 53.2.

Clinical utility of BNP or NT-proBNP includes supporting or excluding the existence of HF in patients presenting with acute dyspnoea and ambiguous signs and symptoms of HF; the negative predictive value is >90%. Screening for cardiac dysfunction in asymptomatic patients is not recommended.

Initial investigations for suspected heart failure

Every patient with suspected HF should undergo an ECG, CXR and echocardiogram, even if physical signs are normal.

ECG: An ECG provides useful information about heart rhythm and electrical conduction that may be the causative or contributing factors for HF. ECG changes are commonly seen in patients with HF. The negative predictive value of a normal ECG to exclude left ventricular systolic dysfunction exceeds 90%. On the other hand, the presence of anterior Q waves and a left bundle branch block or myocardial ischaemia (ST-segment depression) in patients with IHD are good predictors of a decreased EF.

CXR: Can reveal features suggestive of HF, such as cardiomegaly, pulmonary oedema, pleural effusions and upper lobe diversion, and exclude other causes of breathlessness (Figures 53.1 and 53.2).

Echocardiography: The imaging modality of choice in confirming the diagnosis and assessing the severity of HF (Figure 53.3). It can be used to assess chamber volume, wall thickness, left ventricular systolic and diastolic function, right ventricular function and valvular status.

Systolic function of the left ventricle is quantified by measuring left ventricular EF (LVEF). An LVEF above 50% is normal, with degrees of severity being mild (40–50%), moderate (30–40%) or severe (<30%). Regional variation in left ventricular wall motion, either at rest or during stress, is strongly suggestive of IHD. Establishing a diagnosis of HF-PEF can be challenging and requires the following:

1 signs or symptoms of heart failure
2 normal systolic left ventricular function;
3 evidence of diastolic left ventricular dysfunction by echocardiography or by left ventricular end-diastolic pressure mean pulmonary capillary wedge pressure measurement.

Exercise or pharmacological stress echocardiography may be useful for detecting ischaemia as a cause of dysfunction and in determining the viability of akinetic myocardium.

Further investigation

Cardiac MRI

Cardiac MRI may be useful in patients for whom echocardiographic images are suboptimal or the aetiology of HF remains unclear. It is helpful when inflammatory and infiltrative diseases are suspected. Cardiac MRI provides the most accurate and reproducible measures of volume, mass and wall motion.

Coronary angiography

Coronary angiography should be considered for evaluating the presence of coronary artery disease, especially if the patient is a potential revascularisation candidate. Monitoring of haemodynamic parameters by means of a Swan–Ganz catheter may be useful in directing treatment in selected patients. Endomyocardial biopsy may be useful in selected patients with unexplained HF.

Other investigations

Routine screening for haemochromatosis, HIV, amyloid and familial cardiomyopathy is not recommended if clinical history is not suggestive. Measurements of lung function are of little value in diagnosing HF. However, they are useful in excluding respiratory causes of breathlessness. Coexisting conditions are common in patients with HF and may influence prognosis and affect treatment decisions.

54 Peripheral arterial disease

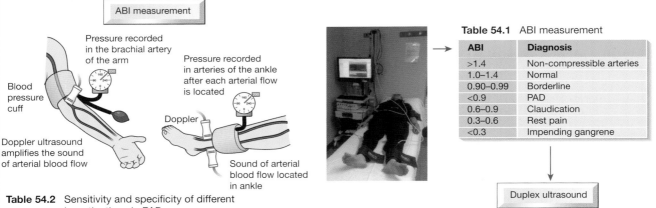

ABI measurement

Pressure recorded
in the brachial artery
of the arm

Pressure recorded
in arteries of the ankle
after each arterial flow
is located

Blood
pressure
cuff

Doppler

Doppler ultrasound
amplifies the sound
of arterial blood flow

Sound of arterial
blood flow located
in ankle

Table 54.1 ABI measurement

ABI	Diagnosis
>1.4	Non-compressible arteries
1.0–1.4	Normal
0.90–0.99	Borderline
<0.9	PAD
0.6–0.9	Claudication
0.3–0.6	Rest pain
<0.3	Impending gangrene

Duplex ultrasound

Table 54.2 Sensitivity and specificity of different
investigations in PAD

WHO classification	Sensitivity (%)	Specificity (%)
Edinburgh claudication questionnaire	56	>90
Examination: absence of both pedal pulses	72	>90
Examination: femoral bruit	28	>90
ABI	77	>95
Duplex arterial ultrasound	96	>95

Figure 54.1 (a) Normal peripheral arterial waveform. (b) Duplex ultrasound
shows high-velocity flow across stenosis (peak systolic velocity 3× compared
with adjacent segment)

(a)

(b)

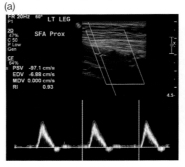
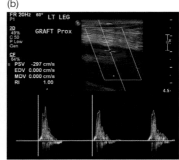

CTA or MRA, depending on renal function

Figure 54.2 CTA shows diffuse
narrowing by atherosclerotic
disease of the left superficial
femoral artery

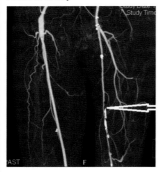

Figure 54.3 MRA showing right iliac
artery occlusion on the picture on the
left; the picture in the middle shows
bilateral superficial femoral artery
and tibial artery disease; picture on
the right shows tibial artery disease

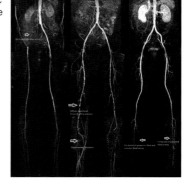

Figure 54.4 DSA of the left foot
shows patent anterior tibial and
posterior tibial artery at the level
of the ankle.

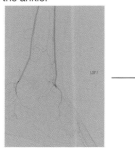

Investigate vascular risk factors

Full blood count

Anaemia, polycythaemia and thrombocytosis can
aggravate PAD.

Biochemistry, blood glucose level, lipid levels

May reveal diabetes and/or chronic kidney disease.
Lipid and glycaemic status is important to ensure
adequate management of these risk factors.

Thrombophilia screen

Patients <50 years of age should have a
thrombophilia screen and serum homocysteine
levels checked.

Electrocardiography

Key points

• ABI is a non-invasive and cost-effective method
of detecting PAD.
• Colour-assisted duplex arterial ultrasound is
non-invasive and can accurately define sites of
stenosis or occlusion.
• CTA and MRA both have good sensitivity and
specificity for diagnosing PAD, but the risks of
iodinated and gadolinium contrast need to be
considered.

Clinical Investigations at a Glance, First Edition. Jonathan Gleadle, Jordan Li and Tuck Yong. © 2017 John Wiley & Sons, Ltd. Published 2017 by John Wiley & Sons, Ltd.

Peripheral arterial disease (PAD) is a spectrum of disorders in which there is impairment of blood flow to the extremities usually as a result of atherosclerotic occlusive disease. Focal atherosclerotic stenoses develop with a predilection for anatomic sites in the distal abdominal aorta, iliac, femoral and infrapopliteal arteries. The patient can be asymptomatic or present with symptoms, including claudication, rest pain, ulcers or even gangrene. Both asymptomatic and symptomatic PAD patients have a high risk of death from cardiovascular disease. Mortality in claudicants at 5 years, 10 years and 15 years is 30%, 50% and 70% respectively, and 25% of critical limb ischaemia patients will die within a year of diagnosis.

Acute limb ischaemia is a sudden decrease in arterial perfusion in the limb, due to thrombotic or embolic causes and threatening limb viability, and requires urgent revascularisation.

Ankle–brachial index (ABI)

ABI is a symptom-independent, non-invasive and cost-effective method of detecting PAD. ABI is calculated by dividing the higher of the posterior tibial or dorsalis pedis artery systolic pressure in the one leg and the higher of the right and left brachial artery systolic pressure. The value of ABI and the probable diagnosis and severity of PAD is summarised in Table 54.1.

The diagnostic value of ABI is limited in diseases that cause arterial calcification and non-compressibility, such as in advanced diabetes mellitus, renal failure and the very elderly. The ABI is a strong marker of cardiovascular disease and is predictive of cardiovascular events and mortality.

Duplex arterial ultrasound

Colour-assisted duplex arterial ultrasound is non-invasive, non-expensive and is the first-line and often the only imaging required to plan endovascular interventions (Table 54.2). It is useful to define sites of stenosis or occlusion, and indicate the degree of stenosis and length of an occlusion (Figure 54.1).

CT angiography (CTA)

CTA (Figure 54.2) can be used to confirm and localise suspected PAD (especially where intervention is being considered) with good sensitivity and specificity compared with arteriography. Renal function must be checked before CTA is performed to prevent contrast nephropathy. Results can be difficult to interpret in the presence of heavily calcified arteries.

Magnetic resonance angiography (MRA)

Like CTA, MRA has good sensitivity and specificity for diagnosing PAD (Figure 54.3). Renal function should be assessed prior to MRA due to the association of nephrogenic systemic fibrosis with exposure to gadolinium in patients with renal insufficiency. Unlike CTA, MRA is not affected by vascular calcification. Previous arterial stents cause signal dropout, making assessments of patency or in-stent stenosis difficult.

Arteriography

While arteriography is the gold standard for imaging peripheral arteries, it is rarely used for diagnosis because of its invasive nature and the availability of other less invasive modalities, such as duplex ultrasonography, CTA or MRA. However, some surgeons still prefer arteriography for planning open revascularisation procedures. A catheter is introduced into the 'normal' femoral artery and guided retrogradely into the aorta. The risks of the procedure include haemorrhage, arterio-venous fistula and false aneurysm formation at the site of injection and subintimal tearing.

In acute lower limb ischaemia, arteriography will demonstrate whether embolism or thrombosis is the cause or whether there is an occluded popliteal aneurysm as well as show which distal vessels are patent.

Digital subtraction angiography (DSA)

DSA allows the electronic processing of the radiological image, 'subtracting' any bony image and enhancing the arteriographic profile and producing an image of contrast-filled vessels only. Large numbers of collaterals can be anatomically visualised quickly (Figure 54.4) and in one session compared to the challenge of mapping collaterals accurately with duplex ultrasound. It can also be used repeatedly for disease follow-up or for morphological screening of arteries where conventional arteriography might not be justified. However DSA lacks the resolution of conventional arteriography.

Investigating vascular risk factors

Inflammatory markers

Raised CRP may be suggestive of an inflammatory process, such as giant cell arteritis.

Biochemistry, fasting blood glucose level and lipid levels

Can reveal diabetes and renal impairment. Evaluation of lipid and glycaemic status is important to ensure adequate management of these risk factors in order to prevent the progression of atherosclerosis.

Thrombophilia screen

Patients under 50 years of age should also have a thrombophilia screen (Chapter 128) and serum homocysteine levels taken.

ECG

Some 60% of patients with intermittent claudication have ECG evidence of pre-existing coronary heart disease.

Screening

Screening for PAD using the ABI or questionnaire is currently not recommended and has not been shown to be beneficial in randomised controlled trials.

55 Infective endocarditis

In patients with features of infection, such as fever and known cardiac disease or new cardiac murmurs, always consider the diagnosis of IE

Antibiotics should be given after blood culture

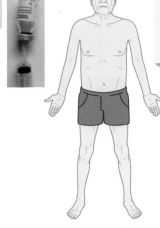

Figure 55.3 TTE shows normal mitral valve

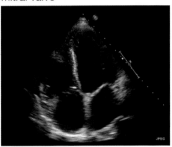

Key points

- Blood cultures should be performed before antibiotics in any patient suspected of having IE. The causative microorganism is identified in about 75% of cases of IE when the optimal blood culture techniques have been used.
- TTE should be performed in every patient with suspected IE.
- TOE has superior sensitivity and specificity and is recommended when the results of TTE are negative and there is a high clinical suspicion, the presence of prosthetic valves or an intracardiac device.

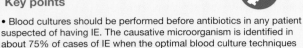

The most important test is blood culture.
Take three sets from both arms, and before antibiotics are given

Figure 55.1 Blood culture   **Figure 55.2** Blood culture positive for *S. aureus*

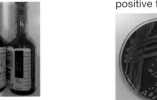

Figure 55.4 TTE shows vegetation in the mitral valve

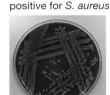

Box 55.1 Duke criteria for diagnosing IE

Major criteria
- Positive blood culture with typical IE microorganism, defined as one of the following.
- Typical microorganism consistent with IE from two separate blood cultures, as follows:
  – Viridans-group streptococci, or
  – *Streptococcus bovis*, including nutritional variant strains, or
  – *Haemophilus* species, *Aggregatibacter actinomycetemcomitans, Cardiobacterium hominis, Eikenella corrodens* and *Kingella kingae* (HACEK) group, or
  – *Staphylococcus aureus*, or
  – Community-acquired enterococci, in the absence of a primary focus.
- Microorganisms consistent with IE from persistently positive blood cultures, defined as:
  – Two positive cultures of blood samples drawn >12 hours apart, or
  – All of three or a majority of four separate cultures of blood (with first and last samples drawn 1 hour apart)
  – *Coxiella burnetii* detected by at least one positive blood culture or antiphase I immunoglobulin G antibody titre >1 : 800
- Evidence of endocardial involvement with positive echocardiogram, defined as:
  – Oscillating intracardiac mass on valve or supporting structures, in the path of regurgitant jets, or on implanted material in the absence of an alternative anatomic explanation, or
  – Abscess, or
  – New partial dehiscence of prosthetic valve or new valvular regurgitation (worsening or changing of pre-existing murmur not sufficient).

Minor criteria
- Predisposing factor: known cardiac lesion, recreational drug injection
- Fever >38 °C
- Evidence of embolism: arterial emboli, pulmonary infarcts, Janeway lesions, conjunctival haemorrhage
- Immunological problems: glomerulonephritis, Osler's nodes
- Positive blood culture (that does not meet a major criterion) or serologic evidence of infection with organism consistent with IE but not satisfying major criterion.

Figure 55.5 TOE shows vegetation on the mitral valve

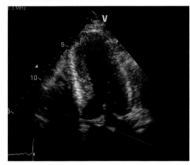

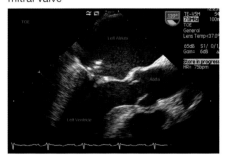

Clinical Investigations at a Glance, First Edition. Jonathan Gleadle, Jordan Li and Tuck Yong. © 2017 John Wiley & Sons, Ltd. Published 2017 by John Wiley & Sons, Ltd.

The annual incidence of infective endocarditis (IE) is three to nine cases per 100,000 of the population. The highest rates are observed among patients with prosthetic valves, intracardiac devices, unrepaired cyanotic congenital heart diseases or a previous history of IE. Other risk factors include chronic rheumatic heart disease and degenerative valvular heart lesions, haemodialysis and intravenous drug use. However, up to half of the cases of IE develop in patients with no prior history of valve disease. IE is a life-threatening disease with substantial morbidity and mortality (approximately 20%), and early diagnosis and treatment will have a significant impact on its outcomes.

In patients with features of infection, such as fever, and known cardiac disease or new cardiac murmurs, always consider the diagnosis of IE. It is critical to seek the presence of causative organisms in blood cultures.

The diagnosis of IE is generally dependent on clinical, microbiological and echocardiographic findings. For diagnosis, the Duke criteria can be applied; these have a sensitivity 72–80% and specificity of 80–90%. Clinically definite IE by the Duke criteria requires the presence of two major criteria, one major criterion and three minor criteria, or five minor criteria (Box 55.1). Fever is the commonest presenting feature (80%). Other presentations include sepsis, unexplained heart failure, septic pulmonary emboli, stroke, back pain, and acute peripheral arterial occlusion.

General investigations

Laboratory investigation

Routine blood testing will reveal a mild to moderate normochromic, normocytic anaemia in half of patients, a neutrophil leucocytosis in 90%, a raised CRP in 90% and haematuria on urinalysis in half of patients.

ECG

An ECG is mandatory for patients with suspected IE and is useful for assessing the extent and severity of the infection. The presence of significant conduction abnormalities demonstrated on the ECG may indicate the need for temporary pacing and is classically seen in the presence of aortic root abscesses due to *S. aureus* infection. Arrhythmias may be due to myocarditis or to ischaemia due to coronary emboli. Atrial fibrillation is common.

CXR

A CXR is useful to see whether there is evidence of cardiomegaly and heart failure. Furthermore, in tricuspid valve endocarditis in intravenous drug abusers or in patients with serious permanent pacemaker infection, infective pulmonary emboli and pulmonary abscesses may be demonstrated.

Microbiologic investigations

Identifying the microorganism involved in the IE is the most important step in diagnosing the condition and guiding antimicrobial treatment. Therefore, blood cultures (Figure 55.1) should be performed before the administration of antibiotics in any patient suspected of having IE. The microorganism is identified in about 75% of cases when the optimal blood culture techniques have been used.

Three sets of blood cultures should be obtained at intervals >1 hour within the first 24 hours before commencing antibiotic treatment. Optimal aseptic technique is essential to avoid false-positive cases due to contaminating organisms from the skin. Each set of blood cultures should be taken via a separate venepuncture, with at least 10 mL of blood into each bottle. If a stable patient has suspected IE but is already on antibiotic treatment, consideration should be given to stopping treatment and performing three sets of blood cultures off antibiotics. Streptococci and staphylococci account for 80% cases of IE (Figure 55.2), with proportions varying depending on the type of valve (native versus prosthetic), source of infection, patient age and coexisting conditions.

Blood culture can be negative in about 10% of IE cases, and the common causes include patients who have received antibiotics before a blood culture has been taken, cases in which IE may be caused by fastidious microorganisms and fungi, or when the endocarditis might be non-infectious (marantic or Libman–Sacks endocarditis).

Anatomical investigations

Echocardiography

Transthoracic echocardiography (TTE; Figures 55.3 and 55.4) should be performed in every patient with suspected IE. Transoesophageal echocardiography (TOE; Figure 55.5) has superior sensitivity and specificity and is recommended when the results of TTE are negative and there is a high clinical suspicion, poor imaging quality, and the presence of prosthetic valves or an intracardiac device.

Combined TTE and TOE shows vegetation in 90% of cases and valve regurgitation in 60%. In patients with negative findings on echocardiography, repeat examination should be performed if IE continues to be suspected. False-positive results from TTE or TOE studies may occur due to previous scarring, severe myxomatous change and even normal structures.

Multislice CT

ECG-gated CT offers an alternative cardiac imaging in patients suspected with IE. It provides more accurate anatomical information regarding the perivalvular extent of abscesses/pseudoaneurysms and the coronary bed.

Cardiac MRI

MRI has been used in identifying valvular and perivalvular damage in patients with IE. Cerebral complications that include ischaemic and haemorrhagic stroke, transient ischaemic attack, silent cerebral embolism, mycotic aneurysm, brain abscess and meningitis are the most severe and frequent extra-cardiac complications of IE. MRI seems to be of most value in the identification of silent cerebral complications.

56 Aortic disease

The aim of investigations:
- To confirm the diagnosis
- To provide detailed information for surgical intervention
  - tear location and disease extent
  - classification of aortic dissection
  - assess flow in false and true lumen
  - assess side branch involvement (including coronary arteries)
  - detect and grade aortic regurgitation
  - detect extravasation (periaortic or mediastinal haematoma, pleural or pericardial effusion)
- To assess myocardial ischaemia
- To assess organ failure due to impaired flow in abdominal arteries

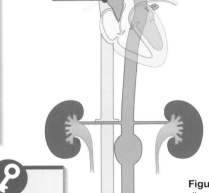

Type A ascending aorta is affected

Type B ascending aorta is not affected

All patients suspected to have aortic dissection should have an ECG and CXR

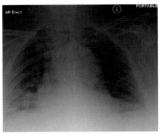

Figure 56.1 CXR shows a widened mediastinum

Key points

- In aortic dissection an ECG may be abnormal with 20% of patients with type A dissection having signs of acute ischaemia.
- A CXR is abnormal in over 60% of patients with aortic dissection, but the sensitivity and specificity of ECG and CXR are too low to definitively establish or exclude the diagnosis.
- CTA is usually the first choice for diagnostic imaging of suspected dissection, but echocardiography, MRI and angiography are all useful and accurate.
- Ultrasound is a cheap, non-invasive and reliable tool for diagnosing and measuring AAAs, but CT should be used if there is any suspicion of leakage from an AAA.

Figure 56.2 CT aortogram: (a) normal; (b) aortic dissection with true lumen and false lumen separated by an intimal flap

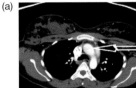
(a)

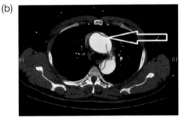
(b)

Table 56.1 The 12-month risk of rupture of an AAA according to diameter of aneurysm

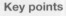

Diameter of AAA (cm)	Risk of rupture (%/year)
3.0–3.9	0
4.0–4.9	1
5.0–5.9	1–10
6.0–6.9	10–22
>7.0	30–50

Table 56.2 Indications for intervention in AAA

Men with AAA >5.5 cm
Women with AAA >5.0 cm
AAA growth >1.0 cm/year
Symptomatic AAA (pain, tenderness, distal embolisation)

Table 56.3 Recommended surveillance intervals of AAA

Diameter of AAA (cm)	Surveillance interval (months)
3.0–3.9	24
4.0–4.5	12
4.6–5.0	6
>5.0	3

Figure 56.3 TTE shows ascending aortic dissection

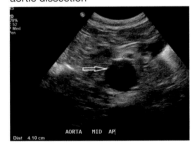

Figure 56.4 Ultrasound shows a 4.1 cm diameter AAA

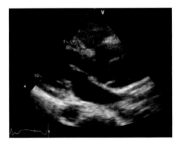

Figure 56.5 CT shows a 5.6 cm diameter infra-renal AAA

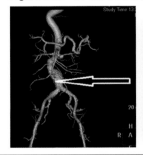
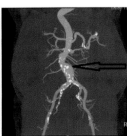
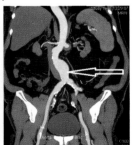

Clinical Investigations at a Glance, First Edition. Jonathan Gleadle, Jordan Li and Tuck Yong. © 2017 John Wiley & Sons, Ltd. Published 2017 by John Wiley & Sons, Ltd.

Aortic dissection is a tear in the intima of the aorta, which allows blood to enter the aortic wall, forming a haematoma that separates the intima from the adventitia and creates a false lumen. Mortality is high, with 20% of patients dying before reaching hospital and 30% during hospital admission.

In the Stanford classification, aortic dissection is categorised by the area affected:

- type A – ascending aorta affected;
- type B – ascending aorta not affected.

Although patients usually present with chest pain, the presentation of aortic dissection is diverse, and 10% do not experience pain. Hypotension or shock is seen in 25% of patients with acute type A dissection at presentation, while hypertension is a more common finding in those with type B dissection. A high index of suspicion is required, and early accurate diagnosis is important because urgent surgical intervention may be life-saving.

Initial investigations

An ECG **must** be performed in all suspected aortic dissection patients. This test helps to distinguish acute myocardial infarction (AMI), for which thrombolytic therapy may be life-saving, from aortic dissection, in which thrombolytic therapy may be detrimental. The dissecting membrane can extend into a coronary ostium, which may induce AMI with ECG changes. 20% of patients with type A dissection have ECG evidence of acute ischaemia. Patients with suspected aortic disease and ECG evidence of ischaemia must undergo diagnostic imaging before thrombolytic therapy is administered.

If the patient is stable, a CXR should be performed. The CXR is not sufficient to exclude aortic dissection, but an enlarged mediastinum may indicate an aortic dissection (Figure 56.1). A CXR is abnormal in 60–90% of cases of aortic dissection. Overall, the sensitivity and specificity of an ECG and CXR are too low to definitively establish or exclude the diagnosis.

Diagnostic imaging

CT angiography (CTA)

CTA is the first choice for diagnostic imaging. The study is relatively non-invasive and can confirm the diagnosis of aortic dissection (Figure 56.2). It can also reveal the extent of the dissection and the status of major vessels. CTA has a high sensitivity (96%) and specificity (98%).

Echocardiography

Transthoracic echocardiography (TTE)/transoesophageal echocardiography (TOE) can be performed in the intensive care unit or in the operating theatre. It can give an indication of site and extent of dissection, haemopericardium, pleural effusion, the aortic valve and left ventricular haemodynamics (Figure 56.3). However, it is limited in the assessment of the aortic arch. Sensitivity and specificity of TTE for ascending aorta dissection range from 77% to 80% and 93% to 96%, respectively.

MRI

MRI has the highest accuracy and sensitivity (98%) as well as specificity (nearly 100%) for detection of all forms of dissection. MRI is often reserved for patients with stable chronic aortic dissection for follow-up.

Angiography

Angiography has a sensitivity of 88% in the diagnosis of aortic dissection. It is rarely used because of the availability of other non-invasive modalities. Angiography is still recommended in patients in whom visceral malperfusion is suspected or percutaneous interventions are being considered, and angiography might form part of concurrent endovascular therapy.

Abdominal aortic aneurysms (AAA)

An aneurysm is a permanent and irreversible dilatation of an artery that is >1.5 times the expected diameter. Aneurysms are most commonly found in the abdominal aorta but may also occur in the thoracic aorta. AAA is rare in adults aged <50 years, but prevalence rises sharply with increasing age. AAA affects 4–7% of men and 1–2% of women over 65 years. Rupture of an aortic aneurysm is a catastrophic event with a very high mortality.

The 'normal' diameter of the abdominal aorta is 2 cm; it increases with age. An abdominal aneurysm is defined as an aortic diameter exceeding 3 cm. The natural history of AAA is ongoing expansion, with increased risk of rupture as the aneurysm enlarges (Table 56.1). Aneurysms <5.5 cm expand at an average rate of 2–3 mm each year, with a greater rate of expansion for larger aneurysms. Aneurysms >5.5 cm in men and >5.0 cm in women are at significant risk of rupture and should be considered for repair. AAAs arise from below the renal arteries, but can involve the renal ostia and arise supra-renally.

AAAs are often found incidentally as a pulsatile mass on abdominal examination, as calcification on plain AXR, CT or ultrasound scanning for other purposes.

Imaging investigation of AAAs

Ultrasound is a cheap, non-invasive and reliable tool for diagnosing and measuring AAAs (Figure 56.4). It can provide information on the relation of the aneurysm to the renal arteries and involvement of the iliac arteries. Obesity and bowel gas may limit visualisation, but an AAA can nearly always be confirmed or excluded by ultrasound.

CT is used to detect any leakage from an AAA in haemodynamically stable patients with an acute abdomen, to delineate anatomy for treatment planning either by surgery or endovascular intervention, and to monitor progress following treatment (Figure 56.5). It is the investigation of choice when considering surgical repair. Its limitations include the need for high doses of intravenous contrast which can cause contrast nephropathy in patients with CKD.

Screening with ultrasound in men over the age of 65 years has been demonstrated to reduce aneurysm-related mortality. The current indications for screening include:

- men ≥65 years old and women ≥70 years old with cardiovascular risk factors;
- men and women over 50 years of age with a family history of AAA.

Surveillance–The majority of AAAs detected by screening are below the threshold for intervention (Table 56.2) but will require surveillance, usually by ultrasound. Suggested surveillance intervals are listed in Table 56.3.

Ruptured AAA–A clinical diagnosis of ruptured AAA should be considered:

- in patients >50 years old presenting with abdominal/back pain and hypotension;
- in patients with a known AAA and symptoms of either abdominal/back pain or hypotension/collapse.

Urgent investigations including FBC, urea and electrolytes, amylase, cross-match, imaging.

57 Hypertension

The aims of investigation in hypertension:
- Confirm diagnosis of hypertension
- Identify end organ damage
- Assess the cardiovascular risk factors
- Exclude secondary causes

Basic blood tests
 Serum electrolyte, blood glucose level
 Serum creatinine
 Lipid study
Blood tests for screening secondary causes
 Renin : aldosterone ratio
 Plasma metanephrines
 Thyroid function test

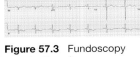

Figure 57.1 ECG shows left ventricular hypertrophy

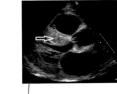

Figure 57.3 Fundoscopy examination shows hypertensive retinopathy

 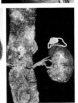

Figure 57.4 CT renal artery angiogram shows: (a) patent right renal artery; (b, c) left renal artery stenosis

(a) (b)

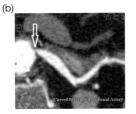

(c)

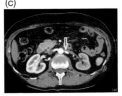

Urine microscopy examination

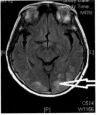

Figure 57.5 MRI brain shows posterior reversible encephalopathic changes

24 hours urine collection for
- proteinuria
- fractionated metanephrines
- cortisol level

Urine dipstick

Figure 57.2 Echocardiogram shows septal and left ventricular hypertrophy

Table 57.1 Target organ damage in hypertension

Target organ	Manifestations	Investigations
Heart	Left ventricular hypertrophy	12-lead ECG (Figure 57.1), echocardiography (Figure 57.2)
Eye	Retinopathy	Examine the fundi (Figure 57.3)
Kidney	Elevated urinary albumin CKD	Albumin : creatinine ratio Test for haematuria Serum electrolytes, creatinine, eGFR

Table 57.2 Suggestive symptoms and signs, investigations for the common causes of secondary hypertension

Cause	Symptoms and signs	Investigations
Renal artery stenosis	Renal bruit, history of flash pulmonary oedema, young females (fibromuscular dysplasia), history of atherosclerotic disease	• CT renal angiography (Figure 57.4) • Doppler ultrasound scan of renal arteries • MR angiography renal artery • Radionuclide renal perfusion scan
Renal parenchymal disease	Nocturia, oedema, raised serum creatinine	• Urine microscopy for haematuria • Measure proteinuria, nephritic, nephrotic, vasculitic screen • Renal ultrasound
Primary hyperaldosteronism	Fatigue, hypokalaemia	• Renin, aldosterone levels and aldosterone/renin ratio
Phaeochromocytoma	Flushing, headaches, labile BP, palpitations, sweating	• 24-hour urinary fractionated metanephrines • Plasma-free metanephrines
Cushing syndrome	Buffalo hump, central obesity, moon facies	• 24-hour urinary cortisol • Late-night salivary cortisol • Low-dose dexamethasone suppression
Thyroid disease	Weight loss or gain, bradycardia/tachycardia, cold/heat intolerance, constipation/diarrhoea	• Thyroxine, thyroid-stimulating hormone
Obstructive sleep apnoea	Apnoeic events during sleep, daytime sleepiness, snoring, obesity	• Polysomnography (sleep study)
Coarctation of the aorta	Arm to leg systolic BP difference >20 mmHg, delayed or absent femoral pulses, murmur	• MRI, echocardiography

Key points in investigating hypertension

- ABPM is useful to confirm the diagnosis of hypertension and exclude the possibility of 'white coat' hypertension.
- Investigate for secondary causes of hypertension in patients with severe, resistant or early-onset hypertension and in those with hypokalaemia.
- ECG, fundoscopy, urinalysis and echocardiography are useful in investigating any end-organ injury related to hypertension.

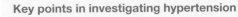

Clinical Investigations at a Glance, First Edition. Jonathan Gleadle, Jordan Li and Tuck Yong. © 2017 John Wiley & Sons, Ltd. Published 2017 by John Wiley & Sons, Ltd.

Hypertension is a persistent rise in arterial blood pressure (BP) that increases the risk for coronary heart disease, stroke, heart failure, peripheral vascular disease and renal failure. Hypertension is one of the most important preventable causes of premature morbidity and mortality.

Diagnosis

Diagnosis of hypertension is based on several BP measurements taken on separate days. If the patient's BP in clinic is persistently above 140/90 mmHg, the diagnosis of hypertension can be made. Ambulatory BP monitoring (ABPM) can confirm the diagnosis of hypertension and exclude the possibility of 'white coat' hypertension, where BP can be raised during a consultation but not on ABPM or at home. If a person is unable to tolerate ABPM, home BP monitoring (HBPM) is a suitable alternative to confirm the diagnosis of hypertension. When using HBPM to confirm a diagnosis of hypertension, ensure that two consecutive BP measurements are taken, at least 1 minute apart and with the person seated, and BP is recorded twice daily, in the morning and evening for 7 days.

The correlation between ABPM and those taken in the clinic is modest. Furthermore, the diagnosis of hypertension can be missed by office BP measurements in some patients who are truly hypertensive, referred to as masked hypertension.

Investigations for target organ damage and cardiovascular risk factors

Target organ damage in hypertension and the required investigations are summarised in Table 57.1. Evidence of target organ damage will help support a diagnosis of poorly controlled hypertension and may influence decisions about an appropriate treatment target. Patients with hypertension should have their glycaemic and lipid status assessed.

Investigations for secondary hypertension

Most patients have no clear aetiology and are classified as having essential hypertension. However, 5–10% patients have secondary hypertension, in which there is an underlying, potentially correctable aetiology. Secondary hypertension should be considered in patients with:
- resistant hypertension;
- symptoms and signs suggestive of secondary hypertension (Table 57.2);
- early or late onset of hypertension;
- severe hypertension.

And the following preliminary biochemical tests should be conducted:
- serum electrolytes, creatinine and eGFR;
- plasma glucose;
- plasma renin and aldosterone levels;
- 24-hour urinary metanephrine or normetanephrine (for phaeochromocytoma);
- urine analysis – micro- or macroalbuminuria.

Potentially treatable secondary causes and investigations for secondary hypertension are listed in Table 57.2.

Resistant hypertension

Resistant (or refractory) hypertension is BP that is persistently higher than target (>140/90 mmHg, or >130/80 mmHg for patients with diabetes or CKD) despite prescription of three different antihypertensive drug classes at optimal or best tolerated doses, including a diuretic. Before a patient is considered to have treatment-resistant hypertension, apparent or pseudo-resistant hypertension must be excluded. This is where there is inadequate BP control in a patient receiving appropriate treatment who does not actually have resistant hypertension. Most often, pseudo-resistant hypertension arises from (a) poor office BP measurement technique, (b) the 'white-coat' effect, (c) poor patient adherence with prescribed therapy, (d) suboptimal antihypertensive regimen or (e) excessive consumption of sodium, liquorice or alcohol.

Hypertensive emergencies

A hypertensive emergency (formerly called 'malignant hypertension') is defined as severe hypertension (BP ≥180/110 mmHg) with an acute impairment of one or more organ systems (especially the central nervous system, cardiovascular system and/or the renal system). Immediate BP reduction (not necessarily to normal values) is required to prevent or limit target-organ damage.

Hypertensive encephalopathy is defined as delirium (acute encephalopathy) occurring as a result of failure of the upper limit of cerebral vascular autoregulation. Clinical features of this disorder include acute or subacute onset of lethargy, confusion, headache, visual disturbance (including blindness) and seizures. If not adequately treated, hypertensive encephalopathy can progress to cerebral haemorrhage, coma and death. MRI of the brain may show characteristic posterior reversible encephalopathic changes affecting the white matter of the parietal–occipital regions (Figure 57.5). The changes on imaging are usually bilateral, but they can be asymmetrical.

Important immediate investigations include measurement of FBC (including peripheral blood smear for evidence of haemolysis), electrolytes, urea, creatinine and urinalysis. An ECG and CXR should be performed. CT or MRI head can be considered in the presence of neurological symptoms and signs.

58 Hyperlipidaemia

Performing a risk factor analysis prior to obtaining screening blood test results is recommended

Table 58.1 Major classes of lipoprotein

Lipoprotein	Primary functions	Composition	Apo-proteins		
Chylomicrons	Exogenous triglycerides	90% triglycerides	A, B	Triglyceride rich	Atherogenic
Very low density lipoprotein (VLDL)	Endogenous triglycerides	55% triglycerides	B, C, E		
Intermediate density lipoprotein	Transient form	—	—		
Low-density lipoprotein (LDL)	Transport cholesterol to tissue	55% cholesterol	B	Cholesterol rich	
High-density lipoprotein (HDL)	Transport cholesterol from tissue to liver	50% proteins	A, C, E		Anti-atherogenic

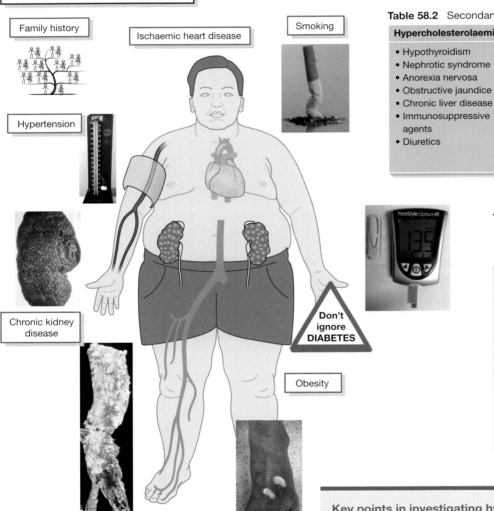

Family history

Ischaemic heart disease

Smoking

Hypertension

Chronic kidney disease

Peripheral vascular disease

Don't ignore DIABETES

Obesity

Gout

Table 58.2 Secondary causes of hyperlipidaemia

Hypercholesterolaemia	Hypertriglyceridaemia
• Hypothyroidism	• Obesity
• Nephrotic syndrome	• Uncontrolled diabetes mellitus
• Anorexia nervosa	• Chronic kidney disease
• Obstructive jaundice	• Hypothyroidism
• Chronic liver disease	• Excessive alcohol intake
• Immunosuppressive agents	• Drug induced
• Diuretics	• Antiretroviral agents
	• Corticosteroids
	• Beta-blockers
	• Oral contraceptives

Table 58.3 Indications for investigating or screening hyperlipidaemia

- Recent acute coronary syndrome
- History of IHD
- Diabetes mellitus
- Hypertension
- Gout
- Metabolic syndrome
- Current smoker
- Chronic kidney disease
- Chronic liver disease
- Hypothyroidism
- Solid organ transplant recipient
- Family history of premature IHD
- Family history of dyslipidaemia
- Signs of hypercholesterolaemia (xanthomas)
- Age (male: >45; female: >55)

Key points in investigating hyperlipidaemia

- Lipid profiles should be done after the patient has fasted for 10–12 hours.
- Repeat lipid profiles can be performed 3 months after initiation of therapy or change in medication dose.
- Familial forms of hyperlipidaemia can be investigated with genetic testing.

Clinical Investigations at a Glance, First Edition. Jonathan Gleadle, Jordan Li and Tuck Yong. © 2017 John Wiley & Sons, Ltd. Published 2017 by John Wiley & Sons, Ltd.

Hyperlipidaemia is characterised by an increase in the concentrations of cholesterol, triglycerides or both. It is a major and modifiable risk factor for developing atherosclerosis and cardiovascular disease (CVD). Lipids are transported in the blood by lipoproteins. There are five major classes of lipoprotein (Table 58.1).

When serum cholesterol is elevated, it is almost always due to an elevation of LDL-cholesterol. Occasionally it is due to a high concentration of HDL-cholesterol, but these patients are not at increased risk of CVD. As LDL-cholesterol accounts for 60–70% of the total cholesterol and is atherogenic, it is the main target of treatment in patients with hypercholesterolaemia. When triglycerides are elevated, this is usually associated with an elevation of VLDL-cholesterol. When fasting triglyceride levels are >1.5 mmol/L, the risk of CVD increases significantly.

Primary hyperlipidaemias are genetically based (single-gene defects or polygenic disorders), but the genetic defects are known for only a minority of patients. Secondary hyperlipidaemia may be the result of other diseases (Table 58.2).

Indications for investigation or screening hyperlipidaemia

Hypercholesterolaemia is generally asymptomatic. Patients may be incidentally diagnosed on routine blood testing, or when presenting with CVD. It is important to carry out a systemic review for CVD, focusing on symptoms of ischaemic heart disease (IHD), cerebrovascular disease and peripheral arterial disease. It is also helpful to take a detailed family history for early-onset IHD and hyperlipidaemia in first-degree relatives, and ask the patient about their level of exercise and diet. The indications for investigating or screening hyperlipidaemia are summarised in Table 58.3. Recent national guidelines have emphasised the importance of assessing cholesterol levels in the context of cardiovascular risk.

Hypertriglyceridaemia is generally asymptomatic until triglyceride levels are sustained above 11 mmol/L – symptoms then may include eruptive xanthomas and pancreatitis.

The patient should be examined for signs of hypercholesterolaemia, such as eyelid xanthelasmas, arcus corneae (with onset before 45 years of age) and xanthomata. Tendinous xanthomas at the Achilles, elbow and knee tendons, and over metacarpophalangeal joints, are characteristic of heterozygous and homozygous forms of familial hypercholesterolaemia (FH).

Screening asymptomatic individuals without any of the aforementioned risk factors should be done every 5 years. Patients with one of the aforementioned risk factors should have a lipid study annually. Performing a risk factor analysis prior to obtaining screening blood test results is recommended.

Serum lipid profile tests include:
- total cholesterol
- triglycerides
- HDL-cholesterol

- calculated LDL-cholesterol: LDL-cholesterol = Total cholesterol − HDL-cholesterol − (TG/5), where TG is triglycerides; direct LDL-cholesterol measurements do not offer any advantages, except in patients with marked hypertriglyceridaemia.

These tests should be done after the patient has fasted for 10–12 hours. Fasting allows diet-derived chylomicrons to be cleared. While not fasting has little impact on LDL levels, it has some effect on HDL and a dramatic effect on triglycerides. Alcohol should be avoided the evening prior to measurement of triglycerides.

Serum lipid levels vary from day to day. Therefore, at least two or three measurements should be made days or weeks apart before initiating therapy. Measurements should be deferred for 2–3 weeks after minor illness and 2–3 months after major illness, surgery or trauma because an acute event has a profound effect on circulating lipids, with a 30% fall in total cholesterol and 50% rise in triglycerides. These effects are maximal at 7 days and take approximately 3 months to resolve. Following an acute myocardial infarction it is generally accepted that the plasma cholesterol is reliable if measured within 24 hours of the onset of symptoms.

Lipoprotein electrophoresis is indicated only if the triglyceride level is >4 mmol/L. Apolipoprotein A1 and B can be measured instead of HDL- and LDL-cholesterol, but there is no advantage in doing so unless familial hyperapolipoproteinaemia B (normal LDL-cholesterol, increased apolipoprotein B) is suspected. Plasma lipoprotein (a) is an independent risk factor for atherosclerosis and may be indicated in patients with a personal or strong family history of atherosclerosis, with normal LDL- and HDL-cholesterol.

Additional tests may be indicated by the history and examination findings to identify secondary causes (Table 58.2) and complications of hypercholesterolaemia. ECG, echocardiography, cardiac stress testing, Doppler examination or ankle–brachial indices may be useful to investigate cardiovascular complications.

Genetic causes

FH is an autosomal dominant disorder. The diagnosis of both homozygous and heterozygous FH is based on severe LDL-cholesterol elevations (>15.6 mmol/L in homozygous FH) in the absence of secondary causes, with triglyceride and HDL-cholesterol levels within the reference range. Definitive diagnosis can be made only with gene or receptor analysis. LDL receptor analysis can be used to identify the specific LDL receptor defect.

Familial hypertriglyceridaemia appears to be transmitted as an autosomal dominant disorder. In the diagnosis of familial hypertriglyceridaemia, secondary causes of hypertriglyceridemia should be excluded (Table 58.2).

Familial combined hyperlipidaemia is transmitted as an autosomal dominant disorder. Concomitant hypercholesterolaemia and hypertriglyceridaemia occurs in this disorder.

59 Pneumonia

The goal of investigations is to:
- Establish the diagnosis
- Assess the severity of pneumonia and the need for hospitalisation or intensive care unit admission
- Identify the causative organism
- Identify complications
- Guide treatment

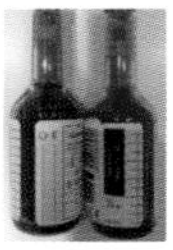

General laboratory investigations
- Full blood count
- Urea, creatinine and electrolytes
- Liver function tests
- Urinalysis
- Oxygenation saturation and often ABGs
- CRP

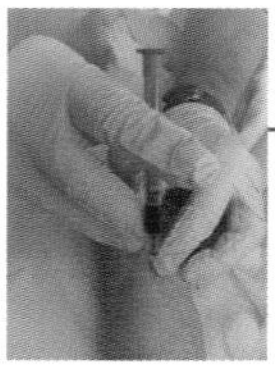

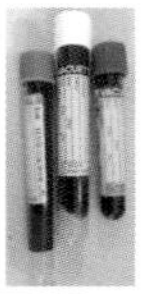

Microbiological tests

Blood cultures

Nasopharyngeal viral PCR

Gram stain
Sputum culture

CXR

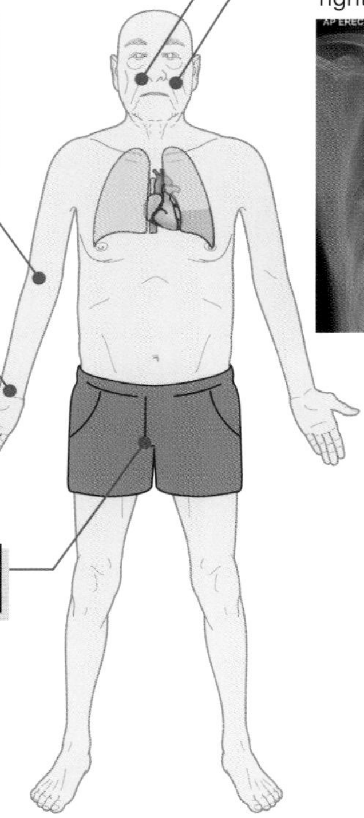

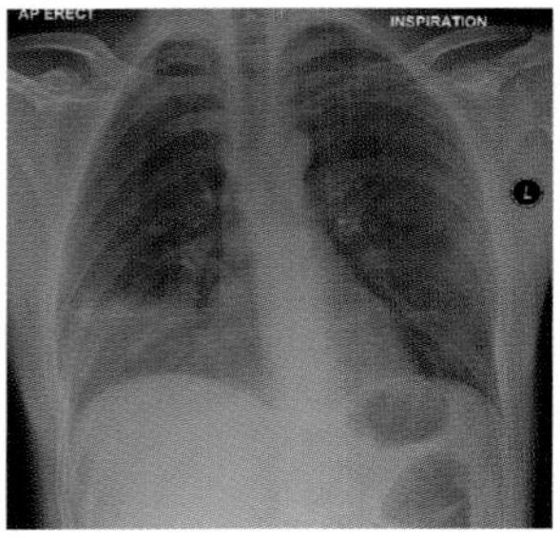

Figure 59.1 CXR shows right middle lobe pneumonia

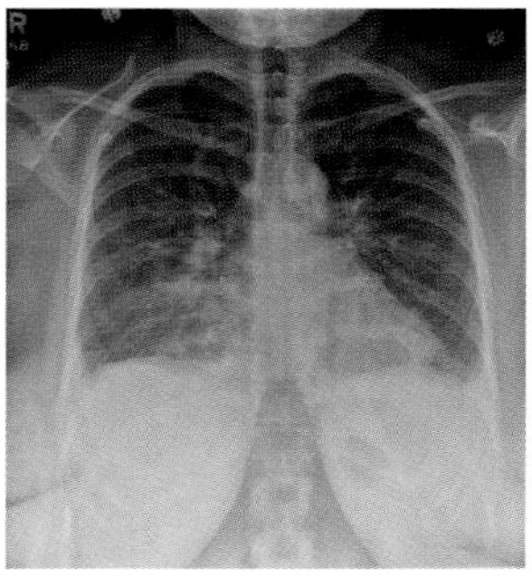

Figure 59.2 CXR shows bronchopneumonia

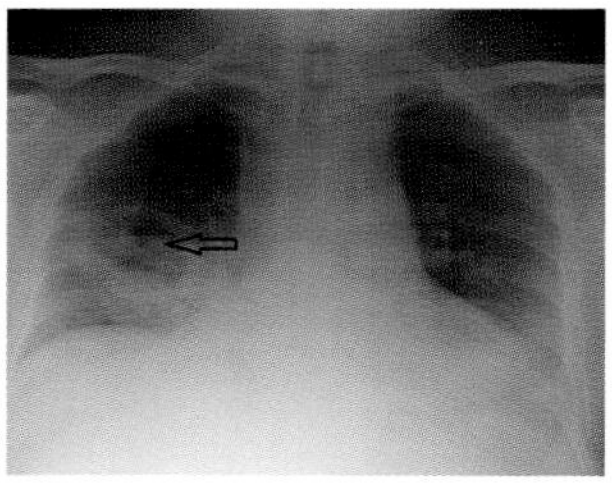

Arterial blood gas

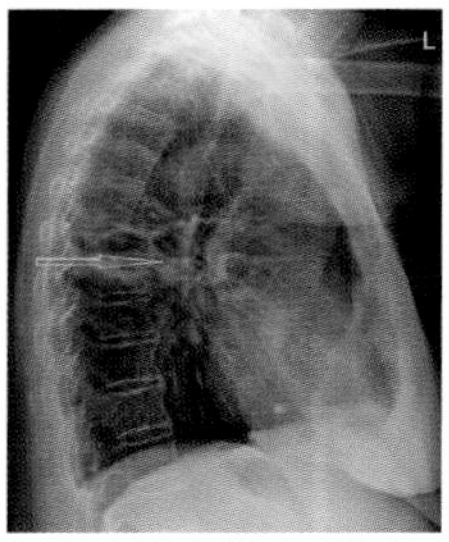

Figure 59.4 CXR lateral view shows right middle lobe pneumonia with cavitation formation

Figure 59.3 CXR shows right middle lobe pneumonia with cavitation formation

Urine antigen tests

CURB-65 pneumonia severity score

	Observation	Score
C	Confusion	1
U	Urea >7 mmol/L	1
R	Respiratory rate = 30/min	1
B	Systolic = 90 mmHg or diastolic = 60 mmHg	1
65	Age >65 years	1

PSI scoring system

	Points
Age	
Men	Years
Women	Years – 10
Nursing home resident	10
Co-morbidity	
Neoplastic disease	20
Liver disease	10
Congestive cardiac failure	10
Cerebrovascular disease	10
Renal disease	10
Clinical observation	
Altered mental state	20
Respiratory rate = 30/min	20
Systolic blood pressure <90 mmHg	20
Temperature <35 or >40	15
Pulse rate >125/min	10
Investigations	
Arterial pH < 7.35	30
Urea = 11 mmol/L	20
Na <130 mmol/L	20
Glucose =14 mmol/L	10
Haematocrit <30%	10
PaO_2 <60 mmHg or SaO_2 (air) <90%	10
Pleural effusion	10

PSI and mortality

PSI score	30-day mortality (%)
70	0.6
71–90	0.9
91–130	9.3
>130	27.0

CURB-65 and mortality

CURB-65 score	30-day mortality (%)	Management
0--1	1.5	Treat as outpatient
2	9.2	Require hospitalisation
3–5	22	Manage as severe pneumonia

Key points

- Infiltrate or consolidation on CXR is required to confirm the diagnosis of pneumonia.
- Microbiologic identification should be limited to patients who are at high risk or have complications (immunocompromised, asplenia, failure to respond to therapy).
- ABG, biochemistry parameters such as urea, sodium and glucose levels, and the finding of pleural effusion are useful to determine the severity of pneumonia.

Clinical Investigations at a Glance, First Edition. Jonathan Gleadle, Jordan Li and Tuck Yong. © 2017 John Wiley & Sons, Ltd. Published 2017 by John Wiley & Sons, Ltd.

Pneumonia is an acute infection of the lung presenting with respiratory symptoms and accompanied by acute infiltrate changes on CXR. Pneumonia is common especially among the elderly and is the leading cause of death.

Nosocomial pneumonia or hospital-acquired pneumonia (HAP) is pneumonia not present on admission but developed in a patient hospitalised for >48 hours. Intubation greatly increases the risk of HAP. Hospitalised patients frequently develop colonisation of the oropharynx with aerobic Gram-negative bacilli and may also be exposed to multiresistant hospital pathogens such as methicillin-resistant *Staphylococcus aureus*.

The clinical manifestations of pneumonia may include cough, sputum, rigors, fever, pleuritic or non-pleuritic chest pain, shortness of breath and confusion. In elderly people, fever may be absent and new-onset delirium is common.

General laboratory investigations

An elevated CRP may aid diagnosis and be predictive of severe pneumonia. Failure of the CRP to fall is a useful indicator of treatment failure. Arterial blood gas (ABG) analysis is used to determine the severity of pneumonia. While non-invasive monitoring of pulse oximetry is simple, it is no substitute for ABG analysis as it gives no indication of ventilatory adequacy and blood pH, carbon dioxide or bicarbonate concentrations.

Various tools to assess the severity of community acquired pneumonia (CAP) and risk of death exist, including the pneumonia severity index (PSI), CURB-65 system and SMART-COP score.

Microbiological tests

Microbiological tests to identify pathogens should be performed on patients with moderate to severe CAP. A microbiological diagnosis can be made on routine microbiological tests in only 15% of inpatients. *Streptococcus pneumoniae* is the most frequently identified pathogen in CAP. Other common organisms include *Mycoplasma pneumoniae*, *S. aureus*, *Haemophilus influenzae* and influenza viruses. A raised incidence of *S. aureus* is found during influenza epidemics.

The Gram stain can be performed quickly on a well-expectorated specimen (not salivary, >25 neutrophils and <10 epithelial cells per high-power field). A Ziehl–Neelsen stain can be performed to look for acid-fast bacilli to help exclude tuberculosis.

Sputum culture is a sensitive means of identifying the bacteria if the patient has not had prior antibiotic treatment and a good-quality specimen can be obtained. However, a pathogen is not identified in up to 50% of patients. Sputum cultures for *Legionella* should always be attempted for patients who are legionella urine antigen positive in order to provide isolates for epidemiological typing and comparison with isolates from putative environmental sources.

Virus detection

PCR tests for an extended range of respiratory viruses and atypical pathogens, such as influenza, parainfluenza, adenovirus, respiratory syncytial virus, metapneumovirus, *Mycoplasma pneumonia*, and *Legionella* in nose, throat swab and nasopharyngeal aspirate, are rapid and sensitive and preferred to serological investigations.

Blood cultures

Overall, blood cultures show poor sensitivity in pneumonia but should be undertaken in severely ill patients.

Urine antigen tests

Urine testing for *Streptococcus pneumoniae* and *Legionella* serogroup 1 is recommended in severe pneumonia. For pneumococcal pneumonia, the advantages of antigen tests are rapidity (~15 minutes), simplicity, reasonable sensitivity of 50–80% and specificity of >90% in adults.

For *Legionella*, urinary antigen assays detect only *Legionella pneumophila* serogroup 1, which accounts for 80–95% of community-acquired cases of legionnaires' disease. but have a sensitivity of 70–90% and a specificity of nearly 99% for detection. The urine is positive for antigen on day 1 of illness and continues to be positive for weeks.

Serologic testing

The diagnosis of infection with atypical pathogens, including *Chlamydophila pneumoniae*, *M. pneumoniae*, and *Legionella* species, relies on acute- and convalescent-phase serologic testing. Where available, paired serology tests can be considered for patients with severe CAP where no microbiological diagnosis has been made by other means, who fail to improve, and/or where there are particular epidemiological risk factors.

CXR

A CXR is crucial to making the diagnosis of pneumonia. There are three distinct radiological patterns:
- *Lobar pneumonia* or focal pneumonia is manifested as homogeneous consolidation involving one, or less commonly, multiple lobes. Larger bronchi often remain patent with air, creating the characteristic air bronchogram (Figure 59.1). In aspiration pneumonia, X-ray findings may be seen in the gravity-dependent portions of the lungs; the right lung is affected twice as often as the left.
- *Bronchopneumonia*, also known as multifocal or lobular pneumonia, is radiographically identified by its patchy appearance, with peribronchial thickening and poorly defined air-space opacities (Figure 59.2). In *S. aureus* pneumonia, abscesses, cavitations (with air–fluid levels) (Figures 59.3 and 59.4) and pneumatoceles are commonly seen, and 30–50% of patients develop pleural effusions, half of which are empyema. Cavitation and associated pleural effusions are also observed in anaerobic infections, Gram-negative infections and tuberculosis.
- *Parapneumonic effusion*. 40% of patients with pneumonia have a pleural effusion, but the amount of fluid is usually small. Ultrasound is useful in evaluating especially if septations are present within the fluid collection that may not be visible on CT scans. Refer to Chapter 62 on pleural effusion for further investigations of parapneumonic effusion.

Chest CT

Chest CT currently has no routine role in the investigation of pneumonia. For inpatients, CT scanning may identify pulmonary infections earlier than CXR and may be useful in subjects where the diagnosis is in doubt.

Bronchoscopy

Bronchoscopy should be considered in patients with severe pneumonia. and persisting signs, symptoms and progressive radiological abnormalities despite appropriate treatments. The other indications are immunocompromised patients with pneumonia. The bronchoscopy will include bronchoalveolar lavage (BAL), protected specimen brushing and/or lung aspiration.

Hospital-acquired pneumonia

In patients with suspected HAP, sputum or BAL for culture, blood culture (two sets) and an endotracheal aspirate sample should be obtained prior to antibiotic therapy. Urine testing for *Legionella* antigen and PCR and nose/throat swabs for respiratory viral PCR should also be considered. Non-infective causes for consolidation should always be considered.

60 Asthma

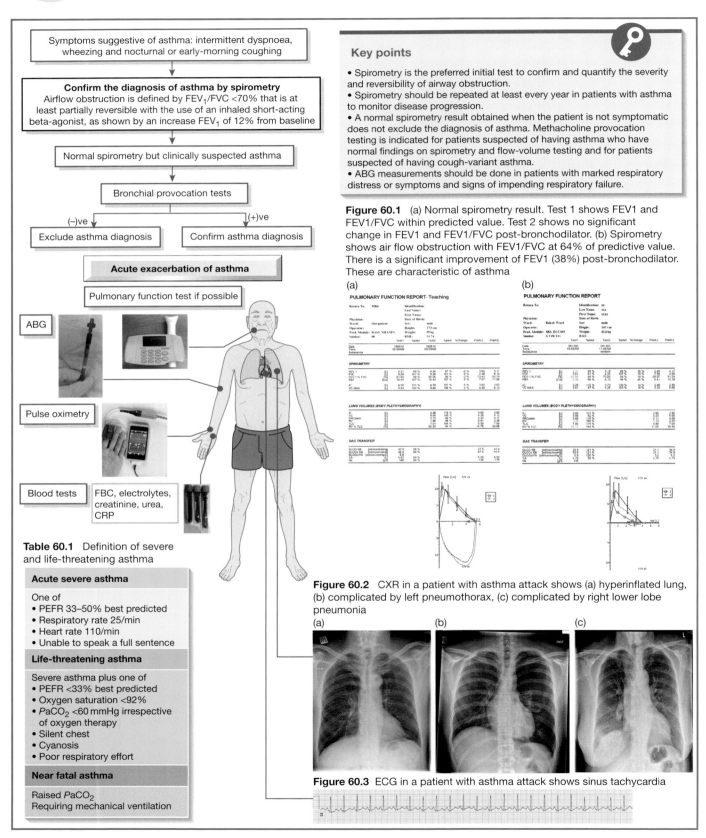

Symptoms suggestive of asthma: intermittent dyspnoea, wheezing and nocturnal or early-morning coughing

Confirm the diagnosis of asthma by spirometry
Airflow obstruction is defined by FEV$_1$/FVC <70% that is at least partially reversible with the use of an inhaled short-acting beta-agonist, as shown by an increase FEV$_1$ of 12% from baseline

Normal spirometry but clinically suspected asthma

Bronchial provocation tests

(–)ve → Exclude asthma diagnosis

(+)ve → Confirm asthma diagnosis

Acute exacerbation of asthma

Pulmonary function test if possible

ABG

Pulse oximetry

Blood tests — FBC, electrolytes, creatinine, urea, CRP

Table 60.1 Definition of severe and life-threatening asthma

Acute severe asthma

One of
• PEFR 33–50% best predicted
• Respiratory rate 25/min
• Heart rate 110/min
• Unable to speak a full sentence

Life-threatening asthma

Severe asthma plus one of
• PEFR <33% best predicted
• Oxygen saturation <92%
• PaCO$_2$ <60 mmHg irrespective of oxygen therapy
• Silent chest
• Cyanosis
• Poor respiratory effort

Near fatal asthma

Raised PaCO$_2$
Requiring mechanical ventilation

Key points

• Spirometry is the preferred initial test to confirm and quantify the severity and reversibility of airway obstruction.
• Spirometry should be repeated at least every year in patients with asthma to monitor disease progression.
• A normal spirometry result obtained when the patient is not symptomatic does not exclude the diagnosis of asthma. Methacholine provocation testing is indicated for patients suspected of having asthma who have normal findings on spirometry and flow-volume testing and for patients suspected of having cough-variant asthma.
• ABG measurements should be done in patients with marked respiratory distress or symptoms and signs of impending respiratory failure.

Figure 60.1 (a) Normal spirometry result. Test 1 shows FEV1 and FEV1/FVC within predicted value. Test 2 shows no significant change in FEV1 and FEV1/FVC post-bronchodilator. (b) Spirometry shows air flow obstruction with FEV1/FVC at 64% of predictive value. There is a significant improvement of FEV1 (38%) post-bronchodilator. These are characteristic of asthma

Figure 60.2 CXR in a patient with asthma attack shows (a) hyperinflated lung, (b) complicated by left pneumothorax, (c) complicated by right lower lobe pneumonia

Figure 60.3 ECG in a patient with asthma attack shows sinus tachycardia

Asthma is a chronic inflammatory airways disease characterised by airway inflammation, hypersensitivity and variable reversible obstruction. It can present with symptoms of intermittent dyspnoea, wheezing and nocturnal or early-morning coughing.

Diagnosis

The diagnosis of asthma is based on the presence of typical symptoms of airflow obstruction or airway hyperresponsiveness and the objective confirmation of variable airflow limitation that is at least partially reversible.

Airflow obstruction is defined by a ratio of forced expiratory volume in 1 second (FEV_1)/forced vital capacity (FVC) of less than 70% that is at least partially reversible with the use of an inhaled short-acting beta-agonist, as shown by

• an increase FEV_1 of ≥12% from baseline;
• an increase in peak expiratory flow rate (PEFR) of ≥20% (or 60 L/min) from baseline;
• diurnal variation of PEFR (measured twice daily) of more than 10%.

Measurement of airflow

Spirometry

Spirometry is the preferred test for initial confirmation of asthma as it provides clearer identification of airway obstruction than PEFR. Spirometry is less effort dependent and is repeatable. It measures the whole volume that may be expelled in one breath (FVC). It also permits the calculation of the percentage exhaled in the first second, FEV_1 and forced expiratory flow from 25 to 75% vital capacity (FEF25–75). FEF25–75 is less reproducible than FEV_1 but it is a more sensitive indicator of airflow limitation. Three maximal forced expirations should be measured and the best reading of the three should be used as the final measurement. It also offers good confirmation of reversibility in subjects with pre-existing obstruction of the airways where a change of >400 mL in FEV_1 is found after short-acting bronchodilator and/or corticosteroid therapy are trialled. Spirometry may be normal in asymptomatic individuals and does not exclude asthma. It should be repeated, ideally when symptomatic. However, a normal spirometry when symptomatic does make asthma unlikely.

An obstructive airway is defined by a ratio of FEV_1/FVC of less than 70% (Figure 60.1). The severity can be determined by using FEV_1/FVC ratio:

• >70% – normal
• 60–70% – mild
• 50–60% – moderate
• <50% – severe.

Significant reversibility, defined by a 20% improvement in any two of FEV_1, FVC and FEF25–75 after inhalation of a bronchodilator, is diagnostic of asthma (Figure 60.1). Similar variability, either spontaneously or after treatment with oral corticosteroids, is also diagnostic of asthma.

Peak expiratory flow rate (PEFR)

PEFR is a simple test using hand-held devices. It measures the maximum expiratory flow rate over the first 10 ms. PEFR is reduced by airway narrowing (e.g. in asthma), expiratory muscle weakness and sub-maximal effort. Therefore, PEFR is not an adequate test in the initial diagnosis of asthma, but it has an important role in the monitoring and management of established asthma.

Bronchial provocation tests

Asthma patients' airways are hyperresponsive to a wide range of non-specific stimuli. Therefore, for patients with normal lung function test, bronchial provocation test with inhaled methacholine or an exercise test may be useful for excluding asthma. A variability of FEV_1 or PEFR of greater than 15% during a provocation test confirms the diagnosis of asthma.

Methacholine is a known asthma trigger. Increasing concentrations of methacholine are inhaled and changes in FEV_1 or PEFR are measured after each dose. A concentration–response curve can be constructed. An increase in bronchial responsiveness indicates the patient has asthma. The sensitivity is 100% and specificity is 80%.

Tests for allergens

Skin testing or in-vitro testing is recommended to identify indoor allergens that may contribute to asthma symptoms in patients with relevant exposure.

Other tests

CXR, high-resolution CT of lungs and CT of sinuses can identify any structural abnormalities or alternative diagnosis that can cause or aggravate asthma. Sputum eosinophils may present when asthma symptoms develop.

Investigations during an exacerbation of asthma

Patients presenting with an acute exacerbation of asthma should be evaluated quickly to assess severity and the need for urgent intervention. Clinicians should look for signs of life-threatening asthma, such as altered mental state, paradoxical chest or abdominal movement or absence of wheezing. The goal of investigation is to define the severity of the acute asthma attack (Table 60.1).

The measurement of FEV_1 or PEFR can be helpful for assessing the severity of an exacerbation, and the response to treatment but should not delay treatment. The following laboratory and imaging studies should be performed.

• pulse oximetry monitoring;
• arterial blood gas (ABG) to assess hypoxia, hypercapnoea and acidosis, which are suggestive of fatigue and impending respiratory failure;
• FBC;
• CXR to exclude pneumothorax and pneumonia (Figure 60.2);
• ECG to identify arrhythmias secondary to beta-agonist and those with heart disease (Figure 60.3).

After treatment in the emergency department for 2–4 hours, patients who have an incomplete or poor response, defined as an FEV_1 or PEFR of less than 70% of the personal best or predicted value, should be evaluated for admission to the hospital. Patients who have an FEV_1 of <40%, persistent moderate-to-severe symptoms, drowsiness, confusion, or a $PaCO_2$ of 42 mmHg or more should be admitted. Patients may be discharged if the FEV_1 or PEFR after treatment is 70% or more of the personal best or predicted value and if the improvements in lung function and symptoms are sustained for at least 60 minutes.

61 Chronic obstructive pulmonary disease

The goals for investigation in COPD include confirming the diagnosis, assessing the severity and investigating the presence of comorbidities

Confirm the diagnosis of COPD

COPD should be suspected in any patient who has dyspnoea, chronic cough and sputum production, and a history of exposure to risk factors for COPD

Spirometry is required to demonstrate airflow limitation that is not fully reversible in order to make a diagnosis of COPD

The presence of a post-bronchodilator FEV_1/FVC ratio <0.7 in a patient with dyspnoea, cough and/or sputum production and a history of relevant exposure confirms the diagnosis of COPD

Assess the severity of COPD

Figure 61.1 Portable spirometer

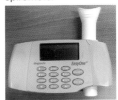

Figure 61.2 Spirometry shows FEV_1 of 0.82 (41% predicted) and FEV_1/FVC of 51%. There is no significant improvement after bronchodilator. This is characteristic of COPD

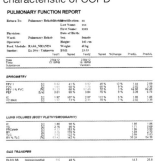

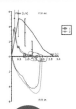

- Hypoxaemic respiratory failure (type I): PaO_2 <60 mmHg with a normal or low $PaCO_2$
- Hypercapnic respiratory failure (type II): $PaCO_2$ >50 mmHg. Hypoxemia is common in patients with hypercapnic respiratory failure who are breathing room air.
- Hypoxaemia is defined as a PaO_2 of 60–79 mmHg

Table 61.1 Stage and severity of COPD according to post-bronchodilator spirometry

COPD stage and severity	Definition
Stage 1 – mild	FEV1/FVC <0.70; FEV1 80% of predicted value
Stage 2 – moderate	FEV1/FVC <0.70; FEV1 50–79% of predicted value
Stage 3 – severe	FEV1/FVC <0.70; FEV1 30–49% of predicted value
Stage 4 – very severe	FEV1/FVC <0.70; FEV1 <30% of predicted value or FEV1 <50% of predicted value plus chronic respiratory failure

Adapted from the Global Initiative for Chronic Obstructive Lung Disease.

Key points

- Reductions of FEV1, FVC and the ratio of FEV 1/FVC are the hallmark of COPD.
- When the FEV1 falls below 1 L, patients develop dyspnoea with activities of daily living; when the FEV1 falls below 0.8 L, patients are at risk of hypoxemia, hypercapnia and cor pulmonale.
- ABG is important to assess acid–base status, arterial partial pressure of oxygen and carbon dioxide.
- CXR and CT chest are useful for evaluation of other concomitant conditions present with COPD, such as malignancy, pneumonia, pneumothorax or pulmonary oedema.

Radiology

Figure 61.3 CXR of COPD, hyper-inflated lung, flattened diaphragm and decreased lung markings

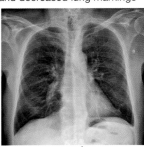

Figure 61.4 CXR of COPD with bullous formation in the right upper zone

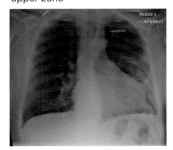

Figure 61.5 CT chest shows COPD with paraseptal and centrilobular emphysematous changes

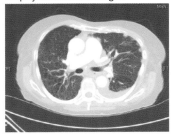

Echocardiogram

Assess the complications of COPD

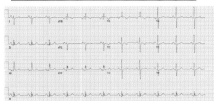

Figure 61.6 ECG shows right ventricular hypertrophy and biatrial enlargement in a patient with COPD

Figure 61.7 Echo shows right heart failure and pulmonary hypertension

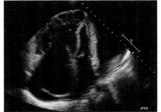

Arterial blood gas analysis

Clinical Investigations at a Glance, First Edition. Jonathan Gleadle, Jordan Li and Tuck Yong. © 2017 John Wiley & Sons, Ltd. Published 2017 by John Wiley & Sons, Ltd.

Chronic obstructive pulmonary disease (COPD) is a spectrum of lung diseases characterised by persistent airflow limitation due to combinations of small airways disease (obstructive bronchiolitis) and emphysema. It is a major cause of morbidity, disability and mortality with a prevalence of about 10% in adults above 40 years. Smoking is the most important cause for COPD, though a significant proportion of patients with COPD are non-smokers.

Investigation for patients with suspected COPD

COPD should be suspected in any patient who has dyspnoea, chronic cough, sputum production and a history of exposure to risk factors for COPD.

Spirometry

Spirometry is required to demonstrate airflow limitation that is not fully reversible in order to make a diagnosis of COPD (Figure 61.1). The presence of a post-bronchodilator forced expiratory volume in 1 second (FEV1) to forced vital capacity (FVC) ratio (FEV1/FVC) of <0.7 in a patient with dyspnoea, cough and/or sputum production and a history of relevant exposure(s) confirms the diagnosis of COPD (Figure 61.2). A normal value for spirometry effectively excludes the diagnosis of clinically relevant COPD. This definition is widely accepted, but its use may lead to overdiagnosis in the elderly, as FEV1 declines more rapidly with age than does FVC, and underdiagnosis in younger adults. The severity of COPD is classified according to the FEV1, as a percentage of the predicted normal value (Table 61.1). The main differential diagnosis is asthma. In some patients with chronic asthma, a clear distinction from COPD is not possible using current investigations. Once a diagnosis of COPD has been established, there are few reasons to repeat spirometry at subsequent visits, but serial measurements at annual intervals may provide prognostic information.

Pulmonary function tests (PFTs)

Full PFTs allow for the simultaneous measurement of flow and volume during maximal expiration. Reduced expiratory flows at mid and low lung volumes are the earliest indicators of airflow limitation in COPD and may be abnormal even when FEV1 is within the normal range (>80%) (Figure 61.2).

Oximetry and arterial blood gas (ABG)

Oximetry can be performed annually or in patients with severe disease to identify those with chronic hypoxaemia who will benefit from long-term domiciliary oxygen therapy. ABG should be performed in patients with severe disease, and this should be done when the patient is clinically stable, at rest and breathing ambient air. If the partial pressure of arterial oxygen (PaO_2) is ≤55 mmHg, or if the arterial oxygen saturation (SaO_2) is ≤88%, domiciliary oxygen therapy should be considered.

Six-minute walk test

Tests of walking distance can evaluate the functional ability of patients in an easy and familiar way. The patient is asked to walk a known length for 6 minutes, while observed by a technician who measures SaO_2 and pulse rate. The test is highly reproducible after the first practice walk. A fall in SaO_2 on exercise that occurs at low work load indicates a ventilation–perfusion mismatch that can be seen in both obstructive and restrictive lung diseases.

Radiology

A CXR should be obtained to rule out other pulmonary diseases, but it is not sensitive enough to diagnose COPD. Findings of COPD on CXR are non-specific and show increased bronchovascular markings (Figure 61.3). Emphysema manifests as lung hyperinflation with flattened hemidiaphragms, a small heart, and possible bullous changes (Figure 61.4).

Chest CT is unnecessary unless another diagnosis is suspected. In COPD, bronchial wall thickening may be seen in addition to enlarged vessels. Emphysema is evidenced by alveolar septal destruction and airspace enlargement, which may occur in a variety of distributions. Centrilobular emphysema is predominantly seen in the upper lobes, with panlobular emphysema predominating in the lower lobes. Paraseptal emphysema tends to occur near lung fissures and pleura (Figure 61.5).

Genetic testing

Testing for α_1-antitrypsin deficiency should be considered if COPD develops at a relatively young age or if there is a strong family history.

Investigations of comorbidities

COPD is associated with comorbidities such as osteoporosis, hypertension, ischaemic heart disease (IHD) and depression, which are probably related to smoking. An ECG (Figure 61.6) should be performed in COPD patients. Common findings are atrial tachycardia and atrial fibrillation. Echocardiography is useful if cor pulmonale is suspected, when breathlessness is out of proportion to the degree of respiratory impairment or when IHD, pulmonary embolus and congestive cardiac failure are suspected (Figure 61.7).

Investigations for acute exacerbations of COPD

An exacerbation of COPD is defined as an acute worsening of the patient's respiratory symptoms that is beyond normal day-to-day variations and necessitates a change in medications. The following investigations should be undertaken:

1 *FBC and biochemistry.*

2 *Spirometry.* This should be performed in a patient with exacerbation of COPD unless patient is confused or comatose. An FEV1 <1 L or <40% predicted is indicative of a severe exacerbation.

3 *ABG.* Hypoxaemia is a common finding in acute exacerbation of COPD. Worsening of ventilation–perfusion matching is the most important determinant of hypoxaemia in this setting. The pH is the best marker of severity and reflects acute deterioration in alveolar hypoventilation compared with the chronic stable state. Hypercapnia indicates the presence of alveolar hypoventilation. This may be caused by depression of respiratory centres, paralysis of respiratory muscles or severe airway obstruction. Hypoxic (type I) respiratory failure is defined as PaO_2 <60 mmHg (8 kPa) and the $PaCO_2$ is normal. Hypercapnic (type II) respiratory failure is defined as $PaCO_2$ >50 mmHg (6.7 kPa) and invariably this will be accompanied by a reduced PaO_2 unless corrected with supplemental oxygen.

4 *CXR.* This will determine if there is any other lung disease, such as pneumonia. An ECG helps to identify alternative diagnoses, such myocardial ischaemia. Routine sputum culture in exacerbation is unhelpful. It is used only when the infection is not responding to antibiotic treatment or when a resistant organism is suspected.

62 Pleural effusion

Pleural effusion investigation

Physical examination suggestive of pleural effusion

CXR to confirm and examine the extent of pleural effusion

The goal of investigation is to
• Determine if the pleural effusion is transudate or exudate
• Determine its cause

Figure 62.1 (a) Normal CXR. (b) Bilateral small pleural effusion. (c) Moderate right pleural effusion. (d) Large left pleural effusion

(a)
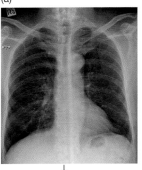
(b)
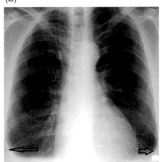
(c)
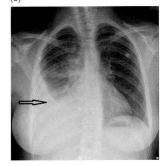
(d)
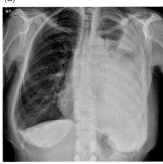

Aspiration

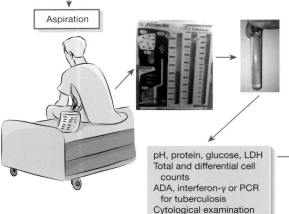

pH, protein, glucose, LDH
Total and differential cell counts
ADA, interferon-γ or PCR for tuberculosis
Cytological examination

Table 62.1 Light's criteria for distinguishing between pleural exudates and transudates and sensitivity and specificity of each criterion to distinguish between transudative and exudative effusions

	Sensitivity for exudates (%)	Specificity for exudates (%)
Light's criteria (fluid is an exudate if two or more of the following three criteria are met)	98	83
Ratio of pleural fluid protein level to serum protein level >0.5	86	84
Ratio of pleural fluid LDH level to serum LDH level >0.6	90	82
Pleural fluid LDH greater than two-thirds the upper limit of normal for serum LDH level	82	89

Table 62.2 Common causes for an exudate and a transudate

Exudate	Transudate
• Lung cancer	• Congestive heart failure
• Pneumonia	• Liver failure
• Pulmonary embolism	• Nephrotic syndrome
• Tuberculosis	
• Rheumatoid arthritis	
• Systemic lupus erythematosus	
• Mesothelioma	

Consider CT chest, bronchoscopy, video-assisted thoracoscopic pleural biopsy

Figure 62.2 CT chest shows large right pleural effusion

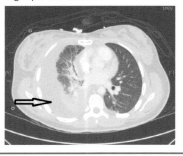

Figure 62.3 Video-assisted thoracoscopic pleural biopsy

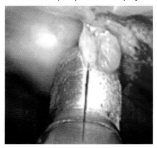

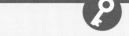

Key points

• CXR is the first test to confirm the presence of pleural effusion.
• Chest CT is valuable for investigating underlying lung parenchyma diseases or masses especially after pleural fluids drained.
• Analysis of the aspirated pleural fluid is useful in distinguishing between transudate and exudate. Light's criteria correctly identify almost all exudates but can wrongly identify about 20% of transudates as exudates.

Pleural effusion is accumulation of fluid in the pleural space. Investigation of a pleural effusion begins with careful history-taking and physical examination. It is typically followed by a CXR, aspiration and analysis of pleural fluid. A history of cardiac or liver failure can suggest a transudative effusion. A history of cancer can point to a malignant pleural effusion. A history of recent or current pneumonia suggests the focus of the investigation is to differentiate a parapneumonic effusion from empyema. Physical findings such as elevated jugular venous pressure, a third heart sound or peripheral oedema would suggest congestive heart failure.

Initial investigations

CXR

The initial investigation is a CXR, but this does not characterise the biochemical nature of the fluid. Small effusions may not be visualised on frontal views. Fluid accumulating posteriorly can be seen on the lateral view before it becomes visible on the frontal view. When the fluid is slightly above the level of the upper portion of the diaphragm, blunting of the lateral costophrenic angle is seen (Figures 62.1a and b). A small amount of pleural fluid (about 250 mL) is required to produce detectable blunting, but as much as 500 mL of fluid can be present without apparent changes on the frontal view. A large free pleural effusion appears as a dependent opacity with lateral upward sloping of a meniscus-shaped contour (Figure 62.1c). The diaphragmatic contour is partially or completely obliterated, depending on the amount of the fluid (silhouette sign). A very large pleural effusion appears as an opaque hemithorax with a mediastinal shift to the contralateral side (Figure 62.1d).

Ultrasound

Ultrasound scan is used to confirm an effusion in a patient with abnormal CXR, such as loculated pleural effusion, and to guide interventional procedures (e.g. thoracentesis, biopsy, placement of chest drains). Ultrasound is helpful in differentiating pleural effusions and pleural thickening.

Thoracentesis

The initial thoracentesis is usually performed for diagnostic purposes; however, in patients who are short of breath at rest, removal of up to 1.5 L of fluid may provide therapeutic relief. Once aspirated, fluid is sent for biochemical, microbiological and cytological analyses. Biochemical analyses include determination of protein, pH, LDH, glucose and albumin levels.

Pleural fluid analysis

Differentiating transudates from exudates

The first step in the analysis of the pleural fluid is to determine whether an effusion is transudative or exudative. Transudates can be differentiated from exudates according to Light's criteria, by measurement of the levels of protein and LDH in the pleural fluid and in the serum (Table 62.1). The level of LDH in the pleural fluid correlates with the degree of pleural inflammation. Leading causes of transudate and exudate are listed in Table 62.2.

pH

Measurement of the pleural fluid pH with the use of a blood-gas machine is indicated if a parapneumonic or malignant effusion is suspected. A pleural fluid pH below 7.20 indicates infection or empyema and the need for drainage. A low pH can also occur in oesophageal rupture and rheumatoid arthritis.

LDH

Elevated levels of LDH occur in lymphoma and tuberculosis; levels >1000 U/L are associated with empyema. An elevated amylase in the pleural fluid is seen with pancreatic disease and oesophageal rupture.

Glucose

The presence of low glucose (<3.3 mmol/L) in the pleural fluid indicates complicated parapneumonic or malignant effusion. Other causes of low glucose pleural effusion are haemothorax, tuberculosis, rheumatoid arthritis and lupus pleuritis.

Total and differential cell counts

A predominance of neutrophils in the pleural fluid (>50% of the cells) indicates an acute process such as pulmonary embolism, parapneumonic effusion or acute tuberculosis. A predominance of mononuclear cells indicates a chronic process, while a preponderance of small lymphocytes can be related to coronary artery bypass surgery, cancer or tuberculous pleuritis. Gram and Ziehl–Nielson staining and culture for both aerobic and anaerobic bacteria will identify infected pleural fluids. The yield is increased if blood culture bottles are inoculated with the pleural fluid.

Markers of tuberculosis

Measurement of adenosine deaminase (ADA), interferon-γ or PCR for mycobacterial DNA can be used to establish the diagnosis of tuberculous pleuritis. An ADA level >40 U/L has a sensitivity of over 90% and a specificity of 85% for the presence of tuberculosis.

Cytological examination

Cytological examination of the pleural fluid is a fast, efficient and minimally invasive means for establishing a diagnosis of cancer. Cytology can establish the diagnosis in approximately 60% more of metastatic adenocarcinoma cases, but the yield is lower in other types of cancers. If lymphoma is suspected, flow cytometry can establish the diagnosis by demonstrating the presence of a clonal cell population in the pleural fluid.

Further investigations

Chest CT

CT scanning may help define the cause of the pleural effusion. Contrast enhancement is helpful in separating an effusion from an adjacent lung process (airspace disease or atelectasis) and can show pathological pulmonary changes, such as pneumonia, tumour, pleural thickening and nodularity, that may be amenable to percutaneous biopsy (Figure 62.2).

Pleural biopsy

If the results of fluid analysis and radiology are not sufficient for diagnosing a persistent unexplained exudative effusion, then a pleural biopsy is indicated. Thoracoscopy is the procedure of choice for patients with suspected cancer and negative results on cytological examination (Figure 62.3). This technique allows close visual examination of the pleura and accurate biopsy of abnormal tissue and is diagnostic in approximately 90% of cases.

Bronchoscopy

Bronchoscopy is not routinely recommended in the investigation of pleural effusion unless the patient has haemoptysis or radiological features of malignant neoplasm, such as a mass, massive pleural effusion, or a shift in the midline toward the side of the effusion.

63 Pneumothorax

Figure 63.1 (a) Normal CXR. (b) CXR shows left pneumothorax with collapse of left lung

(a)

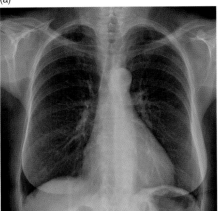

(b)

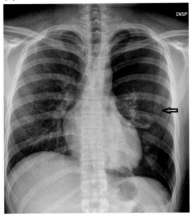

Figure 63.2 CXR shows the completely collapsed left lung with mediastinum and heart compressed to the right, consistent with a left tension pneumothorax

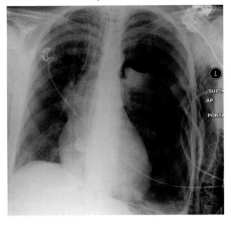

Figure 63.3 (a) CXR shows pneumomediastinum with crisp heart border bilaterally and extension of mediastinal air into the base of the neck. (b) CXR lateral view shows pneumomediastinum

(a)

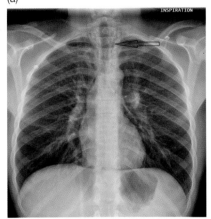

(b)

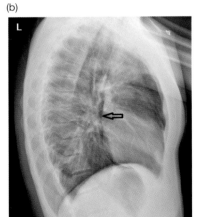

Figure 63.4 CT chest shows pneumomediastinum

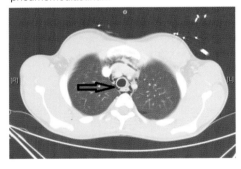

Key points

- On CXR, radiolucent air and the absence of lung markings between a lung edge and the parietal pleura are diagnostic of pneumothorax.
- CT chest is the 'gold standard' in the detection of small pneumothoraces and useful for size estimation.
- Pneumomediastinum can be confirmed by CXR and followed by CT chest.

Clinical Investigations at a Glance, First Edition. Jonathan Gleadle, Jordan Li and Tuck Yong. © 2017 John Wiley & Sons, Ltd. Published 2017 by John Wiley & Sons, Ltd.

Pneumothorax is the presence of air within the pleural space with consequent collapse of the respective lung. Tension pneumothorax is a life-threatening condition that occurs due to the progressive accumulation of intrapleural air in the thoracic cavity as the result of a valve effect during inspiration/expiration. It exerts a positive mass effect on the mediastinum (compressing veins, and the heart) and the opposite lung, which leads to cardiorespiratory arrest.

Pneumothorax is usually suggested by clinical history and physical examination. Radiological investigation of the chest is needed to establish the diagnosis.

CXR

Standard erect CXR on inspiration is recommended for the initial diagnosis of pneumothorax. When assessing the CXR for pneumothorax, a systematic approach should be used. First, always assess the rotation of the film, which can obscure a pneumothorax and mimic a mediastinal shift. In a non-loculated pneumothorax, air generally rises to the non-dependent portion of the pleural cavity. Therefore, the apices of an upright CXR should be examined carefully, and the costophrenic and cardiophrenic angles on a supine CXR evaluated.

Finding of pneumothorax on CXR may include the following (Figure 63.1):
• A linear shadow of visceral pleura with lack of lung markings peripheral to the lung parenchymal may be observed.
• An ipsilateral lung edge may be seen parallel to the chest wall.
• In supine patients, deep sulcus sign (very dark and deep costophrenic angle) with radiolucency along costophrenic sulcus may help to identify occult pneumothorax.
• Small pleural effusions are commonly present and can increase in size if the pneumothorax does not re-expand.
• Mediastinal shift toward the contralateral lung may be apparent.
• Airway or parenchymal abnormalities in the contralateral lung suggest causes of secondary pneumothorax.
• A suspected pneumothorax that is not readily observed on standard postero-anterior radiograph can be demonstrated by obtaining a lateral decubitus film with the involved hemithorax positioned uppermost.

In addition to diagnosis, repeat CXRs are often used to estimate the size of the pneumothorax after aspiration or thoracostomy.

CXRs have the following limitations in detecting a pneumothorax:
• In patients with underlying pulmonary disease, the classic visceral pleural line may be harder to detect, because the lung is hyperlucent, and little difference exists in the radiographic density between the pneumothorax and the emphysematous lung.
• Large bullae can mimic pneumothorax on a CXR.
• Skin folds, the scapula and bed sheets can mimic the pleural line, falsely suggesting a pneumothorax on the CXR. Unlike pneumothoraces, skin folds usually continue beyond the chest wall and lung markings can be seen peripheral to the skin fold line.

Tension pneumothorax

Tension pneumothorax is a clinical diagnosis, a medical emergency and requires immediate treatment. In rare instances when a CXR can be obtained safely, findings of tension pneumothorax can include ipsilateral lung collapse at the hilum, increased thoracic volume, deviation of trachea and mediastinum to the contralateral side, widened intercostal spaces on the affected side and heart border ipsilateral flattening (Figure 63.2).

Pneumomediastinum

Mediastinal emphysema appears as a thin line of radiolucency that outlines the cardiac silhouette, as well as thin, lucent, vertically oriented streaks of air within the mediastinum (Figure 63.3). The aorta and other posterior mediastinal structures are highlighted, and a well-defined lucency around the right pulmonary artery ("ring around the artery" sign) may be seen.

Chest CT

Chest CT is the most reliable imaging study for the diagnosis of pneumothorax, but it is not recommended for routine use in pneumothorax. A CT scan can help to achieve the following:
• distinguish between a pneumothorax and a large bulla;
• indicate underlying emphysema or emphysema-like changes;
• determine the exact size of the pneumothorax, especially if it is small;
• confirm the diagnosis of pneumothorax in patients with head trauma who are mechanically ventilated;
• detect occult/small pneumothoraces and pneumomediastinum (Figure 63.4) (but the clinical significance of these occult pneumothoraces is unclear).

Ultrasound

Ultrasound is increasingly used in the acute care setting as a readily available bedside tool, especially in the intensive care unit and emergency department. This modality provides a rapid imaging option for diagnosis of pneumothorax. Ultrasound has high sensitivity (96%) and specificity (100%) for pneumothorax when using CT as the criterion standard.

Other investigations

Arterial blood gas (ABG)

The ABG measures the degrees of hypoxaemia, acidaemia and hypercarbia. The presence of underlying lung disease along with the size of pneumothorax decides the severity of hypoxaemia. ABG measurements are frequently abnormal in patients with pneumothorax with the arterial oxygen tension (PaO_2) being less than 80 mmHg in 75% of patients, together with a degree of carbon dioxide retention in 16% of patients.

Laboratory investigations

These should include FBC, electrolytes, urea, creatinine, liver function test and CRP.

If vomiting is the precipitating event for a pneumothorax, an oesophagogram should be obtained to evaluate for oesophageal tear, which has a high mortality rate.

64 Pulmonary embolism

Table 64.1 Risk factors for PE

Inherited risk factors

- Protein C or S deficiency
- Antithrombin III deficiency
- Homozygous or heterozygous factor V Leiden
- Homozygous or heterozygous prothrombin gene mutation

Acquired risk factors

- Previous PE or/and deep vein thrombosis (DVT)
- Surgery
- Orthopaedic surgery (hip and knee replacement)
- Major surgery (abdominal surgery, bariatric surgery, spinal surgery)
- Major trauma (fracture neck of femur, pelvic rami, low leg)
- Pregnancy
- Oral contraceptive pill
- Hormone replacement therapy
- Prolonged immobilization (>3 days)
- Malignancy
- Acquired thrombophilia
- Antiphospholipid syndrome, nephrotic syndrome
- Central venous line
- Chronic heart or respiratory failure
- Paralytic stroke
- Obesity
- Increasing age

Figure 64.1 ECG shows classical deep S wave in lead I with Q in III and T wave inversion in lead III, sinus tachycardia that is suggestive of PE

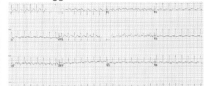

Figure 64.2 Echo shows dilated right heart and hypokinesis in a patient with saddle PE

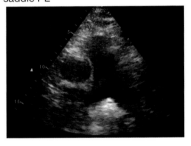

Table 64.2 Clinical prediction rules for PE: the Wells score

Wells score	Points
Variable	
• Predisposing factors	
o Previous DVT or PE	+1.5
o Recent surgery or immobilization	+1.5
o Cancer	+1
• Symptoms	
o Haemoptysis	+1
• Clinical signs	
o Heart rate >100 beats/min	+1.5
o Clinical signs of DVT	+3
• Clinical judgement	
o Alternative diagnosis less likely than PE	+3
Clinical probability (3 levels)	
• Low	0–1
• Intermediate	2–6
• High	≥7
Clinical probability (2 levels)	
• PE unlikely	0–4
• PE likely	>4

Figure 64.3 CTPA shows bilateral multiple PEs

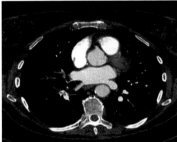

Table 64.3 CXR finding in patients with PE

- Basal atelectasis or infiltrate (65–70%)
- Pleural effusion (about 45–50%)
- Pleural-based opacity (35%)
- Elevated diaphragm (24%)
- Decreased pulmonary vascularity (21%)

Box 64.1 ECG abnormalities in acute PE

- Unexplained sinus tachycardia.
- Non-specific ST segment and T-wave changes.
- Manifestations of acute cor pulmonale, such as an S1, Q3, T3 pattern, new right bundle-branch block, P-wave pulmonale or right axis deviation.

The following ECG abnormalities in patients with PE are associated with poor prognosis:

- atrial arrhythmias
- new right bundle branch block
- inferior Q-waves
- precordial T-wave inversion and ST-segment changes (which may correlate with more severe RV dysfunction).

Key points in investigating pulmonary embolism

- A negative D-dimer in a low-probability case of suspected PE rules out the diagnosis and no further investigation is required.
- A CXR is useful to exclude diagnoses that mimic PE before further investigations.
- If pre-test probability is high or if D-dimer is positive, CTPA (or V/Q scanning when CT contrast is contraindicated) should be performed.

Pulmonary embolism (PE) is associated with significant morbidity and mortality (fatality rate 7–11%). Prompt investigation and diagnosis is of paramount importance because immediate treatment is effective and can reduce the risk of subsequent embolism. PE usually presents with nonspecific chest pain, dyspnoea, tachycardia and sometimes as shock, but some patients with PE have no symptoms at presentation. Therefore, PE cannot be diagnosed by history and physical examination alone.

If PE is suspected, assessment of the known risk factors is needed (Table 64.1). Clinical prediction scores-Wells scores can provide a pre-test probability of PE (Table 64.2). This clinical score stratifies patients into three levels of clinical probability of PE and is particularly valuable in defining low-risk patients in whom PE may be safely excluded by simple non-invasive tests. The prevalence of PE increases with increasing clinical probability (low, 9%; moderate, 30%; high, 68%). Initial investigations include ABG, ECG, CXR, and D-dimer. Further studies, such as CT pulmonary angiography (CTPA), ventilation–perfusion (V/Q) scintigraphy, ultrasonography of leg veins and echocardiography, should be considered in the evaluation of suspected PE.

Arterial blood gas (ABG)

ABG in patients with acute PE usually shows hypoxaemia and elevated alveolar-arterial (A-a) oxygen gradient. However, the partial arterial oxygen pressure (PaO_2) and the A-a oxygen gradient may be normal in patients with PE. A PaO_2 between 85 and 105 mmHg exists in about 18% of patients with PE. A normal A-a gradient is seen in about 6% of patients with PE. ABG analysis alone is therefore of limited diagnostic utility in suspected PE, but significant abnormalities require investigation.

D-dimer

D-dimer is an indicator of coagulation activation and is produced during polymerisation of fibrinogen as it forms fibrin. D-dimer has a sensitivity of 95–98% in the diagnosis of PE but limited specificity. Any thrombotic process, infection, cancer, trauma and inflammatory states will elevate the D-dimer level. D-dimer results can be used in combination with clinical prediction scores to provide a likelihood of PE.

In patients with low or moderate pre-test probability, a negative D-dimer infers a very low likelihood of PE and precludes the need for further imaging studies. The negative predictive value for diagnosis of PE in patients with low pre-test probability is between 90 and 98%. However, in patients with a high pre-test probability, negative D-dimer test is insufficient to exclude PE, and CTPA or V/Q scan should be performed.

Other biomarkers

Troponin levels may be elevated in patients with massive acute PE, and it is used in risk stratification in patients with established PE. It is not sensitive as a diagnostic tool when used alone. Elevated troponin levels are associated with sixfold higher mortality even in haemodynamically stable patients.

Plasma brain natriuretic peptide (BNP) level may be elevated in PE with increase in ventricular stretching, reflects the severity of right ventricle (RV) dysfunction and provides prognostic information. However, BNP has a poor sensitivity (60%) and specificity (62%) for diagnosis of PE because it can be increased in conditions such as heart failure and pulmonary hypertension.

ECG

ECG changes (Box 64.1) occur infrequently in PE (Figure 64.1). ECG alone has no adequate sensitivity or specificity to rule in or rule out PE. Its main value is in finding alternative diagnoses, such as myocardial infarction.

Echocardiography

Echo cardiography is used to stratify the risk of patients with established PE and providing guidance for treatment (Figure 64.2). Only 30–40% of patients with PE have the following echo abnormalities:

- RV dilatation
- decreased RV function
- tricuspid regurgitation.

These abnormalities are more likely in patients with massive PE. Therefore, echo is not an element of diagnostic strategy in haemodynamically stable patients with suspected PE. However, in a patient with shock or hypotension, an urgent echo showing no RV dysfunction practically excludes PE as a cause of shock.

CXR

CXR is often normal in patients with PE, though pleural effusions, basal atelectasis and infiltrates are common (Table 64.3). The additional benefit of the CXR in the assessment of suspected PE is that it might uncover an alternative diagnosis.

CTPA

CTPA is the imaging of choice for suspected PE. CTPA showing a thrombus up to the segmental level is adequate evidence of PE. CTPA has high sensitivity (83%) and specificity (96%) for detecting emboli in the main, lobar or segmental pulmonary arteries (Figure 64.3) when compared with the gold standard of pulmonary angiography. The advantages of CTPA over V/Q scan include speed and characterisation of non-vascular structures, revealing alternative pulmonary abnormalities responsible for patients' symptomatology. However, caution is required in AKI or CKD because of contrast-induced nephropathy.

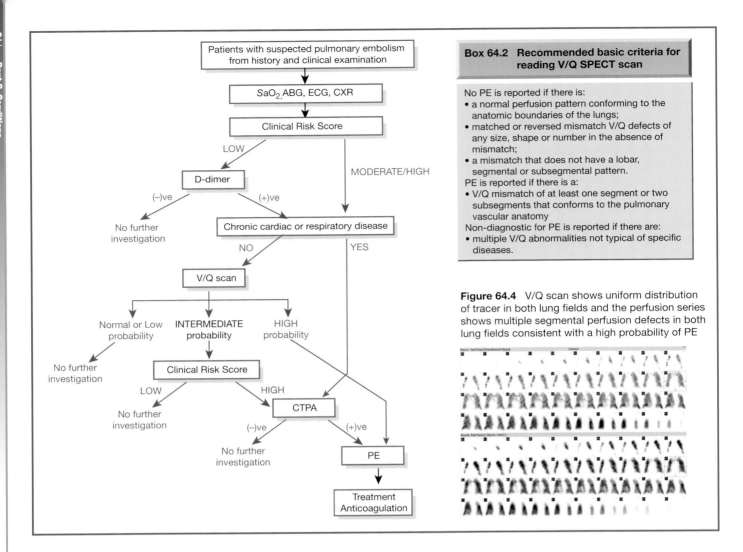

Figure 64.4 V/Q scan shows uniform distribution of tracer in both lung fields and the perfusion series shows multiple segmental perfusion defects in both lung fields consistent with a high probability of PE

Ventilation–perfusion scintigraphy

V/Q scan is a well-established and safe diagnostic test for suspected PE. It is an alternative to CTPA when contrast is a contraindication due to allergy or significant renal impairment. V/Q scan is most likely to be diagnostic in the absence of cardiopulmonary disease. V/Q scan results can be classified into four categories: normal, low, intermediate (non-diagnostic) and high probability.

A normal V/Q scan effectively rules out acute PE. A high probability scan (Figure 64.4) is considered diagnostic unless clinical suspicion is low or there is a history of PE with an identical previous scan. Patients with high clinical probability of acute PE and a high-probability V/Q scan have a 95% likelihood of having PE. On the other hand, patients with low clinical probability of acute PE and a low-probability V/Q scan have only a 4% likelihood of having PE.

The new ventilation–perfusion single-photon emission computed tomography (V/Q SPECT) has higher sensitivity and specificity than a V/Q scan. The recommended basic criteria for reading a V/Q SPECT scan are listed in Box 64.2.

Pulmonary angiography

Pulmonary angiography is the gold standard for diagnosing PE. It reveals direct evidence of a thrombus, either a filling defect or amputation of a pulmonary arterial branch. Thrombi, as small as 1 mm within the subsegmental arteries can be visualized. It is now rarely employed because CTPA offers similar or better information. Furthermore, pulmonary angiography is invasive and associated with morbidity as well as mortality.

Magnetic resonance angiography (MRA)

There is growing evidence that MRA may be an alternative diagnostic tool in cases of suspected acute PE (sensitivity 78%, specificity of 99% for main or lobar PE).

Lower extremity venous ultrasound

PE and DVT are two clinical presentations of venous thromboembolism (VTE). PE is a consequence of DVT in most cases (90%). Among patients with proximal DVT, about 50% have a PE. In about 70% of patients with PE, DVT can be detected by duplex ultrasound. Therefore, the diagnosis of proximal DVT by lower extremity venous ultrasound in a patient with suspected PE is considered sufficient to rule in PE. This is especially useful in patients who have contraindications to CTPA. There are two limitations to this approach that clinicians need to be aware of. First, false-positive venous ultrasound studies can result in unnecessary anticoagulation. Second, many patients with PE are likely to be missed if venous ultrasound is used alone because about 30% of patients with PE, as determined by CTPA or V/Q scan, have no lower extremity DVT.

Considerations in pregnant patients

Women who are pregnant or those in the post-partum period are at increased risk of VTE. In pregnant women with suspected PE, D-dimer should not be used to exclude PE. A CXR should be the first investigation. If the CXR is normal, a V/Q scan is recommended as the next imaging test instead of CTPA. If the V/Q is non-diagnostic or if the woman has an abnormal CXR, CTPA is recommended as the next imaging test. The fetal radiation exposure is similar in V/Q scan and CTPA and presents no measurably increased risk of fetal development and malformation. However, the maternal radiation exposure is lower in V/Q scan. Iodinated contrast, classified as category B by the US Food and Drug Administration, crosses the placenta and enters both the fetal circulation and the amniotic fluid. There is no evidence that it cause neonatal hypothyroidism or teratogenicity.

65 Pulmonary hypertension

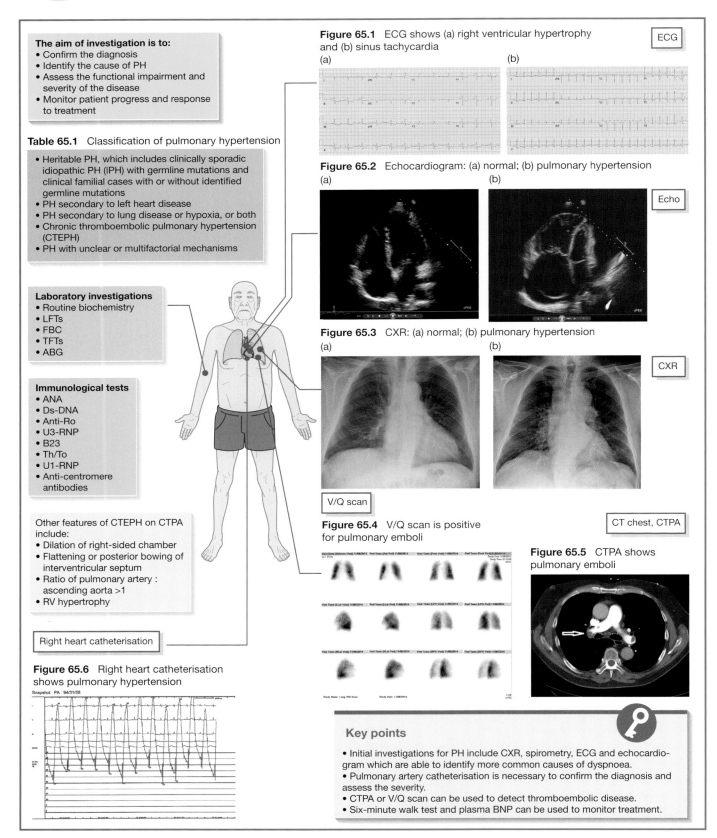

The aim of investigation is to:
- Confirm the diagnosis
- Identify the cause of PH
- Assess the functional impairment and severity of the disease
- Monitor patient progress and response to treatment

Table 65.1 Classification of pulmonary hypertension

- Heritable PH, which includes clinically sporadic idiopathic PH (IPH) with germline mutations and clinical familial cases with or without identified germline mutations
- PH secondary to left heart disease
- PH secondary to lung disease or hypoxia, or both
- Chronic thromboembolic pulmonary hypertension (CTEPH)
- PH with unclear or multifactorial mechanisms

Laboratory investigations
- Routine biochemistry
- LFTs
- FBC
- TFTs
- ABG

Immunological tests
- ANA
- Ds-DNA
- Anti-Ro
- U3-RNP
- B23
- Th/To
- U1-RNP
- Anti-centromere antibodies

Other features of CTEPH on CTPA include:
- Dilation of right-sided chamber
- Flattening or posterior bowing of interventricular septum
- Ratio of pulmonary artery : ascending aorta >1
- RV hypertrophy

Right heart catheterisation

Figure 65.1 ECG shows (a) right ventricular hypertrophy and (b) sinus tachycardia
(a)   (b)

ECG

Figure 65.2 Echocardiogram: (a) normal; (b) pulmonary hypertension
(a)   (b)

Echo

Figure 65.3 CXR: (a) normal; (b) pulmonary hypertension
(a)   (b)

CXR

V/Q scan

Figure 65.4 V/Q scan is positive for pulmonary emboli

CT chest, CTPA

Figure 65.5 CTPA shows pulmonary emboli

Figure 65.6 Right heart catheterisation shows pulmonary hypertension

Snapshot: PA : 94/31/58

Key points

- Initial investigations for PH include CXR, spirometry, ECG and echocardiogram which are able to identify more common causes of dyspnoea.
- Pulmonary artery catheterisation is necessary to confirm the diagnosis and assess the severity.
- CTPA or V/Q scan can be used to detect thromboembolic disease.
- Six-minute walk test and plasma BNP can be used to monitor treatment.

Pulmonary hypertension (PH) is a group of diseases characterised by a progressive increase of pulmonary vascular resistance leading to right ventricular failure and premature death. It is defined as a mean pulmonary artery pressure (PAP) of ≥25 mmHg on cardiac catheterisation. PH most commonly presents with progressive breathlessness. As right ventricular failure (RVF) develops, patients may experience exertional dizziness and syncope. Oedema and ascites occur late in the disorder. PH is classified into five clinical groups (see Table 65.1).

Laboratory investigations

Routine biochemistry, liver function tests (LFTs), haematology and thyroid function tests (TFTs) are required in all patients with suspected PH. Haemoglobin may reveal anaemia as a contributor to dyspnoea. LFTs may be deranged with liver congestion as a consequence of RVF. Up to 2% of individuals with cirrhosis and/or portal hypertension will manifest PH.

Immunological testing should be considered in the clinical context. Up to 40% of patients with idiopathic pulmonary hypertension (IPH) have elevated ANA, usually in low titre (1 : 80). Systemic sclerosis is the most important disorder to exclude because this condition has a high prevalence of PH. Anti-centromere antibodies are typically positive in limited scleroderma, as are other ANAs, including dsDNA, anti-Ro, U3-RNP, B23, Th/To and U1-RNP. In the diffuse variety of scleroderma, U3-RNP is typically positive. Thrombophilia screening, including antiphospholipid antibodies, lupus anticoagulant and anticardiolipin antibodies, should be performed in CTEPH.

Arterial blood gas (ABG) should be performed to exclude hypoxia and acidosis as contributors to PH. It is important to note that normal resting oxygenation does not exclude exertional or nocturnal oxygen desaturation. Exercise and overnight oximetry should also be performed in all patients with PH. Polysomnography should be performed if sleep-disordered breathing is a suspected cause of PH.

ECG

An ECG is useful in evaluating PH by providing signs of right ventricular hypertrophy (87% in IPH), right axis deviation (79% in IPH), right heart strain and tachyarrhythmia, most commonly atrial flutter (Figure 65.1). An ECG by itself cannot diagnose PH, and a normal ECG does not exclude the diagnosis of PH.

Echocardiography

Echocardiography should always be performed in suspected PH. It can be used to estimate systolic PAP (sPAP); together with other echocardiographic features of PH, the likelihood of PH can be determined as follows:
- unlikely – if sPAP ≤36 mmHg with no other features of PH;
- possible – if sPAP ≥36 mmHg with other features of PH or sPAP 37–50 mmHg;
- likely – if sPAP ≥50 mmHg.

Other echocardiographic features suggestive of PH include:
- dilated right sided chambers (Figure 65.2);
- reduced right ventricle (RV) function;
- RV hypertrophy;
- enlarged pulmonary artery;
- abnormal interventricular septal motion.

It is important to realise that PH is defined by mean PAP (measured by right heart catheterisation) and not sPAP (estimated by echocardiography). Furthermore, systolic estimates are less accurate in respiratory disease and during intercurrent illness.

Pulmonary function tests

Spirometry may be mildly deranged and gas transfer is reduced in IPH. The 6-minute walk test can provide functional and prognostic information in PH as well as being used to monitor treatment response. Cardiopulmonary exercise testing can be done in selected patients to obtain more detailed physiological and prognostic information.

CXR

CXR may show prominent pulmonary arteries or/and enlarged RV (Figure 65.3), but a normal CXR cannot exclude the diagnosis. In 90% of patients with IPH, CXR is abnormal at the time of diagnosis. CXR may identify associated lung disease. The extent of CXR abnormalities does not correlate with the severity of PH.

Ventilation–perfusion lung scan (V/Q scan)

A V/Q scan has high sensitivity for CTEPH and a normal scan excludes the diagnosis with a sensitivity of 90–100% and a specificity of 94–100% (Figure 65.4), whereas increased renal isotope uptake may identify right to left shunts and explain hypoxaemia.

HRCT and CTPA

HRCT provides detailed views of the lung parenchyma and facilitates the diagnosis of interstitial lung disease and emphysema. CTPA is used to visualise the pulmonary arterial tree and provide useful additional diagnostic information related to chronic thromboembolic disease. Direct thromboembolic features include occlusions, stenosis and intraluminal web (Figure 65.5). Other features of CTEPH on CTPA are listed on the opposite page.

Cardiac MRI and pulmonary angiography

MRI provides a radiation-free approach of quantitatively assessing cardiac structure and function, prognosis and response to treatment. It provides a direct evaluation of RV size and morphology. Pulmonary angiography is usually carried out at the time of the right heart catheterisation to select CTEPH patients for pulmonary endarterectomy.

Right heart catheterisation

If non-invasive investigations are suggestive of PH, right heart catheterisation is needed to confirm the diagnosis by directly measuring PAP (Figure 65.6). It can also measure cardiac output and estimate left atrial pressure using pulmonary arterial wedge pressure. Haemodynamic parameters (such as right atrial pressure, cardiac index and pulmonary vascular resistance), pulmonary artery saturations and the vasoreactivity of the pulmonary circulation can be measured and have prognostic value. Changes in oxygen saturations between right-sided cardiac chambers may suggest an intracardiac shunt. Complications include those related to central venous access, catheter-related infection, venous or intracardiac thrombus formation, infective endocarditis and pulmonary infarction. Ectopic activity may occur, but ventricular arrhythmias are rare. Overall, this procedure has low morbidity (1.1%) and mortality (0.05%) rates.

66 Pulmonary nodules

The main goal of SPN investigation is to determine if the SPN is malignant.

Table 66.1 Common causes of SPN

Malignant causes	Benign causes
• Adenocarcinoma • Squamous cell carcinoma • Small cell lung cancer • Metastasis • Carcinoid tumour	• Non-specific granuloma • Hamartoma • Infectious granuloma • Aspergillosis • Tuberculosis

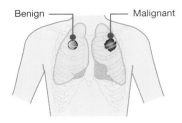

Benign —— Malignant

Table 66.2 Clinical features suggestive of malignant SPN

Patient age >50 years old (three times higher risk than those below this age)
History of smoking
Occupational exposure, such as asbestos exposure
Family history of malignancy
Previously diagnosed malignancy

• High-risk patient is defined by presence of features listed in Table 66.2.
• Low-risk patient is defined by absence of the noted risk factors.
• This summary is not suitable for patients who are young (under the age of 35 years), have extrathoracic malignancy or have unexplained fever.

Table 66.3 Summary of evaluation of SPN

Nodule size (mm)	Low-risk patient	High-risk patient
≤4	No follow-up or optional follow-up	Repeat CT at 12 months; if stable, no further follow-up
>4–6	Repeat CT at 12 months; if stable, no further follow-up	Repeat CT at 6–12 months then at 18–24 months if stable
>6–8	Repeat CT at 6–12 months then at 18–24 months if stable	Repeat CT at 3–6 months then at 9–12 months and 24 months if stable
>8–30	Repeat contrast-enhanced CT at 3, 6, 12 and 24 months, consider FDG-PET scan and CT-guided fine-needle aspiration	FDG-PET scan, CT-guided fine-needle aspiration, and/or bronchoscopy, VATS and frozen section, if malignant for lobectomy

Figure 66.1 CXR shows a 2.5 cm pulmonary nodule in the right upper lobe with irregular and spiculated borders, which is suggestive of malignant nodule

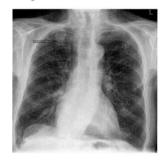

Figure 66.2 CT chest shows a pulmonary nodule in the right upper lobe with irregular and spiculated borders suggestive of malignant nodule: (a) coronal view; (b) axial view

(a)

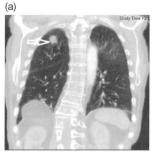

(b)

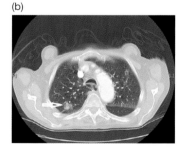

Figure 66.4 Lung biopsy shows squamous cell lung cancer

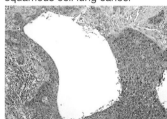

Figure 66.3 FDG-PET scan shows the pulmonary nodule is metabolically active and takes up FDG avidly, which is indicative of malignancy

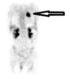

Key points

• CT with thin slices is the initial investigation of choice for the evaluation of the solitary lung nodule. It can distinguish lung nodules from lesions of the chest wall, pleura and artefact.
• CT chest can identify features of the nodule that suggest a benign or malignant process.
• The follow-up interval for a pulmonary nodule with potential for malignancy is dependent on the clinical and radiological risk of malignancy.
• PET has a sensitivity of 97% and specificity of 78% for the detection of malignancy in lung nodules and masses.

Clinical Investigations at a Glance, First Edition. Jonathan Gleadle, Jordan Li and Tuck Yong. © 2017 John Wiley & Sons, Ltd. Published 2017 by John Wiley & Sons, Ltd.

Pulmonary nodules are small, focal, radiographic opacities that may be solitary or multiple. A solitary pulmonary nodule (SPN) is a round or oval opacity ≤3 cm in diameter that is completely surrounded by pulmonary parenchyma and is not associated with lymphadenopathy, atelectasis or pneumonia. Nodules >3 cm have a substantially increased risk of malignancy and are referred to as a mass. SPN is a commonly encountered clinical problem, predominately due to incidental findings on CXR or CT of the chest and abdomen for other purposes. The estimated prevalence of SPN in asymptomatic individuals ranges from 8 to 51%. Causes of an SPN can be benign or malignant (Table 66.1). In clinical practice, most cases of SPN are benign and the incidence of malignant SPN ranges from 3 to 6%.

The initial diagnostic assessment is to evaluate the clinical and radiological features. Clinical features that increase the likelihood of an SPN being malignant are summarized in Table 66.2. Radiological features that determine the likelihood of SNP being malignant include:

- *Size.* A larger lesion is more likely to be malignant than a smaller lesion. A nodule <3 mm has a 0.2% likelihood of being malignant, whereas a nodule >20 mm has a 50% likelihood.
- *Border.* Irregular and spiculated borders are more likely to be associated with malignant lesion (Figure 66.1); benign lesions tend to have a relatively smooth and discrete border.
- *Calcification.* The presence of calcification does not exclude malignancy. However, certain patterns of calcification, namely 'popcorn', laminated (concentric), central and diffuse homogeneous, are more suggestive of a benign lesion.
- *Density.* Increased density indicates a lower likelihood of malignancy.
- *Growth.* An SPN whose size has increased rapidly is more likely to be malignant, while one that has remained stable for a prolonged duration is likely to be benign. For a spherical mass, a 30% increase in diameter corresponds to a doubling of overall volume. Doubling time between 1 month and 1 year suggests malignancy.

Investigations for a solitary pulmonary nodule

Chest CT

In any patient with a newly discovered SPN on CXR, a CT of the chest (preferably thin-slice CT) should be performed (Figure 66.2). The CT examination can potentially identify additional nodules, lymphadenopathy, pleural effusion or chest wall involvement. Serial CT scans are used to monitor a nodule that has a low probability of being malignant, and this may be done at various intervals for up to 2 years depending on the nature of the nodule (Table 66.3).

18-Fluorodeoxyglucose PET scan

FDG-PET scan is a useful investigation to distinguish between benign and malignant SPN because malignancy is metabolically active and takes up FDG avidly (Figure 66.3). The sensitivity and specificity of FDG-PET for malignancy is estimated to be 95% and 78% respectively. Therefore, a negative FDG-PET will exclude malignancy in most cases.

Bronchoscopy

Bronchoscopy is an option for diagnostic evaluation of large, central nodules but is less useful for small or peripheral ones. During bronchoscopy, specimens can be obtained by washing or lavage of the airway supplying the lesion or by direct sampling of the lesion by brushings or transbronchial biopsy. The yield for diagnosing peripheral nodules of <2 cm in size by brushing or biopsy was 33%, whereas the yield for lesions >2 cm increases to 68%.

Percutaneous needle aspiration or biopsy

Percutaneous needle aspiration or biopsy can be performed through the chest wall using CT guidance. Percutaneous needle aspiration can detect malignancy with a sensitivity and specificity of about 90% and 97% respectively (Figure 66.4). The false positive is low, but a negative result does not completely exclude malignancy. With a needle biopsy, up to 97% of patients with a malignant or benign lung nodule will obtain a definitive diagnosis. The complications are haemorrhage and pneumothorax, especially in patients with chronic obstructive pulmonary disease.

Surgical resection

If the SPN has clearly grown on serial imaging tests, the likelihood of malignancy is high, the nodule is FDG-avid on PET or it is proven to be malignant on tissue sampling, surgical excision is indicated. This can be performed by thoracotomy or video-assisted thoracic surgery (VATS) if the nodule is sufficiently close to the pleura.

67 Interstitial lung disease

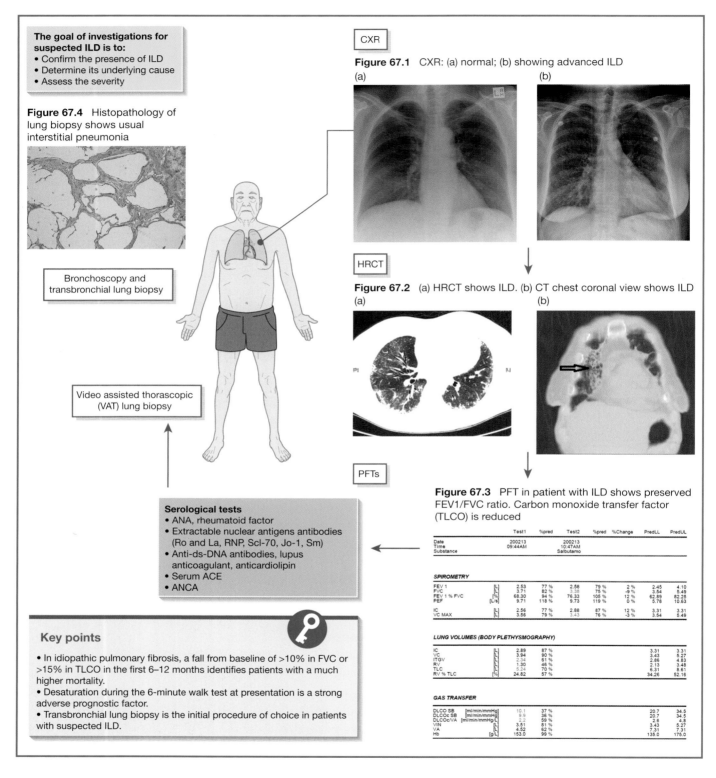

The goal of investigations for suspected ILD is to:
- Confirm the presence of ILD
- Determine its underlying cause
- Assess the severity

Figure 67.4 Histopathology of lung biopsy shows usual interstitial pneumonia

Bronchoscopy and transbronchial lung biopsy

Video assisted thorascopic (VAT) lung biopsy

Serological tests
- ANA, rheumatoid factor
- Extractable nuclear antigens antibodies (Ro and La, RNP, Scl-70, Jo-1, Sm)
- Anti-ds-DNA antibodies, lupus anticoagulant, anticardiolipin
- Serum ACE
- ANCA

CXR

Figure 67.1 CXR: (a) normal; (b) showing advanced ILD
(a)   (b)

HRCT

Figure 67.2 (a) HRCT shows ILD. (b) CT chest coronal view shows ILD
(a)   (b)

PFTs

Figure 67.3 PFT in patient with ILD shows preserved FEV1/FVC ratio. Carbon monoxide transfer factor (TLCO) is reduced

		Test1	%pred	Test2	%pred	%Change	PredLL	PredUL
Date		200213		200213				
Time		09:44AM		10:47AM				
Substance				Salbutamo				
SPIROMETRY								
FEV 1	[L]	2.53	77 %	2.58	79 %	2 %	2.45	4.10
FVC	[L]	3.71	82 %	3.38	75 %	-9 %	3.54	5.49
FEV 1 % FVC	[%]	68.30	94 %	76.33	105 %	12 %	62.89	82.25
PEF	[L/s]	9.71	118 %	9.73	119 %	0 %	5.78	10.63
IC	[L]	2.56	77 %	2.88	87 %	12 %	3.31	3.31
VC MAX	[L]	3.56	79 %	3.43	76 %	-3 %	3.54	5.49
LUNG VOLUMES (BODY PLETHYSMOGRAPHY)								
IC	[L]	2.89	87 %				3.31	3.31
VC	[L]	3.94	90 %				3.54	5.27
ITGV	[L]	2.34	61 %				2.86	4.83
RV	[L]	1.30	46 %				2.13	3.48
TLC	[L]	5.24	70 %				6.31	8.61
RV % TLC	[%]	24.82	57 %				34.26	52.16
GAS TRANSFER								
DLCO SB	[ml/min/mmHg]	10.1	37 %				20.7	34.5
DLCOc SB	[ml/min/mmHg]	9.9	36 %				20.7	34.5
DLCOc/VA	[ml/min/mmHg/L]	2.2	59 %				2.6	4.8
VIN	[L]	3.51	81 %				3.43	5.27
V.A	[L]	4.52	62 %				7.31	7.31
Hb	[g]	153.0	99 %				135.0	175.0

Key points

- In idiopathic pulmonary fibrosis, a fall from baseline of >10% in FVC or >15% in TLCO in the first 6–12 months identifies patients with a much higher mortality.
- Desaturation during the 6-minute walk test at presentation is a strong adverse prognostic factor.
- Transbronchial lung biopsy is the initial procedure of choice in patients with suspected ILD.

The interstitial lung diseases (ILDs) are a group of parenchymal lung disorders that are classified according to specific clinical, radiological and histopathological features. Patients with ILD often present with breathlessness, chronic cough, inspiratory crackles on auscultation and abnormal spirometry.

If ILD is suspected, a detailed medical history and examination are essential. An accurate prognosis and optimal treatment strategy for ILD depend on an accurate diagnosis. It is accepted now that diagnosis of ILDs requires a multidisciplinary approach with reconciliation of clinical, radiological and histological information.

CXR

The CXR can be normal in early ILD. By the time the disease is clinically apparent CXR will usually be abnormal (Figure 67.1). Abnormalities include:

- decreased lung volumes;
- subpleural reticular opacities;
- peripheral migratory air space shadowing;
- mediastinal or hilar lymph node enlargement.

The CXR may also help to identify lung cancer, infection or pneumothorax, which may be associated with interstitial disease. CXR has limited sensitivity and lacks specificity for diagnosing subtypes of ILD; high-resolution computed tomography (HRCT) is significantly superior to CXR in identifying and determining the correct diagnosis of ILD and the optimal site of biopsy.

High-resolution chest CT

Typical reasons for HRCT in suspected ILD are to:

- detect ILD in patients with normal or equivocal CXR findings;
- focus the differential diagnosis in patients with obvious but non-specific CXR abnormalities;
- guide the type and site of lung biopsy;
- evaluate disease reversibility;
- preclude the need for bronchoalveolar lavage (BAL) or lung biopsy if the HRCT appearance is sufficiently characteristic.

Characteristic features of ILD on HRCT (Figure 67.2) include bilateral and symmetrical bibasal pulmonary reticular shadowing with destroyed and fibrotic lung tissue that contains numerous cystic airspaces with thick fibrous walls (honeycombing). The reticular pattern reflects a combination of interlobular septal thickening and intralobular opacities. As the fibrosis progresses, traction bronchiectasis is often present. Ground-glass opacity is often present in ILD, and in the absence of adjacent fibrosis it is associated with response to treatment and longer survival.

Pulmonary function tests (PFTs) and ABG

All patients with suspected ILD should have formal PFTs. ILDs typically display a 'restrictive' pattern on spirometry, as the forced expiratory volume in 1 second (FEV_1) and the forced vital capacity (FVC) are both reduced, which results in a preserved or sometimes increased FEV_1/FVC ratio (Figure 67.3). Carbon monoxide transfer factor (TLCO) or diffusing capacity of the lung for carbon monoxide (D_{LCO}) is typically reduced in patients with ILD, secondary to thickening of the alveolar–capillary barrier impairing gas exchange. A spuriously raised transfer factor measurement can occasionally result from minor pulmonary haemorrhage from a systemic vasculitis or, conversely, from anaemia in the context of an ILD.

Exercise tests (6-minute walk test) enable evaluation of disease severity. It records oxygen saturation before, during and after exercise and measures the total distance walked. Some patients with ILD may appear deceptively well at rest, with normal oximetry and spirometry, but become profoundly hypoxic when walking. Oxygen desaturation associated with exercise significantly correlates with pulmonary hypertension, and patients who have these features merit more detailed assessment for pulmonary artery hypertension, including echocardiography.

Bronchoscopy, bronchoalveolar lavage (BAL) and transbronchial lung biopsy

Fibre-optic bronchoscopy enables visualisation of proximal airways and sampling of more distal lung by using transbronchial biopsy, and BAL to exclude infectious causes. Biopsy of lymph nodes adjacent to the airways can be performed via endobronchial ultrasound-guided transbronchial needle aspiration. It is particularly useful in sarcoidosis, with diagnostic yields of up to 90%.

Lung biopsy

The site of surgical biopsy is best informed by chest HRCT. Video-assisted thoracoscopic (VAT) surgery is now used routinely rather than open thoracotomy. Since a range of interstitial patterns may be seen within the same lung, best-practice guidelines encourage sampling from at least two lobes (Figure 67.4). The risks of VAT surgery include persistent air leak (approximately 10–15%) – which results in delayed re-expansion of the lung following the procedure – perioperative bleeding and sepsis.

Other investigations

Laboratory investigations

All patients with suspected ILD should have the following investigations:

- FBC including differential blood cell count;
- serum biochemistry profile (including renal and liver function tests, calcium, glucose, thyroid function, CRP);
- urine analysis and urine protein quantification;
- ECG.

Serological tests

These tests are largely dependent upon clinical context, especially if a connective tissue disease is suspected:

- ANA, rheumatoid factor;
- extractable nuclear antigens antibodies (Ro and La, RNP, Scl-70, Jo-1, Sm);
- anti-ds-DNA antibodies, lupus anticoagulant, anticardiolipin;
- serum angiotensin-converting enzyme (ACE);
- antineutrophil cytoplasmic antibody (ANCA).

If an environmental factor is suspected, specific serum immunoglobulin G antibody screens can be performed for relevant antigens (such as *Saccharopolyspora rectivirgula*, *Thermactinomycetes vulgaris*, *Aspergillus* for mouldy hay).

Echocardiography

Pulmonary hypertension should be considered in patients with ILD who have either breathlessness or lung dysfunction (reduced D_{LCO} or desaturation on exercise). Echocardiography should be performed.

68 Sleep disorders

Table 68.1 Major categories of sleep disorders

| Insomnia |
| Sleep-related breathing disorders |
| Hypersomnias of central origin |
| Circadian rhythm sleep disorders |
| Parasomnias |
| Sleep-related movement disorders |
| Isolated symptoms and normal variants |
| Other sleep disorders |

Key points

• The diagnosis of OSA and other sleep-disordered breathing is confirmed with polysomnography.
• Portable diagnostic tools can be used to diagnose OSA by providing a value for AHI/RDI.
• To diagnose causes of CSA, brain or brainstem imaging may be indicated.

Figure 68.1 A polysomnogram is a colour-coded representation of sleep state throughout the study; dark blue shows instances of arousal above the timescale. The multicoloured graph shows the timescale related to body position; below this is the pulse oximetry. Apnoea can be central (Cn.A), obstructive (Ob.A) or mixed (Mx.A). Obstruction can cause hypoventilation (Hyp) without causing complete apnoea

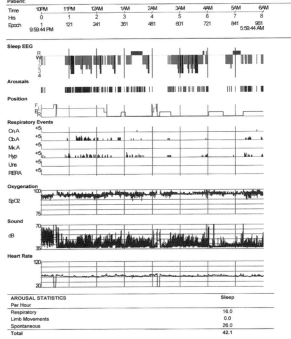

AROUSAL STATISTICS	Sleep
Per Hour	
Respiratory	16.0
Limb Movements	0.0
Spontaneous	26.0
Total	**42.1**

Arousal Definition (adapted from ADSA 1992 and the International Classification of Sleep Disorders):
An arousal is defined as an "abrupt shift in EEG frequency", and may include theta, alpha and/or frequencies > 16 Hz but not spindles; usually of < 15 seconds of alpha activity or waking EEG pattern. It may or may not be associated with detectable body/limb movement or elevation of chin EMG

Figure 68.2 Summary of the sleep study

Patient:

Sex: Male	**Date of birth:**
Weight: 92 kg	**Height:** 162 cm
BMI: 35.1	

SLEEP STATISTICS

Report time from 21:59:44 to 05:59:43		= 480 min
Time available for sleep (lights out)		= 480 min
Sleep latency		= 0 min
REM latency		= 194 min
Sleep period from 21:59:44 to 05:59:13		= 479 min
Total time awake during sleep period		= 210 min
Stage 1 = 3 min 1.1%	Total Sleep	= 269 min
Stage 2 = 156 min 58.1%	NREM Sleep	= 226 min 84.0%
Stage 3 = 34 min 12.6%	REM Sleep	= 43 min 16.0%
Stage 4 = 33 min 12.2%	Sleep Efficiency	= 56.1%

RESPIRATORY / SLEEP STATISTICS

	NREM			REM		
	Back	Other	All	Back	Other	All
SaO_2 min average	93	94	94	-	94	94
SaO_2 lowest	91	89	89	-	88	88
Total duration (min)						
Central Apnoea	0	0	0	0	0	0
Obstructive Apnoea	3	15	19	0	0	0
Mixed Apnoea	1	0	0	0	0	0
Hypopnoea	5	18	23	0	3	3
Apnoea+Hypopnoea	9	33	43	0	4	4
RDI						
Central Apnoea	3.1	0.0	0.3	0.0	1.4	1.4
Obstructive Apnoea	55.4	23.2	26.0	0.0	4.2	4.2
Mixed Apnoea	0.0	0.0	0.0	0.0	0.0	0.0
Hypopnoea	76.9	23.2	27.8	0.0	16.7	16.7
Apnoea+Hypopnoea	135.4	46.4	54.0	0.0	22.3	22.3
			54.0			22.3

Total RDI	**= 49.0**
SaO_2 awake average	= 96 %
Total sleep time with SpO_2 < 90%	= 0.4 min
Mean Apnoea / Hypopnoea duration	= 13 sec
Longest Apnoea	= 21 sec
Longest Hypopnoea	= 25 sec

HEART RATE SUMMARY	
Average Heart Rate during Sleep	64
Number of Bradycardic Periods	0
Number of Tachycardic Periods	0

Figure 68.3 Formal report of the sleep study

TECHNICAL COMMENTS FOR DIAGNOSTIC STUDY:

Epworth Sleepiness Score[1]: 12 out of 24.

ECG: Average heart rate when asleep was 64 bpm, in sinus rhythm.

Blood Pressure: Evening – 123/79; Morning – 144/84.

Snoring: Mild to moderate snoring was noted frequently during the study.

Patient's Impression of Sleep: The patient rated his sleep as worse than his usual sleep experience at home.

Leg index: Abnormal leg movements were not noted.

Rhinomanometry[2]: The total inspiratory flow at 150kPa was estimated at 356ml/second, indicating a severe impairment in baseline nasal airflow. There was a severe reduction in airflow via both nasal airways, resulting in a 1.0 times flow differential between the 2 sides.

Sleep Architecture: The sleep and REM latencies were unable to be calculated as the patient fell asleep prior to calibrations. The sleep architecture was characterised by light NREM sleep, with several short REM bouts achieved. The total arousal index was 42 per hour and the sleep efficiency was 56%.

Respiratory Function in Sleep: Hypopnoeas and apnoeas were noted during both REM and NREM sleep, especially when supine. These events were associated with significant O_2 desaturation (to a nadir of 88%) and EEG arousal. The overall RDI was 49 events per hour.

Technician: David Tickner (Overnight Technician) / Eloise Sheridan (Scoring Technician)

CLINICIAN'S REPORT:
Technical quality of the study is satisfactory and the patient reported worse sleep than usual. No alcohol or sedating medication was consumed prior to the study. Baseline nasal airflow was severely impaired and snoring was heard frequently during the night. No periodic limb movements were seen. Sleep was fragmented with elevated arousal index at 42/hr and reduced sleep efficiency to 56%. There was severe sleep-disordered breathing with total RDI of 49/hr, associated with mild oxygen desaturation episodes to nadir of 88%.

CONCLUSION: Severe OSA (RDI = 49/hr). CPAP titration is recommended.

Clinical Investigations at a Glance, First Edition. Jonathan Gleadle, Jordan Li and Tuck Yong. © 2017 John Wiley & Sons, Ltd. Published 2017 by John Wiley & Sons, Ltd.

Sleep disorders are chronic disturbances in the quantity or quality of sleep that interfere with a person's ability to function normally. Sleep disorders are common (affecting up to 15% of the population) and associated with poor health outcomes. There is a relationship between sleep disorders and hypertension, depression and cardiovascular disease. Sleep disorders can be classified into eight major categories (Table 68.1).

Sleep apnoea

Sleep apnoea is a condition in which the patient stops breathing while asleep. Apnoea is the complete cessation of respiration, and hypopnea is a partial decrease in respiration. Both can cause hypoxaemia and then arousal, which results in fragmented sleep. These arousals are an important contributor to the excessive daytime sleepiness (EDS). Two types of sleep apnoea are recognised: obstructive sleep apnoea (OSA) and central sleep apnoea (CSA).

OSA

In OSA, the primary event is the obstruction of the upper airway leading to diminished airflow in the presence of an effort to breathe. It is defined by an apnoea–hypopnoea index (AHI; the total number of episodes of apnoea and hypopnoea per hour of sleep) of 5 or higher in association with EDS. Severity assessment of EDS can be obtained subjectively by a questionnaires – Epworth Sleepiness Scale.

Patients with history of loud snoring and EDS and in whom apnoeas may have been witnessed should be suspected to have OSA and further investigation is required. A number of screening and clinical prediction tools have been used to identify patients at risk of OSA who may benefit from more urgent investigation and treatment. The important features include snoring and gasping, breathing cessation, obesity, age and sex, increased neck circumference, hypertension, and witnessed apnoeas.

CSA

CSA is characterised by recurrent episodes of apnoea during sleep resulting from temporary loss of ventilator effort due to central nervous system or cardiac dysfunction.

Narcolepsy

Narcolepsy is a rare disorder characterised by abnormalities of rapid-eye movement (REM) sleep and the presence of excessive daytime sleepiness. The three classic features of narcolepsy with cataplexy include excessive sleepiness, sleep paralysis (the patient wakes up with atonia and is unable to move), hypnagogic hallucinations (vivid dreams while awake) and cataplexy (attacks of atonia that are precipitated by emotion). On average, healthy subjects fall asleep in about 10–15 minutes, whereas people with narcolepsy often fall asleep in <8 minutes. The naps of patients with narcolepsy often include REM sleep, and the presence of two or more naps containing REM sleep (known as sleep-onset REM periods) are an essential feature of narcolepsy.

Restless leg syndrome

Restless leg syndrome (RLS) is a neurologic disorder characterised by unpleasant leg sensations that usually occur at rest or before sleep and are temporarily relieved by movement.

RLS has both a familial and a sporadic form. Early onset is a pointer towards a familial aetiology. Secondary causes of RLS include pregnancy, end-stage kidney disease on dialysis and iron deficiency. Therefore, where indicated, investigations for these conditions should be performed.

Diagnostic investigations

The mainstay investigation in sleep disorders is a sleep study, which may be divided into two broad categories:
- polysomnography (PSG);
- limited channel sleep studies.

The current 'gold standard' for diagnosing OSA is laboratory full-night PSG that includes recording of EEG, electro-oculography (to determine REM sleep versus non-REM sleep, and the depth of non-REM sleep) and chin electromyography (EMG) to identify sleep stage, as well as airflow, respiratory effort, body position, limb movements, ECG and oxygen saturation (Figures 68.1, 68.2 and 68.3). An episode of apnoea is defined as cessation of airflow ≥10 seconds. A hypopnoea is a reduction in airflow of ≥10 seconds associated with an EEG arousal or desaturation. The AHI is the number of apnoeas and hypopnoeas per hour of sleep, and is the key measure used to assess disease severity:

Normal	AHI <5 events
Mild	AHI 5–15 events per hour
Moderate	AHI 15–30 events per hour
Severe	AHI more than 30 events per hour

The respiratory disturbance index (RDI) is a formula used in reporting polysomnography. Like the AHI, it reports on apnoea–hypopnoea during sleep, but unlike the AHI it also includes respiratory-effort-related arousals (RERAs). RERAs are arousals from sleep that do not technically meet the definitions of apnoeas or hypopneas, but do disrupt sleep. They are abrupt transitions from a deeper stage of sleep to a shallower one. A RERA is characterised by increasing respiratory effort for 10 seconds or more leading to an arousal from sleep, but one that does not fulfil the criteria for a hypopnea or apnoea. Studies have found that a high RDI was significantly correlated with EDS and that this correlation was stronger than that for the frequency of oxygen saturation decreases below 85%:

Normal	RDI <15
Mild	RDI 15–30
Moderate	RDI 30–45
Severe	RDI ≥45

An increasing number of portable sleep monitoring systems are in use without the need for an attending sleep technician. It records a minimum of airflow, respiratory effort and oximetry and can be used as an alternative to PSG for diagnosis of OSA in patients with a high pretest probability of moderate to severe OSA and without significant medical comorbidities, in conjunction with a comprehensive evaluation by a qualified sleep specialist. Portable monitors should not be used in patients who have congestive heart failure, cerebrovascular disease or respiratory failure. Oximetry lacks the specificity and sensitivity to be used as an alternative to PSG.

The diagnosis of CSA requires a PSG study, with the key finding of recurrent apnoeas (≥5 central apnoeas per hour of sleep) that are not accompanied by respiratory effort.

69 Ascites

Clinical Investigations at a Glance, First Edition. Jonathan Gleadle, Jordan Li and Tuck Yong. © 2017 John Wiley & Sons, Ltd. Published 2017 by John Wiley & Sons, Ltd.

? Cardiac cause: CXR, echo

Figure 69.1 (a) CXR shows congestive heart failure. (b) Echo examination
(a)   (b)

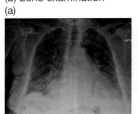

? Portal hypertension, hepatic cause: liver ultrasound scan

Figure 69.2 Liver ultrasound scan: (a) normal; (b) showing heterogeneous texture and irregular surface, consistent with cirrhosis
(a)   (b)

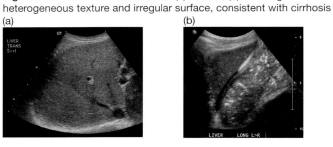

? Any underlying malignancies: CT abdomen and MRI

Figure 69.3 CT abdomen shows large-volume ascites and nodular liver surface due to cirrhosis

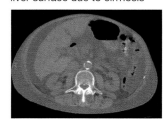

Blood tests
Urine dipstick and urine protein
FBC
Electrolytes, urea, creatinine
Liver function tests
Coagulation studies

Liver biopsy is the gold standard for diagnosis of cirrhosis

Paracentesis
SAAG, transudate versus exudate
? Any evidence of infection
? Any evidence of malignancy

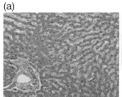
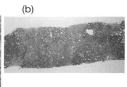

Figure 69.4 Liver biopsy: (a) normal; (b) showing cirrhosis with scar tissue sounding the disarranged regenerative liver cells
(a)   (b)

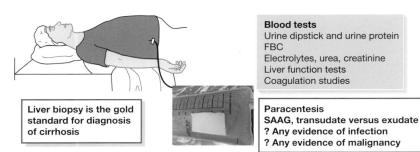
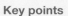

Key points

- Abdominal ultrasound should be used to confirm the presence of ascites.
- Paracentesis and analysis of the ascitic fluid can provide useful biochemical and microbiological information to help differentiate ascites related to portal hypertension from those that are not.
- SAAG has a 97% accuracy in categorising ascites.

Table 69.1 Ascitic fluid analysis

Ascites tests	Results	Results
Appearance	Bloody	Malignancy or a recent invasive test or traumatic tap
	Turbid	Infection
	Milky	Chylous ascites
Count	0–300 mononuclear cells/mm³	Normal
	>500 cells/mm³ or >250 polymorphs/mm³	Spontaneous bacterial peritonitis (SBP)
	Lymphocytes predominance	Tuberculosis or malignancy
SAAG	≥11 g/L	Ascites related to portal hypertension which is indicative of cirrhosis in most cases and heart failure
	<11 g/L	Ascites due to peritonitis, peritoneal carcinomatosis, tuberculous peritonitis, pancreatitis
Protein	≥30 g/L	Exudate due to malignancy, infection, Budd–Chiari syndrome, pancreatitis
	<30 g/L	Transudate due to congestive cardiac failure
LDH	Elevated	SBP and malignancy
Amylase	Elevated	Pancreatic ascites or bowel perforation
Gram and Ziehl–Neelsen stain	Positive	SBP, Acid-fast bacilli smear with Ziehl–Nielsen stain should be performed if tuberculous peritonitis is suspected
Cytology	Positive	Malignancy
Culture	Positive	Infection

Figure 69.5 Endoscopy showing (a) normal oesophagus and (b) oesophageal varices
(a)

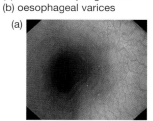

(b)

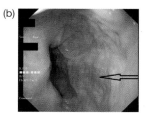

Ascites is the pathological accumulation of free fluid in the peritoneal cavity. Approximately 1500 mL of ascites can be present before flank dullness is detected. If no flank dullness is present, the patient has <10% chance of having ascites. Abdominal ultrasound should be used to determine the presence of ascites. A proper history and clinical examination may reveal the underlying cause, but the following general and specific investigations are to be carried out to identify the possible aetiology and the presence of complications of ascites.

General laboratory investigations

Urine dipstick: a simple and cheap test that will be strongly positive for protein in nephrotic syndrome. If so, a 24-hour urine collection for protein (or albumin:creatinine ratio) should be undertaken.

FBC: raised WBC count may indicate infection; pancytopenia may indicate hypersplenism complicating cirrhosis.

Electrolytes, urea, creatinine: elevated urea and creatinine may indicate a renal aetiology for ascites; but it can be due to hepatorenal syndrome.

LFTs: liver function may be deranged in the presence of liver disease. The serum albumin will indicate hypoalbuminaemia.

Coagulation studies: disturbed coagulation (e.g. prolonged prothrombin time) is suggestive of liver disease as a potential cause of ascites.

Thrombophilia screen: patients with Budd–Chiari syndrome should have a thrombophilia screen.

Ascitic fluid analysis

Paracentesis is performed to obtain ascitic fluid for diagnostic evaluation. This can be part of the management of large-volume ascites. Ultrasound guidance may help with this procedure in difficult cases. Complications such as bowel perforation, haemorrhage and infection are very rare (<0.1%). Paracentesis is indicated in any new onset of ascites. If a cirrhotic patient who is known to have ascites develops general deterioration, fever, abdominal pain, worsening encephalopathy or worsening renal function, paracentesis and ascitic infection should be considered. The common observations and tests on ascitic fluid are listed in Table 69.1. Serum-ascites albumin gradient (SAAG) is calculated as follows:

SAAG = serum albumin concentration − ascites albumin concentration

SAAG has a 97% accuracy in categorising ascites. In terms of Gram stain, the yield is low unless bowel perforation is present. Acid-fast bacilli smear with Ziehl–Neelsen stain should be performed if tuberculous peritonitis is suspected. For cytology examination, sensitivity is increased by centrifuging a large volume of ascites. Ascitic fluid culture is performed with inoculation of aerobic and anaerobic blood culture bottles.

Radiological investigations

CXR

CXR may reveal the presence of congestive cardiac failure (Figure 69.1a).

Abdominal ultrasound

Ultrasound is very sensitive in detecting a small amount of ascitic fluid (as small as 10 mL). It can also indicate an underlying cause, such as portal hypertension, cirrhosis (Figure 69.2), pelvic or other malignancies. Ultrasound can confirm the diagnosis of portal hypertension by showing ascites, splenomegaly and portosystemic collateral veins. Colour Doppler technique enables assessment of blood flow. Doppler ultrasound is the technique of choice for initial investigation of Budd–Chiari syndrome. It has a sensitivity and specificity of ≥85% when Budd–Chiari syndrome is suspected.

CT

Abdominal CT is indicated if ultrasound cannot reveal the underlying cause. It is the better imaging modality for the demonstration of malignant ascites, peritoneal tumour plaques or intra-abdominal lymphadenopathy (Figure 69.3).

MRI

MR venography is now the investigation of choice for the delineation of the portal venous system prior to surgery or transjugular intrahepatic portosystemic shunt. MRI is better for visualising the whole length of the inferior vena cava and may permit differentiation of the acute form of Budd–Chiari syndrome from the subacute and chronic forms.

Portal to hepatic venous pressure gradient

Portal to hepatic venous pressure gradient (portal-vein pressure minus the infrahepatic vena caval pressure) can be measured with a transhepatic fine needle under fluoroscopy. This gradient can be useful in determining the likelihood that portacaval shunting will be successful.

Liver biopsy

Liver biopsy is the gold standard for diagnosis of cirrhosis (Figure 69.4) and the sequential histological grading of inflammation and staging of fibrosis can assess risk of progression. Biopsy can establish the cause of cirrhosis in up to 20% of patients whose cause was previously unknown.

Endoscopy

Upper GI endoscopy is sometimes performed to look for varices (Figure 69.5) as further evidence for the presence of portal hypertension.

Echocardiography

Echocardiography can reveal a cardiac causes of ascites. Cardiac failure will manifest as poorly contractile ventricle with a reduced ejection fraction (Figure 69.1b). A pericardial effusion is visible as an echo-free space between the left ventricle and the pericardium. In some patients, echocardiography may be needed to assess for tricuspid regurgitation and constrictive pericarditis.

70 Intestinal obstruction

The goals of investigation
- To confirm the presence of intestinal obstruction
- To determine if the obstruction is mechanical or functional
- To identify the approximate site of the obstruction
- To determine whether it is simple or strangulated obstruction
- To identify the underlying cause
- To identify complications arising from the obstruction

AXR erect and supine is the first line in imaging investigation

Figure 70.1 Normal AXR: (a) erect; (b) supine
(a)   (b)

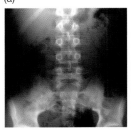

Figure 70.2 (a) AXR (supine) shows LBO. (b) AXR (decubitus film) shows LBO with large fluid levels and gas lying uppermost
(a)   (b)

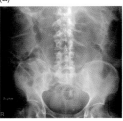
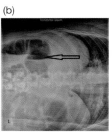

Figure 70.3 AXR (erect) shows SBO; there is a small amount of air and faecal material seen in the rectum. (b) AXR (decubitus film) shows SBO with multiple air and fluid levels
(a)

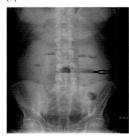

(b)

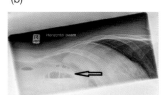

Questions that should be kept in mind when reviewing AXR:
- Are there abnormally dilated bowel loops or/and air–fluid level?
- Is this a SBO or LBO?
- Is there gas throughout the entire length of colon?
- Is there evidence of strangulation?
- Is there massive distention of colon, especially caecum or sigmoid?
- Are there biliary calculi or air in the biliary tree?
- Is there any gas under the diaphragm?
- Is there ileus (functional bowel obstruction) or mechanical obstruction?

Laboratory investigations
Full blood count
Electrolytes, urea, creatinine and liver function tests, lipase, lactate level

CT can confirm or refute bowel obstruction and may define the approximate level and the cause

Figure 70.4 CT abdomen shows SBO with multiple dilated small bowel loops

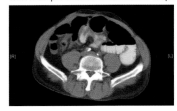

Figure 70.6 Small bowel contrast fluoroscopy studies show SBO

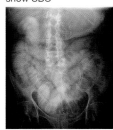

Figure 70.5 CT abdomen shows LBO

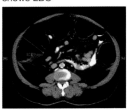

Table 70.1 Difference between SBO and LBO

LBO	SBO
Peripheral	Central
Diameter >5 cm	Diameter 2.5 cm
Presence of haustration	Presence of valvulae conniventes
Presence of solid faeces	Absence of colonic gas or collapsed large bowel

Key points in investigating bowel obstruction

- In patients with suspected bowel obstruction perform a plain erect and supine AXR and CXR.
- If there remains uncertainty about the presence of obstruction undertake a CT abdomen, which has an accuracy in diagnosing intestinal obstruction of 95–98%.
- In LBO, undertake rigid sigmoidoscopy, which may reveal a carcinoma, inflammatory stricture or sigmoid volvulus (which may be corrected).

Intestinal obstruction is the failure of forward progression of intestinal contents as a result of intrinsic or extrinsic compression or gastrointestinal paralysis. Adynamic (functional) intestinal obstruction or paralytic ileus describes temporary disruption of normal peristaltic activity without mechanical blockage, most commonly after abdominal surgery.

The cardinal features of intestinal obstruction are pain, vomiting, abdominal distension and absolute constipation (obstipation). These features vary according to the level, completeness and cause of obstruction. The most acute presentation is proximal small bowel obstruction (SBO), which manifests within hours of onset. In contrast, distal large bowel obstruction (LBO) is often more chronic and may be present for a day or two before symptoms are apparent.

Laboratory investigations

All patients suspected to have intestinal obstruction should have the following basic tests.

FBC

A raised WBC count may indicate infection. A raised haematocrit (or haemoglobin) may indicate haemoconcentration due to dehydration; a decreased haematocrit may signify blood loss.

Electrolytes, urea, creatinine and liver function tests

These tests need to be performed to determine any electrolyte disturbances. Dehydration can result in raised serum urea and creatinine. Some electrolyte disturbances, such as hypokalaemia, can promote or prolong ileus. Lactate levels should be measured, especially if there is suspicion of ischaemic bowel.

Radiological investigations

A plain erect and supine AXR and CXR are mandatory for a patient suspected to have intestinal obstruction (Figure 70.1). Plain films will confirm obstruction and define the approximate site in the majority of cases. The important questions that should be kept in mind when reviewing these images are listed on the opposite page.

AXR

Erect and supine AXR will usually reveal multiple dilated and air-fluid filled bowel loops. It is important to attempt to distinguish between SBO (Figure 70.2) and LBO (Table 70.1, Figures 70.2 and 70.3), though in practice it can sometimes be difficult. In most cases, plain films will not reveal the cause of the obstruction, but specific findings may be present in gallstone ileus, incarcerated hernia, closed-loop obstruction,

volvulus and ischaemic bowel. Thickened small bowel loops, mucosal thumb printing and pneumatosis are evidence of strangulation. In LBO, it is important to note the degree of caecal distension, because marked distension will point to the need for urgent decompression to prevent perforation. Dilatation occurs in LBO when the ileocaecal valve remains competent.

CXR

CXR is useful to identify any gas under the diaphragm indicating perforation of a viscus and any lung parenchyma changes resulting from aspiration of vomitus.

CT

AXR can be normal in patients with complete, closed-loop or strangulation obstruction. Therefore, if the patient's clinical features are consistent with intestinal obstruction, CT of the abdomen with oral and intravenous contrast should be performed (Figures 70.4 and 70.5). CT can confirm or refute bowel obstruction and may define the approximate level and the cause. CT may show mass lesion, inflammatory disease, hernia, volvulus or closed-loop obstruction. CT may also detect other pathology, such as acute appendicitis, diverticulitis and ischaemic bowel. The accuracy of CT in diagnosing intestinal obstruction is 95–98%.

Small bowel contrast fluoroscopy studies

Enteroclysis is a small bowel intubation and direct injection of barium study. It is accurate in diagnosing intestinal obstruction and determining the level, grade and sometimes the cause (Figure 70.6). It is the most sensitive method to distinguish between ileus and partial mechanical SBO. The disadvantages of these studies in complete SBO include the time required for the contrast to reach the obstruction and the dilution of contrast in the bowel. In addition, such studies are limited in demonstrating extrinsic causes of obstruction. There is no evidence that injection of barium causes partial obstruction to progress to complete obstruction.

Sigmoidoscopy

In LBO, sigmoidoscopy may reveal a cancer, sigmoid volvulus or inflammatory stricture. Flexible sigmoidoscopy is relatively contraindicated due to the risk that the insufflation required may worsen obstruction or precipitate a perforation. However, rigid sigmoidoscopy can be accomplished without insufflation and is useful in excluding a rectal obstruction, evaluating a rectosigmoid or rectal obstructing tumour, and confirming a sigmoid volvulus. In sigmoid volvulus, rigid sigmoidoscopic detorsion of sigmoid volvulus is successful in 80–90% of cases and allowing avoidance of emergency surgery.

71 Malabsorption

The goals of investigation
- To confirm the presence of malabsorption
- To identify the cause of malabsorption
- To evaluate the consequences of the malabsorption
- To monitor the response to treatment

Blood tests
FBC
Iron study, vitamin B12, folate
Serum albumin
Vitamin D levels
Electrolytes
INR
Lipid profile

Is this coeliac disease? → Serological tests

Table 71.1 Sensitivity and specificity and positive and negative predictive value of serological tests for untreated coeliac disease

Serological tests	Sensitivity (%)	Specificity (%)	Predictive value (%) Positive	Predictive value (%) Negative
IgA antigliadin antibodies	75–90	82–95	28–100	65–100
IgG antigliadin antibodies	69–85	73–90	20–95	41–88
IgA antiendomysial antibodies	85–98	97–100	98–100	80–95
Tissue transglutaminase antibodies (ELISA)	95–98	94–95	91–95	96–98

Upper gastrointestinal endoscopy with a small intestinal biopsy is the gold-standard diagnostic method for coeliac disease

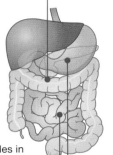

Figure 71.1 Fat globules in stool slide

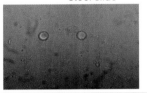

Figure 71.2 Endoscopy shows (a) normal duodenum. (b) Reduction in the circular folds in the descending duodenum, scalloping of folds and a mosaic appearance to the mucosa that is characteristic of coeliac disease. (c) Normal duodenum biopsy. (d) Duodenum biopsy shows absent villi and hyperplastic crypts. There are increased intraepithelial lymphocytes and plasma cells and lymphocytes in the lamina propria, consistent with coeliac disease

(a)   (b)   (c)   (d)

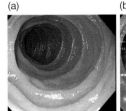 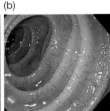 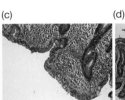 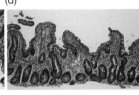

Stool screening tests
1. Stool culture: to detect bacterial infection
2. Ova and parasite examination: to detect parasites
3. Faecal occult blood test: to detect bleeding in the digestive tract
4. Stool smear with fat stain: to detect fat malabsorption (Figure 71.1)

Key points

- Endoscopy with a small intestinal biopsy is the gold-standard diagnostic test for coeliac disease.
- Pancreatic exocrine function can be tested directly (pancreatic secretion via duodenal intubation) or indirectly (faecal elastase measurement).
- Aspiration of duodenal or jejunal contents during endoscopy and estimation of total bacterial count is the 'gold standard' for diagnosing small bowel bacterial overgrowth.

Investigations that can confirm malabsorption

Table 71.2 Characteristic findings of investigations in malabsorption

Investigation	Coeliac disease	Bacterial overgrowth	Whipple's disease	Terminal ileal disease	Chronic pancreatitis
Serum folate	Low (in >50%)	Normal to high	Low	Normal	Normal
Schilling's test	Normal (except ileal involvement)	Abnormal	Normal	Abnormal	Abnormal occasionally
14C trolein breath test	High	High	High	High	Very high
14C glycocholate breath test	Normal	Abnormal	Normal (early peak)	Abnormal	Normal (late peak)
14C D-xylose breath test	Low	High	Low	Normal	Normal
Small-bowel biopsy (proximal)	Subtotal or total villous atrophy	Normal (>10⁵ organisms on jejunal fluid culture)	Flattening of villi, PAS-positive macrophages	Normal	Normal

Is this pancreatic malabsorption?

For clinically suspected pancreatic malabsorption, imaging is the first investigation of choice.

Imaging	Sensitivity
Abdominal ultrasound	50–60%
CT abdomen	75–90%
Endoscopic retrograde cholangiopancreatography (ERCP)	Gold standard
Magnetic resonance imaging abdomen	Equivalent to ERCP

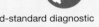

Clinical Investigations at a Glance, First Edition. Jonathan Gleadle, Jordan Li and Tuck Yong. © 2017 John Wiley & Sons, Ltd. Published 2017 by John Wiley & Sons, Ltd.

M

Malabsorption is defective mucosal uptake and transport of adequately digested nutrients, including vitamins and trace elements. The consequence is usually malnutrition. The clinical features suggestive of malabsorption include unintentional weight loss, lethargy, chronic diarrhoea and steatorrhoea.

Initial laboratory investigations

The initial investigations should include:
- stool screening tests;
- FBC with particular attention to red cell indices (e.g. mean corpuscular volume);
- iron studies, serum vitamin B12 and red cell folate;
- serum albumin;
- 25-hydroxy-vitamin D, calcium, phosphate, magnesium, alkaline phosphatase and parathyroid hormone;
- abnormal INR due to vitamin K deficiency;
- lipid studies.

These tests also evaluate the consequences of malabsorption.

Further investigations for underlying cause

Coeliac disease

The availability of highly sensitive and specific serological markers for coeliac disease has greatly assisted diagnosis (Table 71.1). They are also used to monitor adherence and response to a gluten-free diet. Tests for IgA and IgG antigliadin antibodies have moderate sensitivity but are far less specific than tests for IgA antiendomysial antibodies. Test for IgG antigliadin antibody is useful in 2–10% of patients with coeliac disease with coexisting IgA deficiency. Levels of IgA antigliadin, IgA antiendomysial and IgA tissue transglutaminase antibody all become undetectable in patients who are on a strict gluten-free diet. Testing IgA antigliadin antibody is useful to monitor dietary compliance because this antibody is the easiest to quantify.

When the clinical index of suspicion for coeliac disease is low, a negative test for antiendomysial antibodies or tissue transglutaminase has a high negative predictive value. When the index of suspicion is moderate to high (patients with gastrointestinal symptoms and a family history), antiendomysial (or tissue transglutaminase) antibodies and a small-bowel biopsy should be performed.

Radiological investigations are usually not required for the diagnosis of coeliac disease. However, small bowel barium studies and/or CT of the abdomen and pelvis may be required in refractory cases or where complications such as lymphoma, carcinoma or ulcerative jejunoileitis are suspected. Thickening of the small bowel may suggest the presence of lymphoma.

Upper GI endoscopy with a small intestinal biopsy is the gold-standard diagnostic test for coeliac disease. Specimens should be obtained from the distal duodenum. Endoscopic signs of villous atrophy include a reduction in the circular folds in the descending duodenum, scalloping of folds, mucosal fissures and a mosaic or nodular appearance to the mucosa (Figures 71.2a and c). The classic lesion in patients with untreated coeliac disease is absent villi and hyperplastic crypts (Figures 71.2b and d). There are increased intraepithelial lymphocytes and plasma cells and lymphocytes in the lamina propria.

Chronic pancreatitis/pancreatic malabsorption

Pancreatic exocrine function can be tested directly or indirectly. Direct tests involve collecting pancreatic secretions via duodenal intubation while the pancreas is stimulated with exogenous hormones or intestinal nutrients. Although direct tests are the most sensitive and specific methods for assessing pancreatic exocrine function, their cost and invasive nature limit their routine use. Indirect tests of pancreatic exocrine function are less expensive and easier to administer but are less sensitive and less specific. A faecal elastase level <200 μg/g stool indicates mild pancreatic enzyme insufficiency and a level of <100 μg/g stool indicates severe insufficiency. Concentration may be lowered in voluminous watery faeces, resulting in false-positive results. Serum trypsinogen levels <20 ng/mL are reasonably specific for pancreatic enzyme insufficiency. Fat malabsorption tests are also used as indirect tests of pancreatic exocrine function.

Small bowel bacterial overgrowth

Aspiration of duodenal or jejunal contents during endoscopy and estimation of total bacterial count is the 'gold standard' of diagnosing small bowel bacterial overgrowth. In the duodenum and jejunum, the normal total bacterial count is $<10^4$–10^5 colony-forming units (cfu)/mL, while in the ileum the normal count is $<10^5$–10^9 cfu/mL. This investigation has a high specificity, but sensitivity is <60%. Hydrogen breath test or ^{14}C D-xylose breath test are non-invasive tests for small bowel bacterial overgrowth.

Whipple's disease

In patients with classic Whipple's disease, endoscopic examination of the postbulbar region of the duodenum and jejunum may reveal pale yellow, shaggy mucosa alternating with eroded, erythematous or mildly friable mucosa. The classic tool for diagnosing Whipple's disease is periodic acid–Schiff (PAS) staining of small-bowel biopsy specimens, which on light microscopy show magenta-stained inclusions within macrophages of the lamina propria. Polymerase chain reaction assays can detect *Tropheryma whipplei* from a variety of tissues and body fluids.

Investigations that can confirm malabsorption

Fat malabsorption tests

- ^{14}C *triolein breath test:* The sensitivity is 92% in severe pancreatic insufficiency and 46% in mild or moderate insufficiency.
- *Acid steatocrit test:* The steatocrit is a measure of the amount of fat in faeces. It is a more convenient alternative to the 72-hour faecal fat test as it requires only a single stool sample. There is a reasonable correlation between steatocrit and 72-hour faecal fat measurements, and the steatocrit is a reliable screening test for steatorrhoea.

Carbohydrate malabsorption tests

- ^{14}C *D-xylose breath test*: This test uses the principle that, in bacterial overgrowth, ^{14}C D-xylose is metabolised by aerobic Gram-negative bacteria to $^{14}CO_2$, which is absorbed and excreted in the breath. This test is more sensitive and specific for bacterial overgrowth than the ^{14}C glycocholate breath test.
- ^{14}C *glycocholate breath test:* Normally very little deconjugation of bile acid occurs and the bile acid is absorbed intact in the terminal ileum. However, in small bowel bacterial overgrowth, deconjugation by anaerobic bacteria occurs, liberating ^{14}C glycine that is rapidly absorbed and metabolised in the liver to $^{14}CO_2$, which can be detected in the breath (early peak) (Table 71.2). Sensitivity is similar to glucose hydrogen breath test.

72 Inflammatory bowel disease

Symptoms suggestive of IBD: abdominal pain, rectal bleeding, diarrhoea, urgency, tenesmus, malaise, weight loss, extra-intestinal manifestations and fever

Table 72.1 Key features of UC and CD

Feature	UC	CD
Site		
Colon	Exclusively	2/3 of patients
Ileum	Backwash ileitis only	2/3 of patients
Jejunum	Never	Infrequent
Stomach or duodenum	Never	Infrequent
Oesophagus	Never	Infrequent
Intestinal complications		
Stricture	Rare	Common
Fistulas	Absent	Common
Toxic megacolon	Occasional	Absent
Perforation	Unknown	Uncommon
Cancer	Common	? Uncommon
Endoscopic findings		
Friability	Very common	Fairly common
Aphthous and linear ulcer	Absent	Common
Cobblestone appearance	Absent	Common
Rectal involvement	Very common	Fairly common
Radiological findings		
Distribution	Continuous	Segmented
Ulceration	Fine, superficial	Deep, with submucosal extension
Fissures	Absent	Common
Strictures or fistulas	Rare	Common
Ileal involvement	Dilated ('backwash ileitis')	Narrowed, nodular
Laboratory findings		
pANCA	70% of patients	Occasional
ASCA	Occasional	≥50% of patients

Laboratory investigations
FBC
Electrolytes, urea, creatinine
Liver function tests
Iron study, vitamin B12, folate, vitamin D levels
CRP
Serological tests

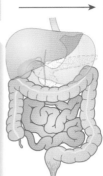

Consider CT abdomen first if if patient is unstable, unable to tolerate colonscopy, other suspected surgical conditions

Figure 72.1 Abdominal CT showing: (a) thickening of the terminal ileum, suggestive of CD; (b) dilatation throughout the large bowel with colonic wall thickening and pericolic fat stranding suggestive of UC

(a)

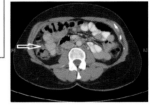

(b)

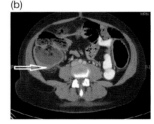

Consider colonoscopy or sigmoidoscopy if patient is stable and can tolerate this procedure or to perform biopsy after CT abdomen

Figure 72.2 Colonoscopy showing: (a) normal colonic mucosa; (b) severe ulcerations with intervening small area of normal mucosa, consistent with CD; (c) loss of vascular appearance of the colon, erythema and friability of the mucosa and superficial ulcerations, consistent with UC

(a)

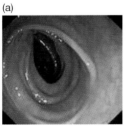

(b)

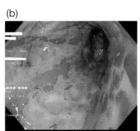

(c)

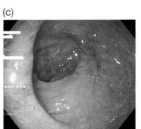

Figure 72.3 (a) Biopsy of small bowel shows transmural inflammation and lymphoid aggregates, consistent with CD. (b) Biopsy of colon shows acute inflammatory infiltrate of the mucosa and submucosa. There is loss of the surface epithelium but no fissuring or granulomas. This is typical for UC

(a)

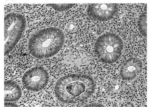

(b)

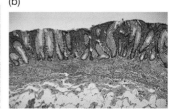

Key points in investigating IBD

- CRP is a good marker in IBD: levels correlate with clinical, endoscopic and histologic disease activity, and persistent elevation is associated with a higher relapse rate.
- In acute colitis, AXR is used to exclude toxic dilatation.
- Ileocolonoscopy and biopsy is the gold standard for diagnosis of UC and CD.
- Risk of CRC in UC is increased in patients with long-standing disease. It is recommended that patients undergo a screening colonoscopy after 8 years of disease.

Clinical Investigations at a Glance, First Edition. Jonathan Gleadle, Jordan Li and Tuck Yong. © 2017 John Wiley & Sons, Ltd. Published 2017 by John Wiley & Sons, Ltd.

Ulcerative colitis (UC) and Crohn's disease (CD) are the two main forms of inflammatory bowel disease (IBD). Clinical features of IBD are non-specific and may include rectal bleeding, diarrhoea, urgency, tenesmus, abdominal pain, malaise, weight loss, extra-intestinal manifestations and fever in severe cases. The incidence of UC is 10–20 per 100,000 per year and CD 5–10 per 100,000 per year. Inflammation in UC is characteristically restricted to the mucosal surface (Table 72.1). The disorder starts in the rectum and generally extends proximally in a continuous manner through the entire colon. CD is typically characterised by rectal sparing, aphthous ulcers, skip lesions (areas of inflammation alternating with normal mucosa), a cobblestone pattern and longitudinal, irregular ulcers (Table 72.1). Indeterminate colitis affects approximately 10% of patients who have colitis with features of both CD and UC.

Laboratory investigations

General tests

FBC with differential count should be assessed for anaemia, leucocytosis and thrombocytosis. Electrolytes, urea, creatinine and liver function tests should be measured. Primary sclerosing cholangitis (PSC) is associated with IBD, so liver function tests may indicate an associated liver disorder. Stool culture and detection of *Clostridium difficile* toxin can rule out an infectious cause. Iron studies, folate, vitamin B12 and 25-hydroxy-vitamin D should be assessed in case of deficiency arising from malabsorption.

Inflammatory markers

CRP is a good inflammatory marker: levels correlate with clinical, endoscopic and histologic disease activity, and persistent elevation is associated with a higher relapse rate and better response to infliximab. However, some patients will not have a CRP response to intestinal inflammation.

Serological tests

A positive test for anti-*Saccharomyces cerevisiae* antibody (ASCA) or perinuclear antineutrophil cytoplasmic antibody (pANCA) is not diagnostic of UC because of the limited sensitivity and specificity of these investigations. It can be used as 'supportive evidence' when the diagnosis is uncertain. However, when they are performed in combination, the results may help to differentiate between UC, CD and indeterminate colitis (Table 72.1).

Radiological investigations

CT of the abdomen and pelvis is useful in assessing acute colitis (Figure 72.1), abdominal collections and abscesses. However, CT appearances of sterile and infected fluid collections are non-specific, and a definitive diagnosis often requires aspiration. AXR is used to exclude toxic dilatation. Small bowel barium studies are too insensitive and unreliable and have been replaced by enterography (where contrast is swallowed) or enteroclysis (where the contrast is infused via a nasogastric tube) with CT or MRI. Ultrasound is a very sensitive way of detecting and localising fluid collections in the upper abdomen and the pelvis and can guide diagnostic aspiration. Transrectal and endoscopic ultrasound can assess perianal complications seen in CD.

Internal fistula is best assessed with a barium study; that is, a follow-through examination for small bowel or an enema for large bowel disease. Fistula draining externally can be assessed with an ultrasound. Enteroclysis combined with CT (CTE) can detect fistulas, but a major disadvantage is high radiation exposure. MRI can be combined with enteroclysis, as an alternative to CTE.

Endoscopic investigations

Colonoscopy

Ileocolonoscopy (Figure 72.2) and biopsy (Figure 72.3) is the gold standard for diagnosis of UC and CD and in most patients can help distinguish between UC and CD. In UC, the histological appearance can help determine the severity of disease. If stricture is detected, multiple biopsies are mandatory to rule out malignant disease.

Risk of colorectal cancer (CRC) in UC is increased in patients with long-standing disease compared with the general population. Therefore, guidelines recommend that patients undergo a screening colonoscopy, with several biopsies throughout the entire colon, after 8 years of disease. In patients with a concomitant diagnosis of PSC, risk of CRC is up to four times higher than in those without. Surveillance programmes should be done ideally during quiescent phases of the disease because reactive atypia can be confounded with dysplasia in the presence of active inflammation. Chromoendoscopy with methylene blue dye-spray-targeted biopsies can improve detection of dysplasia.

Sigmoidoscopy

Sigmoidoscopy allows the inspection and biopsy of the rectal mucosa. UC always involves the rectum, and diseased bowel is always accessible to sigmoidoscopic evaluation. A rectal biopsy should be taken for histology even if there are no macroscopic changes.

Video capsule endoscopy (VCE)

VCE or 'pillcam' is useful for diagnosing CD and defining anatomical distribution and severity in those with established disease. VCE evaluation in patients with established CD detects new proximal small bowel lesions in half of patients. VCE is equivalent or superior to other methods of small bowel testing in evaluating suspected or confirmed CD.

The potential for capsule retention because of stricture CD requires caution, with retention rates varying from 5 to 13% in patients with established CD and 1–2% in those with suspected disease.

73 Irritable bowel syndrome

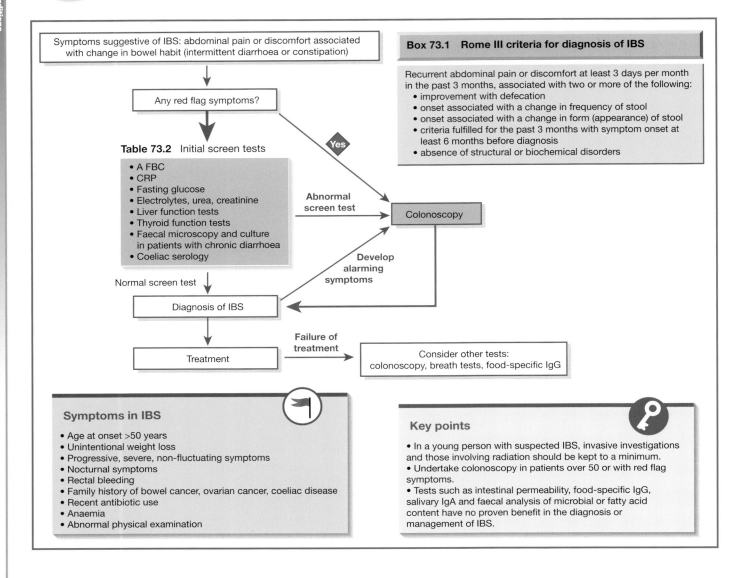

Symptoms suggestive of IBS: abdominal pain or discomfort associated with change in bowel habit (intermittent diarrhoea or constipation)

Any red flag symptoms?

Table 73.2 Initial screen tests

- A FBC
- CRP
- Fasting glucose
- Electrolytes, urea, creatinine
- Liver function tests
- Thyroid function tests
- Faecal microscopy and culture in patients with chronic diarrhoea
- Coeliac serology

Yes

Abnormal screen test

Normal screen test

Colonoscopy

Develop alarming symptoms

Diagnosis of IBS

Treatment

Failure of treatment

Consider other tests: colonoscopy, breath tests, food-specific IgG

Box 73.1 Rome III criteria for diagnosis of IBS

Recurrent abdominal pain or discomfort at least 3 days per month in the past 3 months, associated with two or more of the following:
- improvement with defecation
- onset associated with a change in frequency of stool
- onset associated with a change in form (appearance) of stool
- criteria fulfilled for the past 3 months with symptom onset at least 6 months before diagnosis
- absence of structural or biochemical disorders

Symptoms in IBS

- Age at onset >50 years
- Unintentional weight loss
- Progressive, severe, non-fluctuating symptoms
- Nocturnal symptoms
- Rectal bleeding
- Family history of bowel cancer, ovarian cancer, coeliac disease
- Recent antibiotic use
- Anaemia
- Abnormal physical examination

Key points

- In a young person with suspected IBS, invasive investigations and those involving radiation should be kept to a minimum.
- Undertake colonoscopy in patients over 50 or with red flag symptoms.
- Tests such as intestinal permeability, food-specific IgG, salivary IgA and faecal analysis of microbial or fatty acid content have no proven benefit in the diagnosis or management of IBS.

Clinical Investigations at a Glance, First Edition. Jonathan Gleadle, Jordan Li and Tuck Yong. © 2017 John Wiley & Sons, Ltd. Published 2017 by John Wiley & Sons, Ltd.

Irritable bowel syndrome (IBS) consists of a triad of abdominal pain or discomfort associated with change in bowel habit (intermittent diarrhoea or constipation) in the absence of a structural or biochemical disorder. IBS can be further defined on the basis of the modified Rome criteria (Box 73.1). It is part of a spectrum of functional gastrointestinal disorders. IBS affects 5–11% of the population worldwide. Prevalence peaks in the third and fourth decades, with a female predominance. It has considerable impact on quality of life. However, IBS is not associated with the long-term development of any serious disease, and there is no evidence that IBS is linked to excess mortality.

Symptom onset is usually gradual, and extra-intestinal symptoms such as headache and fatigue are common. The pathophysiology of IBS is not completely understood.

Diagnostic investigations should be guided by the patient's age and the presence/absent of 'red flag' symptoms (see red flag box). There is no objective diagnostic test for IBS.

Initial investigations

IBS has long been mistakenly taught to be a diagnosis of exclusion; in other words, it can only be diagnosed once all other possible conditions such as bowel cancer or inflammatory bowel disease (IBD) have been entirely excluded, implying the necessity to thoroughly investigate every patient with suspected IBS if the diagnosis is to be made. This is inappropriate and unnecessary in a straightforward case of IBS in a young person. Invasive investigations and those involving irradiation should be kept to a minimum. Patients should be warned from the outset that investigations are likely to be normal, hoping to avoid the possibility that negative results will lead to the demand for ever more invasive and unnecessary tests.

The initial tests that should be performed in all patients suspected with IBS at first presentation are listed in Table 73.2. Tissue transglutaminase antibodies have a sensitivity of 79% and a specificity of 98% in diagnosing coeliac disease in the IBS population where the incidence of coeliac disease is low (0–3%). However, in areas of high incidence of coeliac disease, such tests should be performed because the diagnosis of coeliac disease radically alters treatment over a lifetime and may otherwise easily be missed.

Second-line investigations
Colonoscopy
In patients older than 50 years or with the red flag symptoms given in Table 73.1, colonoscopy is indicated. In patients with diarrhoea, multiple biopsy specimens should be obtained from the mucosa of the descending colon to rule out IBD and microscopic colitis. As IBS patients have no increased risk of colon cancer, advice on screening for this is no different from the general population.

Breath tests
Hydrogen breath test for diagnosis of lactose and fructose intolerance can be considered in patients with abdominal pain, bloating or diarrhoea.

Other tests
Intestinal permeability, food-specific immunoglobulin (Ig)G, salivary IgA and faecal analysis of microbial or fatty acid content are other tests used in IBS. These tests are relatively expensive, have a dubious underlying rationale and validity, and no proven benefit in guiding management.

74 Colorectal cancer

Colonoscopy is the first choice; consider CTC if the patients cannot tolerate colonoscopy

Figure 74.1 Colonoscopy: (a) normal; (b, c) showing a colon cancer

(a)

(b)

(c)

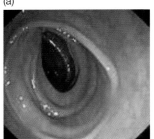
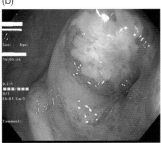
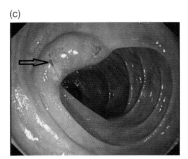

Figure 74.2 CTC: (a) normal; (b) showing a colonic polyp

(a)

(b)

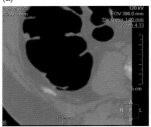
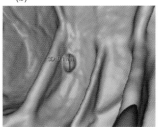

Figure 74.3 CT abdomen shows sigmoid colon abnormal wall thickening and enhancement with large and small bowel dilatation proximal to this level in keeping with an obstructive colorectal carcinoma of the sigmoid colon

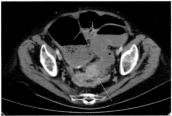

Staging investigation

Contrast-enhanced CT of the chest, abdomen and pelvis to assess the stage of disease should be performed in all patients diagnosed with CRC unless contraindicated

Figure 74.4 CT abdomen shows multiple hepatic metastases from colon cancer

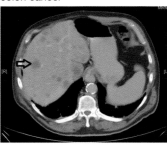

Figure 74.5 PET scan shows intense fluorodeoxyglucose uptake in the liver consistent with widespread hepatic metastases from CRC

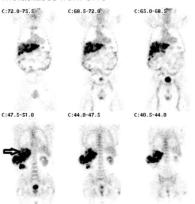

Molecular biomarker

Figure 74.6 Microsatellite instability analysis from a colon cancer sample

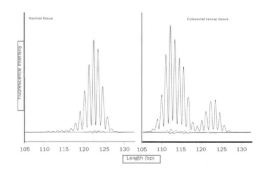

Table 74.1 Colonoscopy surveillance post-polypectomy

Polyps	Recommended colonoscopy interval
Small, rectal, hyperplastic polyps	10 years or yearly faecal occult blood test
1–2 low-risk adenomas	5–10 years
3–10 low-risk adenomas or any high-risk adenoma	3 years
>10 adenomas	<3 years
Inadequately resected adenomas	2–6 months

Key points

- Colonoscopy is first-choice investigation in patients with suspected CRC.
- CTC is reserved for patients with obstructing CRC, who have had incomplete colonoscopy or with significant comorbidity.
- CEA test can be useful in surveillance following intended curative treatment but is not a useful screening test.
- CRC screening is commonly recommended from 50 to 75 years of age for individuals with annual or biannual faecal occult blood immunochemical tests, flexible sigmoidoscopy every 5 years, or colonoscopy every 10 years. A positive faecal immunochemical test has to be followed up by colonoscopy.

Presentations of colorectal cancer (CRC) are influenced by the location of the tumour. Carcinoma of the right half of the colon can present as abdominal pain/discomfort, weight loss, anaemia and bowel obstruction. Carcinoma of the left half of the colon and rectum tends to present with alteration in bowel habit, large bowel obstruction and rectal bleeding. Other less common presentation includes mass, perforation and distant metastases. Whilst any patient with these symptoms and signs should undergo investigation to confirm or rule out a diagnosis of CRC, fewer than 10% of patients are diagnosed with the condition.

Diagnostic investigations

Colonoscopy

Colonoscopy is the gold standard for diagnosing CRC. It detects cancer, pre-malignant adenomas and other symptomatic colonic diseases. Colonoscopy also has the facility to take a biopsy from any lesion, thereby increasing diagnostic accuracy and permitting removal of most benign lesions.

Patients with suspected CRC but without major comorbidity should be offered colonoscopy to confirm a diagnosis of CRC (Figure 74.1). If a lesion suspicious of cancer is detected, perform a biopsy to obtain histological proof of diagnosis. Complete colonoscopy is mandatory to detect synchronous cancers that are present in about 2–4% of patients. If this is not possible preoperatively, complete visualisation of the colon should be done within 6 months after curative resection.

Sigmoidoscopy

Only offer flexible sigmoidoscopy for patients with major comorbidity. Sigmoidoscopy is highly sensitive and specific for neoplasms within reach of the instrument but misses about 50% of lesions that are proximal or right-sided.

CT colonoscopy (CTC)

A CTC involves examination of a computerised image of the colon constructed from data obtained from abdominal CT. CTC is not the first-line investigation for patients suspected with CRC. CTC is used in the following situations:

* patients with obstructing colon cancer;
* patients who have had incomplete colonoscopy;
* patients with significant comorbidity.

CTC has 90% sensitivity and 86% specificity for identifying patients with adenomas 10 mm or larger (Figure 74.2). The negative predictive value is 99% for polyps 10 mm or larger. If a lesion suspicious of cancer is detected on CTC, offer a colonoscopy with biopsy to confirm the diagnosis. Extracolonic findings (extracolonic cancers, abdominal aortic aneurysms, adrenal adenomas, lung nodules, and renal, ovarian, hepatic and splenic cysts) are identified in 6–8% of asymptomatic individuals during CTC, and this adds to the cost of CTC.

Staging investigation

Contrast-enhanced CT of the chest, abdomen and pelvis to assess the stage of disease should be performed (Figure 74.3) in all patients diagnosed with CRC unless contraindicated. If intracranial disease is suspected, offer contrast-enhanced MRI of the brain. About 20% of patients with newly diagnosed CRC present with distant metastases, most commonly the liver (Figure 74.4). If the CT scan shows the patient may have extrahepatic metastases that could be amenable to further radical surgery, a PET-CT scan of the whole body is appropriate. There is no evidence to support routine use of PET-CT (Figure 74.5), bone scan or MRI in patients without suspected metastatic disease.

For rectal cancer, exact local staging at the time of diagnosis is essential and is the basis for requirement of neoadjuvant treatment. Apart from the exact distance from the anal verge, definition of the local tumour extent is important. Endoscopic ultrasound is accurate for determination of the tumour (T) staging of rectal cancer, especially when MRI is contraindicated. The most accurate method to define stages of rectal cancer is MRI.

Molecular biomarker

Microsatellite instability analysis (Figure 74.6) can provide valuable information about the prognosis and therapy response of patients. Patients with high-level microsatellite instability CRC have a better prognosis than patients with low-level microsatellite stability. Mutations of the *KRAS* oncogene render affected cells unresponsive to treatment with anti-epidermal growth factor receptor antibodies, thus lowering response rates from monotherapy from 20% to almost 0% in patients with metastatic CRC.

Surveillance after curative treatment

Surveillance after curative treatment of CRC includes carcinoembryonic antigen (CEA) test, diagnostic imaging and colonoscopy (see Meyerhardt et al, 2013). Compared with the general population, patients with a prior sporadic CRC have a risk of a second primary colorectal tumour that is increased by a factor of 1.5 to 3. Serum CEA level is high in about 60% of CRC, especially in advanced disease (80–100% in liver metastases). However, it may also be elevated in lung cancer, breast cancer and non-malignant conditions such as inflammatory bowel disease (IBD), liver disease and heavy smoking. Therefore, it is inadequately sensitive or specific for screening CRC. A rising level after a potentially curative procedure may suggest recurrence.

All patients with rectal cancer should be offered MRI to assess local recurrence, determined by anticipated resection margin, tumour and lymph node staging.

Colorectal screening

Most international screening guidelines recommend CRC screening starting at 50 years of age until 75 for individuals at average risk, with use of either annual or biannual faecal occult blood immunochemical tests, flexible sigmoidoscopy every 5 years or colonoscopy every 10 years. A positive faecal immunochemical test has to be followed up by colonoscopy. If adenomas, serrated adenomas, large hyperplastic polyps (>1 cm), hyperplastic polyps located in the proximal colon and mixed polyps are detected at sigmoidoscopy or colonoscopy, complete removal of these lesions is mandatory. Depending on the characteristics of the polyp, surveillance colonoscopy is warranted (Table 74.1).

First-degree relatives of individuals diagnosed with CRC at young ages should begin screening at age 40 years or 10 years before the youngest case in the immediate family. For high-risk groups (familial adenomatous polyposis, hereditary nonpolyposis CRC or IBD), specialised and much more rigorous prevention programmes starting in early life are recommended.

75 Liver mass

Table 75.1 Characteristics of different liver masses on ultrasound, CT and MRI

Investigation	Ultrasound	CT	MRI
Metastasis (Figures 75.1 and 75.2)	Multiple hypoechoic lesion with internal heterogeneity	Hypovascular or hypervascular lesions depend on metastasis origin	Multiple hypointense lesions on T1-weight images, hyperintense lesions on T2 images
HCC (Figure 75.3)	Round lesion with sharp, smooth border, varying echogenicity	Arterial phase, rapid vascular enhancement; venous phase, hypodense lesion	Hypointense on T1 and hyperintense on T2 images, intense enhancement with gadolinium contrast
Haemangioma (Figure 75.4)	Well-demarcated lesion with echogenic spot	Early phase: hypodense with peripheral enhancement; delay phase: contrast-filled mass	Hyperintense lesion in T2 image
Adenoma (Figure 75.5)	Often in the right lobe of the liver and hyperechoic lesion	Well-demarcated, isointense lesions with peripheral enhancement	Hyperintense lesions on T1-weighted images
Focal nodular hyperplasia (Figure 75.6)	Lesion with varying echogenicity	Non-contrast phase: low-density lesion; contrast phase: rapid enhancement and wash out with a central scar	Central scar presents with high signal intensity on T2-weighted images, gadolinium produces early enhancement of the lesion and the central scar enhances during the delayed phase on T1-weighted images with sensitivity 70%, specificity 98%
Simple cyst (Figures 75.7 and 75.8)	Anechoic fluid-filled spaces without clear walls with posterior acoustic enhancement	Well-demarcated, water attenuation within lesions, no enhancement with contrast	Well-defined homogeneous lesions with low signal intensity on T1-weighted images and high signal intensity on T2-weighted images; simple cysts do not enhance with gadolinium

Table 75.2 Second-line investigations in patients with hepatomegaly

- Hepatitis B and C serology
- Autoantibodies – primary biliary cirrhosis and autoimmune hepatitis
- Iron studies – haemochromatosis
- Caeruloplasmin – Wilson's disease
- Alpha-1 antitrypsin – alpha-1 antitrypsin deficiency
- AFP – HCC
- Serum protein electrophoresis – amyloidosis

Key points

- More than 70% of masses >1 cm in a cirrhotic liver are HCC. An elevated AFP confirms the diagnosis. If AFP is normal, triphasic CT or MRI is required. If there is still doubt, biopsy might be indicated.
- The gold standard for detection and location of focal lesions is MRI or triple-phase dynamic spiral CT. MRI with gadolinium can differentiate between different lesions in 70% of cases.
- FNA and core biopsy under CT or ultrasonic guidance is safe, accurate and cost-effective with specificity approaching 100% and sensitivity 67–90%.

Figure 75.1 CT abdomen shows multiple hypodense hepatic lesions consistent with metastasis

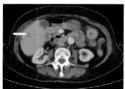

Figure 75.2 MRI shows numerous high T2 lesions consistent with metastasis

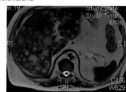

Figure 75.3 Non-contrast CT shows ill-defined hypodense lesion within right lobe of liver that was confirmed HCC by biopsy

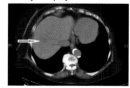

Figure 75.4 Liver ultrasound shows a well-demarcated lesion with tiny echogenic spot that is suggestive of haemangioma

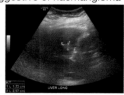

Figure 75.5 Liver ultrasound shows a hyperechoic lesion in the right lobe that is suggestive of adenoma

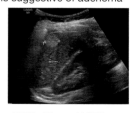

Figure 75.6 Liver ultrasound shows an indeterminate lesion that is confirmed to be a focal nodular hyperplasia by biopsy

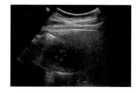

Figure 75.7 Liver ultrasound shows a simple liver cyst

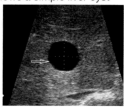

Figure 75.8 Normal USS

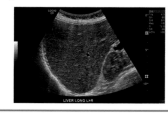

Figure 75.9 Liver biopsy shows typical HCC

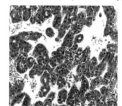

Clinical Investigations at a Glance, First Edition. Jonathan Gleadle, Jordan Li and Tuck Yong. © 2017 John Wiley & Sons, Ltd. Published 2017 by John Wiley & Sons, Ltd.

A liver mass may be palpable on physical examination or detected intentionally or incidentally during liver imaging. The increasing use of imaging modalities for investigation of the abdomen has led to an increase in the detection of liver masses.

The main goal for investigating the liver mass is to determine whether it is malignant or benign. Some benign lesions have malignant potential. Given the broad spectrum of differential diagnoses considered in the evaluation of a focal liver lesion, detailed history, physical examination, LFTs and imaging studies are all essential in making the diagnosis. The size of the liver lesion is important in guiding the investigation. Lesions <1 cm are commonly a benign incidental finding.

Laboratory investigations

The LFTs, coagulation study, FBC and CRP are part of routine investigation. Hepatitis B and C virus serology test may be indicated. Alpha-fetoprotein (AFP) is a major plasma protein in the fetus but is present in very low level in normal non-pregnant adults. Elevated levels occur in >90% of hepatocellular carcinoma (HCC). However, raised levels are also seen in other liver diseases. AFP is used in diagnosis and monitoring of response to treatment of HCC. It is also used for surveillance of HCC in patients with cirrhosis and advanced hepatic fibrosis. With a cut-off point of 20 ng/mL, serum levels of AFP have low sensitivity (25–60%) for detecting HCC and therefore are considered inadequate as the sole means of surveillance. It is usually used in combination with liver ultrasound.

Radiological investigations

Ultrasound

Ultrasound is sensitive in the detection and characterisation of focal liver lesions such as cyst versus solid lesion (Table 75.1). Doppler is helpful to demonstrate vascularity of lesions. Ultrasound features that are specific for a cyst include an echolucent mass with a well-defined thin wall and increased through-transmission. Lesions that show these features need no further evaluation.

Ultrasound of the liver combined with measurement of serum AFP every 6–12 months is required for surveillance of HCC in patients with cirrhosis or advanced hepatic fibrosis irrespective of the cause. Ultrasound has a sensitivity of about 60% and a specificity of 90% for early detection.

CT

CT is indicated if ultrasound is unsatisfactory or indeterminate. It is used for HCC staging and resectability assessment, as HCC can invade portal and hepatic veins. CT is more accurate than good quality ultrasound in the detection of focal lesions. Typical imaging features of HCC on four-phase multidetector CT are early arterial enhancement and delayed washout (less enhancement than the rest of the liver) in the venous or delayed phase. These changes are related to increased vascularity in the HCC, supplied by the hepatic artery.

MRI

MRI is useful in the preoperative assessment of tumour resectability and characterisation of focal lesions in indeterminate cases. It may also be used in the assessment of iron overload in the liver.

Angiography

Angiography is sometimes of value in the diagnosis and staging of suspected primary benign or malignant liver tumours.

Radionuclide scan

Labelled RBCs scan can be used to confirm liver haemangioma. It is also helpful in the assessment of probable focal nodular hyperplasia detected by CT or ultrasound, which will show RBCs uptake.

Biopsy

Ultrasound or CT-guided fine-needle aspiration (FNA) is a safe investigation to obtain samples for cytological or bacteriological examination for focal liver masses with atypical imaging features or discrepant findings on CT or MRI, or for lesions detected in the absence of cirrhosis. A negative biopsy result, though reassuring, does not totally exclude malignancy. The lesion should be further studied at intervals of 3–6 months until it disappears, grows larger or displays characteristics that are diagnostic of HCC. The risk of tumour seeding along the needle track after biopsy in patients with suspected HCC is low (2.7%). Accurate assessment of liver nodules measuring <1 cm is difficult, whether imaging alone or imaging and biopsy are performed. These lesions are probably best monitored with the use of ultrasound at intervals of 3–6 months for 1–2 years. Core biopsies should not be performed unless a satisfactory coagulation profile has been obtained and a vascular tumour has been excluded by a contrast-enhanced CT or prior FNA biopsy.

Hepatomegaly

Hepatomegaly is the enlargement of the liver beyond its normal size. Hepatosplenomegaly is enlargement of both the liver and the spleen. The investigations in patient with hepatomegaly are similar to the investigations of patients with abnormal LFTs. The initial laboratory investigations include LFTs, FBC, serum biochemistry, urea and creatinine. The goal for second-line investigations is to determine the causes of the hepatomegaly and should be guided by the history and physical examination (Table 75.2).

A CXR should be performed to see whether there is evidence of congestive cardiac failure, lymphadenoapthy or sarcoidosis. An ultrasound of the liver can reliably detect a dilated biliary-duct system, which helps distinguish parenchymal liver disease from extrahepatic bile-duct obstruction. Ultrasound can also detect the characteristic texture of a cirrhotic liver, and can guide FNA of the suspected abscesses and tumours. CT can obtain more accurate anatomical information, and is unaffected by obesity or the presence of bowel gases. If the diagnosis remains uncertain, liver biopsy should be considered.

76 Cirrhosis

Table 76.1 Basic investigations for cirrhosis

Investigation	Test	Description	Possible mechanisms
FBC	Haemoglobin	Macrocytic anaemia	Vitamin B12, folate deficiency, alcohol intake
		Normocytic anaemia	Hypersplenism, acute blood loss
		Microcytic anaemia	Iron deficiency, chronic bleeding
	Platelet count	Thrombocytopenia	Hypersplenism, reduced thrombopoietin production
LFTs – liver enzyme	AST, ALT	Normal or moderately, raised, usually increased <3 times of upper limit, except in PBC and PSC	Leakage from damaged hepatocytes; AST/ALT ≥1 is predictive for cirrhosis
	ALP	Raised	Cholestasis
	GGT	Raised	Cholestasis and active alcoholics
	Bilirubin	Raised	Cholestasis, decreased hepatocyte function
LFTs – synthetic function	Albumin	Decreased in advanced cirrhosis	Decreased hepatic production, sequestration into ascites
	INR	Increased in advanced cirrhosis	Decreased hepatic production of factor V/VII; vitamin K deficiency
Electrolyte and renal function	Sodium	Hyponatraemia	Increased activity of ADH
	Creatinine	AKI or CKD	Co-existing CKD, or can develop AKI due to multifactorial causes, including hepato-renal syndrome

Figure 76.1 (a) Liver USS shows heterogeneous echotexture in the liver and surface nodular consistent with cirrhosis. (b) Duplex USS shows retrograde portal venous flow due to portal hypertension

(a)
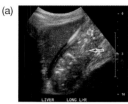

(b)
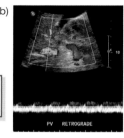

Table 76.2 Child–Pugh score

	1 point	2 points	3 points
Encephalopathy	Absent	Medically controlled	Poorly controlled
Ascites	Absent	Medically controlled	Poorly controlled
Bilirubin (mg/L)	<20	20–30	>30
Albumin (g/L)	<35	28–35	<28
INR	<1.7	1.7–2.2	>2.2

Ultrasound is the first choice of imaging to obtain important information about liver architecture

CT is the second-line investigation which can be used to define the severity of cirrhosis

Figure 76.2 CT abdomen shows cirrhosis, ascites, dilated portal vein and multiple intra-abdominal collaterals consistent with portal hypertension

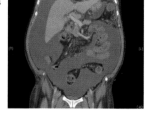

Table 76.3 Investigations for the underlying cause of cirrhosis

Underlying cause of cirrhosis	Laboratory investigations	Features on liver biopsy
HBV	HBsAg, HBeAg, anti-HBc, HBV DNA	
HCV	Anti-HCV, HCV RNA	
HDV	Anti-HDV, HDV RNA, HDAg	
Alcohol hepatitis	AST : ALT = 2, elevated GGT	Mallory bodies, steatosis, granulocytes > hepatic ballooning
NASH	Fasting glucose and triglyceride	Mallory bodies, steatosis, hepatic ballooning > granulocytes
Autoimmune	Autoantibodies (ANA, anti-LKM, anti-SLA),	Bridging necrosis
Primary biliary cirrhosis (PBC)	AMA, increased ALP, GGT and cholesterol	Cholangitis, paucity of bile ducts, granuloma, ductopenia
Primary sclerosing cholangitis (PSC)	pANCA (70%), increased ALP and GGT, beaded intra-hepatic and extra-hepatic bile ducts on imaging	Concentric peri-bile ductular fibrosis, ductopenia
Haemochromatosis	Fasting transferring saturation >60% (men), >50% (women); increased ferritin; HFE mutation	Periportal iron-loaded hepatocytes Quantification of liver iron
Wilson's disease	Increased ceruloplasmin and copper in 24-hour urine	Quantification of liver copper
α1-Antitrypsin deficiency	Reduced α1-antitrypsin; α1-antitrypsin subtyping	α1-Antitrypsin-loaded hepatocytes

MRI sometimes differentiates between regenerating or dysplastic nodules and HCC

Figure 76.3 MRI abdomen shows nodular liver surface, well-defined round low T2, non-enhancing focus representing regenerative nodule

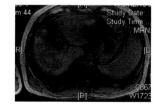

irrhosis is the common pathological endpoint of a wide range of chronic liver diseases. Cirrhosis is defined as the histological development of regenerative nodules surrounded by fibrous bands in response to chronic liver injury, which may lead to portal hypertension and end-stage liver disease. Alcoholic liver disease, viral hepatitis B and C and non-alcoholic steatohepatitis (NASH) disease are the most common causes of cirrhosis.

Cirrhosis is often indolent, asymptomatic and unsuspected until complications of liver disease are present.

The aims of investigations are to:
- establish the diagnosis and severity of cirrhosis;
- identify the cause of cirrhosis;
- assess any complications arising as a result of cirrhosis.

Investigations for establishing diagnosis and severity of cirrhosis

While laboratory investigations do not provide the diagnosis of cirrhosis, they are useful pointers to the diagnosis and assessment of severity. Patients with suspected cirrhosis should have the basic investigations listed in Table 76.1.

The clinical severity of cirrhosis is often assessed by the Child–Pugh scoring system (Table 76.2) and is used to characterise the degree of liver injury and predict the prognosis of patients with cirrhosis on the basis of clinical and laboratory variables. The model for end-stage liver disease, or MELD, is another scoring system for assessing the severity of chronic liver disease. It is mainly used in determining prognosis and prioritising for receipt of a liver transplant instead of the Child–Pugh score:

$$MELD = 3.78 \times \ln[\text{serum bilirubin (mg/dL)}] + 11.2 \times \ln[\text{INR}] + 9.57 \times \ln[\text{serum creatinine(mg/dL)}] + 6.43$$

Radiological investigations

Ultrasound, CT and MRI are not sensitive enough to detect cirrhosis. However, their specificity is high if the cause is obvious and imaging reveals an inhomogeneous hepatic texture or surface, portal vein thrombosis, an enlarged caudate lobe, splenomegaly, ascites or collateral veins. Normal radiological findings do not exclude compensated cirrhosis. The primary role of radiography is for the detection and quantitation of complications of cirrhosis – ascites, hepatocellular carcinoma (HCC), and hepatic vein or portal vein thrombosis.

Ultrasound

Ultrasound is the first choice of imaging to obtain important information about liver architecture. In cirrhosis, nodularity (88% sensitive, 82–95% specificity) and increased echogenicity of the liver are often found (Figure 76.1a). Atrophy of the right lobe and hypertrophy of the left and especially caudate lobe are characteristic signs of cirrhosis. Doppler ultrasound of portal vein with measurement of central vein diameters and velocities are useful tests for assessing portal hypertension and vessel patency (Figure 76.1b).

CT

Nodularity, irregularity, and atrophy are hallmarks of cirrhosis. In advanced disease, the liver appears small and multinodular. CT can be used to define the severity of cirrhosis by determining spleen size, ascites and presence of vascular collaterals (Figure 76.2). Helical CT with contrast is preferred if HCC or vascular lesions are suspected.

CT portal phase imaging can be used to assess portal vein patency, although flow volume and direction cannot be determined accurately.

MRI

MRI sometimes differentiates between regenerating or dysplastic nodules and HCC (Figure 76.3). It is best used as a follow-up study to determine whether lesions have changed in appearance and size. MRI is also useful in determining hepatic iron and fat content in haemochromatosis and liver steatosis respectively.

Transient elastography

Transient elastography (fibroscan) is a novel non-invasive ultrasound-based measure of liver stiffness and it is used to predict the presence of minimal fibrosis or cirrhosis (sensitivities 77–100%; specificities 82–97 %).

Investigating the underlying cause of cirrhosis

Laboratory tests

Table 76.3 summarises laboratory investigations that can be performed to help identify the cause of cirrhosis.

Liver biopsy

Liver biopsy is the gold standard for diagnosis of cirrhosis, and sequential biopsy for histological grading of inflammation and staging of fibrosis can assess risk of progression. A biopsy can establish the cause of cirrhosis in up to 20% of patients with previous unknown aetiology. A liver biopsy sample can be obtained by percutaneous (radiologically guided), transjugular or laparoscopic routes. The main complication is bleeding. If the platelet count is <70 × 10^9 cells/L or if INR is elevated (>1.3) blood products should be given or a transjugular or laparoscopic approach undertaken. Antiplatelet drugs and non-steroidal anti-inflammatory drugs should be stopped at least 1 week before biopsy. Liver biopsy should be considered only after a thorough, non-invasive serologic and radiographic evaluation has failed to confirm a diagnosis of cirrhosis; the benefit of biopsy outweighs the risk; and biopsy result will influence treatment choice.

Investigating complications of cirrhosis

After confirming the diagnosis of cirrhosis, the presence of potential complications should be looked for. Subsequent regular screening aimed at the detection or prevention of complications should be considered. The investigation of portal hypertension and ascites is described in greater detail in Chapter 69.

Key points

- Liver biopsy is the gold standard for diagnosis of cirrhosis.
- Whilst ultrasound, CT and MRI can all detect cirrhosis when changes are advanced, they have limited sensitivity in earlier stages of disease.
- Blood investigations are used to determine the aetiology of cirrhosis and complications associated with decompensated liver failure.
- Transient elastography (fibroscan) is a non-invasive ultrasound-based measure of liver stiffness used to predict the presence of minimal fibrosis or cirrhosis.

77 Liver function tests

Key points

- The commonly used LFTs mainly assess liver injury rather than hepatic function.
- Elevated ALT is relatively specific for liver injury. AST is present in the heart, skeletal muscle, kidneys and pancreas.
- Increased levels of ALP suggest cholestasis. However, it is not specific because ALP consists of several isoenzymes and has a widespread extrahepatic distribution, such as small intestine, kidneys and particularly bone.

Table 77.1 Broad classification of LFT abnormalities

Pattern	Laboratory features	Common causes
Cholestasis	ALP >200 IU/L ALP >3 times ALT GGT highly elevated, >5 times normal limits	Biliary obstruction Drugs (e.g. flucloxacillin, erythromycin, oestrogen) Infiltration (e.g. malignancy)
Hepatocellular damage	ALT >300 IU/L ALT >3 times ALP AST >200 IU/L	Infection (e.g. hepatitis A, B, C; EBV, CMV infection) Alcohol (AST often >2 times ALT) Fatty liver Drugs (e.g. methotrexate, amiodarone) Haemochromatosis Autoimmune hepatitis Ischaemia (LDH usually >1.5 times AST)
Mixed cholestatic and hepatocellular pattern	Raised ALT, AST, GGT and ALP	Acute hepatitis, alcoholic hepatitis, chronic forms of various liver diseases, such as cirrhosis
Isolated hyperbilirubinaemia	Unconjugated Conjugated	Haemolysis Gilbert's syndrome Dubin–Johnson syndrome

Clinical Investigations at a Glance, First Edition. Jonathan Gleadle, Jordan Li and Tuck Yong. © 2017 John Wiley & Sons, Ltd. Published 2017 by John Wiley & Sons, Ltd.

Liver function tests (LFTs) are a panel of blood markers used to evaluate and monitor liver and other diseases. These markers consist of albumin, bilirubin, prothrombin time, gamma-glutamyl transferase (GGT), alkaline phosphatase (ALP), aspartate transaminase (AST) and alanine transaminase (ALT). Abnormal LFTs may be asymptomatic as an incidental finding and may be secondary to other diseases.

Indications for testing

Indications for LFTs are listed opposite. The indications for repeat LFTs will depend on clinical context and results. If the patient is stable, the LFTs usually only need to be repeated every 3–4 days as the half-lives of ALT, AST and GGT are 48 hours, 18 hours and 9 days respectively. ALT and AST have large normal intra-individual variability, such that differences of >30% are significant in serial results. Similarly, a significant change for ALP is >15%, GGT >20% and bilirubin >40%. However, albumin has very low within-subject variation. Almost a third of these abnormalities will return to the reference range on repeat testing, and any persistent abnormality is more likely to be due to significant pathology that requires further investigation. Daily LFT testing may be appropriate for acute toxic or ischaemic insult or if the patient is clinically unstable.

LFTs have various limitations. LFTs can be normal in patients with severe liver disease, and abnormal LFTs can occur in patients without liver disease.

Interpretation of results

Albumin is produced only by liver cells and therefore reflects the synthetic functions of the liver. Low albumin is an indicator of disease severity and poor prognosis in established liver disorder. Low albumin can also occur with other conditions, such as pregnancy, inflammatory disorders, malnutrition and protein-losing disorders.

Abnormal LFT results can be classified into four categories (Table 77.1): (a) cholestatic pattern, implying interruption of bile flow between hepatocytes and the gut; (b) hepatocellular damage pattern; (c) mixed cholestatic and hepatocellular damage pattern; (d) isolated hyperbilirubinaemia.

Bilirubin is a haem metabolite and conjugated in liver. It increases in both cholestatic and hepatotoxic liver disease. In adults, elevated bilirubin is predominantly conjugated. Raised unconjugated bilirubin in adults is usually due to haemolysis or Gilbert's syndrome. Gilbert's syndrome (affecting up to 5% of the population) is a benign condition due to impairment in bilirubin conjugation resulting in bilirubin up to two to three times the upper reference limit but <70 µmol/L. Bilirubin levels increase during acute illness or fasting, and further investigation is unnecessary.

ALP is not specific to the liver because it can be produced in bone, intestine, brain and placenta. Common causes for physiological raised ALP include third trimester of pregnancy, adolescents due to bone growth and familial. A concurrently raised GGT indicates that the liver is more likely a source of the abnormalities, and the common causes are cholestasis and enzyme induction by alcohol or drugs. Isolated ALP elevation is typically due to bone disease, such as primary hyperparathyroidism, Paget's disease of the bone in patients aged >50 years, severe vitamin D deficiency and bone metastasis.

GGT originates from the canalicular (bile) surface of hepatocyte and is a sensitive marker for hepatobiliary disease, but the specificity is very poor. Elevation in GGT is seen in pancreatic disease, renal failure, diabetes and drugs (e.g. carbamazepine, phenytoin and oral contraceptive pill). Elevation of GGT is also associated with excessive alcohol use, but only 70% of isolated raised GGT is due to alcohol excess. Furthermore, 30% of heavy alcohol users will have a normal GGT. GGT levels remain elevated for 2–3 weeks after cessation of heavy alcohol intake or liver injury.

Both ALT and AST originate from hepatocyte cytoplasm, but AST also comes from hepatocyte mitochondria, skeletal and cardiac muscle. On the other hand, ALT most commonly comes from hepatocytes and so it is a more specific marker for liver injury. Raised ALT and AST suggest hepatocellular injury. Large increases (>10 times upper reference limit) usually suggest an acute or severe insult, such as acute viral hepatitis, drugs or ischaemia. Moderate increases (up to five times the upper reference limit) may indicate infection, alcohol, fatty liver or medication.

Careful alcohol and drug history is the first step of investigation. Patients should be asked to abstain from alcohol completely and any suspect medications should be stopped. LFTs should be rechecked in 4 weeks. If the transaminases remain above two times of upper normal limit then further investigation is warranted.

Prothrombin time

Prothrombin time measured by INR is a sensitive marker of hepatic synthetic function. It measures the extrinsic pathway of coagulation and the blood clotting factors are produced by the liver.

78 Acute pancreatitis

The aims of investigations
- Confirm the diagnosis
- Determine the aetiology of pancreatitis
- Assess severity with e.g. APACHE II scale
- Detect complications, and provide guidance for therapy

Blood tests
- FBC with differential
- Urea, creatinine
- Glucose
- Electrolyte
- Calcium level
- Liver function
- Triglycerides

Arterial blood gas

Serum markers for pancreatitis
- Amylase
- Lipase

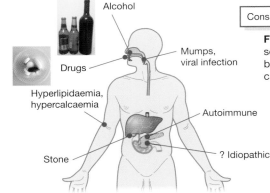

Alcohol

Mumps, viral infection

Drugs

Hyperlipidaemia, hypercalcaemia

Autoimmune

Stone

? Idiopathic

Consider abdominal ultrasound scan first

Figure 78.1 Abdominal ultrasound scan shows a stone in the common bile duct, which is the common cause of acute pancreatitis

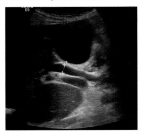

Table 78.1 Serum markers for diagnosing acute pancreatitis

	Time of onset (hours)	Clinical observation/limitations
Amylase	2–12	Sensitivity 47%, specificity 95% when at least twice the upper limit of normal; amylase levels and sensitivity decrease with time from onset of symptoms
Lipase	4–8	Increased sensitivity in alcohol-induced pancreatitis; sensitivity 67%, specificity 97% when at least twice the upper limit of normal; more specific and sensitive than amylase for detecting acute pancreatitis

Consider contrast-enhanced CT, which is the standard imaging modality for diagnosing acute pancreatitis

Figure 78.2 Abdominal CT showing a diffuse enlarged oedematous pancreas with adjacent stranding consistent with acute pancreatitis

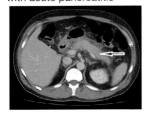

Consider MRCP for better visualisation of peripancreatic inflammation, necrosis, or fluid patient for ERCP

Figure 78.3 MRCP shows gross dilatation of the intrahepatic biliary tree with trace amount of fluid in right subphrenic space

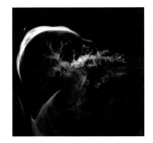

Table 78.2 Comparison of imaging modalities for pancreatitis

Imaging	Effectiveness
Abdominal ultrasound	87–98% sensitivity for the detection of gallstones
EUS	100% sensitivity and 91% specificity for detection of gallstones
Contrast-enhanced CT	78% sensitivity and 86% specificity for detection of severe acute pancreatitis
MRI	83% sensitivity and 91% specificity for detection of severe acute pancreatitis
MRCP	81–100% sensitivity for detecting common bile duct stones; 98% negative predictive value and 94% positive predictive value for bile duct stones

Figure 78.4 ERCP shows extraction of common bile duct stones

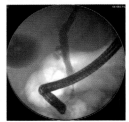

ERCP is indicated in investigating less common causes of pancreatitis and treatment

Box 78.1 Clinical criteria used in severity and prognostic scoring systems for acute pancreatitis

APACHE II scale
Equation includes the following factors: age, rectal temperature, mean arterial pressure, heart rate, PaO2, arterial pH, serum potassium, serum sodium, serum creatinine, haematocrit, white blood cell count, Glasgow coma scale score, chronic health status.
Scoring can be calculated at http://www.sfar.org/scores2/apache22.php.

CT severity index
CT grade:
- A is normal pancreas (0 points)
- B is oedematous pancreas (1 point)
- C is B plus mild extrapancreatic changes (2 points)
- D is severe extrapancreatic changes plus one fluid collection (3 points)
- E is multiple or extensive fluid collections (4 points)
Necrosis score:
- None (0 points)
- Less than 1/3 (2 points)
- More than 1/3 but less than 1/2 (4 points)
- More than 1/2 (6 points)
- Scoring: CT grade + necrosis score

Key points
- Serum markers (lipase or amylase) should be checked if there is a clinical suspicion of acute pancreatitis. Lipase is more specific for pancreatitis, but both enzymes may be increased in renal failure and other surgical conditions, such as perforated ulcer, ischaemic bowel and bowel obstruction.
- Abdominal ultrasound should be done if gallstone pancreatitis is suspected as it can detect gallstones or dilation of the common bile duct.
- CT with intravenous contrast is generally done to identify necrosis, fluid collections or pseudocysts once pancreatitis has been diagnosed.
- ERCP is indicated in severe pancreatitis of proven or suspected gallstone aetiology, presence of cholangitis and presence of jaundice.

Acute pancreatitis is an acute reversible inflammatory process of the pancreas with varying involvement of peripancreatic tissues or more remote organ systems. Acute pancreatitis is most commonly caused by gallstones or alcohol. Acute pancreatitis can be classified as:

• mild acute pancreatitis – minimal or no organ damage, resolves within 24 hours, full recovery;
• severe acute pancreatitis – organ damage, local complications such as necrosis, abscess and pseudocyst formation;
• recurrent acute pancreatitis – episodes of acute pancreatitis with full recovery between episodes.

Laboratory investigations

No single laboratory test is pathognomonic for acute pancreatitis. The initial laboratory evaluation should include lipase or amylase levels, FBC with differential, biochemistry panel (urea, creatinine, glucose and calcium levels), triglyceride level, urinalysis and arterial blood gases.

Elevation of plasma concentrations of lipase and amylase are the most common laboratory tests used to diagnose acute pancreatitis (Table 78.1). Their levels peak early, and decline over 3–4 days. Therefore, the diagnosis of acute pancreatitis should not rely on arbitrary limits of values three or four times greater than normal, but values should be interpreted in light of the time since the onset of abdominal pain.

Elevated amylase and lipase levels can be non-specific, and occur in other intra-abdominal processes and renal insufficiency. Amylase levels may be normal in patients with alcohol-induced acute pancreatitis and elevated in other acute abdominal conditions, such as perforated viscus. Lipase persists longer after the onset of the attack; because the pancreas is the only source of lipase, estimation of plasma lipase has slightly superior sensitivity and specificity and greater overall accuracy than amylase in diagnosing acute pancreatitis. Fasting blood lipids and calcium concentrations should be determined. Early and convalescent viral antibody titres in mumps and Coxsackie B4 may identify a possible viral cause, although no specific therapy will result.

Radiological investigations

There is no role for plain AXR in the diagnosis of acute pancreatitis. Abdominal ultrasound is often unhelpful in diagnosing pancreatitis because bowel gas often limits the accuracy of pancreatic imaging. If the pancreas is visualised (25–50% of patients) the imaging can reveal pancreatic enlargement, echotextural changes and peripancreatic fluid. Ultrasound is the most useful modality to investigate the commonest underlying cause of pancreatitis-cholelithiasis (Figure 78.1). After one negative ultrasound examination, the most sensitive test for diagnosis of gall stones that may have been missed remains a further ultrasound examination.

Endoscopic ultrasound (EUS) is highly accurate in detection of microlithiasis and tumours in the gall bladder or common bile duct stones, especially in obese patients and patients with ileus. It is safer than endoscopic retrograde cholangiopancreatography (ERCP) and can help determine which patient with acute pancreatitis would benefit most from therapeutic ERCP. Furthermore, EUS can assist with endoscopic transmural cyst and abscess drainage.

Contrast-enhanced CT is the standard imaging modality for diagnosing acute pancreatitis. CT is not indicated for patients with mild, uncomplicated pancreatitis and should be reserved for cases that the diagnosis is uncertain or there is deterioration or failure of improvement within 48–72 hours or there is severe abdominal distension and tenderness, leucocytosis or fever. CT is more reliable than ultrasound in showing the entire pancreas, grading severity and detecting complications such as pseudocyst, pancreatic necrosis or abscess formation (Figure 78.2).

MRI is not routinely used but may be indicated if better visualisation of peripancreatic inflammation, necrosis or fluid collections is needed. Magnetic resonance cholangiopancreatography (MRCP) can be used preoperatively to determine which patients would benefit from ERCP. MRCP is as accurate as contrast-enhanced CT in predicting the severity of pancreatitis and identifying pancreatic necrosis. However, unlike ERCP, MRCP does not have interventional capability for stone extraction, stent insertion or biopsy. MRCP is less sensitive for detection of small stones (<4 mm), small ampullary lesions and ductal strictures (Figure 78.3).

The imaging modalities are compared in Table 78.2.

Endoscopic investigations

ERCP is useful in investigating less-common causes of pancreatitis (e.g. microlithiasis, sphincter of Oddi dysfunction, pancreas divisum, and pancreatic duct strictures – which can be benign or malignant) (Figure 78.4). Urgent ERCP is indicated in patients at risk of or with evidence of biliary sepsis, severe pancreatitis with biliary obstruction, ascending cholangitis, and worsening and persistent jaundice because these patients may need immediate surgical intervention. In patients with severe gallstone pancreatitis, morbidity and mortality are reduced with the use of early selective ERCP.

Early evaluation and risk stratification for patients with acute pancreatitis are important to differentiate patients with mild versus severe disease. The Acute Physiology and Chronic Health Evaluation (APACHE II) scale, and the CT Severity Index (Box 78.1) have been developed and validated to predict adverse outcomes, including mortality, in patients with pancreatitis.

79 Acute kidney injury

The purpose of investigations is to:
- Ascertain the severity of the AKI
- Identify the cause or contributing factors
- Assess need for emergency treatments and whether renal replacement therapy is required
- Evaluate any complications related to AKI or the underlying cause(s)

- FBC, blood film
- Serum creatinine, urea
- Electrolytes, LDH
- LFTs, CK
- CRP

1. Blood tests

Tests	Suspected cause for AKI
Haptoglobin, bilirubin, LDH	HUS or TTP
Rhabdomyolysis	CK
Myeloma	Serum electrophoresis, serum free light chains
Goodpasture's syndrome	Anti-GBM
Vasculitis	ANCA
Cryoglobulin-associated vasculitis	Cryoglobulin, hepatitis C serology
Lupus nephritis	ANA, ds-DNA, C3, C4
Post-infectious glomerulonephritis	C3, C4, anti-streptolysin O antibodies

2. Urinary analysis and microscopy

Figure 79.1 Macroscopic haematuria

Figure 79.2 Urine dysmorphic red blood cell

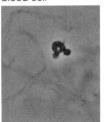

Figure 79.3 Urine red blood cell cast

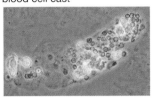

Figure 79.4 Urine granular cast

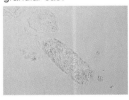

Figure 79.5 Ultrasound scan of the right kidney showing moderate hydronephrosis

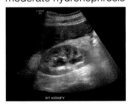

3. Imaging

Figure 79.6 CT urogram shows swelling of the right kidney, dilated collecting system and ureter due to a 5 mm calculus

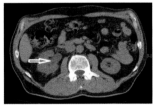

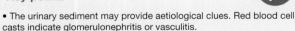

Key points

- The urinary sediment may provide aetiological clues. Red blood cell casts indicate glomerulonephritis or vasculitis.
- Laboratory investigations should pay attention to progressive acidosis, hyperkalaemia, hypocalcaemia and anaemia.
- Ultrasonography of the kidneys is the modality of choice in the initial investigation of AKI and should be performed in all patients, particularly in older men, to rule out obstruction.
- When the cause of AKI is not found and the clinical features are atypical of acute tubular necrosis, renal biopsy may be used to exclude potentially treatable conditions such as granulomatosis with polyangiitis, SLE, Goodpasture's syndrome.

Figure 79.7 Kidney biopsy shows (a) a normal glomerulus and (b) crescentic formation in the glomerulus due to ANCA-associated rapid progressive glomerulonephritis

(a)

(b)

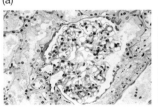

4. Kidney biopsy

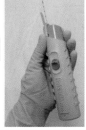

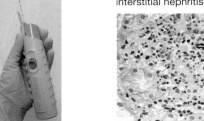

Figure 79.8 Kidney biopsy shows interstitial nephritis

Figure 79.9 Kidney biopsy shows myeloma kidney characterised by cast nephropathy

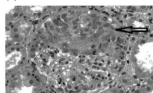

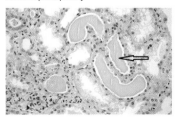

Clinical Investigations at a Glance, First Edition. Jonathan Gleadle, Jordan Li and Tuck Yong. © 2017 John Wiley & Sons, Ltd. Published 2017 by John Wiley & Sons, Ltd.

Acute kidney injury (AKI) is a clinical syndrome characterised by a rapid (hours to days) decrease in renal function, with the accumulation of products of nitrogen metabolism such as creatinine and urea, potassium, acidosis and often fluid overload. The aetiology of acute renal failure is traditionally divided into pre-renal, renal (intrinsic) and post-renal (obstructive).

AKI may be asymptomatic until there is extreme loss of function or there may be findings of the precipitating illness (e.g. sepsis) or those of a systemic disorder (e.g. vasculitis). When a patient presents with a raised serum creatinine, it is important to establish if there is AKI, chronic kidney disease (CKD) or an episode of acute injury superimposed on CKD, and usually the clinical context provides clues.

Clinical and laboratory investigations
Complications of AKI

The laboratory markers of AKI are often increased serum creatinine or urea, or both. However, these markers only rise when glomerular filtration rate decreases substantially and are modified by nutrition, corticosteroids, gastrointestinal bleeding, muscle mass, age, sex, muscle injury and fluid resuscitation.

A dangerous complication of renal failure is hyperkalaemia, which can cause cardiac conduction abnormalities and arrhythmias. In unwell patients with renal failure, or with hyperkalaemia, an ECG should be undertaken looking for signs of hyperkalaemia (peaked T waves, widened QRS, absent P waves, sine wave appearance). If plasma potassium is >6 mmol and/or ECG abnormalities are present, treat with intravenous calcium, insulin and glucose, and Resonium and consider the need for urgent haemodialysis.

Another dangerous complication of renal failure is metabolic acidosis. Patients should have arterial blood gases to establish pH and urgent haemodialysis considered if refractory acidosis pH <7.2.

Marked elevations of urea >35 mmol/L are associated with uraemic complications, such as pericarditis and encephalopathy, which are indications for dialysis treatment.

AKI may be associated with fluid retention, leading to pulmonary and peripheral oedema, and with hypertension. Careful clinical assessment is central to this and may be supplemented by a CXR and sometimes by a central venous line to measure central venous pressure.

Aetiology of AKI

The clinical context will dictate the usefulness of other blood investigations in determining the aetiology of the AKI. If sepsis is suspected, blood cultures are important. If the clinical features or other investigations do not suggest a pre-renal or obstructive cause for AKI, intrinsic renal disease should be considered. FBC and blood film may reveal haemolysis and/or thrombocytopaenia and be a pointer to disseminated intravascular coagulopathy, haemolytic–uraemic syndrome (HUS) or thrombotic thrombocytopaenic purpura (TTP). Haptoglobin, bilirubin, unconjugated bilirubin and LDH are useful for assessing the presence of haemolysis.

Creatine kinase (CK) should be measured to identify possible rhabdomyolysis; levels are usually elevated into the thousands if rhabdomyolysis is the cause of the AKI. Measurement of CRP, cryoglobulin, serum electrophoresis, serum free light chains and antibodies to glomerular basement membrane (anti-GBM), neutrophil cytoplasm (antineutrophil cytoplasmic antibody (ANCA), proteinase 3 and myeloperoxidase) and double-stranded ds-DNA, and complements (C3 and C4) are useful tests to investigate a possible diagnosis of vasculitis, glomerulonephritis or multiple myeloma. Multiple myeloma should be considered in any patient with AKI as it may be a contributory factor combined with other insults, such as dehydration or infection.

Urine examination

Urine microscopy and culture is important in the assessment of AKI. Urinary microscopy showing microscopic haematuria, fragmented red cells, red-cell casts (Figures 79.1, 79.2 and 79.3), white-cell casts or granular casts (Figure 79.4) may indicate an active glomerulonephritis. Urine samples are commonly examined for eosinophils if interstitial nephropathy is suspected, but the sensitivity of the test is poor. Urine microscopy and culture may indicate a urinary tract infection and suggest pyelonephritis.

Urinary albumin and/or protein measurement is useful and suggests a glomerular pathology if significantly elevated.

The presence of uric acid crystals may represent acute tubular necrosis associated with uric acid nephropathy. Calcium oxalate crystals may be present in ethylene glycol poisoning.

Radiological investigations

All patients with AKI should have a renal tract ultrasound. It is particularly helpful in identifying obstruction of the urinary collecting system (Figure 79.5). The number, shape and size of the kidneys is also important. The degree of hydronephrosis found on an ultrasound does not necessarily correlate with the degree of obstruction. Mild hydronephrosis may be observed with early obstruction. Small kidneys suggest CKD.

CT imaging (Figure 79.6), aortorenal angiography and isotope perfusion scans can be helpful in establishing the diagnosis of renal vascular diseases, including renal artery stenosis, renal embolus aortic aneurysm or dissection and some cases of large vessel vasculitis (e.g. polyarteritis nodosa).

Renal biopsy

A renal biopsy can be useful in identifying intrinsic causes of AKI. It may be undertaken if the cause of the AKI is not readily apparent from the clinical context and initial investigations. It may also be undertaken to confirm a diagnosis such as an acute ANCA-associated glomerulonephritis (Figure 79.7) or a tubulointerstitial nephritis (Figure 79.8), or to look for presence and severity of renal disease in conditions such as myeloma (Figure 79.9). A renal biopsy may also be indicated in AKI when renal function does not return for a prolonged period.

80 Chronic kidney disease

The purpose of investigations is to:
- Detect CKD
- Assess stage of CKD
- Identify the cause of CKD
- Monitor the progress of kidney disease
- Assess CKD-related complications, particularly risk of cardiovascular diseases

Indications for screening for CKD
- Age >60 years
- Hypertension
- Diabetes
- History of AKI
- History of renal calculi
- Family history of renal disease
- Exposure to nephrotoxic drugs
- Recurrent urinary tract infection
- History of lower urinary obstruction
- Systemic infection
- Autoimmune diseases
- Other high-risk groups (e.g. Aboriginal people, smokers)

Table 80.1 Stages of CKD

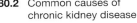

Stage	eGFR (mL/min /1.73 m²)	Description
1	>90	Kidney damage with normal eGFR[a]
2	60–89	Kidney damage with mildly reduced eGFR[a]
3[b]	30–59	Moderately reduced eGFR
4	15–29	Severely reduced eGFR
5	<15	Kidney failure

[a]There must be evidence of chronic (>3 months) kidney damage defined by structural or functional abnormalities (e.g. albuminuria, haematuria or structural abnormalities on imaging).
[b]Stage 3 can be categorised into stage 3a (eGFR 45–59 mL/min/1.73 m³) and stage 3b (eGFR 30–44 mL/min/1.73 m³) to reflect the increased mortality and vascular risk when eGFR <45 mL/min/1.73 m²

Table 80.2 Common causes of chronic kidney disease

Type 1 or 2 diabetes mellitus
Hypertension
Renovascular disease
Glomerulonephritis
Interstitial nephritis
Polycystic kidney disease
Obstructive uropathy
Reflux nephropathy
Recurrent pyelonephritis

Key points
- Microalbuminuria is a sensitive marker of CKD caused by diabetes, hypertension and glomerular diseases.
- Undertake a renal ultrasound in all people with CKD. Patients with CKD may have normal sonographically appearing kidneys.
- The effects of CKD should be investigated, including hypocalcaemia, hyperphosphataemia, metabolic acidosis, anaemia, secondary hyperparathyroidism and renal osteodystrophy.

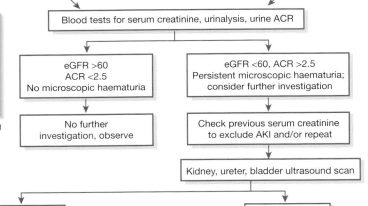

Symptoms and signs suggestive of CKD

Blood tests for serum creatinine, urinalysis, urine ACR

eGFR >60
ACR <2.5
No microscopic haematuria

No further investigation, observe

eGFR <60, ACR >2.5
Persistent microscopic haematuria; consider further investigation

Check previous serum creatinine to exclude AKI and/or repeat

Kidney, ureter, bladder ultrasound scan

No obstruction

Obstruction

Blood tests to detect complications of CKD:
Potassium, bicarbonate
Calcium, phosphate levels
PTH
FBC

Blood tests to detect underlying causes of the CKD (see main text)

Consider kidney biopsy if the cause of CKD remains unclear and there is suspicion of potentially reversible causes, such as lupus nephritis.

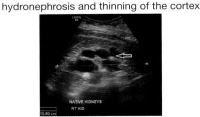

Figure 80.1 Renal ultrasound shows chronic hydronephrosis and thinning of the cortex

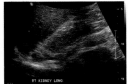

Figure 80.2 (a) Normal kidney ultrasound. (b) Renal ultrasound shows a small echogenic atrophic kidney

(a)　　　　(b)

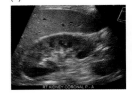

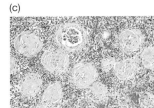

Figure 80.3 Enlarged numerous cysts in both kidneys consistent with polycystic kidneys disease

(d)

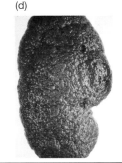

Figure 80.4 (a) Normal kidney biopsy. (b, c) Renal biopsy showing (b) typical diabetic nephropathy and (c) end-stage kidney disease with obsolescent glomeruli. (d) A scarred kidney

(a)

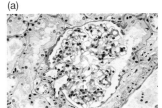

(b)

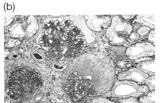

(c)

Clinical Investigations at a Glance, First Edition. Jonathan Gleadle, Jordan Li and Tuck Yong. © 2017 John Wiley & Sons, Ltd. Published 2017 by John Wiley & Sons, Ltd.

Chronic kidney disease (CKD) refers to damage or chronic impairment in the function of the kidney that can arise from a variety of disease processes. The definition of CKD is based on evidence of kidney injury (albuminuria or proteinuria) and/or decreased kidney function eGFR <60 mL/min/1.73 m²) for 3 months or more. End-stage kidney failure can be defined as an eGFR <15 mL/min/1.73 m² or needing renal replacement therapy (dialysis or transplantation) (Table 80.1). Symptoms of kidney failure are rare until eGFR falls significantly.

Laboratory investigations

Creatinine and creatinine-based eGFR

Creatinine is used as a surrogate marker of kidney function but it is insensitive because it is affected by muscle mass, diet and renal tubular secretion. Serum creatinine begins to rise above the normal reference range only after at least 50% of kidney function is lost. Creatinine clearance can be calculated using 24-hour urine collections. However, incomplete urine collection is common and GFR determined in this way shows significant variability and inaccuracy.

Equations to estimate GFR use serum creatinine and a combination of age, sex, ethnic origin and body size and are more accurate for estimation of GFR than creatinine alone. If an elevated creatinine is newly discovered, it is important to ensure that this does not represent an episode of potentially treatable AKI by clinical assessment and repeating the creatinine after a short interval.

Sodium, potassium and bicarbonate

Hyperkalaemia or low bicarbonate levels may be present, occurring with increasing prevalence as renal function declines.

Serum albumin

Serum albumin can be low (<30 g/L) in nephrotic syndrome and chronically unwell malnourished patients with CKD.

Calcium, phosphate, 1,25-hydroxycholecalciferol, parathyroid hormone and urate

Phosphate retention and deficiency of 1,25-hydroxycholecalciferol (due to inadequate renal 1-alpha hydroxylation) are common with increasing renal insufficiency, leading to hypocalcaemia and secondary hyperparathyroidism. Urate is often elevated and may predispose to gout.

FBC

In patients with significant renal impairment, normocytic anaemia develops due to inadequate erythropoietin production by the kidneys, is often exacerbated by deficiencies in iron stores and/or anaemia of chronic disease. Other causes of anaemia, should be considered, particularly if the severity of anaemia is disproportionate to the level of renal impairment.

Lipid studies

A lipid profile should be performed because of the high risk of cardiovascular disease. Both proteinuria and impaired GFR are strong risk factors for cardiovascular disease and mortality.

Others

The following tests may be appropriate as part of the evaluation of patients with CKD. In patients with rapid decline in GFR, the diagnosis should be carefully considered and renal obstruction, autoimmune causes and drug toxicity considered.
- HbA₁C in patients with diabetes mellitus.
- Serum and urine protein electrophoresis and serum and urine free light chains and urine Bence Jones protein to investigate for multiple myeloma.
- Serum immunoglobulin (Ig)A is elevated in a proportion of patients with IgA nephropathy.
- ANA and double-stranded DNA antibody levels for SLE.
- Serum complement levels may be depressed with active SLE and in occasional glomerulonephritides.
- Serology for hepatitis B and C and HIV.
- Cytoplasmic and perinuclear pattern antineutrophil cytoplasmic antibody levels to assist in the diagnosis of vasculitis.

Urine investigations

Urine microscopy can identify RBCs, WBCs and casts. Dysmorphic RBCs in the urine can be identified with phase-contrast microscopy and suggest glomerular origin for haematuria.

Albuminuria can be assessed with dipstick, 24-hour collection or by measurement of urine albumin : creatinine ratio (ACR). The absence of albuminuria or any other abnormality in the urine sediment should prompt review of whether the CKD is arising from obstruction or pre-renal causes.

Microalbuminuria can occur in poorly controlled hypertension, obesity or in the early stages of diabetic nephropathy. It is useful for diagnosis, for assessing prognosis and for monitoring patients.

Macroalbuminuria can be seen in many diseases. In contrast, nephrotic-range albuminuria (ACR >300 mg/mmol; ≥3 g/day proteinuria) indicates glomerular disease. The diagnosis of nephrotic syndrome requires oedema and low serum albumin (<30 g/L) (and often a high serum cholesterol level (>6 mmol/L)). The level of proteinuria is prognostic of subsequent renal decline and cardiovascular mortality.

Radiological investigations

Renal ultrasound is useful to examine for hydronephrosis (Figure 80.1) due to obstruction and to establish the size and symmetry of the kidneys. In advanced CKD small echogenic kidneys are usually seen (Figure 80.2). Structural abnormalities, such as polycystic kidneys (Figure 80.3), may be seen. CT and MRI can define renal masses, cysts and calculi but are not routinely used in the investigation of CKD. Contrast studies should be used with caution in CKD because of the risk of contrast nephropathy and the risk of nephrogenic systemic fibrosis with gadolinium.

Kidney biopsy

It is desirable to know the underlying cause of CKD (Figure 80.4); if this remain unclear after initial non-invasive investigation or if renal function is declining, renal biopsy can be considered provided the kidneys are not too small.

81 Metabolic acid–base disorders

The purpose of investigation is to:
- Determine the cause of the metabolic acidosis
- Determine whether metabolic acidosis is present alone or with a coexisting respiratory disturbance
- Measure the severity

Anion gap, defined as $[Na^+] - ([Cl^-] + [HCO_3^-])$

Table 81.1 Common causes of metabolic acidosis

High anion gap metabolic acidosis	Normal anion gap metabolic acidosis with normal or high serum potassium	Normal anion gap metabolic acidosis with low serum potassium
• AKI and CKD • Diabetic ketoacidosis • Alcoholic ketoacidosis • Fasting ketoacidosis • Lactic acidosis • Salicylate intoxication • Toxic alcohol intoxication (methanol, ethylene glycol)	• CKD • Adrenal insufficiency • RTA type 4 • Drugs (spironolactone, amiloride, trimethoprim, cyclosporine) • Ingestions/infusion: hydrochloric acid, or precursors • Administration of cationic amino acids: lysine, arginine HCl	• Acute diarrhoea • RTA type 1, type 2 • Carbonic anhydrase inhibition: acetazolamide • Urine diversions: ureterosigmoidostomy vesico-colic fistula • Intestinal, pancreatic or biliary fistulae

Table 81.2 Investigations for high anion gap metabolic acidosis

Essential investigations	Investigations in selected patients
• Serum and urine ketones • Serum creatinine, urea • Glucose and alcohol levels • Serum lactate • Urine microscopy for crystals • Serum osmolality and osmolal gap	• Serum salicylates • Serum levels of toxic alcohols • Urine organic acids levels

Table 81.3 Investigations for normal anion gap metabolic acidosis

Serum potassium
Serum creatinine
Urine pH, electrolytes, osmolality
Fractional excretion of bicarbonate
Urine urea, glucose

Table 81.4 Common causes of metabolic alkalosis

Potassium depletion/ mineralocorticoid excess	Chloride depletion
• Primary or secondary hyperaldosteronism • Drugs: liquorice as a confection or flavouring • Adrenal corticosteroid excess: primary, secondary, exogenous • Severe hypertension: malignant, accelerated • Liddle syndrome • Bartter and Gitelman syndromes and their variants • Laxative abuse	• Gastric losses: vomiting, mechanical drainage, bulimia • Diuretics: thiazide, bumetanide • Chronic diarrhoea: villous adenoma • Cystic fibrosis (high sweat chloride) • Hypercalcaemia of malignancy • Milk-alkali syndrome • Bicarbonate ingestion (massive) • Recovery from starvation • Hypoalbuminaemia

Key points

- Initial laboratory investigation of acid–base disorders includes arterial blood gas, serum electrolytes and calculation of anion gap.
- Metabolic acidosis is categorised into high or normal anion gap.
- High anion gap acidosis is most often due to ketoacidosis, lactic acidosis, renal failure or certain toxic ingestions.
- Normal anion gap acidosis is most often due to gastrointestinal or renal bicarbonate loss.

Disturbances in acid–base are common and important in unwell patients. These disturbances do not usually have specific signs and symptoms, and this emphasises the importance of testing for acid–base disturbance in patients who are acutely unwell by undertaking an arterial blood gas.

Metabolic acidosis

Metabolic acidosis is characterised by a reduction in blood pH and a decrease in the serum concentration of bicarbonate. There is often a compensatory reduction in $PaCO_2$ due to respiratory hyperventilatory compensation. Acute metabolic acidosis is common among seriously ill patients. Metabolic acidosis can be acute (lasting minutes to several days) or chronic (lasting weeks to years). The main causes of metabolic acidosis are shown in Table 81.1.

Acute metabolic acidosis can affect a number of organ systems, and confusion, lethargy and circulatory shock can occur. Chronic metabolic acidosis mostly affects the musculoskeletal system and can produce or exacerbate pre-existing bone disease and accelerate muscle degradation.

Anion gap

The serum anion gap, defined as $[Na^+] - ([Cl^-] + [HCO_3^-])$ (concentrations in millimoles per litre), is a useful diagnostic tool as the disorders that produce metabolic acidosis can affect the serum anion gap differently. The normal range is 6–10 mmol/L. The most common cause of an elevated serum anion gap is the accumulation of organic or inorganic anions. Several other factors can alter the serum anion gap:
• serum albumin – for every 10 g/L decrease in serum albumin concentration, serum anion gap is reduced by 2.3 mmol/L;
• accumulation of cationic paraproteins – can lower the anion gap or render it negative;
• accumulation of anionic paraproteins – can raise the serum anion gap;
• hyperphosphataemia – most cases of a very high serum anion gap (>45 mmol/L) are associated with severe hyperphosphataemia.

Investigations for high anion gap metabolic acidosis

These investigations are listed in Table 81.2. The measurement of serum and urinary ketones will usually detect ketoacidosis, but the test for ketones usually recognises only acetoacetate. Therefore, in alcoholic ketoacidosis or in cases where lactic acidosis coexists, β-hydroxybutyrate level should be checked.

A serum lactate >5 mmol/L will identify patients with type A lactic acidosis, which is caused by tissue hypoxia in respiratory failure, severe anaemia, shock, haemorrhage, hypotension and congestive cardiac failure. In type B lactic acidosis there is no tissue hypoxia and can be due to diabetes, liver failure, seizures, thiamine deficiency, ethanol, methanol, ethylene glycol, salicylate and paracetamol overdose. The routine test for lactate detects only the L-isomer; a specialised test is required to detect the D-isomer in D-lactic acidosis.

Osmolal gap

The difference between the estimated serum osmolality and the measured osmolality is the osmolal gap and is usually ≤10 mOsm/L (≤10 mmol/kg). Serum osmolality can be estimated using the following:

$$\text{Serum osmolality (mOsm/L)} = 2 \times [Na^+](\text{mmol/L}) + [\text{Urea}](\text{mmol/L}) + [\text{Glucose}](\text{mmol/L})$$

The metabolites of certain toxic alcohols produce metabolic acidosis and their accumulation elevates serum osmolality and causes an increase in the osmolal gap. A small increase in the osmolal gap can be seen in ketoacidosis, lactic acidosis and CKD. However, a serum osmolal gap >20 mOsm/L (>20 mmol/kg) suggests the accumulation of one of the toxic alcohols or ethanol.

Investigations for normal anion gap

The underlying cause of the normal anion gap metabolic acidosis usually requires further laboratory investigations (Table 81.3).

The measurement of serum potassium level is helpful because some disorders impair potassium excretion, thereby causing hyperkalaemia, whereas others cause urinary or gastrointestinal potassium wasting, which results in hypokalaemia (Table 81.4).

Indices of renal acidification can determine whether the kidney contributes to generation of the acidosis. There are two simple methods:
1 Measurement of urine pH in the presence of hypobicarbonataemia, with a urine pH <5.5 indicating normal acidification and a value ≥5.5 indicating impaired acidification.
2 Measurement of urinary ammonium excretion.
A low urinary ammonium excretion in the presence of a urine pH ≥5.5 is consistent with distal RTA, including aldosterone resistance.

Metabolic alkalosis

Metabolic alkalosis is a characterised by an elevated blood pH and an increase in serum bicarbonate (HCO_3^-) concentration. This occurs due to loss of acid from the extracellular fluid or a net gain in HCO_3^-.

When alkalosis is severe, low ionised plasma calcium may occur and compensatory hypoventilation may cause hypoxia.

Clinical investigation

The cause of chronic metabolic alkalosis is often evident on the initial assessment of the patient with a careful history and physical examination.

Urinary chloride and potassium measurements before therapy are useful. Low urinary chloride (<10 mmol/L) occurs with alkalosis in which chloride depletion predominates unless a chloruretic diuretic is present. A urinary potassium concentration of >30 mmol/L in the presence of hypokalaemia establishes renal potassium wasting, which is indicative of an intrinsic renal defect, diuretics or high circulating aldosterone. Conversely, a urinary potassium concentration of <20 mmol/L suggests extrarenal potassium loss. When metabolic alkalosis due to potassium depletion is suggested, a severe alkalosis should prompt a search for causative factors, such as chloride depletion or base ingestion. If the cause of the alkalosis is not readily apparent, the urine should be screened for diuretics.

For patients with suspected primary hyperaldosteronism, further investigations are required to confirm the diagnosis (see Chapter 101, on primary hyperaldosteronism). Surreptitious induction of alkalosis, as with diuretics or vomiting (bulimia), can be difficult to detect.

82 Potassium disorders

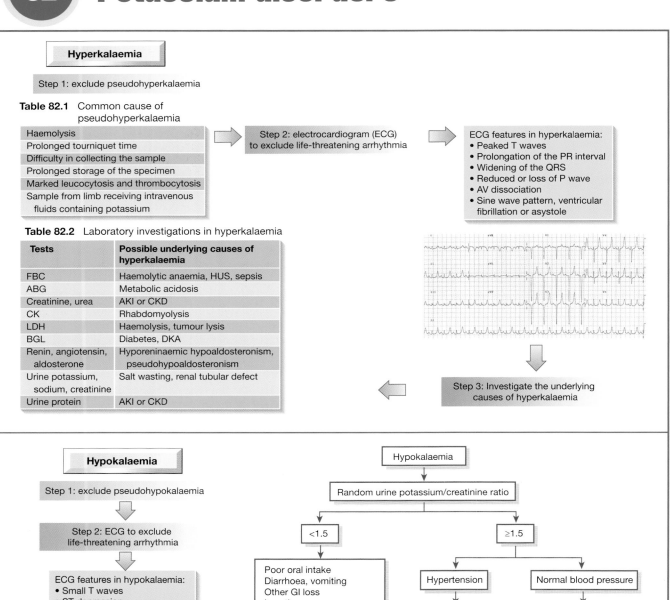

Hyperkalaemia

Step 1: exclude pseudohyperkalaemia

Table 82.1 Common cause of pseudohyperkalaemia

Haemolysis
Prolonged tourniquet time
Difficulty in collecting the sample
Prolonged storage of the specimen
Marked leucocytosis and thrombocytosis
Sample from limb receiving intravenous fluids containing potassium

Step 2: electrocardiogram (ECG) to exclude life-threatening arrhythmia

ECG features in hyperkalaemia:
- Peaked T waves
- Prolongation of the PR interval
- Widening of the QRS
- Reduced or loss of P wave
- AV dissociation
- Sine wave pattern, ventricular fibrillation or asystole

Table 82.2 Laboratory investigations in hyperkalaemia

Tests	Possible underlying causes of hyperkalaemia
FBC	Haemolytic anaemia, HUS, sepsis
ABG	Metabolic acidosis
Creatinine, urea	AKI or CKD
CK	Rhabdomyolysis
LDH	Haemolysis, tumour lysis
BGL	Diabetes, DKA
Renin, angiotensin, aldosterone	Hyporeninaemic hypoaldosteronism, pseudohypoaldosteronism
Urine potassium, sodium, creatinine	Salt wasting, renal tubular defect
Urine protein	AKI or CKD

Step 3: Investigate the underlying causes of hyperkalaemia

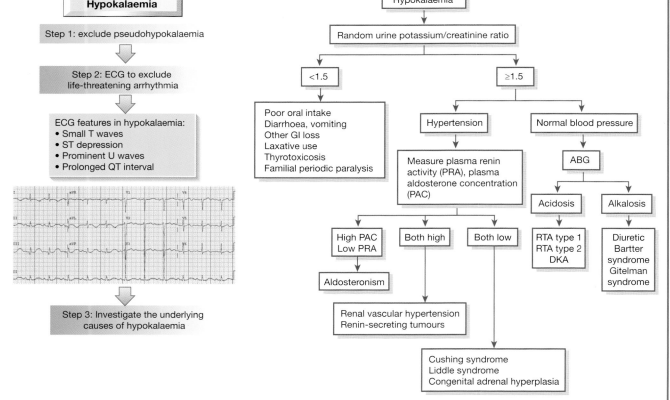

Hypokalaemia

Step 1: exclude pseudohypokalaemia

Step 2: ECG to exclude life-threatening arrhythmia

ECG features in hypokalaemia:
- Small T waves
- ST depression
- Prominent U waves
- Prolonged QT interval

Step 3: Investigate the underlying causes of hypokalaemia

Hypokalaemia

Random urine potassium/creatinine ratio

<1.5

Poor oral intake
Diarrhoea, vomiting
Other GI loss
Laxative use
Thyrotoxicosis
Familial periodic paralysis

≥1.5

Hypertension

Measure plasma renin activity (PRA), plasma aldosterone concentration (PAC)

High PAC
Low PRA

Both high

Both low

Aldosteronism

Renal vascular hypertension
Renin-secreting tumours

Cushing syndrome
Liddle syndrome
Congenital adrenal hyperplasia

Normal blood pressure

ABG

Acidosis

Alkalosis

RTA type 1
RTA type 2
DKA

Diuretic
Bartter syndrome
Gitelman syndrome

Clinical Investigations at a Glance, First Edition. Jonathan Gleadle, Jordan Li and Tuck Yong. © 2017 John Wiley & Sons, Ltd. Published 2017 by John Wiley & Sons, Ltd.

Hyperkalaemia

Hyperkalaemia is defined as serum potassium >5.5 mmol/L and it is a potentially life-threatening metabolic disorder. Hyperkalaemia can be classified into mild (5.5–6.5 mmol/L), moderate (6.5–7.5 mmol/L) and severe (>7.5 mmol/L). Hyperkalaemia can be caused by the following factors or a combination of them:

1 Inability of the kidneys to excrete potassium.

2 Impairment of the potassium move from the circulation into the cells.

3 A shift from the intracellular to the extracellular space.

4 Pseudohyperkalaemia.

The first step in the investigation of hyperkalaemia is to exclude pseudohyperkalaemia, which occurs when laboratory reports of potassium do not reflect actual values. The common causes of pseudohyperkalaemia are listed in Table 82.1. Haemolysis in a venesection specimen is most common. Pseudohyperkalaemia can be excluded by repeating the sample collection and obtaining serum and plasma potassium levels.

The second step is to investigate the causes of hyperkalaemia. Introduction of a medication affecting potassium homeostasis, sepsis, trauma, dehydration and renal failure are the main causes for development of hyperkalaemia. In patients with diabetic nephropathy, hyperkalaemia may be caused by the syndrome of hyporeninaemic hypoaldosteronism. Patients can be asymptomatic or present with muscular weakness or ileus.

Laboratory investigations

Laboratory tests should be directed towards causes suggested by the history and physical examination (Table 82.2).

A spot urine test for potassium, creatinine and osmolality should be obtained to calculate the fractional excretion of potassium and the transtubular potassium gradient. Hyporeninaemic hypoaldosteronism should be considered in patients with diabetes and hyperkalaemia, who generally have a low serum aldosterone.

ECG

Severe hyperkalaemia is associated with ECG changes and arrhythmias (see illustrations).

Hypokalaemia

Hypokalaemia is defined as serum potassium <3.5 mmol/L and is commonly graded as mild (3.1–3.5 mmol/L), moderate (2.5–3.0 mmol/L) and severe (<2.5 mmol/L). Hypokalaemia is relatively common in hospital populations. The causes of hypokalaemia and their associated features are shown in Table 82.5.

Mild hypokalaemia is often asymptomatic and discovered on routine blood tests, but severe hypokalaemia is associated with life-threatening arrhythmias and sudden cardiac death. Other manifestations of hypokalaemia may include muscle weakness, syncope or palpitations.

Laboratory investigations

The main laboratory investigations are assessment of serum and urine electrolytes and acid–base balance. In mild hypokalaemia with an obvious cause, laboratory investigations can be limited to monitoring potassium and magnesium concentrations. If hypokalaemia is moderate or severe, or the cause is unclear, investigations should include sodium, creatinine, urea, magnesium, glucose and bicarbonate. Spurious hypokalaemia may occur due to in vitro redistribution such as potassium uptake by large numbers of abnormal white cell in leukaemia when the sample is left at room temperature.

Acutely, bicarbonate is low in metabolic acidosis and high in metabolic alkalosis, but interpretation can be difficult in chronic compensated acid–base disorders. In the latter situation, analysis of ABG enables complete evaluation of metabolic and respiratory components of the acid–base disturbance.

A spot urine potassium, 24-hour urine potassium, and urine potassium : creatinine ratio (KCR) can be used to assess renal potassium loss. Urine KCR performs better than a random urine potassium concentration alone, without the need for 24-hour urine collection, and is the most practical way to assess renal potassium loss.

Diuretics are the most common cause of hypokalaemia caused by excessive renal potassium loss. Other rare causes include renal tubular acidosis (RTA) or hereditary renal tubular disorders.

Measurement of serum magnesium is important because hypokalaemia and hypomagnesaemia often coexist, and treatment of hypokalaemia is unlikely to be successful without correction of hypomagnesaemia.

Other investigations

Plasma aldosterone-to-renin ratio is the initial investigation of choice for suspected primary hyperaldosteronism. This ratio is raised in primary hyperaldosteronism (see Chapter 101 on hyperaldosteronism).

Patients with features of Cushing's syndrome should have either 24-hour urinary cortisol, overnight dexamethasone suppression test or midnight salivary cortisol tested. Thyroid function test should be checked if thyrotoxic periodic paralysis is suspected.

ECG

The initial assessment of moderate or severe hypokalaemia should immediately include ECG, which may show small T waves, ST depression, prominent U waves or a prolonged QT interval. Patients with rapid onset of hypokalaemia with coexisting risk factors, especially digoxin therapy, left ventricular hypertrophy or heart failure, are at increased risk of serious arrhythmias.

Key points

- The presence of typical ECG changes or a rapid rise or drop in serum potassium indicates that hyper- or hypokalaemia is potentially life threatening.
- Patients with severe potassium disorders need continuous cardiac monitoring.
- A normal ECG does not exclude risk for arrhythmia as life-threatening arrhythmia can occur without warning.

(83) Sodium disorders

Table 83.1 Common causes of hyponatraemia

Hypovolaemia hyponatraemia
Decreased TBW and sodium, with a relatively greater decrease in sodium
• Gastrointestinal (GI) loss – diarrhoea, vomiting
• Third space losses – burns, bowel obstruction, pancreatitis, peritonitis
• Renal losses – diuretics, salt-losing nephropathy, Addison's disease

Euvolaemia hyponatraemia
Increased TBW with near-normal total body sodium
• Drugs – carbamazepine, oxycodone
• Pain, stress
• Post-operation
• Hypothyroidism
• Syndrome of inappropriate antidiuretic hormone secretion (SIADH)

Hypervolaemic hyponatraemia
Increased TBW and sodium, with a relatively greater increase in TBW
• Congestive heart failure
• CKD or acute kidney injury (AKI)
• Nephrotic syndrome
• Cirrhosis

Table 83.2 Causes of SIADH

Malignant tumours
Lung cancer Bowel cancer Prostate cancer Thymoma Lymphoma
CNS disorders
Encephalitis or meningitis Stroke Tumours Head injury Subdural haematoma Hydrocephalus
Drugs

Tricyclic antidepressants
Selective serotonin re-uptake inhibitors
Carbamazepine
Antipsychotic drugs
Non-steroidal anti-inflammatory drugs
3,4-Methylenedioxy-methamphetamine ('ecstasy')
ADH analogues:
    desmopressin
    oxytocin

Pulmonary disorders
Bacterial or viral pneumonia Pulmonary abscess Tuberculosis Aspergillosis Asthma
Other causes
Hereditary Idiopathic

Table 83.3 Diagnostic criteria for SIADH

Plasma sodium concentration <135 mmol/L
Plasma osmolality <280 mOsmol/kg
Urine osmolality >100 mOsmol/kg
Urinary sodium concentration >40 mmol/L with normal dietary salt intake
Clinically euvolaemic
Absence of clinical or biochemical features of adrenal and thyroid dysfunction
No recent use of diuretic
Serum creatinine <120 µmol/L

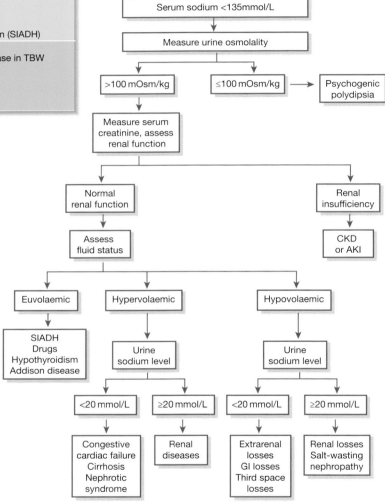

The purpose of investigation in hyponatraemia is to:
• Confirm the diagnosis and the severity
• Investigate the underlying causes

Serum sodium <135 mmol/L → Measure urine osmolality

>100 mOsm/kg / ≤100 mOsm/kg → Psychogenic polydipsia

Measure serum creatinine, assess renal function

Normal renal function / Renal insufficiency → CKD or AKI

Assess fluid status

Euvolaemic: SIADH, Drugs, Hypothyroidism, Addison disease

Hypervolaemic: Urine sodium level
<20 mmol/L → Congestive cardiac failure, Cirrhosis, Nephrotic syndrome
≥20 mmol/L → Renal diseases

Hypovolaemic: Urine sodium level
<20 mmol/L → Extrarenal losses, GI losses, Third space losses
≥20 mmol/L → Renal losses, Salt-wasting nephropathy

Key points

• Plasma sodium and osmolality, urine sodium and osmolality, exclusion of diuretic use and evaluation of thyroid and adrenal function are important in diagnosing SIADH.
• Other investigations to determine the cause of SIADH should be guided by the clinical presentation.
• In hypernatremia, a high urine osmolality (>700 mOsm/kg) in a setting of a low urine sodium level usually indicates an extrarenal hypotonic loss of free water. Urine osmolality that is 'inappropriately' low in the setting of hypernatremia suggests renal free-water loss.

Clinical Investigations at a Glance, First Edition. Jonathan Gleadle, Jordan Li and Tuck Yong. © 2017 John Wiley & Sons, Ltd. Published 2017 by John Wiley & Sons, Ltd.

Hyponatraemia

Hyponatremia is a serum sodium concentration <135 mmol/L. Symptoms often do not occur until the serum sodium concentration <125 mmol/L and are more severe with rapid-onset hyponatremia. Neurologic symptoms including headache, fall, confusion and seizures are the main clinical manifestations, due to an osmotic shift of water into brain cells causing oedema. The purpose of investigation in hyponatraemia is to confirm the diagnosis, severity and underlying causes.

Hyponatremia indicates an excess of total body water (TBW) relative to total body sodium, which is reflected by extracellular fluid (ECF) volume status; therefore, the causes of hyponatremia (Table 83.1) must be considered along with ECF volume: hypovolaemia, euvolaemia and hypervolaemia.

Clinical evaluation

As the clinical manifestations are nonspecific, hyponatremia is diagnosed after serum electrolyte measurement. If hyponatraemia is present, translocational hyponatremia due to severe hyperglycaemia or pseudohyponatraemia with normal serum osmolality in severe hyperlipidaemia or extreme hyperproteinaemia should be excluded first. The history and volume status often point to a cause such as new drugs or severe vomiting (Table 83.1).

Laboratory investigation

Serum sodium concentration and serum osmolality that are low and urine osmolality that is inappropriately high (>100 mmol/L) with respect to the low serum osmolality suggest volume overload, volume contraction or syndrome of inappropriate antidiuretic hormone secretion (SIADH). Volume overload and volume contraction are differentiated clinically. When neither volume overload or volume contraction appears likely, SIADH is considered. In patients with hypovolemia and normal renal function, sodium reabsorption results in a urine sodium <20 mmol/L. Urine sodium >20 mmol/L in hypovolaemic patients suggests mineralocorticoid deficiency or salt-losing nephropathy. Euvolaemic patients should have thyroid and adrenal function tested.

SIADH

SIADH is characterised by inappropriate secretion of antidiuretic hormone (ADH) leading to water retention, and increase in urine osmolality due to urine concentration and subsequent hyponatraemia. The clinical presentation of SIADH varies from an incidental finding to headache, difficulty concentrating, impaired memory, muscle weakness and falls with mild hyponatraemia to confusion, hallucinations, seizures, coma and respiratory arrest when severe (serum sodium <110 mmol/L).

It is important to recognise that increased secretion of ADH may be appropriate or physiological if there is hypovolaemia, nausea, vomiting and pain. There are many causes of SIADH grouped as related to malignant tumours, pulmonary diseases, central nervous system (CNS) disorders, medications and others (Table 83.2).

Investigations for establishing diagnosis

See Table 83.3 for criteria for diagnosis of SIADH.

The serum sodium measurement indicates the severity of the hyponatraemia. Hypouricaemia and low urea may be seen with SIADH but are not diagnostic. Potassium concentration is usually normal and there is usually no acid–base disturbance. ADH level is not recommended because urinary osmolality >100 mOsm/kg is indicative of excess of circulating ADH. To make the diagnosis of SIADH, urine osmolality must exceed 100 mOsm/kg when the effective plasma osmolality is low. In SIADH, urinary sodium is usually >40 mmol/L with normal salt intake.

Thyroid function tests should be undertaken. If there is any suspicion of adrenal insufficiency a short Synacthen test should be performed before SIADH is diagnosed.

SIADH diagnosis is based on the exclusion of other causes of hyponatraemia and of appropriate secretion of ADH. Once hypotonic hyponatraemia has been established and there is a urine sodium >40 mmol/L and osmolality >100 mOsm/kg, with euvolaemia, SIADH should be considered. SIADH is commonly overdiagnosed. It is important to ensure the patient is not fluid overloaded or deplete. Iatrogenic post-operative hyponatraemia (as a result of the injudicious use of isotonic dextrose), pain and nausea, or diuretic-induced hyponatraemia are often misdiagnosed as SIADH.

Investigating the cause

Other investigations to determine the cause of SIADH include a CXR to determine if there is an underlying pulmonary disorder. Further investigations, such as CT or MRI of head, chest and abdomen, should be guided by the clinical presentation. SIADH may be difficult to distinguish from cerebral salt wasting, a syndrome of hyponatremia and ECF volume depletion in patients following insults to the CNS.

Hypernatraemia

Hypernatremia is primarily due to a defect in water intake and usually implies impairment in the thirst mechanism or a lack of access to adequate fluid intake. The common causes of hypernatraemia include:

1 **Primary hypodipsia.** This is a defect of thirst usually associated with destruction of the hypothalamic thirst centre secondary to primary or metastatic tumours, granulomatous disease, vascular disease or trauma.

2 **Diabetes insipidus.** This is a defect in the secretion or action of ADH, which may be hypothalamic (central) or nephrogenic.

3 **Inadequate fluid intake in the setting of increased free-water loss.** Pure water loss is frequently seen in patients with fever and diabetes insipidus. Hypotonic loss is seen related to GI loss, burns and diuretic therapy.

The clinical manifestations of hypernatremia are non-specific and often subtle. The first step is a detailed clinical history, including a careful review of the patient's weight, intake and output, and a critical analysis of fluid, nutrition and nursing care. Measurements of spot urine/plasma osmolality and urine sodium levels may help in more difficult cases.

A high urine osmolality (>700 mOsm/kg) in a setting of a low urine sodium level usually indicates an extrarenal hypotonic loss of free water. Urine osmolality that is 'inappropriately' low in the setting of hypernatremia suggests renal free-water loss. A urine osmolality that is <150 mOsm/kg indicates diabetes insipidus in the setting of hypernatremia and polyuria. Sophisticated and more dangerous dehydration testing is rarely necessary and reserved for more difficult cases of diabetes insipidus.

84 Calcium disorders

Initial investigations in hypercalcaemia:
- PTH, FBC, CRP
- Renal function, serum electrolytes: phosphate, magnesium, liver function tests, PSA
- Serum and urine protein electrophoresis, urine Bence Jones protein, serum free light chains (for myeloma)
- CXR for lung cancer or metastases, sarcoidosis or tuberculosis

Table 84.1 Clinical manifestations of hypercalcaemia

Gastrointestinal symptoms
Nausea, vomiting, anorexia
Constipation
Abdominal pain, pancreatitis
Urinary tract symptoms
Nephrolithiasis or/and nephrocalcinosis
Polyuria and polydipsia
Dehydration
Central nervous system symptoms
Impaired concentration and memory
Confusion, stupor, coma
Musculoskeletal system symptoms
Muscle weakness
Bone pain
Pathological fracture

Table 84.2 Causes of hypercalcaemia

Parathyroid hormone (PTH) related
• Primary hyperparathyroidism
• Multiple endocrine neoplasia I and II
Malignancy related
• Humoral hypercalcaemia of malignancy – mediated by PTH-related protein (PTHrP)
• Local osteolysis – mediated by cytokines (e.g. multiple myeloma)
• Ectopic PTH
Vitamin D related
• Vitamin D intoxication
• Granulomatous disease (e.g. sarcoidosis and lymphoma)
Medications related
• Thiazide diuretics
• Lithium
• Milk-alkali syndrome (excessive intake of calcium from calcium antacids)
Other causes
• Genetic disorders – familial hypocalciuric hypercalcaemia (FHH)
• Immobilisation
• Paget's disease – high bone turnover
• Hyperthyroidism

Table 84.3 Common causes of hypocalcaemia

Hypoparathyroidism
Vitamin D deficiency
Renal tubular acidosis
Advanced renal failure
Magnesium
Acute pancreatitis
Drugs including anticonvulsants (e.g. phenytoin)
Transfusion of >10 units of citrate-anticoagulated blood

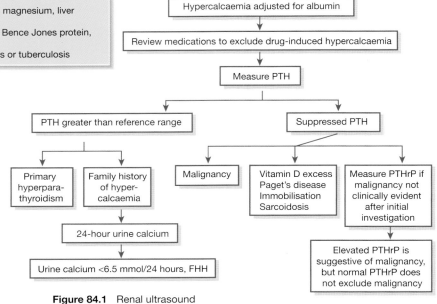

Hypercalcaemia adjusted for albumin
↓
Review medications to exclude drug-induced hypercalcaemia
↓
Measure PTH

PTH greater than reference range → Primary hyperparathyroidism / Family history of hyper-calcaemia → 24-hour urine calcium → Urine calcium <6.5 mmol/24 hours, FHH

Suppressed PTH → Malignancy / Vitamin D excess, Paget's disease, Immobilisation, Sarcoidosis / Measure PTHrP if malignancy not clinically evident after initial investigation → Elevated PTHrP is suggestive of malignancy, but normal PTHrP does not exclude malignancy

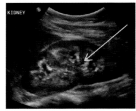

Figure 84.1 Renal ultrasound shows nephrocalcinosis

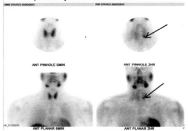

Figure 84.2 Sestamibi parathyroid scan shows parathyroid adenoma

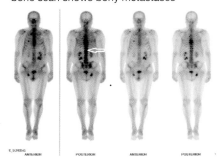

Figure 84.3 Whole-body radionuclide bone scan shows bony metastases

Key points

- Total calcium should always be corrected for albumin concentration. Serum calcium concentration can be falsely elevated by prolonged use of tourniquet.
- Measurement of intact PTH levels helps differentiate PTH-mediated hypercalcemia (e.g. caused by hyperparathyroidism or FHH), in which PTH levels are high or high–normal, from non-PTH-mediated causes.
- 24-hour urine calcium excretion is helpful to differentiate between primary hyperparathyroidism and FHH.
- Low serum concentrations of magnesium, phosphate and potassium are frequently (20–30%) detected in association with hypocalcaemia, and these abnormalities should be corrected. In patients with hypocalcaemia, a PTH below the reference range is virtually diagnostic of hypoparathyroidism.

Hypercalcaemia

Hypercalcaemia is a raised serum total calcium >2.60 mmol/L and is a common clinical problem requiring investigation to discover the underlying cause. Mild hypercalcaemia (calcium levels 2.60–3.00 mmol/L) can be asymptomatic and often found incidentally on blood testing. Severe hypercalcaemia (calcium level >3.0 mmol/L) is usually associated with acute symptoms and signs. Measurement of calcium is important in any acutely unwell patient and considered in patients with unexplained gastrointestinal, musculoskeletal, urinary tract symptoms or weakness. Symptoms of hypercalcaemia are listed in Table 84.1.

The causes of hypercalcaemia can be divided into five categories (Table 84.2). The most common cause of hypercalcaemia in ambulatory care and young patients is primary hyperparathyroidism (90%). However, in hospitalised or elderly patients the most common cause is malignancy (65%).

Initial investigations

About 50% of serum calcium is bound to albumin, and the remaining calcium is ionised, physiologically 'active' and under hormonal regulation. The ionised or 'corrected calcium' should therefore be determined. Corrected calcium is calculated from total calcium and serum albumin:

Corrected calcium (mmol/L) = measured calcium (mmol/L)
+ {0.02 × [40 – albumin (g/L)]}

When hypercalcaemia is present, it is important to repeat the measurement to ensure it is not an artefact. Serum calcium concentration can be falsely raised because the patient was not fasting, there has been a prolonged use of tourniquet or a laboratory error. Determine if hypercalcaemia is drug related. Drugs to be considered include calcium supplements, calcium-containing antacids (which can cause milk-alkali syndrome), vitamin D or vitamin D analogues (which may last for many weeks after cessation of vitamin D intake since 25-hydroxyvitamin D (25-OHD) has a 10–20 day half-life), thiazide diuretics and lithium.

The next useful investigation is measurement of serum parathyroid hormone (PTH level). As the physiological response to hypercalcaemia is to suppress production of PTH, a raised PTH level or an inappropriately 'normal' level is diagnostic of primary hyperparathyroidism, whereas a reduced concentration indicates other causes of hypercalcaemia, such as malignancy. Other initial investigations are listed on the opposite page. Hyperparathyroidism and hypercalcaemia due to malignancy often occur with hypophosphataemia caused by the inhibition of proximal phosphate reabsorption in the renal tubule. Serum phosphate is normal or elevated in granulomatous diseases, vitamin D intoxication, immobilisation, milk-alkali syndrome, thyrotoxicosis and metastatic bone disease.

Other investigations

24-hour urine calcium

A normal (<7.5 mmol/day) or raised value is typical in primary hyperparathyroidism and hypercalcaemia of malignancy, and a raised value increases the risk of renal calculi. However, there are three disorders in which an increase in renal calcium reabsorption leads to relative hypocalciuria:
- milk-alkali syndrome
- thiazide diuretics
- familial hypocalciuric hypercalcaemia (FHH).

FHH is an autosomal dominant condition presenting with hypercalcaemia. This diagnosis should be considered especially in younger patients and those with a family history of hypercalcaemia.

Renal ultrasonography

Primary hyperparathyroidism is associated with an increased incidence of nephrolithiasis (15–20% of all patients), which is an indication for parathyroid surgery; renal ultrasonography may also identify asymptomatic stones or nephrocalcinosis (Figure 84.1). Renal ultrasonography has a sensitivity of 64% and a specificity of >90% for detecting renal calculi.

Parathyroid imaging

Sestamibi parathyroid scan and neck ultrasonography is not indicated for the diagnosis of primary hyperparathyroidism but it is useful for disease localisation before planned parathyroidectomy. It may also localise ectopic parathyroid glands (Figure 84.2).

Parathyroid-hormone-related protein (PTHrP)

Elevation of PTHrP is the primary mediator of humoral hypercalcaemia of malignancy. Measurement of PTHrP is often **not** necessary for diagnosis since most patients have clinically apparent malignancy. PTH is usually appropriately suppressed in these patients.

Radionuclide bone scan

If metastatic bone disease is suspected, a whole-body radionuclide bone scan is useful (Figure 84.3). It has a sensitivity of 77% and a specificity of 96% for detecting bone metastases.

25-Hydroxyvitamin D and 1,25-dihydroxyvitamin D (1,25-OHD) level

Raised concentrations of 25-OHD may indicate vitamin D toxicity. Very high concentrations (>150 nmol/L) suggest exogenous sources of vitamin D. 1,25-OHD concentrations are high in sarcoidosis and other granulomatous diseases, primary hyperparathyroidism.

Hypocalcaemia

Hypocalcaemia is total serum calcium concentration <2.10 mmol/L in the presence of normal plasma protein concentrations or a serum ionised calcium <1.10 mmol/L. The common causes of hypocalcaemia are listed in Table 84.3. Manifestations include paraesthesia, muscle spasm/pain, tetany, and, when severe, seizures and encephalopathy. Hypocalcaemia is often found incidentally. Because low plasma protein can lower total, but not ionised, serum calcium, ionised calcium should be estimated based on albumin concentration.

Serum electrolytes, creatinine, vitamin D and PTH levels should be checked in patients with hypocalcaemia. Patients with renal failure and hypocalcaemia usually present with hyperphosphataemia and high PTH. Hypophosphataemia develops in patients with vitamin D deficiency and hungry bone disease. Hypomagnesaemia may contribute to hypocalcaemia. Low PTH occurs in patients with hereditary or acquired hypoparathyroidism.

An ECG should be performed as acute hypocalcaemia can cause prolongation of the QT interval, which may lead to ventricular dysrhythmias. Imaging studies may include plain radiography or CT scans. Rickets or osteomalacia presents with the pathognomonic Looser zones in the pubic ramus, upper femoral bone and ribs. Radiography may also disclose osteoblastic metastases from breast or prostate or lung cancer, which can cause hypocalcaemia.

85 Proteinuria

The purposes of investigation for proteinuria are:
- Establish that the dipstick result is a true positive
- Quantify the severity of proteinuria
- Exclude serious causes
- Decide the need for further investigation
- Investigate the underlying causes of proteinuria

Figure 85.1 Urine dipstick test for proteinuria

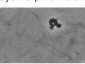

Figure 85.2 Urine microscopy shows dysmorphic RBCs

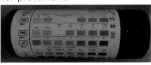

Figure 85.3 Urine microscopy showing RBC casts

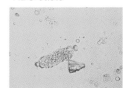

Table 85.1 Common causes of false-positive or -negative results in dipstick proteinuria test

False-positive	False-negative
• Alkaline urine (pH >7.5)	• Dilute urine (specific
• Prolonged immersion dipstick	gravity <1.015)
• Highly concentrated urine	• Non-albumin
• Gross haematuria	• Low molecular weight
• Presence of penicillin,	proteinuria
sulfonamides	
• Contaminated with pus, semen	
or vaginal secretions	

Table 85.2 Interpretation of common findings on urine microscopic examination

Microscopic finding	Pathologic process
Leukocytes, leukocyte casts with bacteria	Urinary tract infection
Normal-shaped RBCs	Suggestive of lower urinary tract lesion
Dysmorphic RBCs, RBC casts	Suggestive of glomerular disease
Fatty casts, free fat or oval fat bodies	Nephrotic range proteinuria (>3.5 g/day)
Waxy, granular or cellular casts	Advanced CKD

Table 85.3 Laboratory investigations for nephrotic syndrome/nephrotic-range proteinuria

Test	Interpretation of finding
FBC	Anaemia may be present in CKD
Serum electrolytes, creatinine, urea	Assess renal function
LFTs and serum albumin	Albumin decreased in nephrotic syndrome
Fasting blood glucose level and HbA1c	Elevated in diabetes mellitus
Lipid profile	Cholesterol level increased in nephrotic syndrome
CRP	If normal, helps to rule out inflammatory and infectious causes
ANA	Elevated in SLE and some autoimmune diseases
Anti-dsDNA antibodies	Elevated in SLE
Complement C3 and C4	Levels are low in glomerulonephritis
HIV, and hepatitis B and C serologic tests	HIV, hepatitis B and C, have been associated with glomerular proteinuria
Serum, urine protein electrophoresis, serum light chains levels	Results are abnormal in multiple myeloma
ANCA	Vasculitis usually presents with a nephritic syndrome rather than typical nephrotic

Table 85.4 Features predisposing to renal disease in patient with non-nephrotic-range proteinuria

Active urine sediment (haematuria, dysmorphic RBCs, RBC casts)
Impaired renal function
Progressive worsening renal function
Hypertension (less suggestive with increasing age)
History suggestive of systemic disorder
Family history of renal disease

Key points

- Patients with more than 1 g of protein/24 hours are likely to have a glomerular disorder and require further investigation to identify the cause.
- Urine ACR can be used to quantify the degree of proteinuria.
- Renal biopsy is often recommended in persons with nephrotic syndrome to establish the diagnosis, to assess disease activity and prognosis.

Clinical Investigations at a Glance, First Edition. Jonathan Gleadle, Jordan Li and Tuck Yong. © 2017 John Wiley & Sons, Ltd. Published 2017 by John Wiley & Sons, Ltd.

Proteinuria is defined as urinary protein excretion >150 mg/day. Proteinuria can be an indication of renal disease or a transient normal finding.

Detecting and quantifying proteinuria

Dipstick tests

Dipstick tests can detect urine protein semi-quantitatively. The results are graded as negative (<10 mg/dL), trace (10–20 mg/dL), 1+ (30 mg/dL), 2+ (100 mg/dL), 3+ (300 mg/dL) or 4+ (1000 mg/dL) (Figure 85.1). This method preferentially detects albumin and is less sensitive to globulins, heavy or light chains. Detection limit is 30 mg/dL. False-positive and false-negative results can occur (Table 85.1). Patients with persistent urine dipstick positive proteinuria should undergo a quantitative measurement of protein.

Urine albumin to creatinine ratio (ACR)

Early morning spot urine is preferred, but a random urine sample is acceptable. Specimens should not be collected during an acute illness or menstruation. Urine ACR correlates well with 24-hour urine protein and 24-hour urine collections may not be necessary.

Urine protein-to-creatinine ratio (PCR)

Urine PCR can be determined in a random urine specimen. Correlation between PCR, ACR and 24-hour protein excretion is reasonable. The ratio is about the same numerically as the number of grams of protein excreted in urine per day. Thus, a ratio of <0.2 is equivalent to 0.2 g/day of protein and is considered normal; a ratio of 3.5 is equivalent to 3.5 g of protein per day and is considered nephrotic-range proteinuria. ACR should be requested in preference to PCR in patients who are being screened for proteinuria and is recommended for diabetic patients.

24-hour urine protein measurement

This method is the gold standard to quantify proteinuria. The 24-hour urinary creatinine concentration should be measured to determine the adequacy of the specimen. Creatinine excretion is relatively constant on a daily basis. A 24-hour proteinuria of >300 mg or 30 mg/mmol creatinine is pathological.

Diagnostic evaluation of proteinuria

Microscopic urinalysis

When proteinuria is found on dipstick urinalysis, the urinary sediment should be examined microscopically (Table 85.2). RBC casts (Figures 85.2 and 85.3) are indicative of glomerular disease. Gross haematuria will cause proteinuria on dipstick urinalysis, but microscopic haematuria will not.

Transient proteinuria

If the results of microscopic urinalysis are normal or inconclusive, the dipstick shows trace to 2+ protein, the test should be repeated on a morning specimen at least twice during the next month. If a dipstick shows 3+ or 4+ protein, work-up should proceed to quantify proteinuria. If two subsequent dipstick results are negative, the patient has transient proteinuria. This condition is not associated with increased morbidity and mortality, and further investigation and follow-up are not indicated.

Persistent proteinuria

When a diagnosis of persistent proteinuria is established by 24-hour urine protein measurement or urine ACR, a detailed history and physical examination should be performed, specifically looking for systemic diseases with renal involvement.

Nephrotic syndrome

The diagnostic criteria of nephrotic syndrome are:
- nephrotic-range proteinuria (>3.5 g/day)
- hypoalbuminaemia (<25g/L)
- peripheral oedema and hypercholesterolaemia may present

The disease process can be a primary or secondary glomerulonephritis.

Laboratory investigations

These tests are listed in Table 85.3.

Renal ultrasound

Ultrasound can determine whether a patient has two kidneys and to demonstrate their echogenicity. Having only one kidney is a relative contraindication to kidney biopsy. Increased renal echogenicity and small-size kidneys by ultrasound is suggestive of intrarenal fibrosis and chronic disease.

Renal biopsy

Adult nephrotic syndrome of unknown origin may require a renal biopsy for diagnosis. Reaching a pathological diagnosis is important because different primary or secondary causes have different treatment options and prognoses. A renal biopsy is not indicated in adults with nephrotic syndrome from an obvious cause. Nephrotic syndrome is likely to be secondary to diabetic nephropathy in a patient with long-standing diabetes and diabetic retinopathy, so kidney biopsy may be unnecessary.

Non-nephrotic-range proteinuria

Patients with non-nephrotic-range proteinuria but proteinuria >1 g/day (or ACR >70, PCR >100 mg/mmol) should also be investigated for underlying causes and tubulointerstitial diseases considered. In the absence of features predisposing to renal disease (Table 85.4), inactive urine sediment, low levels (<1 g protein/day or PCR <100 or ACR<70) or intermittent proteinuria and normal renal function can be managed by regular monitoring of urine ACR or PCR, blood pressure, and serum creatinine. These patients have a 20% risk for renal impairment after 10 years; therefore, regular follow-up is usually suggested.

Orthostatic proteinuria

Patients younger than 30 years who excrete <1 g/day of protein and who have normal renal function and urine microscopic examination should be tested for orthostatic or postural proteinuria. This benign condition occurs in about 3–5% of adolescents and young adults. It is characterised by increased protein excretion in the upright position but normal protein excretion when the patient is supine. To diagnose orthostatic proteinuria, split daytime and overnight urine specimens are obtained. Annual blood pressure measurement and urinalysis are recommended.

86 Renal mass

The goals of investigation in renal mass are to:
- Differentiate between benign and malignant mass/lesion
- Consider the need for biopsy before intervention
- Stage the malignant mass/lesion
- Decide the need for follow-up/surveillance of benign mass/lesion
- Provide surveillance post-nephrectomy

Key points

- Ultrasound scan can elucidate whether a renal mass is solid or cystic.
- CT or MRI is essential for staging renal cancer. It can provide information about perirenal extension, vascular invasion (renal vein and inferior vena cava), nodal and liver involvement.
- Indications for percutaneous biopsy of a renal mass include patients who opt for either active surveillance or ablative therapy and patients with advanced CKD in whom nephrectomy may lead to dialysis.

Table 86.1 Features to distinguish between simple renal cysts and solid masses

	Simple cyst	Solid mass
Margin	Well marginated	Ill defined
Wall	Smooth and thin	Irregular and thick
Ultrasound	Echo free Posterior enhancement No vessels on Doppler	Echogenic, multilocular mass, calcified mass No posterior enhancement Vessels shown on Doppler
CT	−10 to +20 HU No contrast enhancement	+30 to +70 HU Contrast enhancement

HU: Hounsfield units.

Table 86.2 Bosniak classification of cystic lesions

Classification	Malignant (%)	Management/surveillance
I	0	No surveillance
II	1	No surveillance
IIF	5	Follow up
III	35	Surgery
IV	90	Surgery

Figure 85.1 Renal ultrasound showings (a) a normal right kidney, (b) a simple renal cyst and (c) a complex renal cyst

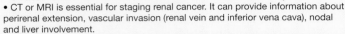
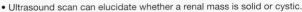

Figure 85.2 (a) Renal ultrasound shows an angiomyolipoma. (b) CT abdomen shows an angiomyolipoma

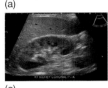 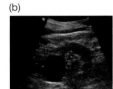 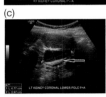

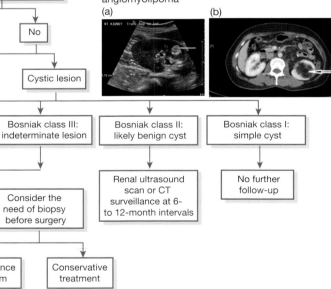

Figure 85.3 (a) Renal ultrasound shows an RCC. (b) CT abdomen shows an RCC

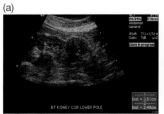 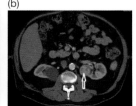

Figure 85.4 CT chest shows pulmonary metastasis of an RCC

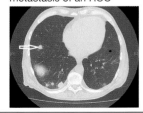

Figure 85.5 CT of pelvis shows bony metastasis of an RCC

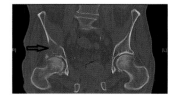

Renal masses rarely present with symptoms of pain, haematuria or systemic symptoms. Increasingly, the widespread use of imaging has resulted in increased findings of small incidental renal cysts and masses. Over 20% of abdominal imaging studies identify a renal lesion incidentally. The common causes of renal masses include:

- simple renal cysts;
- renal cell carcinoma (RCC);
- benign tumours (oncocytoma, angiomyolipoma);
- abscess.

The majority of renal lesions are small, non-enhancing simple cysts. A proportion of small renal masses (25%) are solid tumours or complex cysts that show contrast enhancement on CT imaging and are suggestive of malignancy. The incidence of renal cancer, especially early stage and localised, has more than doubled in the last 30 years and now accounts for 3% of all adult cancers, and most (>90%) are RCCs. The primary goal in investigating a renal mass is to exclude malignancy.

Laboratory investigations

In a patient with a suspected malignant renal mass, the following laboratory investigations should be performed:

- FBC;
- urea, creatinine, calcium, LDH;
- liver function tests;
- urinalysis for haematuria and proteinuria.

Radiological investigations

Ultrasound

Ultrasound is the initial imaging modality of choice. Ultrasound can elucidate whether the mass is solid or cystic (Figures 86.1a and b). Colour Doppler may help to determine the vascularity of the mass. No further investigation is necessary if the cysts have the ultrasonographic characteristics of a simple cyst (Table 86.1) since the possibility of malignancy is very low. If ultrasound is equivocal or complex cyst (Figure 86.1c) or has the following features then consider undertaking a CT scan:

- solid or complex;
- with internal echoes;
- irregular walls;
- calcifications or septae;
- multiple clustered cysts (which may mask underlying carcinoma).

CT

A four-phase (arterial, corticomedullary, nephrographic and excretory) kidney CT scan with intravenous contrast is the next investigation. Simple cysts can be reliably diagnosed on the basis of well-defined radiological criteria (Table 86.1). The Bosniak classification, which uses the lesion's morphology and enhancement characteristics, is used to classify cystic lesions, indicate risk of malignancy and guide management (Table 86.2).

Macroscopic fat within a renal mass, identified by CT or MRI, is highly suggestive of angiomyolipoma (a benign mass) (Figure 86.2), unless calcification is present, which suggests a malignant lesion. The majority of enhancing masses are malignant. No specific findings conclusively identify a mass as malignant or benign. Therefore, a solid enhancing small renal mass must be considered malignant unless proven otherwise.

An enhancing mass is one that is has an increase in density of >15 Hounsfield unit (HU) after contrast administration (Figure 86.3).

The smaller the mass, the greater the chance that it is benign. Masses that show no growth are less likely to be malignant. If a mass is too small to be characterised adequately, a follow-up CT can be performed at 3- to 6-monthly intervals to determine progress.

CT is essential for staging renal cancer. It can provide information about perirenal extension, vascular invasion (renal vein and inferior vena cava), nodal, lung and liver involvement (Figure 86.4).

MRI

MRI is used to evaluate solid masses seen on ultrasound or CT if a patient is unable to receive intravenous contrast. It is useful for both the characterisation of lesions and the assessment of invasion of the renal vein and inferior vena cava. Post-surgical histopathological diagnosis shows that 20% of lesions that were highly suspicious of renal cancer on imaging turned out to be benign at surgery.

Staging

At the time of diagnosis, metastases are present in 1–8% of patients with renal cancers that are 3–4 cm in diameter. CXR, CT chest and bone scanning (Figure 86.5) should be performed to stage.

Renal mass biopsy

The role of percutaneous biopsy in the evaluation of a small renal mass is controversial. There are concerns about its safety, accuracy and sampling errors. Certainly not all patients with small renal masses need biopsy. Indications for biopsy include patients who opt for either active surveillance or ablative therapy and patients with advanced CKD in which nephrectomy may lead to dialysis.

With current biopsy techniques the risk of tumour seeding is negligible and significant bleeding is very rare. Percutaneous needle biopsy under CT guidance has a sensitivity of 80–92% and specificity of 83–100% in detecting cancer. Smaller masses (≤3 cm) may have a higher false-negative rate (negative predictive value of 60%), but the false-negative rate can be reduced by repeat biopsies. In most cases, benign findings of a biopsy specimen cannot rule out cancer in the rest of the mass, but a definitive benign diagnosis may be made with angiomyolipoma, adenoma or focal infection. Biopsy is generally avoided in cystic lesions.

Active surveillance

Active surveillance can be undertaken for small renal masses (<4 cm). This approach is based on the rationale that many small renal masses are either benign or have an indolent nature. Also, for elderly patients or those with extensive comorbidities or limited life expectancy, the risks of treating such lesions may outweigh the survival benefit.

Active surveillance involves serial ultrasound, CT or MRI. CT or MRI is generally preferred over ultrasound because of greater resolution and reproducibility. The recommendation is to repeat imaging at 6- to 12-month intervals, but financial costs and risks of radiation from serial CT should be taken into consideration.

87 Kidney stones

The purpose of investigations is to:
- Confirm the diagnosis of kidney stones
- Identify the type of kidney stones, if possible
- Diagnose any complications related to the kidney stones or associated medical conditions
- Identify any patients who require further metabolic investigation

Table 87.1 Medical conditions and risk factors associated with kidney stones

Medical conditions	Risk factors
• Small bowel resection, ileostomy • Bariatric surgery – duodenal switch, Roux-en-Y gastric bypass • Chronic diarrhoea, malabsorption • Primary hyperparathyroidism • Primary hyperoxaluria • Hypocitraturia • Idiopathic hypercalciuria • Sarcoidosis • Myeloma • Gout • Renal tubular acidosis	• Low fluid intake • Low calcium intake • High salt diet • High animal protein • intake

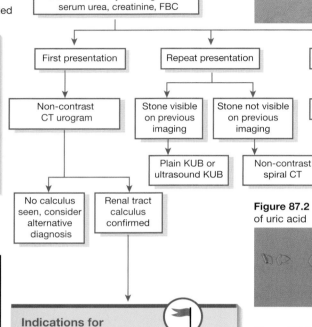

Clinically suspected renal colic

↓

Urine culture and microscopy

↓

Basic laboratory investigations: serum urea, creatinine, FBC

↓

First presentation → Non-contrast CT urogram → No calculus seen, consider alternative diagnosis / Renal tract calculus confirmed

Repeat presentation → Stone visible on previous imaging → Plain KUB or ultrasound KUB / Stone not visible on previous imaging → Non-contrast spiral CT

Pregnant → Ultrasound

Figure 87.1 Urinary crystals of calcium oxalate

Figure 87.3 CT urogram shows: (a) dilated right collecting system and ureter; (b) an obstructing 5 mm calculus in the right ureter at the L3–L4 level

(a)   (b)

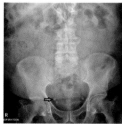

Figure 87.5 KUB plain X-ray shows renal calculi

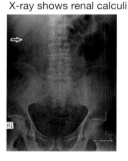

Figure 87.6 KUB plain X-ray shows multiple pelvic phleboliths

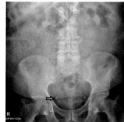

Indications for metabolic investigation

- Recurrent kidney stones
- More than one stone in the past year
- Children <16 years
- Family history of kidney stones
- Residual calculi after surgical treatment
- Initial presentation with multiple calculi, especially bilateral calculi
- Associated with CKD
- Solitary kidney (including renal transplant)
- Associated gastrointestinal disorder (bypass or ileal resection)

Figure 87.2 Urinary crystals of uric acid

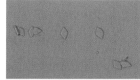

Figure 87.4 Renal ultrasound shows an echogenic focus in the right kidney consistent with renal calculus without obstruction

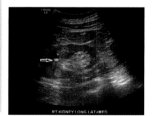

RT KIDNEY LONG LAT>MED

Figure 87.7 Stones in the bladder

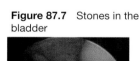
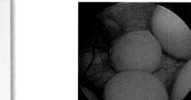

Key points

- Non-contrast CT is the most accurate test for detecting calculi in the renal tract, with a sensitivity of 97% and specificity of 98%.
- Additional metabolic testing should be performed in high-risk or recurrent stone formers.
- KUB plain X-ray has a sensitivity of 45–50% and specificity of 64–77% for detecting ureteric calculi. It can identify radiopaque stones, which are usually calcium-containing, struvite or cystine stones.

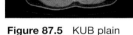
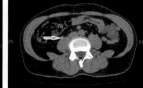

Kidney stones affect 10% of people and the incidence increases with age. Stone formation is associated with increased risk of CKD and hypertension. Although many inherited and systemic diseases are associated with kidney stones (Table 87.1), most kidney stones are idiopathic. The single most important risk factor (Table 87.1) is low fluid intake.

Baseline investigations

All patients presenting with renal colic or suspected kidney stone should have the following baseline investigations.

Urine microscopy and culture

Urine dipstick, microscopy and culture are essential in the investigation of renal calculi as the combination of infection and obstruction in the renal tract can rapidly result in septicaemia and permanent loss of renal function. A negative urine culture does not completely exclude upper tract infection due to complete upper tract obstruction.

Frank haematuria is present in 85% of patients with urinary calculi. Microscopic haematuria occurs in 95% of patients with urinary stones. The lack of microscopic haematuria does not eliminate renal colic as a potential diagnosis. Degree of haematuria is not predictive of stone size or likelihood of passage.

Urinary crystals of calcium oxalate (Figure 87.1), uric acid (Figure 87.2) or cystine may be found on urine microscopy and are clues to the type of renal calculus.

Laboratory investigations

Basic laboratory investigations should include:
- serum urea and creatinine;
- FBC;
- serum calcium and PTH levels should be measured;
- uric acid – hyperuricaemia may suggest uric acid stone;
- potassium – hypokalaemia and decreased serum bicarbonate level suggest underlying type 1 renal tubular acidosis;
- blood culture – if infection is suspected.

Radiological investigations

CT urogram

Non-contrast CT of the kidneys, ureter and bladder (CT urogram) is the investigation of choice for patients presenting or suspected with renal colic (Figure 87.3). CT provides information about the presence, size and location of stones, as well as any anatomical abnormalities. It offers near absolute sensitivity and specificity in the diagnosis of ureteric and renal stones, irrespective of stone type. CT has the potential to diagnose alternate pathology if a stone is not identified (e.g. aortic aneurysm).

Renal ultrasound

Ultrasound is reserved for the assessment of flank pain in pregnant women or for suspected radiolucent uric acid stones, which cannot be seen on a plain kidney, ureter and bladder (KUB) X-ray. Ultrasound can be used in follow-up of hydronephrosis after conservative management of ureteric colic or to monitor stone size in asymptomatic patients. Ultrasonography relies on indirect visualisation clues to identify stones (Figure 87.4). Differentiating an extrarenal pelvis from an obstructed one is sometimes difficult. Intermittent obstruction or mild hydronephrosis can be missed with ultrasonography.

Kidney, ureter and bladder plain X-ray

Plain KUB X-ray is useful for assessing total stone burden, as well as the size, shape, composition and location of urinary calculi in some patients (Figure 87.5). It can be utilised for follow-up imaging and thus reduces radiation dose compared with CT follow-up, but is less sensitive than CT. Only calcium-containing stones (approximately 85% of all upper urinary tract calculi) are radiopaque; pure uric acid, indinavir-induced and cystine calculi are radiolucent and not visualised on plain X-ray. Many calcifications observed on the KUB radiograph are phleboliths (Figure 87.6), vascular calcifications, calcified lymph nodes and granulomas. Differentiation between a phlebolith and an obstructing stone is easier if radiograph demonstrates a lucent centre indicative of phlebolith.

Retrograde pyelography

The most precise imaging method for determining the anatomy of the ureter and renal pelvis and for making a definitive diagnosis of any ureteric calculus is retrograde pyelography. A cystoscope is placed in the bladder; a ureteral catheter is inserted into the ureteral orifice on the affected side. An X-ray is taken while contrast is injected through the ureteral catheter directly into the ureter. It is considered essential when surgery is deemed necessary because of uncontrollable pain, urosepsis with obstruction, a solitary obstructed kidney, a stone ≥8 mm that is unlikely to pass spontaneously or the presence of possible anatomical abnormalities (e.g. ureteral strictures).

Metabolic investigations

Not every patient needs metabolic investigations. Red flag box lists the indications for metabolic investigations. However, all of the 24-hour urine chemistry findings may be within the reference range in patients who actively form stones and who are at high risk for stones.

A 24-hour urine collection is performed to examine volume, calcium, oxalate, uric acid, cystine, citrate, magnesium and sodium levels. Findings can include hypercalciuria, hyperoxaluria, hyperuricosuria, hypocitraturia and low urinary volume. High urinary sodium and low urinary magnesium concentrations may also contribute to stone formation. Urine pH should be measured.

Hypercalciuria can be classified as absorptive, resorptive (e.g. due to hyperparathyroidism) and renal-leak types based on serum calcium, PTH levels and 24-hour urine calcium levels on both regular and calcium-restricted diets. Hyperoxaluria may be primary (a rare genetic disease), enteric (due to malabsorption associated with chronic diarrhoea or short-bowel syndrome) or idiopathic. Hypocitraturia is a common metabolic defect that predisposes to stone formation.

Stone analysis

Analysis of the stone (Figure 87.7), whenever possible, will help in the further investigation and management. The stone types most commonly encountered are calcium oxalate (>80%), followed by urate stones, struvite and the rare cystine stone.

88 Renal artery stenosis

The purpose of investigation is to:
- Confirm the diagnosis, assess the site and severity
- Investigate the underlying cause and assess renal function
- Determine if the stenosis is amenable to or needs revascularisation

Clinical clues for RAS

- The abrupt onset of significant hypertension
- Hypertension associated with CKD, especially if renal function deteriorates after the use of angiotensin-converting enzyme inhibitor or angiotensin II receptor blockers (>30% increase in serum creatinine)
- Accelerated or malignant hypertension
- Hypertension with repeated hospital admission for pulmonary oedema
- Refractory hypertension, defined as blood pressure >140/90 mmHg despite treatment with at least three different classes of anti-hypertensive medications at optimal doses
- Hypertension with abdominal bruit and presence of peripheral vascular disease
- Hypertension in females under 30 years

Figure 88.1 Renal artery angiogram shows RAS with appearance of 'string of beads' that is typical for FMD

Figure 88.2 CT renal angiogram shows left main high-grade RAS

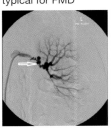

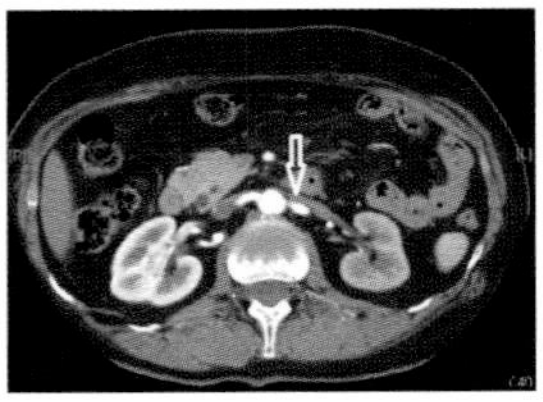

Figure 88.3 Reconstructed CT renal angiogram shows right high-grade RAS

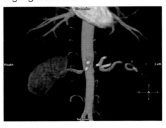

Figure 88.4 MRI renal angiogram shows bilateral high-grade RAS

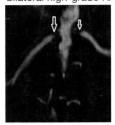

Figure 88.5 DSA shows high-grade left RAS before stent insertion

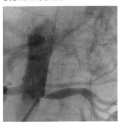

Figure 88.6 DSA shows no residual stenosis and normal nephrogram post-stent insertion

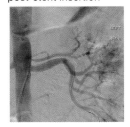

Table 88.1 Diagnostic imaging tests for RAS

	Sensitivity (%)	Specificity (%)	Anatomical assessment[a]	Functional assessment	Potential disadvantages
CTA	90	94	Yes +++	No	Risk of CIN in patients with CKD
MRA	80–90	70–85	Yes ++	Yes +	Suboptimal images
Gadolinium-enhanced MRA	83–96	92–97	Yes ++	Yes +	Risk of NSF in patients with CKD
Arterial DSA	100	100	Gold standard	No	Invasive, risk of CIN in patients with CKD, risk of atheroembolic events, and vascular complications at puncture site
Duplex ultrasound	90	90	Indirect assessment	Yes	Operator dependent, limited by obesity or bowel gas
Captopril radionuclide scan	70	70	No	Yes	CKD and dehydration can reduce reliability

[a] Plus signs indicate how 'good' at each category.

Figure 88.7 Baseline renal perfusion scan shows delayed perfusion to the left kidney, which is smaller than the right

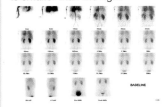

Figure 88.8 Post-captopril renal perfusion scan shows a 13% reduction of the left kidney function compared with baseline, consistent with a functionally significant left RAS

Clinical Investigations at a Glance, First Edition. Jonathan Gleadle, Jordan Li and Tuck Yong. © 2017 John Wiley & Sons, Ltd. Published 2017 by John Wiley & Sons, Ltd.

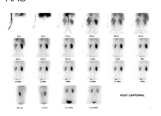

Renal artery stenosis (RAS) is the narrowing of one or both renal arteries or their branches. Haemodynamically significant RAS may cause refractory hypertension and CKD. The prevalence of RAS in patients with mild hypertension is about 1% but may be as high as 30% in severe hypertension and 20% among patients with CKD.

RAS in elderly patients is usually caused by atherosclerosis (90% of cases), while in young females is frequently caused by fibromuscular dysplasia (FMD) (Figure 88.1).

Who should be investigated for RAS?

It is important to recognise that there is no good evidence that treatment of atherosclerotic RAS with angioplasty or stenting significantly affects renal or blood pressure outcomes. Therefore, great care needs to be exercised in deciding whether patients should be investigated at all if detection will not affect patient management. Patients with RAS will commonly have atherosclerotic disease affecting subsequent smaller renal arterial vessels and atherosclerosis in other vessels.

Indications for endovascular intervention are controversial given the lack of benefit in randomised controlled trials but are often considered for patients with failure of optimal medical therapy to control blood pressure, recurrent flash pulmonary oedema or refractory heart failure, bilateral renal artery stenosis. The clinical clues for possible RAS are listed opposite.

Basic laboratory investigations

Basic laboratory investigations include FBC, electrolytes, urea and creatinine. In patients with vascular risk factors, fasting glucose, HbA1c and lipid studies should be performed. Measurement of plasma renin lacks specificity and should not be routinely performed.

Investigations for anatomical assessment of RAS

CT angiography (CTA) and MRI angiography (MRA)

CTA is the first-line investigation for anatomical assessment of suspected RAS if the renal function is normal (Figures 88.1–88.3). MRA can provide reasonable images of the renal arteries and the abdominal aorta in multiple planes without gadolinium contrast in patient with CKD (Figure 88.4). In patients with CKD, the use of MRA and CTA is limited by contrast-induced nephropathy (CIN) or gadolinium-associated nephrogenic systemic fibrosis (NSF).

Angiography

Conventional aortography produces excellent images of the renal artery but requires an arterial puncture and carries a risk of cholesterol emboli and CIN. Intravenous subtraction angiography is sensitive for identifying stenosis of the main renal artery but does not sufficiently demonstrate accessory or branch renal arteries; however, this technique avoids a high volume of contrast, arterial puncture and cholesterol emboli.

Intra-arterial digital subtraction angiography (DSA) has a high diagnostic accuracy (Figures 88.5 and 88.6) compared with conventional angiography and is associated with fewer complications, lower doses of contrast and smaller catheter size. It is the current gold standard for diagnosing RAS (Table 88.1).

Carbon dioxide angiography uses an alternative contrast agent in combination with DSA to avoid the risk of CIN in patients with advance CKD. The image quality is poorer than intra-arterial DSA.

The definition of what degree of narrowing constitutes 'significant' RAS is controversial. Quantification of the degree of an RAS lesion by radiological means is subject to intra-observer variability. Haemodynamic (manometric) measurements via a calibrated electronic measuring device in renal arteries and aorta may be useful.

Ultrasound

Non-invasive duplex ultrasound can assess direct and indirect signs of RAS. Doppler measurement of renal artery velocity (normal <2 m/s) provides a functional assessment of the severity of stenosis; higher velocity correlates with a greater pressure difference across the stenosis. Measurement of the bilateral intra-renal resistive index can aid diagnosis of haemodynamically significant RAS. Duplex ultrasound is highly operator and patient dependent (limited by obesity or bowel gas), technically demanding, time consuming and of low reproducibility. Over 10% false-negative and false-positive results may be expected. Accessory renal arteries can be a diagnostic pitfall.

Investigations for functional assessment

Radionuclide studies

There is no test or finding that can conclusively establish the functional significance of a stenotic lesion or predict response to revascularisation. Radionuclide scans provide indirect evidence of RAS but the sensitivity and specificity are too low for a screening test, particularly in the presence of CKD or bilateral RAS. Captopril radionuclide studies are useful for the assessment of global and differential renal function and help assess potential for salvage.

Baseline study enables visual inspection of kidney size, perfusion, function and drainage (Figure 88.7). After baseline study, a further scan can be repeated an hour after a single dose of 25 mg oral captopril (Figure 88.8). Perfusion pressure is maintained by angiotensin I/II in RAS. Captopril reduces perfusion pressure, leading to a fall in relative function and delayed tracer uptake on the affected side.

Key points

- There is no conclusive evidence that treatment of atherosclerotic RAS with angioplasty or stenting significantly affects renal or blood pressure outcomes.
- Doppler interrogation of the renal arteries is the safest and least expensive but also the least accurate and most operator dependent.
- Nuclear scintigraphy with captopril enables assessment of the functional significance of RAS.
- CT angiography has 95% sensitivity and specificity in detecting RAS. MRA with gadolinium also has a 95% sensitivity and specificity in detecting RAS.

89 Diabetes mellitus: diagnosis

Screening for diabetes

Who should be screened?
Persons 45 years of age or older or with other risk factors should be screened for diabetes

Modifiable risk factors

Obesity/overweight
Physical inactivity
Smoking
Sustained blood pressure of greater
  than 135/80 mmHg
Hypertension
Hyperlipidaemia

Non-modifiable risk factors

A first-degree relative with diabetes
History of gestational diabetes
Polycystic ovarian syndrome
Certain race/ethnicity (African, Indian,
  Asian, Aboriginal and Pacific Islanders)
Age ≥45 years

Methods of screening
Fasting glucose, OGTT or glycated haemoglobin (HbA1c)

Screening interval
• For patient >45 years old with an initial normal fasting glucose test: re-screen every 3 years if no risk factors
• For patient with risk factors: repeat annual screening is warranted

Gestational diabetes mellitus

Screening
The usual approach for detecting gestational diabetes mellitus is to screen all pregnant women by measuring their plasma glucose after a 50-g oral glucose load at 24–28 weeks' gestation. Women are referred for OGTT if the plasma glucose concentration 1 hour later is above 140 mg/dL (7.8 mmol/L).

Diagnosis
75-g OGTT at 24–28 weeks of gestation

Glucose measurement	mmol/L	mg/L
FPG	≥5.1	≥92
or 1-hour plasma glucose	≥10.0	≥180
or 2-hour plasma glucose	≥8.5	≥153

Diagnosis of diabetes

Table 89.1 Criteria for the diagnosis of diabetes mellitus

Test	Normal, mmol/L (mg/dL)	Impaired glucose tolerance, mmol/L (mg/dL)	Type 2 diabetes, mmol/L (mg/dL)
Random plasma glucose	<7.8 (140)	7.8–11.0 (140–199)	>11.1 (200) and symptoms of hyperglycaemia (polyuria, polydipsia, weight loss)
Fasting plasma glucose	<5.5 (100)	5.5–6.9 (100–125)	>7.0 (126)
2-hour OGTT	<7.8 (140)	7.8–11.0 (140–199)	>11.1 (200)
HbA1c	<6%	6–6.5%	>6.5% on two separate tests

Table 89.2 Comparison of diagnostic tests for diabetes mellitus

Test	Sensitivity (%)	Specificity (%)	PPV (%)	NPV (%)
Diabetes risk calculator based on prevalence of 6%	78–88	67–75	6–14	99
Random plasma glucose, mmol/L (mg/dL)				
≥7.8 (140)	55	92	31	97
≥8.3 (150)	50	95	40	97
≥8.9 (160)	44	96	41	96
≥9.4 (170)	42	97	47	96
≥10.0 (180)	39	98	56	96
HbA1c levels (%)				
6.1	63	97	61	98
6.5	43	100	87	97
7.0	28	100	95	96

Key points

• A single random HbA1c result >6.5% (48 mmol/mol) is diagnostic of diabetes.
• In an individual with typical symptoms, diabetes is diagnosed by finding a random plasma glucose concentration >11.0 mmol/L or a fasting plasma glucose concentration >6.5 mmol/L or a plasma glucose concentration >11.0 mmol/L two hours after taking 75 g of glucose in an OGTT.
• In the absence of typical symptoms, diagnosis should not be based on a single glucose determination but requires confirmation by at least one further glucose test result on another day with a value in the range confirming diabetes.
• If the fasting or random glucose concentrations do not fall into the criteria given above, then an OGTT should be performed.

Clinical Investigations at a Glance, First Edition. Jonathan Gleadle, Jordan Li and Tuck Yong. © 2017 John Wiley & Sons, Ltd. Published 2017 by John Wiley & Sons, Ltd.

Diabetes mellitus is a group of metabolic diseases characterised by hyperglycaemia resulting from defects in insulin secretion, in insulin action, or both. Chronic hyperglycaemia due to diabetes is associated with long-term damage and dysfunction of organs including the heart, kidneys, eyes, nerves and blood vessels. There are two major categories of diabetes based on pathogenesis. Type 1 diabetes is characterised by an absolute deficiency of insulin secretion due to cellular-mediated autoimmune destruction of islet β cells, whereas type 2 diabetes arises from a combination of factors including insulin resistance and inadequate insulin secretion. An increasing range of genetic causes of diabetes is also being defined.

Screening

The rationale for screening includes the following.
- Diabetes is a common disease that is associated with significant morbidity and mortality.
- Diabetes has an asymptomatic stage that may be present for many years before diagnosis.
- Diabetes is treatable and testing is simple.
- Early treatment of diabetes identified primarily by symptoms improves microvascular outcomes.

Diagnostic tests

Diabetes can be diagnosed clinically in a symptomatic patient (e.g. polydipsia, polyuria) and confirmed by finding an elevated blood glucose concentration. In an individual presenting with severe hyperglycaemia, the initial assessment should address both the causes and consequences of the hyperglycaemia. This includes recognition and appropriate management of diabetic ketoacidosis and hyperosmolar hyperglycaemia (see Chapter 90).

The majority of patients are asymptomatic. In screening those at risk of diabetes, diagnostic tests include:
- measurement of fasting plasma glucose (FPG);
- oral glucose tolerance test (OGTT) in a person with an equivocal FPG result;
- HbA$_{1c}$.

In the absence of symptoms, an abnormal result in one of the above tests should be confirmed, preferably by the same test on a separate occasion.

The diagnostic criteria for diabetes are listed in Table 89.1. Capillary glucose determination by glucometer is a useful point-of-care test in monitoring diabetes. However, the results from glucometer are usually lower than those from standard FPG and are therefore not recommended for initial diagnosis. OGTT is carried out after an overnight fast, following 3 days of adequate carbohydrate intake (>150 g/day). A 75-g load of oral glucose is given and the diagnosis of diabetes can be made if venous FPG is 7.0 mmol/L or greater or the 2-hour post glucose load is 11.1 mmol/L or greater. However, the test is labour-intensive and time-consuming, taking at least 2 hours and involving three blood glucose samples. The OGTT is unnecessary for diagnosis in people with an unequivocally elevated fasting or random plasma glucose. FPG of 6.1 mmol/L or above but less than 7.0 mmol/L is classified as impaired fasting glucose. Impaired glucose tolerance is defined by a 2-hour glucose level of 7.8 mmol/L or above but less than 11.1 mmol/L after a 75-g glucose load.

Glycated haemoglobin (HbA$_{1c}$) can be used to establish the diagnosis of diabetes (Table 89.2). An HbA$_{1c}$ of 6.5% (48 mmol/mol) or greater is recommended as the cut-off point for diagnosis. The use of HbA$_{1c}$ measurement can simplify the diagnostic process and may lead to earlier diagnosis of more patients with diabetes. The main limitation is that a number of clinical conditions can result in falsely high or low HbA$_{1c}$, for example anaemia.

Investigations to determine type 1 or type 2 diabetes

There is no specific test to determine if an individual has type 1 or 2 diabetes and often the clinical picture suggests the diagnosis (e.g. asymptomatic obese patient likely having type 2 diabetes vs. a younger patient with recent-onset polyuria, polydipsia and weight loss suggesting type 1 diabetes) and further testing is not required. Tests that reflect β-cell function (e.g. C-peptide matched with glucose) or which measure autoantibodies against β-cell autoantigens can help distinguish between type 1 and type 2 diabetes when the clinical picture is not clear. Patients with type 1 diabetes typically have low C-peptide levels because of low levels of endogenous insulin and β-cell function. Patients with type 2 diabetes typically have normal to high levels of C-peptide, reflecting higher amounts of insulin but relative insensitivity to it. More than 90% of individuals with type 1 diabetes have one or more of the following autoantibodies at disease onset: islet cell antibodies, insulin autoantibodies or glutamic acid decarboxylase antibodies.

Monitoring

HbA$_{1c}$ reflects average glycaemia over the preceding 8–12 weeks. In some patients, HbA$_{1c}$ may be measured more frequently than 3-monthly to closely monitor glycaemic control.

HbA$_{1c}$ does not reflect swings in blood glucose, which can be as clinically important as overall glycaemia. Therefore self blood glucose monitoring and HbA$_{1c}$ complement each other.

The level of HbA$_{1c}$ is affected by conditions that affect red blood cell (RBC) survival time or non-enzymatic glycation of haemoglobin. A reduced RBC survival time will lower the HbA$_{1c}$ level and may lead to a false-negative result. RBC survival time is reduced in haemolytic anaemia, CKD, severe liver disease, iron deficiency, vitamin B$_{12}$ and folate deficiencies, and anaemia of chronic disease. Haemoglobinopathies affect glycation to a variable amount, principally due to interference with the laboratory measurement of HbA$_{1c}$. If a patient has had a therapeutic venesection or transfusion, the test should be delayed for 3 months.

Tests for hyperglycaemia during pregnancy

Hyperglycaemia first detected at any time during pregnancy should be classified as gestational diabetes. Hyperglycaemia in pregnancy is associated with adverse effects on both maternal and fetal health. If marked hyperglycaemia is detected in early pregnancy, consideration should be given to the potential of undiagnosed pre-existing diabetes and the complications associated with this. Women not known to have pre-existing glucose abnormalities but with risk factors for hyperglycaemia in pregnancy should be tested early in pregnancy, via either a pregnancy OGTT or an HbA$_{1c}$ level.

All women not previously known to have pre-pregnancy diabetes or hyperglycaemia in pregnancy should undergo a 75-g pregnancy OGTT at 24–28 weeks of gestation. All women with gestational diabetes should be tested for persistent diabetes with a 75-g OGTT 6–8 weeks after delivery. These women have a 30% risk of recurrence of hyperglycaemia in subsequent pregnancies and a risk of developing type 2 diabetes ranging from about 2 to 10% per year.

90 Diabetes mellitus: complications

The aims of investigation in diabetic emergency are to:
- Recognise the common diabetic emergencies: hypoglycaemia, DKA, hyperglycaemic hyperosmolar state
- Recognise and monitor important electrolyte disturbances
- Investigate the precipitants of diabetic emergencies

Table 90.1 Clinical features suggestive of diabetic ketoacidosis

Polyuria and polydipsia
Dyspnoea or hyperventilation
Vomiting
Dehydration
Abdominal pain
Reduced level of consciousness

Table 90.3 Criteria for microalbuminuria and macroalbuminuria: ACR (mg/mmol) of first voided morning urine specimen

	Women	Men
Normal	0–3.5	0–2.5
Microalbuminuria	3.6–35	2.6–25
Macroalbuminuria	>35	>25

Table 90.2 Diagnostic criteria for diabetic ketoacidosis and hyperglycaemic hyperosmolar state

	Diabetic ketoacidosis	Hyperglycaemic hyperosmolar state
Mental state	Alert to stupor/coma	Stupor/coma
Plasma glucose	>13.9 mmol/L (250 mg/dL)	>33.3 mmol/L (600 mg/dL)
Arterial pH	≤7.30	>7.30
Serum bicarbonate	≤18 mmol/L	>15 mmol/L
Anion gap	>10 mmol/L	<12 mmol/L
Urine ketones	Positive	Negative/weak positive
Serum ketones	Positive	Small
Serum osmolality	Variable	>320 mosmol/kg

Figure 90.2 Fasting lipid studies show hyperlipidaemia

Test	Result	Units		Normal Range
Total Triglycerides	6.6	mmol/L	HH	0.3 – 2.0
Total Cholesterol	13.6	mmol/L	H	<5.5
HDL Cholesterol	1.6	mmol/L		1.0 – 2.2
Total Chol/HDL Ratio	8.5		H	<5.0

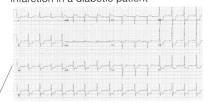

Figure 90.3 ECG shows acute myocardial infarction in a diabetic patient

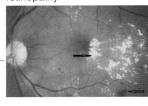

Figure 90.4 Echocardiogram and stress echocardiogram are used in evaluation of coronary artery disease in diabetic patients

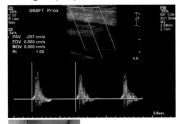

Figure 90.5 Duplex ultrasound to investigate peripheral arterial disease

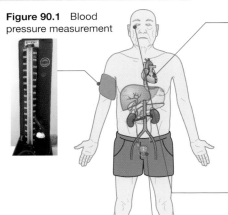

Figure 90.1 Blood pressure measurement

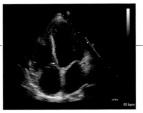

Figure 90.6 Fundoscopy examination shows diabetic retinopathy

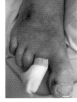

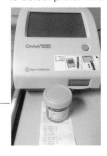

Figure 90.7 Urinalysis to detect proteinuria

Figure 90.8 Electrodiagnostic studies to assess peripheral neuropathy

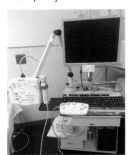

Figure 90.9 Radiopharmaceutical nuclear scan shows prolonged lag phase followed by delay in gastric emptying indicative of gastroparesis

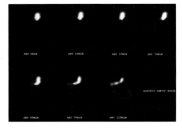

Key points

- Diagnosis of DKA is based on the triad of hyperglycaemia, ketosis and metabolic acidosis.
- Consider hypoglycaemia in any diabetic patient presenting with altered mental status; bedside glucose testing should be performed immediately followed by laboratory confirmation.
- Comprehensive cardiovascular risk assessment includes blood pressure, lipid study, LFTs, urine ACR and eGFR.
- Regular retinal photography and measurement of urine albumin excretion are important in assessing diabetic retinopathy and nephropathy, respectively.

Clinical Investigations at a Glance, First Edition. Jonathan Gleadle, Jordan Li and Tuck Yong. © 2017 John Wiley & Sons, Ltd. Published 2017 by John Wiley & Sons, Ltd.

Investigations for diabetes-related emergencies

Diabetic ketoacidosis (DKA)

DKA occurs predominantly in type 1 diabetes and can be the initial presentation. DKA is characterised by the combination of hyperglycaemia, metabolic acidosis and ketonaemia. All patients presenting with a blood glucose of 11.1 mmol/L or greater and clinical features of DKA (Table 90.1) should have blood ketones measured. If ketones are positive (>0.6 mmol/L), the presence of acidosis should be assessed with arterial blood gases. Urinalysis for ketones is used for initial assessment. The diagnostic criteria for DKA are listed in Table 90.2.

Basic blood investigations

• FBC, blood glucose, urea, creatinine, electrolytes (sodium, potassium, calcium, magnesium, chloride, bicarbonate).
• Blood ketones: β-hydroxybutyrate is the predominant ketone associated with DKA.
• Arterial or venous blood gas.

Investigations for precipitating cause

Blood culture and/or urine culture should be performed if there are symptoms and clinical signs of infection. CXR is required to exclude chest infection.

DKA must be distinguished from other causes of high-anion gap metabolic acidosis, including lactic acidosis, ingestion of drugs such as salicylate, and CKD (which is more typically hyperchloraemic acidosis rather than high-anion gap acidosis). Measurement of blood lactate, serum salicylate and blood methanol level can be helpful in these situations. During initial treatment of DKA, electrolytes, especially potassium, should be checked every 2 hours.

Hyperglycaemic hyperosmolar state

This complication usually occurs in elderly patients with suboptimal control of type 2 diabetes. It is associated with high mortality and can be the first presentation of diabetes. Patients can present with severe polyuria, polydipsia, dehydration and impaired conscious state but respiration is usually normal. The investigations are the same as for DKA except the serum osmolality should be checked. Significant ketosis occurs in up to one-third of patients with hyperglycaemic hyperosmolar state.

Hypoglycaemia

In patients with recurrent hypoglycaemia, adrenal insufficiency as a contributing factor should be considered. In this situation, adrenal function should be tested (see Chapter 97).

Investigations for diabetes-related complications

Macrovascular complications

Diabetes mellitus is a major risk factor for the development of atherosclerosis of major vessels, especially the coronary and aorto-ilio-femoral systems. These arterial diseases are the major cause of premature death in people with diabetes.

Hypertension is common and eventually occurs in over 50% of patients with diabetes (Figure 90.1). Ambulatory blood pressure monitoring can provide useful information on blood pressure profiles over a 24-hour period. Such monitoring should be considered in those with suspected 'white-coat' hypertension or with hypertension resistant to therapy.

Dyslipidaemia (Figure 90.2) is common in patients with diabetes and is usually characterised by a high triglyceride level, low high-density lipoprotein (HDL) and mildly elevated low-density lipoprotein (LDL). All patients with diabetes should have an annual fasting lipid panel measured.

ECG (Figure 90.3) should be obtained in patients with diabetes who are over 50 years old with at least one other vascular risk factor. ECG has low sensitivity and specificity but provides a useful baseline. Patients with diabetes at high risk for macrovascular disease may need to undergo echocardiography (Figure 90.4) and/or stress testing. Peripheral vascular disease is common and duplex ultrasound (Figure 90.5) should be performed in suspicious cases (see Chapter 54).

Microvascular complications

Eye complications

Patients with diabetes are at increased risk of developing eye complications including refractive errors, cataracts, retinopathy and maculopathy. Corrected visual acuity should be assessed and direct ophthalmoscopy (with dilated pupils) performed. Retinal photography (through dilated pupils) should be performed (Figure 90.6).

Nephropathy

Proteinuria (Figure 90.7) is the hallmark of diabetic nephropathy. Once clinical proteinuria occurs, progressive renal damage is likely. Some patients manifest a reduced eGFR without proteinuria. Proteinuria is a cardiovascular risk factor independently from decreased GFR.

Morning first-voided urine albumin/creatinine ratio (ACR) or 24-hour urine protein excretion should be measured at diagnosis. Positive urine samples should be repeated at least twice. Urine ACR should be checked annually to monitor progress of diabetic nephropathy (Table 90.3). Trends in albumin excretion with time are important. An eGFR is a better reflection of renal function than serum creatinine.

Neuropathy

Peripheral neuropathy can be assessed with a 10-g monofilament or 128-Hz tuning fork. Electrodiagnostic studies (Figure 90.8) are useful in painful sensory neuropathy for identifying mononeuropathy (focal nerve entrapment), differentiating multiple mononeuropathy from polyneuropathy, and distinguishing axonal neuropathies from demyelinating neuropathies.

Gastroparesis

Investigations for gastroparesis may include upper gastrointestinal endoscopy to exclude pyloric or other mechanical obstruction, manometry to detect antral hypermotility and/or pylorospasm, and double-isotope scintigraphy to measure solid-phase gastric emptying following ingestion of a solid labelled with radionuclides (Figure 90.9).

Erectile dysfunction

See Chapter 104.

Bladder dysfunction

Investigation for suspected bladder dysfunction should be done for any patient with recurrent urinary tract infection, incontinence or urinary retention. Evaluation should include assessment of kidney function, urine culture, post-void volume and dilation of upper urinary tract on ultrasound. Cystometry and voiding cystometrogram can help measure bladder sensation and volume–pressure changes associated with bladder filling.

91 Diabetes insipidus

Table 91.1 Causes of central and nephrogenic diabetes insipidus

Central diabetes insipidus
Acquired
Head trauma
Tumours
Granulomas: sarcoidosis,
granulomatosis with polyangiitis
Infections: encephalitis, meningitis
Inflammatory: lymphocytic hypophysitis
Vascular: Sheehan's syndrome
Post radiotherapy
Idiopathic
Congenital malformation
Genetic disorders

Nephrogenic diabetes insipidus
Acquired
Drugs: lithium (most common),
amphotericin B
Metabolic: hypercalcaemia
Post-obstructive uropathy
Chronic kidney disease
Vascular: ischaemia (acute tubular
necrosis)
Granulomas: sarcoidosis
Idiopathic
Congenital/genetic

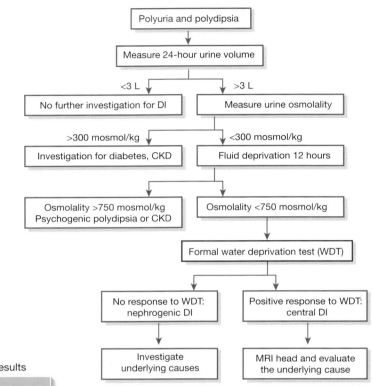

```
Polyuria and polydipsia
        │
        ▼
Measure 24-hour urine volume
   │              │
  <3 L           >3 L
   ▼              ▼
No further       Measure urine osmolality
investigation        │            │
for DI          >300 mosmol/kg   <300 mosmol/kg
                     ▼            ▼
             Investigation for   Fluid deprivation 12 hours
             diabetes, CKD
                     │            │
            Osmolality >750       Osmolality <750 mosmol/kg
            mosmol/kg                      │
            Psychogenic                    ▼
            polydipsia or CKD    Formal water deprivation test (WDT)
                                   │              │
                          No response to     Positive response to
                          WDT:               WDT:
                          nephrogenic DI     central DI
                                   ▼              ▼
                          Investigate        MRI head and evaluate
                          underlying causes  the underlying cause
```

Table 91.2 Interpretation of water deprivation test results

After dehydration osmolality (mosmol/kg)		After AVP osmolality (mosmol/kg)	
Plasma	Urine	Urine	Diagnosis
283–293	>750	>750	Normal
>293	<300	<300	Nephrogenic DI
<293	300–750	<750	Primary polydipsia or partial nephrogenic DI
>293	<300	>750	Central DI
>293	300–750	>750	Partial central DI

Key points

- Diagnosis of DI is made by using a water deprivation test, which can also distinguish between central and nephrogenic DI.
- Patients cannot maximally concentrate urine following dehydration but can concentrate urine after receiving exogenous vasopressin.
- MRI of the pituitary is useful in localising causes of central DI.
- The underlying cause of central and nephrogenic DI should be investigated before attributing it as idiopathic.

Figure 91.1 T1-weighted MRI shows an absent posterior pituitary bright spot in central DI due to sarcoidosis

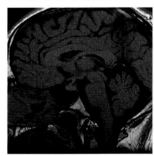

Figure 91.2 MRI with contrast shows an enlarged gadolinium-enhancing pituitary gland in central DI due to sarcoidosis

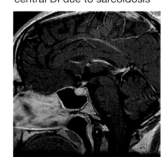

Clinical Investigations at a Glance, First Edition. Jonathan Gleadle, Jordan Li and Tuck Yong. © 2017 John Wiley & Sons, Ltd. Published 2017 by John Wiley & Sons, Ltd.

Diabetes insipidus (DI) is characterised by either relative or absolute deficiency of or insensitivity to the effects of anti-diuretic hormone (ADH) leading to inability to concentrate urine and subsequent polyuria (>50 mL of dilute urine per kilogram per hour), polydipsia and potentially fluid and electrolyte imbalances.

There are two types of DI: central (neurogenic) DI and nephrogenic DI. Central DI is due to inadequate ADH secretion leading to the impairment of urine concentration. Nephrogenic DI is due to resistance to ADH in the kidney. Causes of central and nephrogenic DI are listed in Table 91.1.

DI by itself is usually well tolerated and results in mild symptoms such as polydipsia and polyuria. Nocturia with a large urine volume should raise the suspicion of DI and lead to basic investigations. Laboratory evaluation usually shows a low urine osmolality. Overt disturbances in fluid and electrolytes are uncommon unless there is loss of the normal compensatory mechanism of polydipsia such as with loss of consciousness.

Basic laboratory investigations

• Blood biochemistry including sodium, glucose, calcium and urea.
• Simultaneous serum and urine osmolality.
• Urine specific gravity, sodium, glucose.

A urine specific gravity of 1.005 or less and a urine osmolality less than 200 mosmol/kg is the hallmark of DI. The serum sodium level is usually normal or slightly elevated in central and nephrogenic DI as long as thirst is intact and water is available. In primary or psychogenic polydipsia, sodium may be low as a result of water overload. However, if DI is due to a central lesion that also impairs thirst, the sodium level can exceed 160 mmol/L. Hyperglycaemia must be ruled out but this condition usually exhibits a higher urine osmolality due to glycosuria.

Simultaneous serum and urine osmolality measurement, particularly after mild fluid restriction, may be diagnostic and make the water deprivation test unnecessary. Spot urine osmolality in excess of 750 mosmol/kg indicates good urine concentrating ability and makes DI unlikely. If a patient is dehydrated (plasma osmolality >295 mosmol/kg) and a freshly voided urine sample shows urine osmolality below 700 mosmol/kg, DI is present. In primary polydipsia, plasma osmolality is usually in the low to low-normal range (275–295 mosmol/kg).

Water deprivation test

The purpose of this test is to distinguish primary or psychogenic polydipsia and central and nephrogenic DI by assessing response to dehydration and the effect of arginine vasopressin (AVP). This test is potentially very dangerous and must be undertaken with great care. Patients unable to conserve water may become critically dehydrated within a few hours of water restriction. The last dose of desmopressin, clofibrate or carbamazepine should be taken at least 24 hours before the test and 72 hours allowed after stopping thiazide diuretics.

At the start of the test, plasma and urine osmolality are measured. Blood pressure and weight after voiding are also measured. Urine volume and osmolality are measured on an hourly basis until one of the following end points is reached.

1 Urine osmolality is higher than concurrent plasma osmolality and urine concentration has reached a plateau, i.e. difference between the osmolality of the last three urine specimens is less than 30 mosmol/kg. This is seen in normal individuals, primary polydipsia and many of those with partial ADH deficiency.
2 The maximum urine osmolality is near or below plasma osmolality. In this case, DI (central or nephrogenic) is proven when plasma osmolality is significantly above the reference interval, i.e. above 297 mosmol/kg.

Once one of these end points is reached, desmopressin intranasally or Pitressin intramuscularly is administered and urine is collected for two further half-hour periods. Results obtained can be interpreted using Table 91.2.

The test should be stopped if the patient becomes hypotensive, plasma osmolality exceeds 300 mosmol/kg, or there is weight loss of more than 2 kg or 3% of total body weight. Under such circumstances, if possible, collect spot samples of urine and blood before giving fluid.

Anterior pituitary hormones should be assessed. In patients with suspected nephrogenic DI who are taking lithium, the drug level should be measured.

Radiological investigations

MRI of the head should be performed to exclude tumours and other lesions of the sellar and parasellar region in patients with central DI (Figures 91.1 and 91.2). MRI normally shows an increased signal in the posterior pituitary, which is lost in central DI. However, this sign is not helpful in distinguishing more subtle degrees of DI from other causes.

92 Thyroid disorders

Table 92.1 Common causes of hypothyroidism

Autoimmune lymphocytic thyroiditis: Hashimoto's thyroiditis, atrophic thyroiditis
Post ablative therapy or surgery: radioiodine therapy, thyroidectomy
Transient: subacute thyroiditis, silent thyroiditis, postpartum thyroiditis
Iodine associated: iodine deficiency, iodine induced
Drug-induced: carbimazole, propylthiouracil, iodine, amiodarone, lithium
Infiltrative: fibrous thyroiditis, amyloid disease, infection (e.g. tuberculosis)
Congenital: thyroid agenesis or ectopia
Secondary hypothyroidism: pituitary or hypothalamic disease

Table 92.2 Prevalence of anti-thyroid antibodies

	Thyroperoxidase autoantibody	Thyroglobulin autoantibody	TSH receptor antibody
General population (%)	9–27	5–20	1–2
Graves' disease (%)	50–80	50–70	90–99
Chronic autoimmune thyroiditis (%)	90–100	80–90	10–20

Figure 92.2 CT chest shows a large solitary mass arising from the left lobe of the thyroid with retrosternal extension

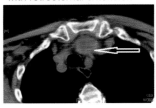

Figure 92.3 Thyroid USS shows a large left thyroid nodule with heterogeneous echotexture

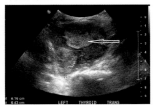

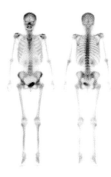

Figure 92.4 Whole-body radioiodine scan demonstrates bony metastatic disease of thyroid cancer

Table 92.3 Common causes of hyperthyroidism

Graves' disease
Toxic multinodular goitre
Toxic adenoma
Over-replacement of thyroxine
Sporadic thyroiditis or postpartum thyroiditis
Painful subacute thyroiditis
Amiodarone-induced thyroiditis

Table 92.4 Common causes of goitre

Autoimmune thyroiditis
Graves' disease
Familial or sporadic multinodular goitre
Iodine deficiency
Colloid nodule or cyst
Thyroid benign tumours or cancer

Table 92.5 Ultrasound features associated with an increased risk of cancer in thyroid nodule

Hypoechogenicity
Microcalcifications
Irregular margins
Increased nodular flow visualised by Doppler
Invasion or regional lymphadenopathy

Table 92.6 Indications for biopsy of thyroid nodules

Nodules >5 mm in patients with high risk of thyroid cancer
Head and neck irradiation
Thyroid cancer in a first-degree relative
Radiotherapy or radiation exposure as a child
Multiple endocrine neoplasia type 2
Elevated calcitonin
All nodules associated with abnormal cervical lymph nodes
Nodules >1 cm with microcalcifications
Solid nodules >1 cm
Mixed cystic/solid nodules >1.5–2.0 cm
Spongiform nodules >2 cm

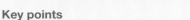

Key points

- Initial testing for patients with suspected hypothyroidism is TSH level.
- It is important to investigate the underlying cause of thyrotoxicosis to guide management. A radionuclide thyroid scan has the highest diagnostic yield.
- Thyroid ultrasound and FNA is useful in the assessment of patients with thyroid nodules.

Clinical Investigations at a Glance, First Edition. Jonathan Gleadle, Jordan Li and Tuck Yong. © 2017 John Wiley & Sons, Ltd. Published 2017 by John Wiley & Sons, Ltd.

Thyroid disorders are common, with a prevalence of 1%. Disorders of the thyroid include both overt and subclinical hypothyroidism and hyperthyroidism, goitre and thyroid cancer. They can present with non-specific symptoms so need to be considered in many clinical situations.

Hypothyroidism

The prevalence of overt hypothyroidism is about 0.5%. Iodine deficiency remains the most common cause of hypothyroidism worldwide. In developed countries, autoimmune chronic lymphocytic thyroiditis is the most common cause (Table 92.1).

Initial investigation of suspected hypothyroidism is by measuring thyroid-stimulating hormone (TSH). If this is elevated, a low free thyroxine (FT4) confirms the diagnosis. If there are convincing clinical features of hypothyroidism, FT4 should be checked even in the absence of TSH elevation to exclude the possibility of central causes of hypothyroidism. Subclinical hypothyroidism is an elevated TSH with normal FT4 levels. It should be confirmed by repeat thyroid function tests (TFTs) after 3 months.

Thyroid autoantibodies

Thyroid autoantibodies (Table 92.2), namely thyroid peroxidase (TPO) and thyroglobulin autoantibodies, are positive in 95% of patients with autoimmune thyroiditis. TPO antibody assay is sensitive and specific in confirming a diagnosis of autoimmune thyroiditis. Positive anti-TPO is seen in 10–15% of the general population and is not an indication for treatment if the patient is euthyroid. Anti-thyroglobulin is non-specific and the use of this test is confined to thyroid cancer follow-up.

Thyroid imaging

Hypothyroidism per se is not an indication for thyroid imaging. Thyroid radionuclide scanning has no role in the work-up of hypothyroidism. Thyroid ultrasound can be performed if there are palpable thyroid nodules. If central hypothyroidism is confirmed, the function of the hypothalamic–pituitary–adrenal axis should be tested and MRI of the pituitary gland obtained.

Hypothyroidism in pregnancy

Maternal thyroid function changes during pregnancy and the thyrotropic activity of β-hCG results in a decrease in TSH in the first trimester. Therefore, trimester-specific reference intervals for TFTs are recommended. Lower TSH targets are used in pregnancy when treating hypothyroidism.

Hyperthyroidism

The prevalence of hyperthyroidism is 0.5%. The most common cause of hyperthyroidism is Graves' disease (50–80%) followed by toxic multinodular goitre (Table 92.3). Graves' disease is an autoimmune disorder due to thyroid-stimulating immunoglobulins directed towards the TSH receptor of the thyroid hormone-producing cell.

The single most important test is serum TSH. If the TSH level is within the reference range, then a diagnosis of hyperthyroidism is effectively ruled out except in TSH-producing tumours of the pituitary and syndromes of thyroid hormone resistance. The presence of a low TSH should prompt measurement of FT4. If FT4 is elevated, then a diagnosis of hyperthyroidism is confirmed and measurement of free triiodothyronine (FT3) is not required. If FT4 is not above the reference range in a patient with low serum TSH, FT3 should be measured to confirm the diagnosis of 'T3 toxicosis', characterised by elevation of serum FT3 but normal FT4. This pattern can be observed in mild cases of toxic nodular hyperthyroidism and early in the course of Graves' disease.

Thyroid autoantibodies

Measurement of TSH receptor antibodies (Table 92.2) is useful for establishing the diagnosis of Graves' disease, especially when a radionuclide thyroid scan cannot be performed due to pregnancy or lactation, when the presentation is atypical (e.g. Graves' ophthalmopathy in a euthyroid individual) or in amiodarone-induced thyrotoxicosis. However, up to 10% of patients with Graves' disease have undetectable TSH receptor antibodies. Second-generation TSH receptor antibody assays have a sensitivity of 90–99% and specificity of 95–100% for Graves' disease.

Thyroid imaging

If the aetiology of hyperthyroidism is not evident or there is a palpable nodule, a radionuclide thyroid scan with technetium-99m (^{99m}Tc) pertechnetate should be performed to assess the activity of the thyroid gland (Figure 92.1). Uptake of the radiotracer is inhibited, resulting in non-diagnostic scans if the patient is taking or exposed to iodine supplementation or thyroxine therapy. Iodine supplements, iodinated contrast or amiodarone can inhibit tracer uptake by the thyroid for up to 9 months. Thyroid scan is contraindicated in pregnancy. Colour-flow Doppler ultrasound can be used to distinguish between Graves' disease (hypervascular) and subacute thyroiditis (low-to-normal vascularity).

Thyroid-associated ophthalmopathy

Ophthalmopathy commonly complicates Graves' disease but can also be associated with Hashimoto's thyroiditis. Measurement of TSH receptor antibody may have diagnostic value because of its high specificity and sensitivity for Graves' disease. Orbital imaging with CT or MRI may show enlargement of extraocular muscles, increase in orbital fibroadipose tissue, or both.

Goitre

Goitre refers to an enlarged thyroid gland. The prevalence of goitre, diffuse and nodular, is dependent on the status of iodine intake of the population. In general, in iodine-sufficient countries the prevalence of clinically palpable goitre is less than 4%. The common causes of goitre are shown in Table 92.4.

Laboratory investigations

Patients with goitre should have TSH measured to determine thyroid function. If TSH is outside the reference interval, FT4 should also be measured. If the patient is hyperthyroid, TSH antibody can be tested.

Imaging

A thyroid ultrasound performed at the time of initial investigation helps with diagnosis and provides a baseline for monitoring the progress of thyroid volume or size of nodules. It helps to determine the need for fine-needle aspiration (FNA) biopsy in patients with thyroid nodules.

Box 92.1 Patterns of radionuclide thyroid scan

- Normal scan (Figure 92.1a).
- Diffuse increased uptake indicating Graves' disease (Figure 92.1b).
- Heterogeneous uptake with suppressed background activity indicating toxic multinodular goitre (Figure 92.1c).
- Solitary autonomous nodule showing intense increased uptake with complete suppression of the surrounding gland (Figure 92.1d).
- Absent tracer uptake is a characteristic of acute thyroiditis, in the absence of taking thyroxine or iodine-rich preparations (Figure 92.1e).
- Cold nodule (Figure 92.1f).

Figure 92.1 (a–f) Patterns of radionuclide thyroid scan

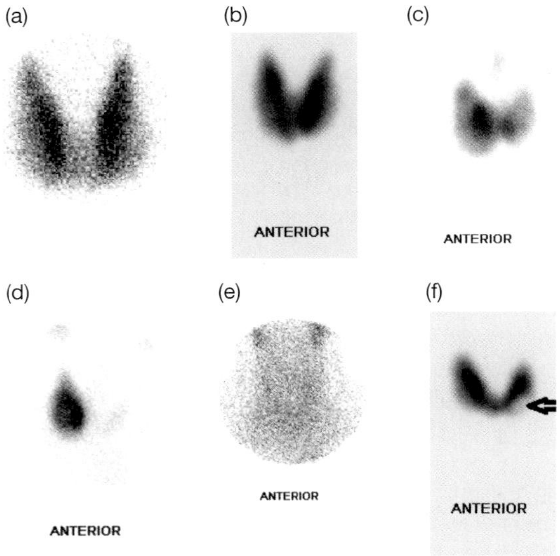

A ^{99m}Tc thyroid scan is indicated in patients with suppressed TSH to determine the functional status of any nodules within the thyroid and elucidate the underlying cause of overt or subclinical hyperthyroidism. Hyperfunctioning ('hot') nodules are rarely malignant and do not require cytological evaluation.

CT of the neck and/or chest is not a routine investigation for goitre but may be performed in patients with significant compressive symptoms or suspicion of retrosternal extension (Figure 92.2). The CT should be done without intravenous contrast due to the risk of contrast-induced hyperthyroidism or hypothyroidism in patients with nodular thyroid disease.

Thyroid nodules

About 4–7% of the general population have a palpable thyroid nodule and 30–50% of adults have a thyroid nodule visible on ultrasound. Therefore the challenge is to determine which of these nodules are malignant because only 1 in 20 clinically identified nodules prove to harbour malignancy.

Laboratory investigations

The first step is to assess thyroid function by measuring serum TSH. A suppressed level of TSH with a solitary nodule usually suggests a benign hyperfunctioning nodule, but the finding of an elevated TSH does not obviate the need for FNA biopsy.

If a patient has a family history of medullary thyroid cancer (MTC) or multiple endocrine neoplasia (MEN) type 2, a basal serum calcitonin level should be measured as an elevated level suggests MTC. Calcitonin level should not be routinely assessed in patients without a relevant family history because only 1 in 250 patients with a thyroid nodule has MTC. Before surgery is performed, investigations for primary hyperparathyroidism and phaeochromocytoma should be performed.

Imaging

Ultrasound can detect non-palpable nodules, estimate the size and number of the nodules, and differentiate simple cysts from solid nodules or mixed cystic and solid nodules (Figure 92.3). Table 92.5 lists the findings on ultrasound which are associated with an increased risk of cancer. However, ultrasonographic features cannot reliably distinguish between benign and malignant nodules.

Fine-needle aspiration biopsy

FNA biopsy provides the most direct and specific evaluation of a thyroid nodule. With two to four passes of the needle, FNA has a diagnostic yield of about 80%. Adequacy of samples obtained increases if aspiration is guided by ultrasound. FNA is safe and inexpensive and can be performed in an outpatient setting. Indications for FNA biopsy of the thyroid are shown in Table 92.6.

If FNA reveals a follicular neoplasm, radionuclide scan should be performed. Approximately 15% of nodules are follicular neoplasms but only 20% prove to be malignant. If the scan shows a functioning nodule, surgery can be avoided because the risk of cancer is negligible. In a cystic lesion or one with a mixture of cystic and solid components, FNA of the solid component should be performed because the risk of cancer is the same as for a solid non-functioning nodule.

Thyroid cancer

Patients with thyroid cancer usually present with a solitary thyroid nodule and should be investigated as above. The measurement of serum thyroglobulin has no role in the diagnosis of thyroid cancer. All new patients with MTC should be tested for the *RET* mutation.

Imaging

For differentiated follicular thyroid cancer, whole-body radioiodine scan is performed several days after adjuvant radioablation therapy in order to detect residual and metastatic disease (Figure 92.4). Undifferentiated and papillary carcinoma may be negative on this scan.

Long-term monitoring

After total thyroidectomy and ^{131}I ablation for thyroid cancer, thyroxine replacement should be sufficient to suppress the TSH to below 0.10 mU/L. Thyroglobulin is produced exclusively by thyroid follicular cells. Therefore, in patients who have been successfully treated with total thyroidectomy and ^{131}I ablation, detectable serum thyroglobulin (>2 µg/L) provides indirect evidence that functional thyroid tissue or tumour is present.

93 Thyroid function tests

The purpose of thyroid function tests are to:
- Identify and classify any disorders of thyroid function
- Monitor the effects of treatment of known thyroid disease

Table 93.1 Indications for thyroid function tests

Clinical findings suggestive of thyroid disease
Autoimmune and endocrine conditions associated with increased risk of thyroid disease
Goitre (diffuse, multinodular or single)
Patients with atrial fibrillation, dyslipidaemia, osteoporosis or subfertility
All patients on amiodarone therapy before commencing treatment, then every 6 months thereafter whilst on treatment and up to 12 months after cessation of therapy
All patients on lithium therapy before commencing treatment, then routinely monitored every 6–12 months whilst on treatment
Thyroid function should be tested yearly in patients treated by external irradiation to the neck
Patients treated with radioiodine or thyroidectomy: TFTs should be assessed 4–8 weeks post treatment, then 3-monthly up to 1 year and annually thereafter

Table 93.2 Risk factors for hypothyroidism

Age over 60 years
Female sex
Goitre
Previous hyperthyroidism
Family history of thyroid disease
History of head or neck cancer, post neck irradiation
Down's syndrome and Turner's syndrome
History of thyroiditis
Other autoimmune diseases
Treatment with lithium or amiodarone
Patient with type 1 diabetes

Table 93.3 Diagnostic pattern of thyroid function tests

TSH (mU/L)	FT4 (pmol/L)	Diagnosis
Increased (>10)	Decreased (<12)	Hypothyroidism
Increased (>5)	Normal (12–23)	Subclinical hypothyroidism
Normal (0.3–4.0)	Normal (12–23)	Normal thyroid function
Decreased (0.02–0.3)	Normal (12–23)	Subclinical hyperthyroidism
Decreased (<0.02)	Increased (>23)	Hyperthyroidism
Decreased (<0.02)	Normal (12–23)	T3 thyroid toxicosis
Increased or decreased (>5 or 0.02–0.3)	Normal (12–23)	Sick euthyroid syndrome

Key points

- TFTs should be performed in patients with depression, cognitive impairment, atrial fibrillation, osteoporosis, dyslipidaemia and hyponatraemia.
- TSH level is the most sensitive indicator of thyroid dysfunction but cannot be used alone in patients with pituitary disease.
- Avoid performing TFTs in patients who are systemically unwell.

The thyroid gland produces two major hormones: triiodo-thyronine (T3) and thyroxine (T4). TSH is released from the pituitary gland and controls the release of T4 from the thyroid. TSH in turn is under negative feedback control by the amount of free thyroid hormone in the circulation.

TFTs are a series of blood tests used to measure how well the thyroid functions. The reference intervals are as follows.
- TSH: 0.3–4.0 mU/L.
- FT4: 12.0–23.0 pmol/L.
- FT3 3.5–6.5 pmol/L.

There is a logarithmic-linear relationship between FT4 and TSH, meaning that a twofold change in FT4 level will normally result in a 10–20 fold change in TSH level. This makes TSH a very sensitive indicator of dysfunction of the thyroid gland. In unselected populations, measurement of serum TSH has a sensitivity of 89–95% and specificity of 90–96% for thyroid dysfunction. Therefore, in most circumstances the initial test of choice is TSH alone. However, in certain conditions the relationship between TSH and FT4 may be disrupted and it is necessary to measure both TSH and FT4. These conditions include:
- hospital inpatients;
- suspected pituitary dysfunction;
- psychiatric illness or dementia;
- investigation of amenorrhoea or infertility;
- treatment with drugs likely to affect thyroid function, e.g. glucocorticoids, amiodarone, phenytoin, lithium or carbamazepine.

Indications for TFTs

TFTs should be performed in the circumstances listed in Table 93.1. Screening for thyroid dysfunction in a healthy adult population is not warranted. Case-finding in women at the menopause or if visiting a doctor in primary care with non-specific symptoms may be justified in view of the high prevalence of mild thyroid failure (Table 93.2).

Interpretation of TFTs for diagnosis of thyroid dysfunction

Primary thyroid failure triggers the release of excess amounts of TSH while thyroid overactivity suppresses TSH release. Hence its measurement can define normality, hypothyroidism (increased TSH) or hyperthyroidism (decreased TSH). If a patient has normal TSH level, thyroid dysfunction is unlikely and no further testing is required. If the TSH is outside the reference interval, FT4 should also be measured. Once TSH and FT4 have been measured, common patterns can be interpreted (Table 93.3).

Monitoring thyroxine treatment

TSH measurement is the mainstay for monitoring thyroxine treatment. If there is pituitary disease or in the first few months after treatment of hyperthyroidism, FT4 should be measured. Measurements should not be made until at least 6 weeks after starting treatment or after changing dose as it takes this long to achieve a steady state. Once a stable dose has been achieved tests should be undertaken two to three times per year. The aim of treatment is to maintain the TSH within the lower half of the reference interval for normal individuals.

Monitoring treatment for hyperthyroidism

FT4 is the mainstay of monitoring and should be measured every 4–12 weeks after commencing treatment until stable, and then annually if used as a long-term treatment. TSH remains low for some time after the normalisation of FT4 and should be measured if the FT4 falls to low normal levels, the thyroid gland enlarges or symptoms suggest hypothyroidism.

Sick euthyroid syndrome

Persons who are seriously ill often have changes in TFTs but this does not usually indicate thyroid dysfunction. Common changes include low TSH (but not fully suppressed), or slight elevation or depression in FT4. These changes can occur in starvation as well as with systemic disease. During recovery from a severe illness the TSH may be transiently elevated. The sick euthyroid syndrome does not usually mimic the changes of frank hyperthyroidism or hypothyroidism.

Pituitary disease

Disorders of the pituitary gland are relatively rare as a cause of thyroid dysfunction. A pituitary cause of hypothyroidism produces a low or normal TSH together with a low FT4. If this is suspected other pituitary hormones should be tested, for example prolactin, luteinising hormone (LH), follicle-stimulating hormone (FSH), cortisol and (in males) testosterone, along with physical examination and pituitary imaging. Pituitary causes of hyperthyroidism are exceedingly rare and the pattern of elevated TSH and FT4 is more likely to be due to thyroid hormone resistance, an inherited defect of the thyroid hormone receptor.

94 Hypopituitarism

Table 94.1 Common causes of hypopituitarism

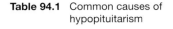

Pituitary tumours
Non-pituitary tumours
Meningiomas
Gliomas
Metastases
Head trauma
Traumatic brain injury
Subarachnoid haemorrhage
Neurosurgery
Irradiation
Infections
Abscess
Meningitis
Encephalitis
Infarction
Apoplexy
Sheehan's syndrome
Autoimmune disorders
Lymphocytic hypophysitis
Infiltrative disorders
Haemochromatosis
Granulomatous diseases
Histiocytosis
Genetic disorders

The aims of investigation of hypopituitarism are to:
• Assess the extent of pituitary hormone deficiency
• Investigate the underlying causes of hypopituitarism

Box 94.1 Indications for screening for pituitary function

• Presence of pituitary or hypothalamic lesions
• Post cranial irradiation
• Unexplained gonadal dysfunction
• Head trauma, brain surgery
• Post neurosurgery
• Inflammatory disorders, granulomatous disease
• Newly discovered empty sella
• Pregnancy-associated haemorrhage
• Refractory postural hypotension, unexplained hypothermia

Basic electrolytes, blood glucose level, creatinine

ACTH, 8 a.m. cortisol, TSH, FT4, FSH, LH, estradiol, testosterone and prolactin

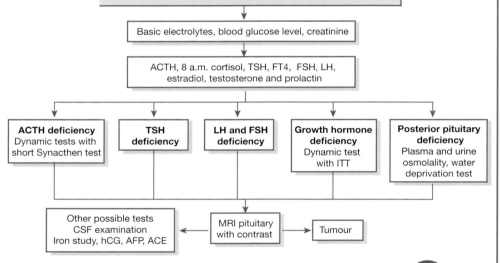

| **ACTH deficiency** Dynamic tests with short Synacthen test | **TSH deficiency** | **LH and FSH deficiency** | **Growth hormone deficiency** Dynamic test with ITT | **Posterior pituitary deficiency** Plasma and urine osmolality, water deprivation test |

Other possible tests
CSF examination
Iron study, hCG, AFP, ACE

MRI pituitary with contrast → Tumour

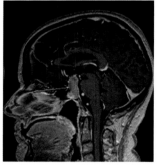

Figure 94.1 Sagittal T1-weighted MRI post contrast shows pituitary macroadenoma extending below into bony clivus

Key points

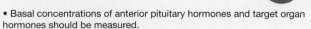

• Basal concentrations of anterior pituitary hormones and target organ hormones should be measured.
• Plasma and urine osmolality are often adequate as the initial investigation of posterior pituitary function.
• Dynamic testing is usually required to confirm the diagnosis of ACTH, GH and ADH deficiency.
• MRI of the pituitary is useful in localising and characterising any lesion causing the hypopituitarism.

Clinical Investigations at a Glance, First Edition. Jonathan Gleadle, Jordan Li and Tuck Yong. © 2017 John Wiley & Sons, Ltd. Published 2017 by John Wiley & Sons, Ltd.

Hypopituitarism is the partial or complete deficiency of anterior or posterior pituitary hormone secretion, or both, and may result from pituitary or hypothalamic disease. Although the clinical symptoms of this disorder are usually non-specific, it can cause life-threatening events and lead to increased mortality. Of the various causes of hypopituitarism in adults (Table 94.1), pituitary adenoma or its treatment by surgery and/or radiotherapy is by far the commonest.

Laboratory investigations

The indications for screening for pituitary function are listed in Box 94.1. Basic biochemistry should be checked first. Diagnosis of hypopituitarism is based on biochemical confirmation of hormone deficits. Each hormone has to be tested separately and there is a variable pattern of hormone deficiency among patients. As a general principle, a combination of low peripheral and inappropriately low pituitary hormones (below the upper level of the reference range) indicates hypopituitarism. However, basal concentrations alone might not be diagnostic owing to pulsatile, circadian or situational secretion of some hormones. The investigations usually include measurement of basal anterior pituitary hormones and their respective target gland hormone levels, namely adrenocorticotrophic hormone (ACTH), cortisol, thyroid-stimulating hormone (TSH), free thyroxine (FT4), free triiodothyronine (FT3), follicle-stimulating hormone (FSH), luteinising hormone (LH), estradiol, testosterone and prolactin.

ACTH deficiency

Secondary adrenal insufficiency can be excluded by finding a morning cortisol concentration in excess of 500 nmol/L and is confirmed by a concentration below 100 nmol/L. ACTH deficiency causes adrenal atrophy and ACTH receptor downregulation. Therefore the standard 250-μg corticotrophin test can be used to establish secondary adrenal insufficiency if done at least 4 weeks after the onset of ACTH deficiency. Stimulated cortisol concentrations at 30 min of 500 nmol/L or less strongly indicate ACTH deficiency, while concentrations above 600 nmol/L rule out the disorder. At values in between, a second test is recommended.

TSH deficiency

Central hypothyroidism is diagnosed when FT4 is decreased and TSH is also low or normal.

LH and FSH deficiency

Before a diagnosis of LH and FSH deficiency, hyperprolactinaemia should be excluded, which might be present because of disturbed hypothalamic inhibition of prolactin release. Diagnosis of female LH and FSH deficiency should be based on clinical findings, supported by laboratory values. Oligomenorrhoea togther with inappropriately low LH and FSH concentrations indicate secondary hypogonadism in premenopausal women. During or after menopause, an absence of rise in LH and FSH shows central hypogonadism. In men, secondary hypogonadism is shown by low testosterone concentrations in combination with inappropriately low gonadotrophins.

Growth hormone (GH) deficiency

An insulin tolerance test (ITT) is the gold standard test. After an overnight fast, intravenous insulin 0.05–0.15 units/kg is injected and samples are taken for blood glucose and GH levels at 0, 30, 60, 90 and 120 min. Definition of a normal GH response to an ITT performed with an appropriate degree of hypoglycaemia (blood glucose 2.2 mmol/L) is a peak of at least 15 mU/L (5 mg/L). Care is needed to carefully monitor and treat possible hypoglycaemia. Contraindications to an ITT include ischaemic heart disease, an abnormal resting ECG, arrhythmias or epilepsy/unexplained syncope. Circulating insulin-like growth factor (IGF)-1 can be helpful in the diagnosis of adult GH deficiency; however, there are alternative causes of a low IGF-1 other than GH deficiency including malnutrition, liver disease, diabetes mellitus and hypothyroidism.

Antidiuretic hormone (ADH) deficiency

ADH deficiency causes polyuria and polydipsia. Before testing, diabetes mellitus as a typical cause of polyuria should be excluded. Diabetes insipidus (DI) is possible if polyuria (≥40 mL/kg per day) is present in combination with a urine osmolality less than 300 mosmol/kg of water and hypernatraemia. For further investigations, see Chapter 91.

Radiological investigations

MRI of the head should be performed in the presence of clinical and biochemical evidence of hypopituitarism (Figure 94.1). When MRI is contraindicated CT with contrast provides a suitable alternative. In central DI the normal high-intensity posterior pituitary bright spot on T1-weighted MRI is generally absent.

Investigations for underlying causes

Depending on the clinical suspicion, other tests such as serum ferritin (haemochromatosis) or antineutrophil cytoplasmic antibody (vasculitis) may provide additional information to elicit the aetiology.

Follow-up investigations

Once hypopituitarism has been diagnosed, adequate hormone replacement should be monitored at regular intervals. After the initial titration, intervals of 6–12 months are usually recommended. If a tumour is the cause, regular visual field assessment and MRI should be undertaken. Endocrine assessment after brain injury should be done initially in the rehabilitation phase (3–6 months after trauma). Since pituitary dysfunction can recover after this phase, but sometimes new deficiencies might become manifest, assessment should be repeated at 1 year after trauma.

95 Acromegaly

Table 95.1 Causes of acromegaly

Primary GH excess

Pituitary adenoma or carcinoma
Extrapituitary tumour
Familial syndromes: multiple
    endocrine neoplasia type 1,
    familial acromegaly,
    McCune–Albright syndrome,
    Carney's syndrome

Extrapituitary GH excess

Pancreatic islet-cell tumour
Lymphoma
Iatrogenic

GHRH excess

Central cause: hypothalamic
    tumour
Peripheral causes: bronchial
    carcinoid tumour, small-cell
    lung cancer

Table 95.2 Common complications in acromegaly

Complications	Tests

Cardiovascular diseases
    Ischaemic heart disease,
    congestive cardiac failure,
    arrhythmias
	CXR, ECG, echocardiogram, lipid profile

Hypertension	24-hour blood pressure monitor
Carpal tunnel syndrome	Nerve conduction test
Arthritis	Plain X-ray
Colonic polyps	Colonoscopy
Glucose intolerance or diabetes	Fasting blood glucose, oral glucose tolerance test (OGTT), HbA1c
Sleep apnoea	Formal sleep study
Vision impairment	Visual fields assessment

Figure 95.1 Sagittal T1-weighted MRI post contrast shows pituitary macroadenoma

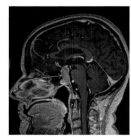

Figure 95.4 The chart shows acromegaly-associated severe obstructive sleep apnoea

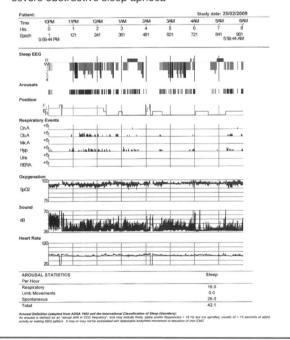

Figure 95.2 X-ray of the pelvis shows severe bilateral osteo-arthritis of the hips, a common complication of acromegaly

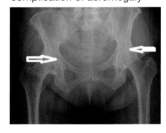

Figure 95.3 Colonoscopy reveals a colonic polyp, common in patients with acromegaly

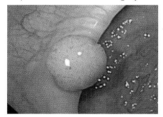

Key points

- Random GH is not useful in the diagnosis of acromegaly because of episodic secretion and short half-life of GH, but low random GH below 0.04 µg/L (1.0 mU/L) makes acromegaly unlikely.
- IGF-1 is the polypeptide target of GH. It is relatively stable and positively correlated with GH. It is excellent for diagnosis and monitoring.
- In acromegaly, there is failure to suppress GH to below 0.04 µg/L (1.0 mU/L) in response to a 75-g oral glucose load (OGTT).
- Once a biochemical diagnosis of acromegaly has been made, MRI of the pituitary gland with contrast should be performed because a pituitary GH-secreting adenoma is the cause in most cases.

Acromegaly is a result of prolonged excessive growth hormone (GH) secretion. The incidence of acromegaly is 3 per million persons per year and the prevalence is about 60 per million. More than 90% of patients with acromegaly have a benign monoclonal GH-secreting pituitary adenoma. Other causes are summarised in Table 95.1. The mortality rate of acromegaly is two to three times higher than that of the general population, with cardiovascular and respiratory complications being the most frequent causes of death. Disease features develop insidiously over decades, often resulting in a delay of 7–10 years in diagnosis after the estimated onset of symptoms. Therefore a high index of suspicion and early investigation are needed.

Diagnostic investigations: assessment of GH

Insulin-like growth factor 1 (IGF-1)

IGF-1 is the most reliable biochemical indicator of acromegaly because of a linear correlation between serum IGF-1 level and 24-hour integrated GH secretion. A random IGF-1 level should be measured and compared with laboratory reference intervals corrected for age in all patients suspected of acromegaly. This can be used as an initial screen test. IGF-1 should be raised in all cases of acromegaly but levels can be reduced by fasting and systemic illness.

Glucose tolerance test

Autonomous secretion of GH can be assessed by measuring GH levels during a 2-hour period after a standard 75-g oral glucose load (0, 30, 60, 90 and 120 min) as well as by changes in IGF-1 levels. If no GH values are below 4 mU/L (or 2 µg/L with most commercial assays), then the diagnosis of acromegaly is confirmed. The production of GH may not be suppressed in patients with liver disease, chronic kidney disease, uncontrolled diabetes, malnutrition or anorexia, in late adolescence, or in those who are pregnant or receiving estrogens. GH release is pulsatile so isolated levels are difficult to interpret; a random GH measurement is not helpful and may be high in normal people.

GH releasing hormone (GHRH)

Most cases (>90%) of acromegaly are due to pituitary tumours. If acromegaly is confirmed and a pituitary tumour is not seen on MRI, a GHRH level should be assessed to exclude ectopic production. Levels above 300 pg/mL usually indicate an ectopic source of GHRH. In pituitary disease, GHRH concentration is normal or suppressed.

Other pituitary-related hormones

About 25% of GH adenomas co-secrete prolactin. Patients can also have loss of other pituitary trophic hormones such as FSH, LH, TSH, ACTH and prolactin. These hormones and their target hormones should be evaluated.

Radiological and visual field investigations

Formal visual perimetry should be performed once the biochemical diagnosis of acromegaly has been confirmed. This is particularly important if the tumour is a macroadenoma (>10 mm on MRI), though restriction of the superior fields may reflect expansion of the supraorbital ridges.

MRI of the pituitary with gadolinium should only be performed after the biochemical diagnosis of acromegaly. It is the most sensitive technique for identifying the source of excess GH (Figure 95.1). Adenomas that are greater than 2 mm in diameter can be visualised together with tumour dimensions, invasive characteristics and optic tract contiguity. At diagnosis, more than 75% of patients with acromegaly have a macroadenoma (>10 mm in diameter) which often extends laterally to the cavernous sinus or dorsally to the suprasellar region. In rare cases, when a non-pituitary cause of excess GH or GHRH is suspected, CT and/or MRI of the chest and abdomen are indicated.

Investigations for monitoring

For follow-up of treated cases of acromegaly, IGF-1 levels and nadir GH in a series of four estimations over 2 hours is a reasonable approach. In patients with biochemically active and clinically inactive disease, the tumour mass should be monitored for growth by 6–12 monthly MRI.

Investigations for coexisting illnesses

Excessive GH and IGF-1 can cause many complications (Table 95.2). Structural and functional cardiac diseases such as arrhythmias, myocardial hypertrophy and diastolic heart failure are common. CXR, ECG and echocardiography are used to evaluate these complications.

Patients with acromegaly have an increased risk of diabetes mellitus and dyslipidaemia and should be investigated with fasting glucose, lipid profile and HbA_{1c}.

Up to 70% of patients have large joint and axial arthropathy (Figure 95.2). Plain X-ray can be used to evaluate these problems.

Compared with the general population, the difference in relative risk of cancer in patients with acromegaly is controversial. However, a colonoscopy should be arranged due to the increased risk of colonic polyps (Figure 95.3) and malignancy; care should be taken because of the frequency of a tortuous megacolon.

Patients with acromegaly are at high risk of developing obstructive sleep apnoea (Figure 95.4), which will elevate their cardiovascular risk. A formal sleep study should be performed in all patients at baseline.

96 Hyperprolactinaemia

Table 96.1 Drugs causing hyperprolactinaemia

Dopamine receptor agonists
Antipsychotics
Antidepressants, e.g. imipramine, SSRIs
Antiemetics, e.g. metoclopramide, domperidone
Antihypertensive agents, e.g. methyldopa, verapamil
High-dose estrogens
Opiates

Table 96.2 Non-drug causes of hyperprolactinaemia

Physiological causes
Pregnancy
Lactation
Hypothalamic–pituitary disorders
Tumours
Pituitary microadenoma and macroadenoma
Craniopharyngioma
Infiltrative disorders
Sarcoidosis
Giant cell granulomas
Others
Cranial radiation
Empty sella
Neurogenic causes
Chest wall lesions
Breast stimulation
Systemic disorders
Primary hypothyroidism
CKD
PCOS
Stress
Idiopathic

Figure 96.1 MRI of the head shows a pituitary adenoma

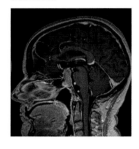

Figure 96.2 Visual field test shows bitemporal hemianopia caused by a pituitary macroadenoma (dark areas indicate the visual field deficits)

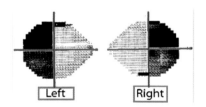

Box 96.1 Indications for measurement of prolactin levels

- Patients with symptoms suggestive of pituitary tumours (headache, visual field deficit)
- Patient with pituitary incidentaloma
- Male and female patients with galactorrhoea
- Male patient with erectile dysfunction
- Female patient with amenorrhoea or oligomenorrhoea
- Female patient with symptoms of premenopausal hypogonadism
- Patient taking antipsychotics for extended period

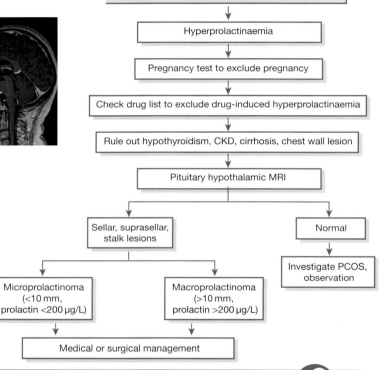

Hyperprolactinaemia

↓

Pregnancy test to exclude pregnancy

↓

Check drug list to exclude drug-induced hyperprolactinaemia

↓

Rule out hypothyroidism, CKD, cirrhosis, chest wall lesion

↓

Pituitary hypothalamic MRI

Sellar, suprasellar, stalk lesions ——— Normal

Normal → Investigate PCOS, observation

Microprolactinoma (<10 mm, prolactin <200 µg/L) — Macroprolactinoma (>10 mm, prolactin >200 µg/L)

↓

Medical or surgical management

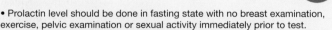

Key points

- Prolactin level should be done in fasting state with no breast examination, exercise, pelvic examination or sexual activity immediately prior to test.
- Other basal anterior pituitary hormones and their target hormones should be evaluated in patients with suspected prolactinoma.
- MRI is useful for identifying microadenoma and assessing the size effects of macroadenoma.
- Visual field testing must be performed in patients with macroadenoma.

Hyperprolactinaemia is the most common endocrine disorder of the hypothalamic–pituitary axis. It is defined as a serum prolactin level above 30 μg/L. Hyperprolactinaemia is physiologically normal during pregnancy and lactation. Drugs that cause hyperprolactinaemia (Table 96.1) should be excluded before further investigating other underlying causes. The common non-drug causes of hyperprolactinaemia include stress, pituitary tumour (microprolactinomas), polycystic ovary syndrome (PCOS) and primary hypothyroidism (Table 96.2). Hyperprolactinaemia is found in 8–10% of women with oligomenorrhoea and 3% of women with unexplained infertility.

Clinical features of hyperprolactinaemia in women include oligomenorrhoea, infertility and galactorrhoea. In men, hyperprolactinaemia leads to impotence, infertility, galactorrhoea, gynaecomastia and decreased libido. If patients present with these symptoms, the serum prolactin level should be checked. The majority of prolactinomas in women are small at the time of diagnosis, so headaches and neurological deficits are rare. However in men, prolactinomas tend to be large at the time of diagnosis and may cause cranial nerve dysfunction, visual loss and hypopituitarism.

Prolactin level and laboratory investigations

A single measurement of prolactin in a blood sample obtained at any time of the day is usually adequate to document hyperprolactinaemia. Because of the pulsatile nature of prolactin secretion and the effect of stress, a concentration between 25 and 40 μg/L should prompt a repeat test before a diagnosis of hyperprolactinaemia is confirmed.

After rechecking an elevated prolactin level for confirmation, a pregnancy test should be performed in women of childbearing age to exclude pregnancy. Then a review of medication should be undertaken to exclude drug-induced hyperprolactinaemia before further investigations. In general, serum prolactin levels parallel tumour size fairly closely.

Serum electrolytes, creatinine, and thyroid and liver function should be assessed. Testing of pituitary function is usually unnecessary in patients with microadenomas because pituitary function is typically normal in such patients. In women with amenorrhoea, serum FSH should be measured to exclude primary ovarian failure, and in men serum testosterone levels should be assessed. Bone densitometry should be done in patients with chronic hyperprolactinaemia.

MRI

Once other possible causes of hyperprolactinaemia have been excluded, the diagnosis of a prolactinoma is confirmed by gadolinium-enhanced MRI (Figure 96.1). MRI is indicated even in cases of mild hyperprolactinaemia to determine tumour size and to rule out the presence of other sellar and stalk lesions. CT with contrast is an alternative but MRI is more effective in revealing small adenomas and the extension of large tumours.

Visual field testing

Patients with macroadenoma adjacent to the optic chiasm or compressing it should undergo formal visual field examination (Figure 96.2) because visual compromise necessitates rapid treatment.

Follow-up investigations

Prolactin levels usually, but do not always, correspond to changes in tumour size. Therefore prolactin levels and tumour size, assessed using MRI, should be checked routinely once a year for the first 3 years and then every 2 years if the patient's condition is stable. However, data regarding optimal follow-up intervals are lacking.

97 Adrenal insufficiency

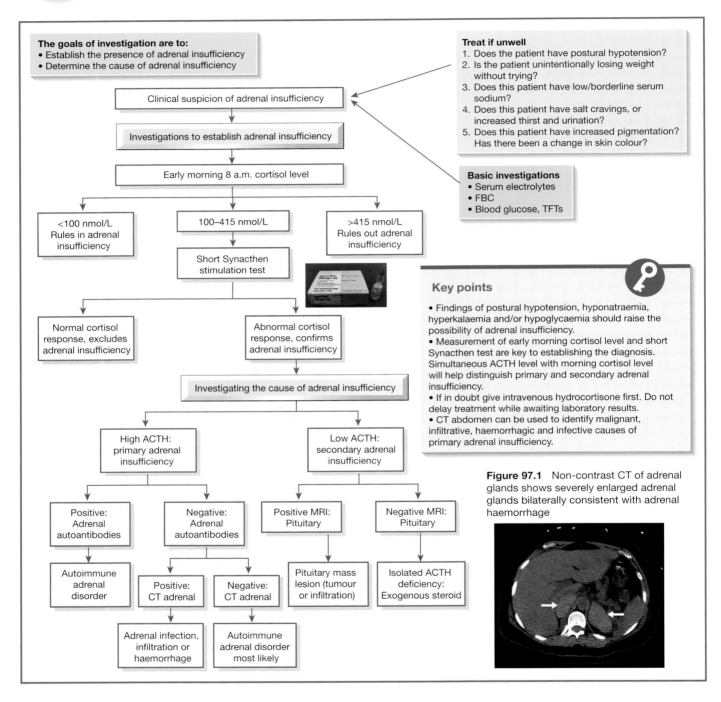

The goals of investigation are to:
- Establish the presence of adrenal insufficiency
- Determine the cause of adrenal insufficiency

Treat if unwell
1. Does the patient have postural hypotension?
2. Is the patient unintentionally losing weight without trying?
3. Does this patient have low/borderline serum sodium?
4. Does this patient have salt cravings, or increased thirst and urination?
5. Does this patient have increased pigmentation? Has there been a change in skin colour?

Basic investigations
- Serum electrolytes
- FBC
- Blood glucose, TFTs

Clinical suspicion of adrenal insufficiency

Investigations to establish adrenal insufficiency

Early morning 8 a.m. cortisol level

<100 nmol/L
Rules in adrenal insufficiency

100–415 nmol/L

>415 nmol/L
Rules out adrenal insufficiency

Short Synacthen stimulation test

Normal cortisol response, excludes adrenal insufficiency

Abnormal cortisol response, confirms adrenal insufficiency

Investigating the cause of adrenal insufficiency

High ACTH: primary adrenal insufficiency

Low ACTH: secondary adrenal insufficiency

Positive: Adrenal autoantibodies

Negative: Adrenal autoantibodies

Positive MRI: Pituitary

Negative MRI: Pituitary

Autoimmune adrenal disorder

Positive: CT adrenal

Negative: CT adrenal

Pituitary mass lesion (tumour or infiltration)

Isolated ACTH deficiency: Exogenous steroid

Adrenal infection, infiltration or haemorrhage

Autoimmune adrenal disorder most likely

Key points

- Findings of postural hypotension, hyponatraemia, hyperkalaemia and/or hypoglycaemia should raise the possibility of adrenal insufficiency.
- Measurement of early morning cortisol level and short Synacthen test are key to establishing the diagnosis. Simultaneous ACTH level with morning cortisol level will help distinguish primary and secondary adrenal insufficiency.
- If in doubt give intravenous hydrocortisone first. Do not delay treatment while awaiting laboratory results.
- CT abdomen can be used to identify malignant, infiltrative, haemorrhagic and infective causes of primary adrenal insufficiency.

Figure 97.1 Non-contrast CT of adrenal glands shows severely enlarged adrenal glands bilaterally consistent with adrenal haemorrhage

Adrenal insufficiency is characterised by a deficiency of adrenal hormones. Primary adrenal insufficiency, known as Addison's disease, is due to failure of the adrenal glands to produce adrenal hormones, while secondary adrenal insufficiency is caused by dysfunction in the hypothalamus or pituitary gland, leading to a decrease in secretion of adrenocorticotrophic hormone (ACTH). Adrenal insufficiency, either primary or secondary, can present as a life-threatening condition requiring prompt investigation and treatment. Addison's disease is most commonly caused by autoimmune disease, which accounts for 70–90% of cases. Of those patients with autoimmune adrenal insufficiency, about 60% have one or more other autoimmune endocrine disorders. Disseminated tuberculosis remains the leading cause of Addison's disease in developing countries.

Fatigue, anorexia, nausea, weight loss, hypoglycaemia, dizziness and postural hypotension are common presenting features. Increased pigmentation may be seen in primary adrenal insufficiency (due to chronic ACTH hypersecretion). Addison's disease is associated with other autoimmune diseases, such as thyroid disease, vitiligo, type 1 diabetes, pernicious anaemia, and coeliac disease. In patients with pre-existing type 1 diabetes, the onset of recurrent hypoglycaemic episodes should raise the suspicion of adrenal insufficiency. Symptoms for adrenal insufficiency are non-specific, often leading to a delay in diagnosis. Investigations must never delay treatment which should be initiated on strong clinical suspicion of adrenal insufficiency. The questions that are helpful in raising suspicion of adrenal insufficiency are shown on the page opposite.

Basic investigations

These should include electrolytes, blood glucose and FBC. Diminished mineralocorticoid activity can result in volume depletion, hyponatraemia, hyperkalaemia and metabolic acidosis. Hyponatraemia is observed in 80% of acute cases whereas less than half present with hyperkalaemia. Serum glucose may be low. If the person is not in adrenal crisis, electrolyte levels may be borderline or normal. In secondary adrenal insufficiency, sodium and potassium may be normal as there is no associated deficiency of mineralocorticoids; aldosterone secretion is under the control of the renin–angiotensin system rather than ACTH. Glucocorticoid deficiency can be associated with normocytic anaemia, lymphocytosis and eosinophilia.

To establish adrenal insufficiency

Early morning cortisol

Serum cortisol levels peak in the early morning. Therefore a low cortisol level (<272 nmol/L or <10 µg/dL) at 8 a.m. is suggestive of adrenal insufficiency and this cut-off is associated with a sensitivity of 62% and specificity of 77%. If the serum cortisol level is below 100 nmol/L, adrenal insufficiency is highly likely and urgent treatment required. Conversely, a high morning cortisol (>415 nmol/L or >15 µg/dL) indicates adrenal insufficiency is unlikely. However, patients with partial adrenal deficiency may demonstrate relatively normal morning values. Random serum cortisol levels have a very low sensitivity for adrenal insufficiency and should not be performed.

Short Synacthen stimulation test

The capacity of the adrenal cortex to respond to ACTH is tested with short ACTH (Synacthen) stimulation test, which measures cortisol level before intravenous or intramuscular injection of 250 µg of ACTH and 30 and 60 min after. An increase to peak concentration above 500 nmol/L (>18 µg/dL) excludes adrenal insufficiency. The short Synacthen test is used to establish hypocortisolism; it does not distinguish between primary and secondary adrenal insufficiency. The adrenal responsiveness to exogenous ACTH is often impaired in chronic secondary adrenal disease due to adrenal atrophy from lack of ACTH stimulation, but with mild deficiency, or soon after an acute pituitary event (e.g. pituitary surgery or bleed), the response to ACTH challenge may be normal.

Other hormonal tests

Secondary adrenal insufficiency may be associated with other pituitary hormone deficiencies. Adrenal androgen deficiency can be present in both primary and secondary adrenal insufficiency.

The cause of adrenal insufficiency

ACTH level

Simultaneous ACTH measurement and cortisol will distinguish primary from secondary of adrenal insufficiency. Primary adrenal insufficiency is confirmed by high ACTH levels, and low (or inappropriately low) levels of ACTH are seen in secondary adrenal insufficiency.

Anti-adrenal antibodies

These are present in 70% of patients with autoimmune adrenal disorder but can also be present without adrenal insufficiency in patients with other autoimmune conditions.

CT or MRI of adrenal glands

If there is no coexisting autoimmune disease and adrenal autoantibodies are negative, imaging of the adrenal glands is warranted. Infiltrative diseases including malignancies and haemorrhage can be identified on CT (Figure 97.1). If disseminated tuberculosis is considered a likely cause, CXR should be performed.

MRI of pituitary

If ACTH is inappropriately low in the presence of cortisol deficiency, MRI of the hypothalamic–pituitary region should be performed. If the hypothalamic–pituitary region is responsible for the cortisol insufficiency, the endocrine pituitary profile needs to be assessed.

Corticotropin releasing hormone (CRH) stimulation test

This investigation can be used to distinguish between secondary (pituitary) and tertiary (hypothalamus) adrenal insufficiency, although from a treatment point of view the distinction is not usually important. After administration of CRH, an exaggerated response is seen with hypothalamic disease but ACTH and cortisol response are minimal or absent with pituitary-related deficiency.

Treatment monitoring

Monitoring of glucocorticoid replacement is based on clinical assessment with the aim of relieving symptoms of glucocorticoid deficiency and avoiding signs and symptoms of glucocorticoid excess. In primary adrenal insufficiency the ACTH concentration may be a useful marker of compliance but can fluctuate between glucocorticoid doses, making it hard to interpret. Normalisation of ACTH levels should not be an aim; low normal or suppressed morning plasma ACTH concentration indicates excessive glucocorticoid replacement in patients with primary adrenal insufficiency. Monitoring of mineralocorticoid replacement includes supine and standing blood pressure, serum sodium and potassium, and plasma renin activity.

98 Adrenal incidentaloma

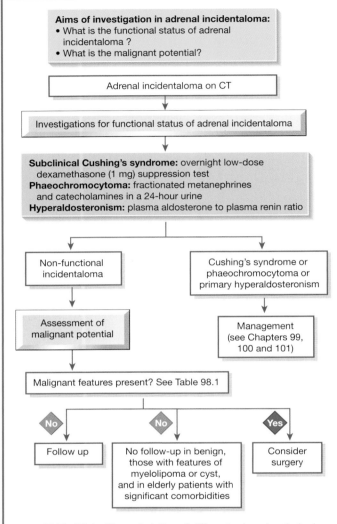

Aims of investigation in adrenal incidentaloma:
- What is the functional status of adrenal incidentaloma ?
- What is the malignant potential?

Adrenal incidentaloma on CT

↓

Investigations for functional status of adrenal incidentaloma

↓

Subclinical Cushing's syndrome: overnight low-dose dexamethasone (1 mg) suppression test
Phaeochromocytoma: fractionated metanephrines and catecholamines in a 24-hour urine
Hyperaldosteronism: plasma aldosterone to plasma renin ratio

Non-functional incidentaloma

Cushing's syndrome or phaeochromocytoma or primary hyperaldosteronism

↓

Assessment of malignant potential

Management (see Chapters 99, 100 and 101)

↓

Malignant features present? See Table 98.1

No → Follow up

No → No follow-up in benign, those with features of myelolipoma or cyst, and in elderly patients with significant comorbidities

Yes → Consider surgery

Figure 98.1 (a) Right adrenal 11-mm mass (15 HU) represents an incidentaloma. (b) Coronal CT shows a low-attenuation right adrenal lesion containing fat (arrow) and higher-attenuation myeloid tissue consistent with benign adrenal myelolipoma. (c) Axial T2-weighted MRI shows intense, high-signal pheochromocytoma (arrow) in right adrenal gland. (d) CT with contrast shows a heterogeneous enhancing right adrenal lesion in a hypertensive patient with raised plasma metanephrines consistent with phaeochromocytoma

(a)　　　　　　　　　(b)

(c)　　　　　　　　　(d)

Key points

- A homogeneous mass with low attenuation (<10 HU) on CT is likely to be a benign adenoma.
- Excess hormonal secretion can initially be evaluated with 24-hour urinary cortisol and catecholamine measurement, and aldosterone/renin ratio if hypertensive or hypokalaemic.
- For patients with adrenal incidentaloma to be managed non-surgically, repeat CT or MRI can be performed at 6 and 12 months.
- In patients with an adrenal mass that remains stable on two imaging studies at least 6 months apart and does not exhibit hormonal hypersecretion over 4 years, further follow-up is usually not required.

Table 98.1 Characteristics of different adrenal pathologies on radiological imaging

	Benign phenotype	Malignant phenotype	Metastasis phenotype	Phaeochromocytoma
Size	≤3 cm	≥4 cm	<3 cm	>3 cm
Margins	Smooth margins	Irregular margins	Irregular margins	Clear margins
Texture	Homogeneous	Heterogeneous	Heterogeneous with mixed densities	Heterogeneous with cystic areas
Laterality	Unilateral	Unilateral	Often bilateral	Unilateral
Hounsfield unit (HU)	≤10 HU	>25 HU	>25 HU	>25 HU
Vascularity	Not vascular	Usually vascular	Usually vascular	Prominent vascular
Contrast washout	≥50% at 10 min	<50% at 10 min	<50% at 10 min	<50% at 10 min
Necrosis, haemorrhage or calcifications	Rare	Common	Occasional haemorrhage	Haemorrhage and cystic areas are common
Growth rate	Stable over time or very slow (<1 cm/year)	Rapid growth (>2 cm/year)	Growth at variable rate	Slow growth (0.5–1.0 cm/year)
T2-weighted MRI	Isointense	Hyperintense	Hyperintense	Markedly hyperintense

An adrenal 'incidentaloma' is an adrenal mass (generally ≥1 cm) discovered during a radiological examination performed for other purposes and for which there are no symptoms or clinical findings suggestive of adrenal disease. The prevalence of adrenal incidentaloma in abdominal CT increases with age, and is approximately 7% in patients over 70 years old. The widespread use of ultrasound, CT and MRI has resulted in the increasing clinical dilemma of how to investigate adrenal incidentalomas.

The majority of adrenal incidentalomas are clinically non-hypersecreting benign adrenocortical adenomas but up to 15% may be hypersecreting hormonally and a small proportion may be malignant, either a primary adrenal cancer or metastatic deposit. Of the tumours that are hormonally active, about 9% are cortisol-secreting, 5% are phaeochromocytomas and 1% aldosterone-secreting.

Evaluation should start with a careful history and physical examination, focusing on the signs and symptoms suggestive of adrenal hyperfunction or malignant disease. Laboratory and imaging studies are used to assess the hormonal status and the potential malignancy of the mass. In elderly asymptomatic patients or those with significant comorbidities, care is needed in deciding whether investigations for hormonal activity and potential malignancy are appropriate. In many such patients, investigations may cause unnecessary anxiety, not improve the patient's health and surgical treatments be inappropriate.

Investigations for functional status of adrenal incidentaloma

Subclinical Cushing's syndrome

Subclinical Cushing's syndrome exhibits clinically significant autonomous production of glucocorticoid in the absence of symptoms and signs of Cushing's syndrome. Subclinical Cushing's syndrome may cause hypertension, obesity, diabetes and osteoporosis. Overnight low-dose dexamethasone (1 mg) suppression test is widely used as a screening test and should be performed in appropriate patients with asymptomatic adrenal incidentalomas. Using a cortisol level of 140 nmol/L (5 µg/dL) as the cut-off value, this suppression test has a specificity of about 91% and sensitivity close to 100%. If the result is abnormal, confirmatory testing should be performed to rule out a false-positive result (see Chapter 99).

Phaeochromocytoma

Not all phaeochromocytomas are symptomatic and patients can be normotensive, so patients with an adrenal incidentaloma should be screened for phaeochromocytoma. This can be done with either 24-hour measurement of fractionated metanephrines and catecholamines (more specific but less sensitive) or fractionated free plasma metanephrines (more sensitive but less specific).

Hyperaldosteronism

Hypertensive patients with adrenal incidentaloma should be screened for hyperaldosteronism. The ratio of ambulatory morning plasma aldosterone to plasma renin activity is the screening test. If this ratio is high, a confirmatory test should be done (see Chapter 101). The measurement of potassium is not reliable in screening.

Sex-hormone secreting mass

Sex-hormone secreting adrenocortical tumours are rare and typically occur in the presence of clinical manifestations (e.g. hirsutism or virilisation). Therefore routine screening for excess androgens or estrogens in patients with adrenal incidentaloma is not warranted.

Assessment of malignant potential

The size of the mass and its appearance on imaging are two major predictors of malignant disease. A diameter greater than 4 cm has a 90% sensitivity for the detection of adrenocortical carcinoma but the specificity is low, with only 24% of lesions over 4 cm being malignant. The features suggestive of malignancy are listed in Table 98.1 and examples shown in Figure 98.1. Features of malignancy or hormonal secretion may be indications for surgical resection. PET scan can be helpful in patients with a history of malignant disease because of its high sensitivity in detecting malignant disease.

Follow-up of adrenal incidentaloma

The optimal frequency and duration of follow-up for patients with adrenal incidentalomas are uncertain and the appropriateness of further imaging needs consideration in the context of the patient's overall health.

For masses that appear benign in appearance and which are non-functioning, repeat imaging and biochemical evaluation is recommended at 1–2 years and one further scan another 12 months later if this remains reassuring. For more indeterminate lesions, repeat imaging to assess growth at 3–12 months is recommended. Subsequent testing would depend on growth. Adrenocortical carcinomas typically have a rapid growth rate (>2 cm per year). The yield and cost-effectiveness of repeated imaging at these intervals are uncertain.

99 Cushing's syndrome

The purpose of investigations in a patient with suspected Cushing's syndrome is to:
- Establish if there is hypercortisolism
- Determine if the hypercortisolism is ACTH dependent or independent
- Determine whether it is a consequence of Cushing's disease or ectopic ACTH production if ACTH-dependent
- Determine the complications of Cushing's syndrome

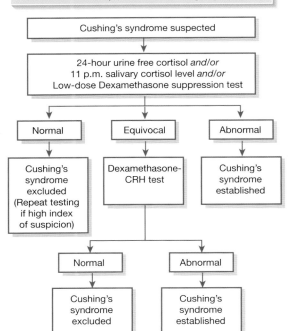

Cushing's syndrome suspected
↓
24-hour urine free cortisol *and/or*
11 p.m. salivary cortisol level *and/or*
Low-dose Dexamethasone suppression test

Normal →
Cushing's syndrome excluded (Repeat testing if high index of suspicion)

Equivocal →
Dexamethasone-CRH test

Abnormal →
Cushing's syndrome established

Dexamethasone-CRH test →
Normal →
Cushing's syndrome excluded

Abnormal →
Cushing's syndrome established

Figure 99.1 (a) T1-weighted MRI of the head post contrast shows normal pituitary; (b) T1-weighted MRI of the head post contrast shows pituitary macroadenoma

(a) (b)

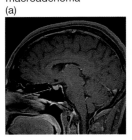

Figure 99.2 CT abdomen showing a right adrenal adenoma with low attenuation in a patient with Cushing's syndrome

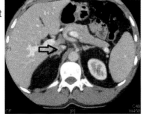

Table 99.1 Causes of Cushing's syndrome

ACTH-dependent
Cushing's disease (pituitary)
Ectopic ACTH syndrome
Ectopic CRH syndrome

ACTH-independent
Adrenal adenoma
Adrenal carcinoma
Micronodular and macronodular hyperplasia

Pseudo-Cushing's syndrome
Major depressive disorder
Alcoholism

Table 99.2 Interpretation of investigations to distinguish causes of Cushing's syndrome

	Pituitary	**Adrenal**	**Ectopic ACTH/CRH**
ACTH	Normal/high	Low	High
CRH test	Response	No response	No response
High-dose (8 mg) dexamethasone	Suppression	No suppression	No suppression
Adrenal CT	Normal/enlarged	Tumour	Normal/enlarged
Pituitary CT/MRI	Tumour	Normal	Normal
Inferior petrosal sinus sampling	Central/peripheral gradient	Not applicable	No central/peripheral gradient

Table 99.3 Example of ACTH levels (pg/mL) in the interior petrosal sinus before and after infusion of CRH, showing no substantial gradient in ACTH levels between the center and the periphery

	Periphery	**Right**	**Left**
Time before infusion			
5 min	142	162	152
2 min	145	158	163
Time after infusion			
2 min	147	159	153
5 min	149	165	168
10 min	159	176	173

Key points

- Diagnosis of Cushing's syndrome is made by elevated nocturnal serum or salivary cortisol levels, 24-hour urinary free cortisol, or a dexamethasone suppression test.
- After confirming the diagnosis of Cushing's syndrome, a serum basal ACTH should be measured to distinguish between ACTH-dependent and ACTH-independent aetiologies.
- High-dose dexamethasone suppression test and CRH test are useful for distinguishing between Cushing's disease and ectopic ACTH secretion.
- MRI with gadolinium localises corticotroph adenomas in up to 80% of cases. A petrosal sinus-to-peripheral ACTH ratio of 2:1 is considered diagnostic for a pituitary source, with accuracy of more than 95%.

Cushing's syndrome is a chronic state of glucocorticoid excess. There are many causes for Cushing's syndrome, which can be separated into adrenocorticotropic hormone (ACTH)-dependent and ACTH-independent causes (Table 99.1). Cushing's disease accounts for two-thirds of the cases of Cushing's syndrome. There are no pathognomonic symptoms for Cushing's syndrome so clinical suspicion should be based on the development of sudden onset of weight gain (truncal obesity), proximal muscle weakness, skin atrophy, purple striae, glucose intolerance and hypertension.

Investigations to confirm hypercortisolism

24-Hour urinary free cortisol

This is the best screening test, with a sensitivity for Cushing's syndrome of 95–100% and a specificity of 94–98%. To assess the adequacy of 24-hour collection, urine creatinine should be measured. Renal function should be verified before testing because urinary free cortisol measurements are not valid in patients with an eGFR <30 mL/min /1.73m². Cushing's syndrome is excluded by a cortisol level below 250 nmol/day.

Salivary cortisol

Cortisol concentration in saliva is highly correlated with free cortisol in plasma and may distinguish patients with Cushing's syndrome from normal individuals when tested late at night (11 p.m.). Saliva can be easily collected at home several times to assess cortisol production over long periods. Late-night salivary cortisol levels consistently above 7.0 nmol/L (>0.25 μg/dL) are diagnostic of Cushing's syndrome. Salivary cortisol levels have a sensitivity and specificity of 90–95% for the diagnosis of Cushing's syndrome.

Midnight plasma cortisol

A single cortisol measurement taken at midnight indicates the presence of Cushing's syndrome when values are above 50 nmol/L, with a sensitivity of 100%.

Low-dose dexamethasone suppression tests

These tests do not provide additional information in patients with very high urinary free cortisol. They should be used for patients with mild hypercortisolism or suspected pseudo-Cushing's syndrome or unable to perform a 24-hour urine collection. The overnight dexamethasone suppression test (1 mg at 11 p.m.) may exclude the presence of Cushing's syndrome when the morning plasma cortisol concentration is below 50 nmol/L, with a sensitivity of 98–100%. In the 2-day test, the patient takes eight doses of dexamethasone 0.5 mg at intervals of 6 hours. A normal response is a morning plasma cortisol below 50 nmol/L. This investigation has a diagnostic accuracy of only 71% in patients with mild Cushing's syndrome.

Investigating the cause of Cushing's syndrome

ACTH measurement

ACTH measurement is the first step and the best way to distinguish ACTH-dependent from ACTH-independent hypercortisolism. In active Cushing's disease, plasma ACTH at 9 a.m. is usually raised. Concentrations below the limit of detection (<1.1 pmol/L, <5 pg/mL) indicate autonomous adrenal hyperfunction. The higher the ACTH concentration, the more likely an ectopic source of the hormone.

High-dose dexamethasone suppression test

This test is used to distinguish pituitary from ectopic ACTH-dependent Cushing's syndrome. In Cushing's disease, high-dose dexamethasone results in suppression of ACTH secretion. An overnight dexamethasone suppression test may be used in which 8 mg of dexamethasone is taken between 11 p.m. and midnight and a single plasma cortisol level is obtained at 8 a.m. the next morning. The cortisol level should be below 140 nmol/L (<5 mg/dL) in patients with Cushing's disease. This test yields a diagnostic sensitivity, specificity and accuracy of 80% when the pre-test probability of Cushing's disease is at least 90%. However, this differentiation is not always reliable because some ectopic ATCH tumours are sensitive to glucocorticoid-negative feedback.

Inferior petrosal sinus sampling

Bilateral inferior petrosal sinus sampling for ACTH is the most reliable approach for distinguishing between pituitary and non-pituitary ACTH-dependent Cushing's syndrome. After catheterisation, blood samples are obtained from each inferior petrosal sinus and a peripheral vein in the basal state and at 2 or 3, 5 and 10 min after Corticotropin-releasing hormone (CRH) (1 μg/kg) is administered intravenously. Ratios of the right and left inferior petrosal sinus to peripheral ACTH are calculated at each time point. A ratio above 3.0 after the administration of CRH is consistent with Cushing's disease. Patients with ectopic ACTH syndrome will have a ratio below 2 before and after CRH administration. A gradient across left and right sides of more than 1.4 can predict the exact site of ACTH hypersecretion with an accuracy of 70–90% (Table 99.3). However, this test is associated with a low rate of complications, which include venous thrombosis and brainstem vascular damage.

Pituitary MRI

MRI of the pituitary gland with gadolinium enhancement should be performed in patients with ACTH-dependent Cushing's syndrome. It will demonstrate a discrete pituitary lesion in about 35–60% of patients (Figure 99.1).

Adrenal CT or MRI

If an adrenal tumour is suspected, CT or MRI helps to localise the mass and distinguish benign and malignant lesions (Figure 99.2). In patients with ACTH-dependent Cushing's syndrome, CT may show bilateral adrenal enlargement, with nodular adrenal hyperplasia in 10–15%, but in up to 30% the adrenal glands are of normal size. In patients with suspected ectopic ACTH production, chest and abdominal CT should be performed to identify any tumours in the lungs or mediastinum which may be the source.

Investigation after pituitary surgery

The treatment of choice for patients with Cushing's disease is trans-sphenoidal microadenomectomy. The criteria for a cure should be an undetectable morning plasma cortisol below 28 nmol/L (<1 μg/mL) and an ACTH below 1.1 pmol/L (<5 pg/mL) 24 hours after the last dose of hydrocortisone, at 4–7 days after surgery.

Other investigations

Cushing's syndrome is associated with neutrophilic leucocytosis, hypokalaemia, hyperglycaemia and hypercholesterolaemia. FBC, serum electrolytes, lipid profile and creatinine should be performed. Patients should have glucose tolerance test and bone mineral density assessed because hypercortisolism is associated with bone loss. Patients with hypertension should have a baseline echocardiogram.

100 Phaeochromocytoma

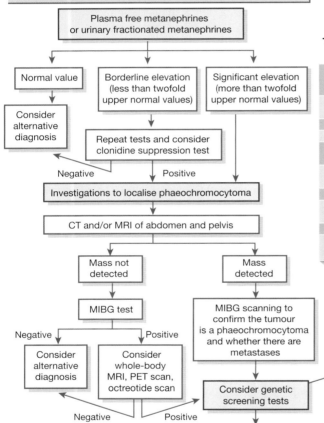

Plasma free metanephrines
or urinary fractionated metanephrines

Normal value

Borderline elevation (less than twofold upper normal values)

Significant elevation (more than twofold upper normal values)

Consider alternative diagnosis

Repeat tests and consider clonidine suppression test

Negative   Positive

Investigations to localise phaeochromocytoma

CT and/or MRI of abdomen and pelvis

Mass not detected

Mass detected

MIBG test

MIBG scanning to confirm the tumour is a phaeochromocytoma and whether there are metastases

Negative   Positive

Consider alternative diagnosis

Consider whole-body MRI, PET scan, octreotide scan

Negative   Positive

Consider genetic screening tests

Consider therapeutic options

Figure 100.1 CT with contrast shows a heterogeneous enhancing right adrenal lesion in a hypertensive patient with raised plasma metanephrines consistent with phaeochromocytoma

Table 100.1 Sensitivity and specificity of biochemical investigations for phaeochromocytoma

	Sensitivity (%)	Specificity (%)
Plasma free metanephrines	99	89
Plasma catecholamines	84	81
Urinary catecholamines	86	88
Urinary fractionated metanephrines	97	96
Urinary total metanephrines	77	93
Urinary vanillylmandelic acid	64	95

Table 100.2 Medications and conditions that affect biochemical investigations for phaeochromocytoma

Medication or condition	Investigation(s) confounded
Tricyclic antidepressants	Urinary catecholamines and metanephrines, plasma free metanephrines
Levodopa	Plasma free metanephrines and catecholamines
Clozapine	Urinary catecholamines and metanephrines
Phenoxybenzamine	Plasma free metanephrines
Calcium channel blockers	Plasma norepinephrine, urinary norepinephrine and urinary epinephrine
β-Adrenergic blockers	Urinary catecholamines and metanephrines, plasma free metanephrines (minor effect)
α1-Adrenergic blockers	Urinary norepinephrine
Sympathomimetics	Urinary catecholamines and metanephrines, plasma free metanephrines
Buspirone	Urinary metanephrines
Major physical and psychological stress	Urinary catecholamines and metanephrines, plasma free metanephrines

Key points

- Plasma free and total metanephrines and urinary metanephrines are equivalent for assessing a phaeochromocytoma. The combination of two of these tests is the best approach for biochemically diagnosing phaeochromocytoma.
- MRI and [123I]-MIBG are useful in the localisation of phaeochromocytoma tumours.
- When appropriate, genetic testing should be performed in patients with phaeochromocytoma.
- High-risk patients should be evaluated for associated conditions (VHL, MEN, NF1).

Phaeochromocytomas are catecholamine-producing tumours originating from chromaffin cells, usually located in the adrenal medulla. Traditional teaching has encouraged the 'rule of 10s', i.e. about 10% of tumours are extra-adrenal, 10% multiple, 10% bilateral, 10% malignant and 10% familial. However, it is being increasingly recognised that a larger proportion of pheochromocytomas are familial. Phaeochromocytoma is a rare condition, with a prevalence of 0.01%. It is frequently investigated because patients who go unrecognised risk significant morbidity and mortality. On the other hand, it is curable if diagnosed correctly and treated properly. Phaeochromocytomas occur in 25–75% of patients with multiple endocrine neoplasia (MEN) type 2, in 25% of those with von Hippel–Lindau (VHL) disease, and in less than 1% of those with neurofibromatosis.

Half of patients are symptomatic. The predominant feature of phaeochromocytoma is paroxysmal or sustained hypertension. The classic triad of headache, sweating and palpitations, seen in up to 20–40% of patients, has high specificity (93.8%) and sensitivity (90.9%) for phaeochromocytoma in hypertensive patients.

Biochemical tests for establishing the diagnosis of phaeochromocytoma

Plasma metanephrine

Plasma metanephrine screening test (sample with the patient in supine position) has high sensitivity (97–99%) but low specificity (85–89%), especially in patients aged over 60 years. However, high plasma normetanephrine/norepinephrine ratio or metanephrine/epinephrine ratio is strongly predictive of phaeochromocytoma. Good correlation has been found between tumour size, location and plasma metanephrine concentrations. Negative values reliably exclude phaeochromocytoma.

Urinary catecholamine metabolites

Historically, 24-hour urine collection for total catecholamines, vanillylmandelic acid (catecholamine metabolite), metanephrines and creatinine are used for diagnosis. The 24-hour urinary fractionated metanephrines have comparable sensitivity (96–97%) and have been recommended as the first investigation in patients with a lower suspicion of phaeochromocytoma. In comparison, a 24-hour urinary collection for catecholamines and metanephrines has a sensitivity of 87.5% and a specificity of 99.7% (Table 100.1). The collection container should be dark and acidified and kept cold to avoid degradation of catecholamines. Optimally, urine should be collected during or immediately after a hypertensive emergency. A number of medications and conditions may cause false-positive results in the biochemical investigation of phaeochromocytoma (Table 100.1).

Clonidine suppression test

This test is useful when plasma catecholamine and metanephrine results are borderline. Plasma epinephrine and norepinephrine are measured before and 3 hours after oral administration of 0.3 mg clonidine. Failure of clonidine to reduce plasma epinephrine and norepinephrine by more than 50% of basal values is highly suggestive of phaeochromocytoma.

Investigations to localise phaeochromocytoma

Localisation should be initiated only after unequivocal biochemical evidence of a phaeochromocytoma and is targeted at locating both primary and metastatic disease. Treatment of phaeochromocytoma depends critically on accurate localisation as it confirms tumour sites and helps in surgical strategy.

CT or MRI

CT has a sensitivity of 93–100% for detecting adrenal tumours of 0.5–1 cm in size, and of 90% for detecting extra-adrenal tumours (Figure 100.1).

MRI is marginally more sensitive than CT and has other advantages. T2-weighted MRI with gadolinium can be used in the pregnant patient and in children and in patients allergic to contrast, and for extra-adrenal, juxtacardiac and juxtavascular phaeochromocytomas. Phaeochromocytomas appear as a hyperdense lesion on MRI. The sensitivity of both MRI and CT decreases to below 91% when the tumour is extra-adrenal, metastatic or recurrent.

Radionuclide scans

^{123}I-labelled metaiodobenzylguanidine (MIBG) scans can detect recurrent or metastatic phaeochromocytoma, extra-adrenal tumours, tumours with fibrosis or distorted anatomy, or in unusual locations. The specificity of MIBG is 95–100%. Labetalol and tricyclic antidepressants can give rise to false-negative results as they prevent uptake of MIBG at sympatho-medullary tissue. These should be withdrawn for five half-life days.

Octreotide scan can localise adrenal phaeochromocytomas, but has a lower sensitivity than MIBG (20–50%). It is only used in cases of negative MIBG scans. In extra-adrenal phaeochromocytomas, MIBG has a lower sensitivity (72%) than octreotide scan (96%), especially in the head and neck.

PET

PET imaging is reserved for cases where biochemical testing is positive and conventional imaging does not locate the tumour.

Genetic testing

The indications for genetic tests are listed in Table 100.2. Germline mutations in five genes are responsible for hereditary phaeochromocytomas and paragangliomas, and are found in 25% of sporadic phaeochromocytomas:

- *RET* proto-oncogene mutations in MEN type 2;
- *VHL* gene mutations leading to VHL syndrome;
- neurofibromatosis type 1 (*NF1*) gene (von Recklinghausen's disease);
- genes encoding succinate dehydrogenase subunits D (*SDHD*) and B (*SDHB*) are associated with familial non-syndromic phaeochromocytomas and paragangliomas.

101 Primary hyperaldosteronism

The goal of investigation in primary hyperaldosteronism is to:
- Provide screening tests in selected patients
- Perform confirmatory investigations in patients with positive screening test
- Classify the subtype of PHA
- Consider genetic test

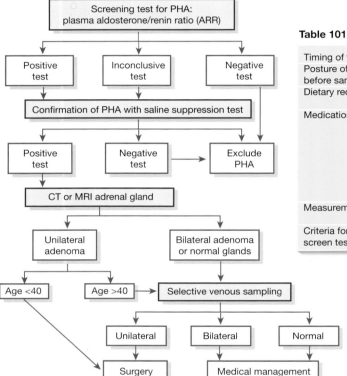

Box 101.1 Indications for screening PHA

- Hypertension with hypokalaemia
- Resistant or severe hypertension (suboptimal control with three antihypertensive medications)
- Adrenal incidentaloma and hypertension
- Onset of hypertension at young age (<40 years old)
- Patients with untreated hypertension who have a low-normal serum potassium level

Table 101.1 Screening test for PHA

Timing of the test	Morning
Posture of the patient before sampling	Seated in ambulant patient
Dietary requirements	None. Do not restrict dietary sodium intake prior to testing
Medications	Diuretics (including spironolactone) are stopped for 4 weeks Beta-blockers and dihydropyridine calcium channel antagonists are stopped for 2 weeks ACE inhibitors and angiotensin II receptor blockers (ARBs) are not routinely withdrawn, but there is the possibility that these agents could produce a false-negative result
Measurement	Plasma aldosterone concentration (PAC)/plasma renin activity (PRA) gives aldosterone/renin ratio (ARR)
Criteria for positive screen test	Increased PAC >8ng/dL, reduced PRA <0.2 ng/mL per hour, and ARR >25

Table 101.2 Effects of drugs on plasma renin activity and aldosterone

Drug	Effect on plasma renin activity	Effect on aldosterone
Diuretics	↑	↑
Spironolactone	↑	Variable
Calcium channel blocker	May ↑	↓
ACE inhibitor/ARB	↑	↓
Vasodilators	↑	↑
Beta-blockers	↓	↓
NSAIDs	↓	↓

Table 101.3 Subtypes of primary hyperaldosteronism

Solitary adrenal adenoma (most common)
Bilateral micronodular or macronodular adrenal hyperplasia
Unilateral micronodular or macronodular adrenal hyperplasia
Adrenal carcinoma (rare)
Glucocorticoid-remediable aldosteronism

Key points

- A high aldosterone/renin ratio is suggestive of PHA.
- Confirmation of autonomous aldosterone production is made by demonstrating the inability to suppress aldosterone level with sodium or volume loading.
- CT or MRI of the adrenals is useful for localising adrenal adenoma but the frequency of adrenal incidentaloma increases with age.
- Adrenal vein sampling is the gold standard for differentiation between unilateral and bilateral aldosterone production.

Primary hyperaldosteronism (PHA) is the excessive autonomous adrenal secretion of aldosterone resulting in secondary hypertension and suppression of renin. The prevalence of PHA in unselected patients with hypertension is 1–2% but rises to 5–10% in patients with resistant hypertension. In contrast to PHA, secondary hyperaldosteronism is driven by high plasma renin and is suppressed by volume expansion.

Basic biochemical investigations

Hypokalaemia is not as prevalent as commonly anticipated in patients with PHA (20–37%) and the absence of hypokalaemia does not exclude PHA. Increased urinary excretion of potassium (>30 mmol/day in the presence of hypokalaemia and the absence of extra potassium intake) points to hyperaldosteronism.

Screening investigations

It is not cost-effective to screen for PHA in all patients with hypertension. The indications for screening investigations are listed in Box 101.1. Determining the ratio of plasma aldosterone level to the plasma renin activity in a subject with hypertension is the widely accepted screening method for PHA (Table 101.1) but requires care with cessation of specific medications (Table 101.2).

Confirmatory investigation

Confirmation of PHA involves demonstration of autonomous aldosterone production that cannot be suppressed by volume expansion (via saline infusion), oral sodium loading, or fludrocortisone suppression or captopril challenge. These confirmatory investigations should be performed when the patient is in an untreated state or after medications have been withheld for an adequate period of time (Table 101.2). If the patient has severe hypertension, prazosin or verapamil treatment is least likely to affect measurements of renin and aldosterone. After oral salt loading (>200 mmol, or about 6 g, per day for 3 days) PHA is unlikely if urinary aldosterone is lower than 10 µg per 24 hours (27.7 nmol/day) in the absence of renal disease. Elevated urinary aldosterone excretion (>12 µg per 24 hours, >33.3 nmol/day) makes PA highly likely.

Subtype investigation

The histopathological expression of PHA is highly variable (Table 101.3). Correctly establishing the subtype is important in guiding therapy, which ranges from curative surgical removal or, in bilateral disease, medical management with mineralocorticoid receptor antagonists. There is considerable overlap between subtypes, and the morphological appearance does not necessarily predict the precise site of aldosterone overproduction. Incidental adrenal adenomas are common (see Chapter 98) and the finding of an adrenal adenoma on CT, particularly in a patient over 40 years old, does not confirm a solitary aldosterone-secreting adrenal adenoma. The aim of investigating is to answer the following questions.

• Does the patient have a large adrenal mass lesion (>4 cm) or with features concerning for cancer? If so, it may warrant removal based on its malignant potential.

• Is aldosterone production confined to one adrenal gland (treated with unilateral adrenalectomy) or is it bilateral (medical management with aldosterone antagonists)?

• Any adrenal mass which is not removed should undergo repeat CT at 6 months, then 12 months (if no change at 6 months) and then at intervals of 3–5 years thereafter.

Subtype determination can be achieved by the following investigations.

CT of the adrenals

CT imaging of the adrenal glands is used to exclude an adrenocorticoid carcinoma. The finding of a large adrenal tumour (>4 cm) or other concerning features (see Chapter 98, Table 98.1) should raise the possibility that the patient has adrenal carcinoma. The CT scan should not be relied on to distinguish between unilateral and bilateral disease.

Adrenal vein sampling

Adrenal vein sampling, if both veins can be catheterised successfully, is the most reliable method of localising the abnormal adrenal gland. Aldosterone and cortisol are measured in the adrenal venous effluent and a sample from the inferior vena cava in order to evaluate the accuracy and success of adrenal venous sampling. If the blood sampling is reliable, it has 95% sensitivity and 100% specificity for detecting unilateral aldosterone excess, which usually suggests the presence of an aldosterone-secreting adrenal adenoma but in some cases the diagnosis may be unilateral adrenal hyperplasia. In contrast, CT has only 78% sensitivity and 75% specificity, and can be misleading by demonstrating unilateral nodules in patients with bilateral disease.

Genetic testing

Glucocorticoid remediable hyperaldosteronism (GRA) is a monogenic form transmitted as an autosomal dominant disease and responsible for less than 1% of PHA. GRA is due to recombination between the genes coding for CYP11B1 (11β-hydroxylase) and CYP11B2 (aldosterone synthase). Diagnosis of GRA is commonly made by genetic testing. Genetic testing for GRA is recommended for patients with onset of PHA before 20 years of age and in those with a family history of PHA or strokes at a young age. Patients with GRA can be treated with low-dose long-acting glucocorticoids, which usually lower the blood pressure to or towards normal.

There are other causes of familial PHA, including autosomal dominant familial hyperaldosteronism type II. The clinical features and management of this condition are identical to those for sporadic PHA but family screening should be considered.

Post-adrenalectomy investigations

In surgically treated PHA, plasma aldosterone and renin activity can be measured after adrenalectomy to determine if the offending lesion has been successfully removed.

Male hypogonadism

The purpose of investigations is to:
- Establish the diagnosis of hypogonadism
- Determine if the hypogonadism is primary or secondary and the underlying cause
- Evaluate suitability for testosterone replacement and monitoring of treatment effects

Indications to screen for hypogonadism
- Pituitary mass, following radiation involving the sellar region and other diseases in the hypothalamic and sellar region
- End-stage renal disease receiving renal replacement treatment
- Treatment with medications that cause suppression of testosterone levels, such as corticosteroids and opiates
- Moderate to severe COPD
- Infertility
- Osteoporosis or low-trauma fractures
- Type 2 diabetes

Symptoms and signs suggestive of hypogonadism
- Erectile dysfunction
- Infertility, low sperm count
- Reduced libido
- Hot flushes and sweats
- Loss of male body hair
- Low-trauma fracture
- Gynaecomastia
- Muscle weakness and wasting

Table 102.1 Causes of primary and secondary hypogonadism

	Congenital	Acquired
Primary hypogonadism	Klinefelter's syndrome Y-chromosome microdeletions Mutations to LH and FSH receptors Myotonic dystrophy Cryptorchidism	Testicular trauma/torsion Orchitis (mumps) Chemotherapy Medications, e.g. ketoconazole Autoimmune testicular failure Haemochromatosis Cirrhosis Excessive alcohol intake
Secondary hypogonadism	Kallmann's syndrome Prader–Willi syndrome	Hyperprolactinaemia Pituitary damage: Tumour Apoplexy Infection Infiltrative disease Head trauma Acute systemic illness Medications, e.g. androgen blockade Morbid obesity or diabetes Idiopathic

Table 102.2 Conditions that can affect serum concentration of SHBG

Increased concentrations	Decreased concentrations
Ageing Hyperthyroidism Hyperestrogenaemia Liver disease HIV Use of anticonvulsants	Obesity Insulin resistance and diabetes mellitus Hypothyroidism Growth hormone excess Glucocorticoids Androgens Progestins Nephrotic syndrome

Flow chart:

Morning total testosterone
- Normal → No further investigation
- Low total testosterone → Repeat total testosterone or check free testosterone + FSH, LH
  - Normal testosterone, LH, FSH
  - Low testosterone, low FSH, LH → Secondary hypogonadism → Prolactin, iron study, TSH and MRI brain
  - Low testosterone, high FSH, LH → Primary hypogonadism → Karyotype Klinefelter's syndrome

Key points
- A morning (9 a.m.) serum testosterone is essential in the evaluation of testicular function because of the diurnal variation in circulating levels.
- Concentrations of SHBG should be taken into account when interpreting a serum testosterone level.
- FSH and LH are elevated in primary testicular failure and inappropriately low in pituitary or hypothalamic hypogonadism.
- Patients on testosterone replacement therapy should undergo repeat testosterone measurements every 3–6 months in the first year and annually thereafter. Haemoglobin and PSA should also be evaluated.

Clinical Investigations at a Glance, First Edition. Jonathan Gleadle, Jordan Li and Tuck Yong. © 2017 John Wiley & Sons, Ltd. Published 2017 by John Wiley & Sons, Ltd.

Male hypogonadism is a clinical syndrome caused by androgen deficiency. Androgens play a crucial role in the development and maintenance of male reproductive and sexual functions. Testosterone levels decrease as a process of ageing, with an average annual decline in circulating testosterone of 0.4–2.0%. Hypogonadism exerts a wide range of effects on various organs, such as decreased muscle formation and bone mineralisation, disturbances of fat metabolism, cognitive dysfunction and quality of life. The incidence of hypogonadism in middle-aged men is about 6%. It is more prevalent in older men, in men with obesity, those with comorbidities, and in men with poor health status and occurs deliberately in the endocrine treatment of prostate cancer. Hypogonadism can be classified as:
- primary hypogonadism, caused by testicular disease;
- secondary hypogonadism, due to dysfunction of the hypothalamic–pituitary axis.

In primary hypogonadism, serum testosterone concentration is substantially lower, spermatogenesis is impaired and gonadotrophin levels are raised. Secondary hypogonadism is characterised by low testosterone, reduced spermatogenesis and low or inappropriately normal levels of gonadotrophins. Both forms can arise from numerous congenital and acquired disorders (Table 102.1).

The clinical features of hypogonadism vary depending on age of onset, severity of testosterone deficiency, and androgen sensitivity of an individual. Postpubertal onset can lead to decreases in libido, spontaneous erections, testicular volume, bone mass and muscle mass.

The diagnosis of male hypogonadism is based on persistent symptoms and signs associated with androgen deficiency as well as consistently low testosterone levels (on at least two occasions).

Confirm the diagnosis of hypogonadism

The best initial test for the diagnosis of hypogonadism is the measurement of total serum testosterone in a morning sample on at least two occasions. Testosterone is secreted in a circadian rhythm, with peaks in the morning and troughs during the evening. Total testosterone includes:
- 58% bound loosely to albumin;
- 40% bound tightly to sex hormone-binding globulin (SHBG);
- 0.5–2.0% circulating in free form, which is the fraction taken to be biologically active.

Bioavailable testosterone refers to free plus albumin-bound testosterone. Total testosterone concentration cannot be measured accurately if SHBG levels are affected by other conditions (Table 102.2). Therefore, measurement of free or bioavailable testosterone is indicated if these conditions are suspected. Reference ranges for the lower normal level of testosterone have been compiled from large community-based samples, suggesting a cut-off of 12.1 nmol/L for total serum testosterone and 243 pmol/L for calculated free testosterone to distinguish between normal levels and levels possibly associated with deficiency.

Differentiate primary and secondary hypogonadism

After the initial diagnosis, gonadotrophins should be measured to determine if the patient has primary or secondary hypogonadism. Raised gonadotrophins would suggest primary hypogonadism. Karyotyping should be used to evaluate for Klinefelter's syndrome (XXY). If gonadotrophins are low or inappropriately normal, secondary hypogonadism should be considered. Serum prolactin and other pituitary hormones should be measured and iron studies done.

Radiological investigation

Patients with hyperprolactinaemia, symptoms of mass effect and panhypopituitarism should undergo MRI of the sella turcica (see Chapters 95 and 97).

Investigations for the consequence of hypogonadism

In men presenting with infertility, semen analysis should be done. Bone densitometry should be performed in men with confirmed hypogonadism.

Investigations before testosterone replacement therapy and treatment monitoring

Testosterone replacement therapy has a number of adverse effects. Therefore, the following tests should be done before commencing replacement therapy and monitored during the treatment.
- Testosterone: titre dose to maintain testosterone levels in the normal range.
- PSA: check at baseline in all men over 60 years, check at 3–6 months after the start of therapy and annually thereafter.
- Haemoglobin: check at baseline as testosterone can stimulate erythropoiesis; haemoglobin levels check at 6-month intervals after the start of therapy and annually thereafter.
- Sleep apnoea: assess symptoms and evaluate with polysomnography.
- Bone density: measure at baseline and repeat every 1–2 years if indicated.

Population screening

Population-level screening for hypogonadism is currently not recommended because its cost-effectiveness and effects on public health are unclear. However in patients with conditions listed opposite, screening for hypogonadism should be performed.

103 Infertility

Table 103.1 Causes of female and male infertility

Causes of female infertility	Causes of male infertility
• Ovulation dysfunctions (25%)	• Abnormal semen production (30–40%)
• Ovulatory disorders (25%)	• Disorders of sperm transport (10–20%)
• Endometriosis (15%)	• Primary hypogonadism (10–15%)
• Pelvic adhesions (12%)	• Seminiferous tubule dysfunction (6–10%)
• Tubal blockage (11%)	• Secondary hypogonadism
• Other tubal abnormalities (11%)	• Drugs
• Hyperprolactinaemia	• Erectile dysfunction
• Systemic diseases	• Systemic diseases
• Genetic disorders	• Genetic disorders
• Idiopathic infertility	• Idiopathic infertility

Table 103.2 Standard semen analysis and normal values

Parameter	Normal reference value
Volume	2–6 mL
pH	>7.2
Concentration	>15 million sperm/mL
Total sperm number	>39 million per ejaculate
Motility	>50% with forward progression
Vitality	>58% live spermatozoa
Morphology	>35% normal
Leucocyte count	<1 million/mL
Microscopy for agglutination	
Search for immature germ cells	

Figure 103.1 Evaluation of female infertility

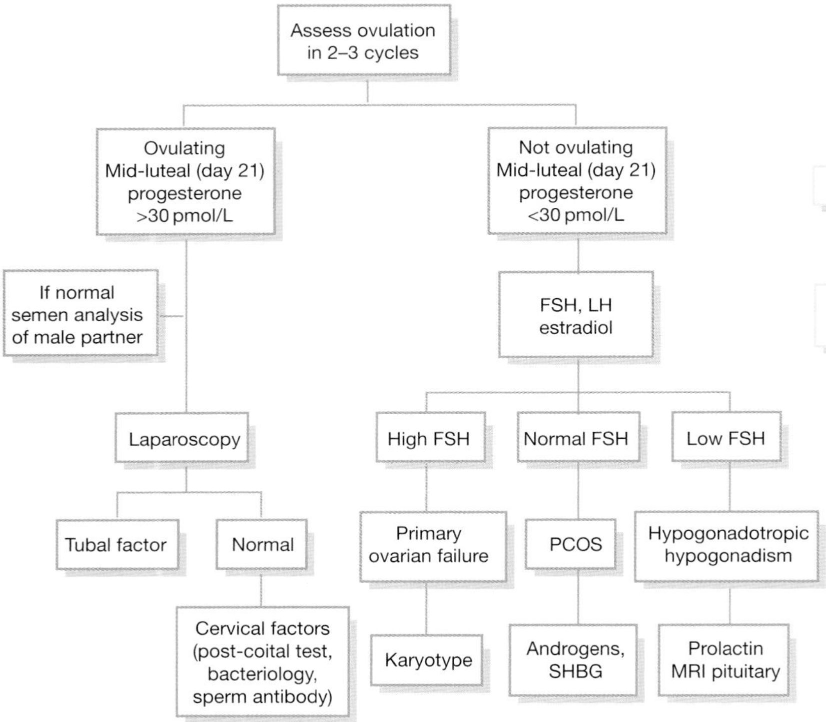

Figure 103.2 Evaluation of male infertility

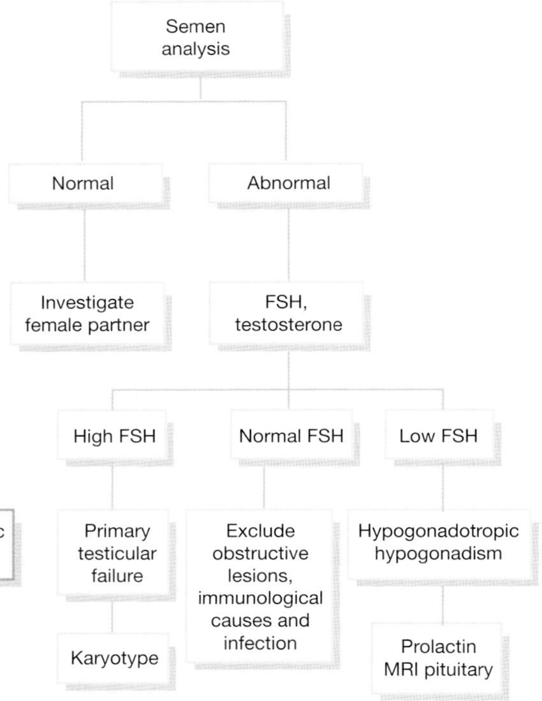

Key points

- In female infertility, evaluation begins with an assessment of ovulatory function by measuring a mid-luteal (day 21) progesterone.
- In male infertility, semen analysis is essential in addition to the clinical assessment.
- Karyotyping may be helpful in females with primary ovarian failure or males with primary testicular failure.
- Pelvic or transvaginal ultrasound is used to assess uterine and ovarian anatomy.

Infertility can be defined as the failure of a couple to conceive after 12 months of frequent intercourse without contraception (Table 103.1).

Initial infertility assessment

The evaluation should be initiated after 6 months of unprotected intercourse in women between the ages of 35 and 40 years and immediate evaluation in those over 40 years. Early evaluation of the male partner may be warranted if there is a history of testicular trauma requiring treatment, adult mumps, impotence or other sexual dysfunction, or chemotherapy and/or radiation. It is very important to evaluate both the female and the male partner, as a diagnosis of infertility can be made only on the basis of the results of assessments of both partners. General medical, reproductive, gynaecological and family history together with physical examination should be performed first as it will point the direction of further investigation. The focus should include:

- factors contributing to ovulatory dysfunction;
- risk factors for tubal infertility;
- assessment of body mass index (BMI) and thyroid function;
- signs of hyperandrogenism such as hirsutism;
- a cervical smear if indicated;
- bimanual examination.

Investigating female infertility (Figure 103.1)

Assessing ovulation

The most appropriate test for detecting ovulation is a serum progesterone concentration. If the menstrual cycle is irregular, a mid-luteal (18–24 days after the onset of menses) serum progesterone should be obtained. A level above 3 ng/mL is diagnostic of ovulation. Lower values suggest either anovulation or inappropriate timing of the blood test. A low concentration should be rechecked by taking two measurements of progesterone a week apart in the next cycle. In patients with amenorrhoea (after excluding pregnancy), a progestin challenge test may be usedd to verify ovarian estradiol production and the presence of a normal outflow tract. A progestin (e.g. medroxyprogesterone acetate 10 mg/day orally for 5 days) is administered and if bleeding occurs in the week after the challenge, then significant estrogen is present and able to affect the endometrium and the outflow tract is patent. Measurement of serum testosterone is sufficient to exclude ovarian or adrenal tumours as a cause of hyperandrogenism and infertility. To evaluate other causes of infertility, prolactin and thyroid function may be measured.

Assessing ovarian reserve

The following investigations can be performed to identify a depleted ovarian reserve, although none is completely accurate.
- Anti-mullerian hormone measurement.
- FSH levels: if the FSH is elevated, ovarian reserve is reduced. FSH level above 20–30 IU/L on day 3 of menstrual cycle suggests ovarian failure, but this test should be repeated on several occasions as the condition of ovarian failure fluctuates remarkably.
- Clomiphene challenge test.

- Ultrasound of the ovaries can determine either ovarian volume or antral follicle count, which is used for estimating a woman's ovarian reserve. The number of antral follicles visible on ultrasound is indicative of the relative number of primordial follicles remaining in the ovary. Ultrasound can also assess the thickness of endometrium and monitor follicle development.

Assessment of tubal patency

Hysterosalpingogram is the initial test for tubal patency and uterine cavity. It has high specificity (83%) for confirming tubal patency but is less sensitive (65%) for diagnosing tubal occlusion due to a high false-positive rate and is unreliable in the evaluation of peritubal adhesions or endometriosis.

Other investigations

Laparoscopy is indicated in women with unexplained infertility and a suspicion of endometriosis or pelvic adhesions due to a history of pelvic pain and/or previous surgery or infection. Hysteroscopy and endometrial biopsy and mycoplasma cultures have limited utility in the investigation of female infertility.

Investigating male infertility (Figure 103.2)

Semen analysis (Table 103.2)

A semen specimen should be produced, after 3 days abstinence from ejaculation, into a clean jar and delivered to the laboratory within 30 min. Because of inherent variability of semen analysis, at least two samples should be collected 1–2 weeks apart. It is difficult to predict pregnancy based on semen analysis alone because there is extensive overlap between the semen parameters of fertile and infertile men. Lack of sperm in the ejaculate does not indicate the absence of testicular sperm production as it may be due to retrograde ejaculation, congenital absence of vas deferens and other causes of obstructive azoospermia.

A low semen volume in the presence of azoospermia (no sperm) or severe oligospermia (severely subnormal sperm concentration) suggests genital tract obstruction. Congenital absence of vas deferens is diagnosed by physical examination and low semen pH, whereas ejaculatory duct obstruction is diagnosed by the finding of dilated seminal vesicles on transrectal ultrasound.

Males with sperm counts below 15 million/mL will have difficulty in being fertile. Sperm motility is evaluated microscopically and is classified as rapid progressive motility, slow progressive motility, non-progressive motility and non-motility. At least 50% of spermatozoa should be motile and at least 25% should have rapid progressive motility. If sperm motility is poor, sperm vitality should be assessed to determine whether the majority of immotile spermatozoa are dead. The distinction between living, non-moving or dead sperm affects the type of assisted reproductive treatment that can be offered.

Other investigations

- Hormone testing: the level of testosterone should be measured as it plays a key role in sexual development and sperm production.
- Testicular biopsy: to determine if sperm production is normal.

104 Erectile dysfunction

The goals of investigation for ED are to:
- Assess the severity of ED
- Determine if it is psychogenic or organic in origin
- Identify significant underlying medical disease or comorbid diseases
- Identify those for whom specific medical therapy may be beneficial
- Assess cardiovascular risk factors and sexual activity

Box 104.1 First and second-line investigations for ED

- Medical, sexual and psychosocial history
- Physical examination with focus on cardiovascular, neurological, gonadal and genital systems
- First-line investigations:
  - FBC
  - Blood glucose level
  - Serum creatinine
  - Liver function tests
  - Lipid study
  - PSA (age >50 years)
  - TSH
- Consider endocrinological hormone tests in appropriate patients:
  - Prolactin
  - Total testosterone
  - SHBG in obese subjects, men aged >60 years, patients affected by endocrine disease
  - LH
- Second-line investigations:
  - History, examination and first-line investigations should guide the second-line investigations
  - PDU
  - Angiography/cavernosography
  - MRI
  - Nocturnal penile tumescence and rigidity testing, ultrasound and neurological testing

Table 104.1 Common organic causes of ED

- Cardiovascular disease
- Diabetes mellitus
- Hypertension
- Hyperlipidaemia
- Hypogonadism
- Chronic kidney disease
- Congestive heart failure
- Spinal cord injury
- Multiple sclerosis
- Parkinson's disease
- Radical prostatectomy
- Medications, alcohol
- Penile injury/anatomical abnormalities (e.g. Peyronie's disease, priapism)

Figure 104.1 Penile Doppler ultrasound

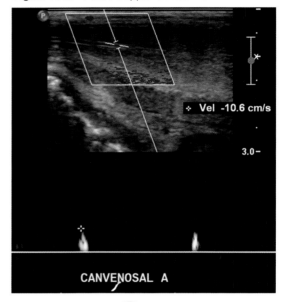

Vel -10.6 cm/s

3.0 —

CANVENOSAL A

Key points

- Baseline investigation of ED should include pituitary–gonadal hormones, thyroid function tests, biochemistry (kidney and liver function) and serum ferritin.
- ED may be an early marker of subclinical metabolic and cardiovascular disease and appropriate investigations (fasting glucose, lipid studies) should be performed.
- Penile duplex ultrasonography has limited diagnostic value for ED.

Clinical Investigations at a Glance, First Edition. Jonathan Gleadle, Jordan Li and Tuck Yong. © 2017 John Wiley & Sons, Ltd. Published 2017 by John Wiley & Sons, Ltd.

Erectile dysfunction (ED) is the inability to obtain or maintain a penile erection sufficient for successful sexual intercourse. ED is the preferred term to impotence. This is a common medical condition affecting approximately 50% of men aged between 40 and 70 years at some stage, with 10% of these affected severely. It is important to distinguish ED from ejaculatory disorders including premature ejaculation. ED is a strong predictor for coronary artery and peripheral vascular disease.

A full history including sexual history and thorough physical examination are needed to confirm that the patient is experiencing ED. ED is considered a disorder with multiple causes. Approximately 80% of ED cases are of organic origin (Table 104.1) and 20% are psychogenic. Clinical examination should include assessment of the external genitalia, endocrine and cardiovascular systems and the prostate gland. ED is a symptom, not a disease.

The degree to which further investigations are required will depend on the patient's history and examination findings. Extensive investigations are not usually justified.

Laboratory investigations

Basic laboratory investigations which should be performed are listed in Box 104.1. Investigations for cardiovascular diseases and risk factors should be performed in patient presenting with ED. The threshold of testosterone to maintain ED is low and ED is usually a symptom of more severe cases of hypogonadism. For levels above 8 nmol/L the relationship between circulating testosterone and sexual function is very low. Further investigations include serum LH and prolactin.

Specific investigations

The routine use of specific investigations in ED is not advisable. Such investigations should be reserved for those patients with little or no response to medications including the phosphodiesterase (PDE)5 inhibitors (e.g. sildenafil).

Penile Doppler ultrasound

Penile Doppler ultrasound (PDU) is the most informative investigation. It can examine penile structure and cavernosal and dorsal penile arteries (Figure 104.1). PDU can also provide information about penile haemodynamics after maximal smooth muscle relaxation has been induced with a vasoactive agent. The aim of this investigation is to differentiate arterial insufficiency and veno-occlusive dysfunction from other causes of ED. Ultrasound can demonstrate alternative pathologies such as plaques, areas of fibrosis and defects in the tunica albuginea once full tumescence has been achieved that may cause ED. Peyronie's disease is a localised benign connective tissue disorder with an unknown aetiology that results in fibrous thickening of the penile tunica albuginea.

Angiography/cavernosography

Catheter angiography is reserved for those patients with a suspected stenotic or occlusive lesion causing arterial insufficiency. It is considered a second-line investigation utilised as an adjunct to ultrasound. Cavernosography is a technique utilising injection of contrast medium into the cavernosa to detect defects in the veno-occlusive mechanism that are causing leaks.

MRI

MRI readily demonstrates penile anatomy, with both the cavernosa and spongiosum displaying intermediate to high signal on T1-weighted sequences and high signal on T2-weighted sequences. Peyronie's disease plaques and haematoma resulting from penile trauma/fracture can also be well visualised. MRI is utilised almost exclusively as a second-line 'problem-solving' modality in those cases where structural abnormality has been demonstrated but requires further characterisation.

Nocturnal penile tumescence and rigidity testing

This evaluates the frequency, duration and rigidity of nocturnal erections. It is considered the gold standard test in distinguishing between psychogenic and organic ED.

105 Amenorrhoea

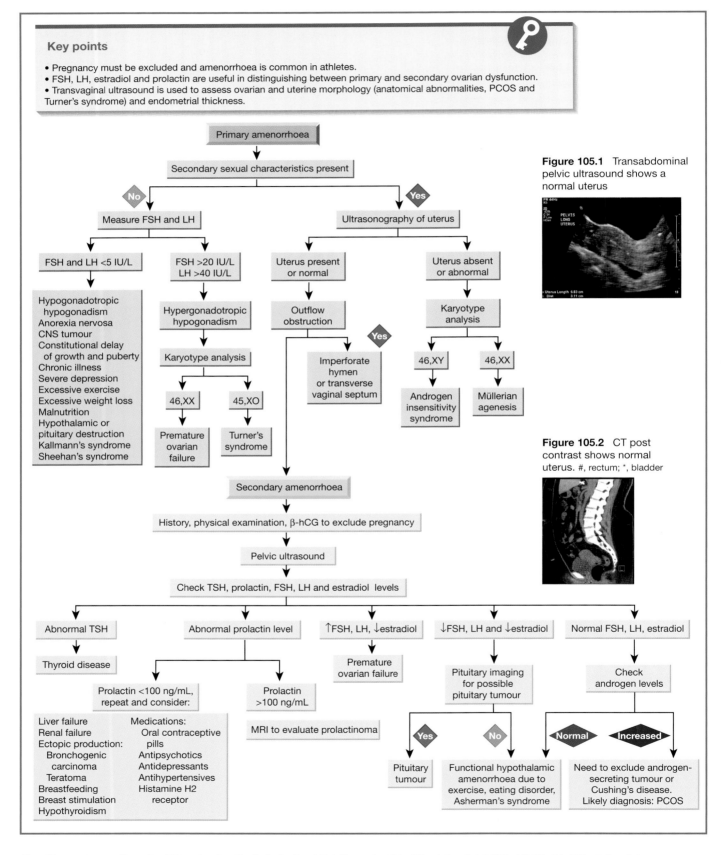

Primary amenorrhoea

Secondary sexual characteristics present

No → Measure FSH and LH

Yes → Ultrasonography of uterus

FSH and LH <5 IU/L

FSH >20 IU/L LH >40 IU/L

Uterus present or normal

Uterus absent or abnormal

Hypogonadotropic hypogonadism
Anorexia nervosa
CNS tumour
Constitutional delay of growth and puberty
Chronic illness
Severe depression
Excessive exercise
Excessive weight loss
Malnutrition
Hypothalamic or pituitary destruction
Kallmann's syndrome
Sheehan's syndrome

Hypergonadotropic hypogonadism → Karyotype analysis

46,XX → Premature ovarian failure

45,XO → Turner's syndrome

Outflow obstruction

Yes → Imperforate hymen or transverse vaginal septum

Karyotype analysis

46,XY → Androgen insensitivity syndrome

46,XX → Müllerian agenesis

Secondary amenorrhoea

History, physical examination, β-hCG to exclude pregnancy

Pelvic ultrasound

Check TSH, prolactin, FSH, LH and estradiol levels

Abnormal TSH → Thyroid disease

Abnormal prolactin level

↑FSH, LH, ↓estradiol → Premature ovarian failure

↓FSH, LH and ↓estradiol → Pituitary imaging for possible pituitary tumour

Normal FSH, LH, estradiol → Check androgen levels

Prolactin <100 ng/mL, repeat and consider:

Prolactin >100 ng/mL → MRI to evaluate prolactinoma

Liver failure
Renal failure
Ectopic production:
  Bronchogenic carcinoma
  Teratoma
Breastfeeding
Breast stimulation
Hypothyroidism

Medications:
  Oral contraceptive pills
  Antipsychotics
  Antidepressants
  Antihypertensives
  Histamine H2 receptor

Yes → Pituitary tumour

No → Functional hypothalamic amenorrhoea due to exercise, eating disorder, Asherman's syndrome

Normal / **Increased** → Need to exclude androgen-secreting tumour or Cushing's disease. Likely diagnosis: PCOS

Figure 105.1 Transabdominal pelvic ultrasound shows a normal uterus

Figure 105.2 CT post contrast shows normal uterus. #, rectum; *, bladder

Amenorrhoea is the absence of menstruation, which can be transient, intermittent or permanent. It is classified as follows.

• Physiological amenorrhoea: before the menarche, after the menopause, in pregnancy, or post hysterectomy.

• Primary amenorrhoea: the absence of menarche by age 16.

• Secondary amenorrhoea: the absence of menses for over 6 months in a woman who has previously menstruated.

Primary amenorrhoea is usually the result of a genetic or anatomical abnormality. All causes of secondary amenorrhoea can also present as primary amenorrhoea. After excluding pregnancy, the causes of secondary amenorrhoea are usually the direct failure of some part of hypothalamic–pituitary–ovarian–uterine axis or other metabolic disease that secondarily affects the function of the axis.

A thorough history and detailed physical examination is essential. In the differential diagnosis of primary or secondary amenorrhea, the most important step in diagnosis is to exclude pregnancy by measurement of serum hCG. After pregnancy is excluded, the next step is to decide whether patient has primary or secondary amenorrhoea.

Primary amenorrhoea

The first task in a patient with primary amenorrhoea is to differentiate a genetic or congenital anatomical abnormality from delayed puberty.

Initial investigations

Initial evaluation of a woman with primary amenorrhoea depends on the findings on physical examination, in particular whether Müllerian structures (vagina, cervix or uterus) are present or absent. If a normal vagina or uterus is absent, pelvic ultrasound should be performed to confirm the presence or absence of ovaries, uterus and cervix and to look for vaginal or cervical outlet obstruction in patients with cyclical pain.

Next line of investigations

Uterus absent

With absence of the uterus, further evaluation should include karyotyping and measurement of serum testosterone. These tests should allow the differentiation of abnormal Müllerian development (46,XX karyotype with normal female serum testosterone level) and androgen insensitivity syndrome (46,XY karyotype and normal male serum testosterone level).

Uterus present (Figures 105.1 and 105.2)

For patients with normal Müllerian structures and no evidence of an imperforate hymen, vaginal septum, congenital absence of the vagina or pregnancy, endocrine investigations should be performed as outlined in the section on secondary amenorrhoea.

Secondary amenorrhoea

The causes of secondary amenorrhoea can be situated at one of four levels: hypothalamic, pituitary, ovarian and uterine. The first step is to assess the length of time that secondary sex characteristics have been present without menses starting. If this is more than 3 years, the focus of investigation should be to confirm the absence of uterus, an obstructing vaginal septum or androgen insensitivity. If secondary sex characteristics are absent, it indicates absence or malfunction of the ovaries or a defect in the higher above-mentioned axis.

Initial laboratory investigations

Prolactin, TFT, LH and FSH should be measured. A high serum FSH concentration indicates ovarian failure or absence. This test should be repeated monthly on three occasions to confirm the persistent elevation. Intermittent follicle development does occur in ovarian failure, resulting in transient normalisation of serum FSH concentrations. If there are signs of hyperandrogenism such as hirsutism, serum dehydroepiandrosterone sulphate (DHEA-S) and testosterone should also be measured.

Next line of investigations

Elevated prolactin

Prolactin secretion can be transiently increased by stress and should be remeasured at least twice before further investigation (see Chapter 97).

Elevated androgen levels

Depending on the clinical setting, high androgen level is highly suggestive of polycystic ovary syndrome (PCOS) or may raise the possibility of an androgen-secreting tumour of the ovary or adrenal gland. Testosterone above 5.2–6.9 nmol/L (150–200 ng/mL) or DHEA-S above 13.6 μmol/L (700 μg/dL) should lead to investigation for an androgen-secreting tumour. A pelvic ultrasound is useful in patients with suspected PCOS.

Persistently elevated FSH

A karyotype should be considered in women with secondary amenorrhoea aged 30 years or younger.

Normal or low gonadotrophin levels and all other tests are normal

This set of results is one of the most common outcomes of laboratory testing in women with amenorrhoea. Women with hypothalamic amenorrhoea (e.g. associated with excessive exercise, weight loss or anorexia nervosa) have normal to low FSH, with FSH typically higher than LH. If the FSH is normal or low in combination with neurological signs or symptoms or other pituitary defects, the hypothalamic–pituitary region should be assessed with MRI or CT. No further testing is required if the onset of amenorrhoea is recent and is easily explained and there are no features suggestive of other disease.

Spontaneous premature ovarian failure

The following tests should be done to evaluate a woman with suspected premature ovarian failure:

• a pregnancy test

• serum prolactin

• serum FSH and estradiol.

Once the diagnosis of premature ovarian failure is made, other evaluation should include:

• karyotyping;

• TFT and anti-thyroid peroxidase antibodies (because of the association between spontaneous premature ovarian failure and hypothyroidism);

• anti-adrenal antibodies to evaluate for the presence of asymptomatic adrenal insufficiency.

106 Hirsutism

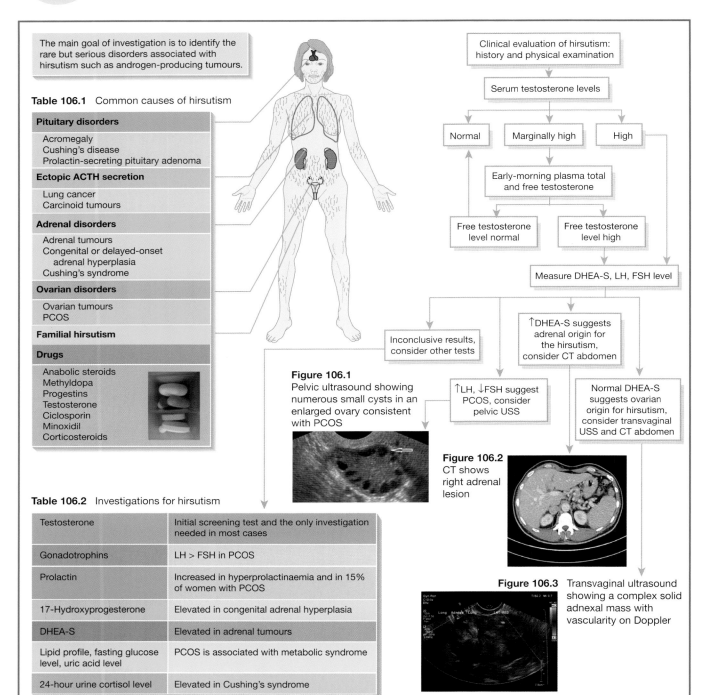

The main goal of investigation is to identify the rare but serious disorders associated with hirsutism such as androgen-producing tumours.

Table 106.1 Common causes of hirsutism

| **Pituitary disorders** |
| Acromegaly |
| Cushing's disease |
| Prolactin-secreting pituitary adenoma |
| **Ectopic ACTH secretion** |
| Lung cancer |
| Carcinoid tumours |
| **Adrenal disorders** |
| Adrenal tumours |
| Congenital or delayed-onset adrenal hyperplasia |
| Cushing's syndrome |
| **Ovarian disorders** |
| Ovarian tumours |
| PCOS |
| **Familial hirsutism** |
| **Drugs** |
| Anabolic steroids |
| Methyldopa |
| Progestins |
| Testosterone |
| Ciclosporin |
| Minoxidil |
| Corticosteroids |

Clinical evaluation of hirsutism: history and physical examination

↓

Serum testosterone levels

↓

Normal → Marginally high → High

Early-morning plasma total and free testosterone

Free testosterone level normal / Free testosterone level high

↓

Measure DHEA-S, LH, FSH level

↓

Inconclusive results, consider other tests

↑DHEA-S suggests adrenal origin for the hirsutism, consider CT abdomen

↑LH, ↓FSH suggest PCOS, consider pelvic USS

Normal DHEA-S suggests ovarian origin for hirsutism, consider transvaginal USS and CT abdomen

Figure 106.1 Pelvic ultrasound showing numerous small cysts in an enlarged ovary consistent with PCOS

Figure 106.2 CT shows right adrenal lesion

Figure 106.3 Transvaginal ultrasound showing a complex solid adnexal mass with vascularity on Doppler

Figure 106.4 CT post contrast shows a complex cystic right mass arising from right adnexa abutting uterine fundus

Table 106.2 Investigations for hirsutism

Testosterone	Initial screening test and the only investigation needed in most cases
Gonadotrophins	LH > FSH in PCOS
Prolactin	Increased in hyperprolactinaemia and in 15% of women with PCOS
17-Hydroxyprogesterone	Elevated in congenital adrenal hyperplasia
DHEA-S	Elevated in adrenal tumours
Lipid profile, fasting glucose level, uric acid level	PCOS is associated with metabolic syndrome
24-hour urine cortisol level	Elevated in Cushing's syndrome

Key points

- Testing for plasma free testosterone is 50% more sensitive than that for total testosterone in detecting androgen excess and is the best single indicator of hyperandrogenism.
- Women with mild hirsutism and normal menses do not require laboratory investigations and can be treated empirically first.
- It is important to investigate whether women with hirsutism have underlying PCOS as treatment can delay or arrest its metabolic sequelae.

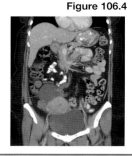

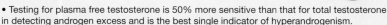

Clinical Investigations at a Glance, First Edition. Jonathan Gleadle, Jordan Li and Tuck Yong. © 2017 John Wiley & Sons, Ltd. Published 2017 by John Wiley & Sons, Ltd.

Hirsutism is excessive hair growth in women that appears in areas usually associated with male sexual maturity, such as on the face, chest, lower back, buttocks and anterior thighs. Hypertrichosis is excessive hair growth all over the body. Hirsutism results from androgenic effects on the pilosebaceous unit and is commonly associated with acne.

About 5% of women of reproductive age suffer from hirsutism. It is usually due to increased androgen production from the ovaries or adrenal glands. Elevated levels of Dehydroepiandrosterone Sulfate (DHEA-S) are virtually always of adrenal origin, while high testosterone levels may be of ovarian or adrenal origin. Regardless of the etiology, women with hyperandrogenism often have irregular menses, anovulation, infertility, and a risk of endometrial hyperplasia or neoplasia.

Virilisation is an extreme degree of hirsutism that may include male pattern baldness and other hyperandrogenic effects on female genitalia and body such as voice deepening, increased muscle bulk and clitoral enlargement. Virilisation is a sign of high and often rapid androgen production, suggesting an androgen-secreting tumour.

More than 90% of women with hirsutism have the relatively benign conditions of idiopathic hirsutism or polycystic ovary syndrome (PCOS). Other causes include hyperprolactinaemia, congenital adrenal hyperplasia, insulin resistance syndromes, Cushing's syndrome, ovarian tumours and adrenal tumours. Medications such as danazol and levonorgestrel can also cause hirsutism (Table 106.1). The investigations needed to thoroughly evaluate the patient for all possible causes of hirsutism are expensive and time-consuming. Therefore, it is neither possible nor necessary to perform all these tests in all patients.

Androgen studies (Table 106.2)

Androgen studies are the first investigation. The finding of only mildly elevated total testosterone provides an assurance that sinister causes such as a tumour or congenital adrenal hyperplasia are unlikely. Further work-up is generally not necessary unless hirsutism progresses despite therapy or features such as menstrual irregularity, obesity or increasing masculinisation. Free testosterone should be measured in patients with such features, even if total testosterone is not clearly increased.

Very high levels of total testosterone (>6.94 nmol/L or >200 ng/dL or 100% above the normal range) or DHEA-S (>19 μmol/L or >700 μg/dL) or testosterone/SHBG ratio three times above normal are regarded as highly suspicious for androgen-producing tumour or congenital adrenal hyperplasia and warrant additional investigations.

Assessment of free testosterone level in the early morning (ideally on days 4–10 of the menstrual cycle in menstruating women) is the most sensitive measure. It is 50% more sensitive than total testosterone in detecting androgen excess and is the single best indicator of hyperandrogenism. However, a level that is measured at random usually suffices.

Routine testing for other androgens is of little use. The level of DHEA-S is increased in about 15% of women with normal levels of total and free testosterone (elevated levels of DHEA-S indicating an adrenal source).

Other investigations (Table 106.2)

If PCOS is suspected, gonadotrophin levels and estradiol should be checked (see Chapter 108). Abdominal and pelvic ultrasonographic and CT examination of adrenals and ovaries as preliminary investigation are relatively inexpensive and non-invasive tests (Figures 106.1–106.4).

If other endocrinological disorders such as Cushing's syndrome, hyperprolactinaemia and acromegaly are suspected, the relevant endocrine tests should be performed (see Chapters 96, 97 and 100).

107 # Polycystic ovary syndrome

Key features for diagnosis of polycystic ovary syndrome:
- Oligo-ovulation or anovulation
- Clinical and/or biochemical hyperandrogenism
- Polycystic ovaries on ultrasound

Box 107.1 Investigations for PCOS

- Initial investigations to exclude other conditions that can mimic PCOS
  - Pregnancy test
  - Thyroid function test
  - Serum prolactin levels
  - 24-hour urine cortisol
- Investigation for oligo-ovulation/anovulation
  - Mid-luteal progesterone levels
  - LH and FSH levels to rule out primary ovarian failure
- Investigation of hyperandrogenism
  - Measure free testosterone, SHBG and DHEA-S
- Ultrasound to confirm polycystic ovaries
- Other investigations
  - Oral glucose tolerance test
  - Lipid studies
  - Sleep study (if there is evidence of sleep-disordered breathing)

Figure 107.1 Ultrasound of the ovary shows multiple follicles in a patient with PCOS

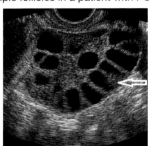

Key points

- Testosterone, SHBG and LH should be measured.
- Transvaginal or pelvic ultrasound is useful to assess ovarian morphology and endometrial thickness.
- Ultrasound findings of PCOS are >12 follicular cysts 2–9 mm in diameter or ovarian volume >10 mL.
- All women with PCOS and obesity should have an annual fasting glucose and lipid profile.

Polycystic ovary syndrome (PCOS) is one of the most common endocrine disorders in women of reproductive age, affecting about 1 in 15 women worldwide. It is estimated that 70% of women with PCOS remain undiagnosed. The pathophysiology of PCOS is unclear. The underlying hormonal imbalance includes a combination of increased androgens and/or hyperinsulinaemia secondary to insulin resistance.

Women with PCOS may present with a wide range of symptoms. In younger women, reproductive symptoms predominate. The prevalence of metabolic features increases with age. The diagnosis of PCOS is now largely based on the Rotterdam criteria, which include the original National Institutes of Health (NIH) criteria and require two of the following three features for diagnosis and exclusion of other aetiologies such as hypothyroidism, hyperprolactinaemia, congenital adrenal hyperplasia, androgen-secreting tumours and Cushing's syndrome:

- oligo-ovulation or anovulation;
- clinical and/or biochemical hyperandrogenism;
- polycystic ovaries on ultrasound.

Chronic anovulation most often manifests as oligomenorrhoea (fewer than nine menses per year) or amenorrhoea. Anovulatory cycles may lead to dysfunctional uterine bleeding and decreased fertility. Manifestations of hyperandrogenism include hirsutism, acne and male-pattern hair loss. A substantial proportion of women with PCOS are overweight or obese.

Initial investigations (Box 107.1)

The diagnosis of PCOS requires the exclusion of all other disorders that can result in menstrual irregularity and hyperandrogenism, including adrenal or ovarian tumours, thyroid dysfunction, congenital adrenal hyperplasia, hyperprolactinaemia and Cushing's syndrome. PCOS is a syndrome and there is not a single diagnostic test. Therefore, the investigations should include the following.

Tests to exclude other possible disorders

- Pregnancy test
- Thyroid function test
- Serum prolactin levels
- 24-hour urine cortisol.

Tests for oligo-ovulation/anovulation

Measurement of luteal progesterone (day 21 in a 28-day cycle) will determine ovulatory status. FSH level should be checked to rule out primary ovarian failure. In patients with PCOS, FSH levels are within the reference range or low while LH levels are elevated for Tanner stage, sex and age. The LH/FSH ratio is usually greater than 3.

Tests to confirm hyperandrogenism

Hyperandrogenaemia is best measured with free testosterone, i.e. calculated free testosterone, free androgen index (FAI) or bioavailable testosterone. FAI is defined as

$$\frac{\text{Total free testosterone}}{\text{SHBG}} \times 100$$

to give a calculated free testosterone level. Hormonal contraceptive pills can affect free testosterone levels. If appropriate, assess after 3 months' cessation. An elevated free testosterone level is a sensitive indicator of androgen excess. Other androgens, such as DHEA-S, may be normal or slightly above the normal range in patients with PCOS. Levels of SHBG are usually low in patients with PCOS. If free testosterone is significantly raised or there is evidence of rapid virilisation, further investigations are required to exclude late-onset congenital adrenal hyperplasia and virilising tumours.

Ultrasound to confirm polycystic ovaries

Ultrasound can check for polycystic ovaries and endometrial thickness. Polycystic ovaries are diagnosed when, in the follicular phase ovary, the presence of 12 or more follicles measuring 2–9 mm or increased ovarian volume (>10 mL) are seen in each ovary (Figure 107.1). A unilateral polycystic ovary is rare but still clinically significant. The role of ultrasound remains controversial in adolescence, when polycystic appearance of the ovaries is very common (70%), potentially leading to overdiagnosis. It has been suggested that transabdominal ultrasound measuring ovarian volume only is sufficient because the criterion based on follicles is less reliable by the abdominal route.

Other investigations for metabolic syndrome

Women with PCOS have a higher risk of metabolic syndrome. A 75-g oral glucose-tolerance test should be performed routinely because of the high prevalence of impaired glucose tolerance and type 2 diabetes mellitus in women with PCOS. Fasting lipids should also be assessed. Repeated measurements of glucose and lipid status should take place more regularly in women with PCOS than in those without the syndrome. Obstructive sleep apnea (OSA) is increased in PCOS and investigations should be performed in patients with clinical manifestations.

108 Pre-eclampsia and hypertensive disorders in pregnancy

The goals of investigation are to:
- Recognise the diagnosis early
- Assess the severity of pre-eclampsia
- Monitor the progression of pre-eclampsia
- Determine the best time of delivery

Table 108.1 Risk factors for pre-eclampsia

Major risk factors	Minor risk factors
• Chronic hypertension • CKD • Pre-eclampsia in a previous pregnancy • Diabetes mellitus (pre-gestational and gestational) • Antiphospholipid syndrome or inherited thrombophilia • Autoimmune diseases	• Age >40 years • Family history of pre-eclampsia • BMI >35 kg/m² • First pregnancy • Multiple pregnancy

Table 108.3 Indications for delivery in women with pre-eclampsia or hypertensive disorders

Maternal indications	Fetal indications
• Gestational age >36 weeks • Uncontrollable severe hypertension (>170/110 mmHg) • Rapid deterioration of thrombocytopenia • Deteriorating liver function • Progressive worsening renal function • Placental abruption • Eclampsia • Clinical evidence of HELLP syndrome • Acute pulmonary oedema	• Severe fetal growth restriction • Non-reassuring fetal status

Box 108.1 Laboratory investigations for pre-eclampsia
- Blood tests
  - FBC and blood film
  - Serum electrolyte, urea and creatinine
  - LFTs
  - Pre-eclampsia panel: urate, LDH, AST, ALT
- Urinalysis and microscopy
- Spot urine protein/creatinine ratio or 24-hour urine protein

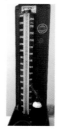

Figure 108.1 Blood pressure monitoring

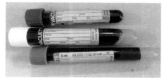

Figure 108.2 Blood tests

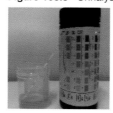

Figure 108.3 Urinalysis

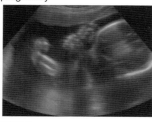

Figure 108.4 Obstetric USS shows a normal 24-week pregnancy

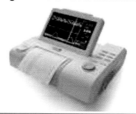

Figure 108.5 CTG monitoring

Pregnant woman with blood pressure >140/90 mmHg

<20 weeks of gestation → | Proteinuria <0.3 g per 24 hours, or stable proteinuria, history of hypertension | New or increased proteinuria, increasing blood pressures |

>20 weeks of gestation → | Proteinuria >0.3 g per 24 hours | Proteinuria <0.3 g per 24 hours |

- Proteinuria <0.3 g per 24 hours, or stable proteinuria, history of hypertension → Chronic hypertension
- New or increased proteinuria, increasing blood pressures → Pre-eclampsia superimposed on chronic hypertension
- Proteinuria >0.3 g per 24 hours → Pre-eclampsia
- Proteinuria <0.3 g per 24 hours → Gestational hypertension

Blood tests and assess severity of pre-eclampsia

Assess fetal well-being: USS, consider CTG

Table 108.2 Clinical features indicative of severe pre-eclampsia

- Severe hypertension (>170/110 mmHg) refractory to three antihypertensive medications
- Pulmonary oedema
- Persistent neurological symptoms: headache/altered mental state/clonus
- Severe epigastric pain and/or vomiting with abnormal LFTs
- Any component of HELLP syndrome
- Serum creatinine >106 μmol/L
- Fetal growth restriction

Table 108.4 Four hypertensive disorders in pregnancy

- Pre-eclampsia
- Gestational hypertension
- Chronic hypertension including primary and secondary hypertension
- Pre-eclampsia superimposed on chronic hypertension

Key points
- All pregnant women should be evaluated for pre-eclampsia at the first prenatal visit and periodically throughout the remainder of the pregnancy by measuring BP and urine dipstick.
- Laboratory tests for patients with mild pre-eclampsia and no progression include fortnightly platelet counts, LFTs, renal function and proteinuria. If disease progression is suspected, testing should be more frequent.
- A baseline ultrasound should be performed at 25–28 weeks of gestation to investigate fetal growth in pregnant women at high risk for pre-eclampsia. Weekly CTG or twice-weekly testing if oligohydramnios or fetal growth restriction is suspected and ultrasound examinations every 3 weeks are commonly recommended.

Clinical Investigations at a Glance, First Edition. Jonathan Gleadle, Jordan Li and Tuck Yong. © 2017 John Wiley & Sons, Ltd. Published 2017 by John Wiley & Sons, Ltd.

Pre-eclampsia

Pre-eclampsia is a multisystem disorder affecting 5% of pregnancies. It remains the leading cause of maternal and perinatal mortality and morbidity worldwide. Pre-eclampsia is characterised by new onset of hypertension and proteinuria (>0.3 g per 24 hours) after 20 weeks of gestation in a previously normotensive woman. Risk factors for pre-eclampsia are shown in Table 108.1.

Initial laboratory investigations

Laboratory investigations should be interpreted using pregnancy-specific ranges, some of which are gestation dependent. The laboratory investigations that should be performed if pre-eclampsia is suspected are listed in Box 108.1. Results of these investigations, combined with clinical evaluation, most notably blood pressure (BP), will provide the necessary information to diagnose and monitor the development of severe pre-eclampsia (Figures 108.1–108.3).

Further investigations in selected patients

• Extended coagulation study (coagulation studies, blood film, LDH, fibrinogen, D-dimer) if suspected disseminated intravascular coagulopathy (DIC).
• Patients with severe early-onset pre-eclampsia warrant investigation for associated conditions such as SLE, CKD, antiphospholipid syndrome or thrombophilia.

Assessment of severity of pre-eclampsia

If the patient has any of the clinical features and investigation results listed in Table 108.2, the patient is classified as having severe pre-eclampsia. Pre-eclampsia usually pursues a course of deterioration; it may evolve from mild to moderate to severe over a period of hours or days, and requires frequent reassessment.

Fetal monitoring in pre-eclampsia

The following investigations are performed to monitor fetal well-being in women with preeclampsia:
• ultrasound assessment of fetal growth, amniotic fluid volume and umbilical artery flow (Figure 108.4);
• cardiotocography (CTG) (Figure 108.5);
• biophysical profile, amniocentesis (to determine the maturation of fetal lungs) in selected cases only.
Ultrasound assessment of fetal growth should be performed every 2–3 weeks in pregnancies complicated by pre-eclampsia. Significant intrauterine growth retardation is a poor prognostic indicator and oligohydramnios should prompt frequent CTG monitoring and ultrasound examination every week.

Determine the timing for delivery in pre-eclampsia

Pre-eclampsia is a progressive disorder that tends to worsen if pregnancy continues. Delivery is the definitive treatment. Prolongation of pregnancy in the presence of pre-eclampsia carries no benefit for the mother but is desirable at early gestations to improve fetal prognosis. The timing of delivery should be individualised and investigations are performed to help in determining the timing of delivery (Table 108.3).

HELLP syndrome

HELLP (haemolysis, elevated liver enzymes and low platelet count) syndrome is a variant of severe pre-eclampsia. Maternal mortality is reported to be 1–2%. In a woman with pre-eclampsia, the presence of any of the following is an indicator of HELLP syndrome:
• thrombocytopenia (platelet count <100,000 × 10^9/L)
• haemolysis
• elevated LFTs (transaminase level or LDH more than double the normal upper limit).
Epigastric or right upper quadrant pain in a woman with pre-eclampsia often represents hepatic involvement. The investigations should include those for pre-eclampsia and also haemolysis (see Chapter 122) and an abdominal ultrasound to exclude gallbladder disorders.

Hypertensive disorders in pregnancy

There are four hypertensive disorders related to pregnancy (Table 108.4). Normal pregnancy is characterised by a fall in BP in the first trimester, reaching a nadir in the second trimester. BP rises towards pre-conception levels near the end of the third trimester. Hypertension is defined as a systolic BP of 140 mmHg or greater and/or a diastolic BP of 90 mmHg or greater.

Detecting a rise in BP from 'booking' or pre-conception BP (>30/15 mmHg) alone cannot be used in diagnosing pre-eclampsia/hypertension when BP is below 140/90 mmHg. Nevertheless, such a rise requires close monitoring.

Gestational hypertension is new onset of hypertension arising after 20 weeks' gestation and no additional features of pre-eclampsia. It resolves within 3 months postpartum.

Identifying superimposed pre-eclampsia in women with chronic hypertension can be challenging, given that BP are high at the start and some women may have proteinuria at baseline.

Investigations

Initial laboratory and radiological investigations for pregnant women with chronic hypertension should include:
• FBC;
• electrolyte, urea, creatinine and glucose;
• LFTs, urate;
• urinalysis, microscopy, culture;
• spot urine protein creatinine ratio (PCR) or 24-hour urine protein, if results of urinalysis are positive for protein;
• 24-hour urinary catecholamines and metanephrine, if clinically indicated;
• ultrasound for the assessment of fetal anatomy;
• ECG.

Investigations for monitoring

The frequency of ongoing monitoring for FBC, electrolytes, creatinine, urate, LFTs and urine PCR should be decided by the severity of the disease. Follow-up ultrasound should be at 26–28 weeks and then every 2–3 weeks to evaluate fetal growth.

Postpartum evaluation

A postpartum evaluation is required at 3 months to check BP, urinalysis and urine microscopy. If BP is still elevated or if there is proteinuria or abnormal urine sediment, further investigations are required.

109 Pregnancy

The aims of investigations in pregnancy are:
- confirm pregnancy and establish an estimated date of confinement
- diagnose and monitor pregnancy-related clinical conditions
- assess fetal well-being

Table 109.1 Indications and timing of early (pre-12 week) USS

Indications	Timing of examination
Threatened abortion	At presentation
Recurrent abortion	Prior to time of previous abortion
Suspected ectopic pregnancy	5–6 weeks
History of fetal or chromosomal anomaly, screening for trisomy 21	10–13 weeks
Severe hyperemesis gravidarum	At presentation
High-risk patient, e.g. diabetes mellitus or history of severe intrauterine growth restriction	8–12 weeks
Pelvic mass >4 cm	At presentation
Suspected uterine abnormality	8–12 weeks
Prior to cervical suture	Late first or early second trimester
Prior to chorionic villous sampling	10–12 weeks
Prior to amniocentesis	14–16 weeks

Table 109.2 Indications and timing of 26-week or later USS

Indications	Timing of examination
Clinical polyhydramnios	At presentation
Suspected IUGR	At presentation
History of IUGR	Earlier than previous presentation
History of intrauterine fetal death	Prior to time of previous death
Multiple pregnancy	26 and 32 weeks
Moderate to severe pre-eclampsia or eclampsia	At presentation
Diabetes mellitus	26 and 32 weeks
Chronic kidney disease or hypertension	26 and 32 weeks
History of low placenta	32–34 weeks
Review of fetal anomaly	26 weeks and on indication
Malpresentation	37+ weeks
Planned vaginal delivery of breech	37+ weeks

Key points

- Serum quantitative β-hCG assays are highly specific for pregnancy.
- Ultrasound is useful for initial diagnosis of pregnancy, assessment of the growing baby and the surrounding intrauterine environment, and for planning delivery.
- Antenatal screening can be performed in the first or second trimester to ascertain whether a baby has an increased risk of Down's syndrome, Edward's syndrome or open neural tube defects.

Box 109.1 Conditions that can cause true-positive serum β-hCG which are non-pregnancy related

- Pituitary hCG: diagnosed by administering oral contraceptive pills, which should suppress hCG levels
- Exogenous administration of hCG
- Trophoblastic neoplasm
- Non-trophoblastic neoplasm: secreted by different cancers such as testicular cancer
- Phantom hCG: caused by heterophilic antibodies that bind the labelled antibodies without hCG being present

Box 109.2 Investigations at different antenatal visits

Investigations at first antenatal visit
- FBC
- Blood group: ABO and Rhesus
- Screen for red cell antibodies
- Rubella immunity
- Screening test for syphilis, hepatitis B
- Urine culture for asymptomatic UTI
- Other investigations such as TFTs, hepatitis C and HIV serology according to medical history
- Varicella antibodies if no history or uncertain history of previous illness

Investigations at 12–20 weeks
- A full ultrasound examination at 15–20 weeks recommended

Investigations at 24–30 weeks
- FBC; if anaemia is detected, iron study should be performed
- Red cell antibodies
- Screening for gestational diabetes mellitus (see Chapter 89)
- Screening for group B streptococcal infection with a low vaginal swab

Figure 109.1 USS (a) early gestation sac (b) gestation at week 20 (c) twin pregnancy, and (d) Placenta previa

(a)
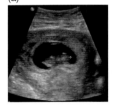

(b)
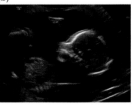

(c)
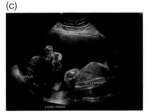

(d)
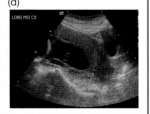

The diagnosis of pregnancy can be reached by history and physical examination, laboratory evaluation and/or ultrasonography. It should be considered in any woman who develops amenorrhoea.

β-hCG

β-hCG is detectable in maternal serum of 5% of women 8 days after conception and in more than 98% of women by day 12.

Levels peak at 10–12 weeks' gestation, then decline rapidly until another more gradual rise begins at 22 weeks which continues until term. β-hCG assays are highly specific and most pregnancy tests can detect levels as low as 25 mIU/mL. Urine testing devices detect hyperglycosylated hCG.

The initial rate of increase, measured by serial quantitative β-hCG, is useful for detecting and monitoring early complications of pregnancy. Failure to achieve the projected rate of rise suggests

Clinical Investigations at a Glance, First Edition. Jonathan Gleadle, Jordan Li and Tuck Yong. © 2017 John Wiley & Sons, Ltd. Published 2017 by John Wiley & Sons, Ltd.

an ectopic pregnancy or spontaneous abortion. β-hCG doubling times can vary during early pregnancy, so interpretation of these values must take into account the assays used and the clinical context. An abnormally high level or accelerated rise should prompt investigation into the possibility of molar pregnancy, multiple gestation or chromosomal abnormalities.

The false-positive serum β-hCG rate is low (0.1%) and usually due to interference by non-hCG substances such as LH, rheumatoid factor or the detection of pituitary hCG. The levels of false-positive results are usually below 150 mIU/mL. If there is suspicion of false-positive results, measurement of urine β-hCG levels is useful because the substances that cause false-positive results have higher molecular weights that are not filtered through the glomeruli; therefore, they do not produce a positive urine hCG result.

The conditions which can cause true-positive serum β-hCG levels but which are non-pregnancy related are listed in Box 109.1. False-negative β-hCG test results are more common in urine than in serum and are due to:

- β-hCG below the sensitivity threshold of the specific test;
- miscalculation in the onset of missed menses, or delayed menses from early pregnancy loss;
- delayed ovulation or implantation.

Progesterone

Serum progesterone is produced by the corpus luteum, which is stimulated by a viable pregnancy. Measurement of serum progesterone can reliably predict pregnancy prognosis but is not routinely used in the diagnosis of pregnancy. Viable intrauterine pregnancy can be diagnosed with 97.5% sensitivity if progesterone levels are above 79.5 nmol/L (>25 ng/mL). Serum progesterone levels below 15.9 nmol/L (<5 ng/mL) confirm the diagnosis of a non-viable pregnancy with virtually 100% sensitivity. If serum progesterone is between 15.9 and 79.5 nmol/L, further testing using ultrasound or additional hormonal assays is warranted to establish the viability of the pregnancy.

Home pregnancy tests

These tests are commonly used in the week after the missed menstrual period (fourth completed gestational week). Urine β-hCG values are extremely variable at this time and can range from 12 to >2500 mIU/mL. This variability continues into the fifth week (range from 13 to >6000 mIU/mL). Both weeks have a proportion of urine β-hCG values below the sensitivities of detection for many home pregnancy tests (range 25–100 mIU/mL). It is important to note the limitations of these tests so that pregnancy detection is not missed.

Ultrasound

Ultrasonography is useful for the diagnosis of early pregnancy when it is used in conjunction with quantitative β-hCG levels. The identification of gestational structures by ultrasound (Figure 109.1a) correlates with specific levels of serum β-hCG. If gestational structures are not seen when β-hCG levels are 3600 mIU/mL or greater, other pathology should be considered.

Routine investigations

Investigations at first visit

The investigations performed in pregnant women at their first antenatal care visit are listed in Box 109.2. The presence of haemoglobin below 110 g/L and/or low MCV should lead to iron study, haemoglobin electrophoresis to detect thalassaemia trait or DNA analysis for alpha-thalassaemia.

Investigations at 15–20 weeks

A full ultrasound examination at 15–20 weeks is usually recommended. It can provide:

- accurate gestational age (Figure 109.1b);
- exclude twin or multiple pregnancy (Figure 109.1c);
- fetal morphology and growth;
- placental localisation (Figure 109.1d);
- volume of amniotic fluid;
- exclude some, but not all, types of abnormality;
- the sex of the baby (if parents wish to know), though the test is not always accurate.

Investigations at 24–30 weeks (see Box 109.2.)

Antenatal tests for Down's syndrome

Antenatal screening can be performed in the first or second trimester to ascertain whether a baby has an increased risk of having Down's syndrome (affects 1 in 500 pregnancies), Edward's syndrome (1 in 3000) or open neural tube defects (1 in 750).

Women/parents must be counselled first as these tests are for risk assessment only and place their pregnancy in an increased or decreased risk category. If the test suggests a high risk, a subsequent diagnostic test that carries a small risk of miscarriage is required to confirm the diagnosis. Women who have had a previous pregnancy with Down's syndrome or with a family history of neural tube defects and women over 35 years of age may choose to proceed directly to a definitive diagnostic test. Women carrying twins can still have screening, but women carrying triplet or higher-order pregnancies cannot be offered antenatal screening.

First trimester combined screening

- Measurement of two biochemical markers: pregnancy-associated placental protein A (PAPP-A) and free β-hCG.
- Ultrasound at 12 weeks to measure nuchal translucency (the thickness of the fluid-filled region at the fetus's neck). A thickness of more than 2.5 mm is suggestive of chromosomal abnormalities. The presence of an ossified nasal bone confers a lower risk for Down's syndrome.

The biomarker results together with nuchal translucency measurements can be used to calculate the risk with commercially validated software. First trimester screening has a detection rate of 95% and a screen positive rate of 2.5%.

Second trimester screening

This involves measurement of maternal serum levels for four markers: AFP, free β-hCG, unconjugated estriol (uE3) and inhibin A.

Then commercial software packages are used to calculate risks for trisomy 21, trisomy 18 and neural tube defects.

Chorionic villous sampling and amniocentesis

Chorionic villous sampling at 12–14 weeks' gestation or amniocentesis after 15 weeks are more definitive diagnostic tests. These tests are performed on an outpatient basis with local anaesthetic, but carry a miscarriage risk of 1–2% and 0.5–1.0%, respectively.

110 Pyrexia of unknown origin

Table 110.1 Common causes of PUO

Sepsis

Abdominal and pelvic abscesses
Extrapulmonary/disseminated tuberculosis
Infective endocarditis
Osteoarticular infections
Typhoid/enteric fevers
EBV or CMV infection
Brucellosis
Prostatitis
Malaria
Rickettsial infections
Dental abscess

Inflammatory disorders

Systemic lupus erythematosus
Adult-onset Still's disease
Autoimmune hepatitis
Systemic vasculitis
Mixed connective tissue disease
Polymyalgia rheumatica
Inflammatory bowel disease
Sarcoidosis

Malignancy

Lymphoma
Hepatocellular carcinoma
Renal cell carcinoma
Leukaemia
Colon cancer
Pancreatic cancer

Other causes

Drug fever
Factitious fever
Mediterranean familial fever
Hyperthyroidism
Thyroiditis

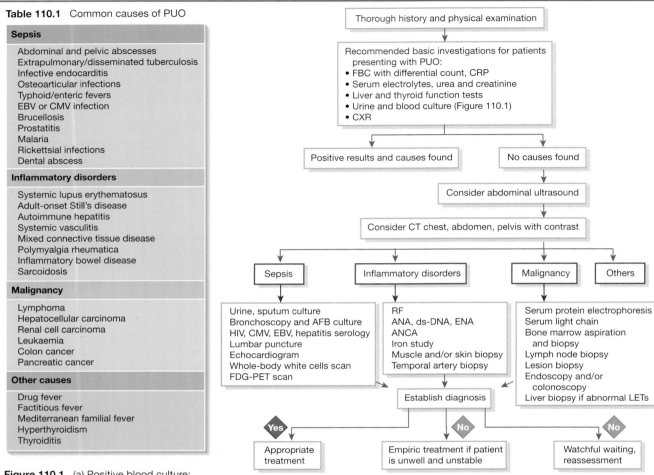

Thorough history and physical examination

↓

Recommended basic investigations for patients presenting with PUO:
• FBC with differential count, CRP
• Serum electrolytes, urea and creatinine
• Liver and thyroid function tests
• Urine and blood culture (Figure 110.1)
• CXR

Positive results and causes found | No causes found

No causes found → Consider abdominal ultrasound

↓

Consider CT chest, abdomen, pelvis with contrast

Sepsis
Urine, sputum culture
Bronchoscopy and AFB culture
HIV, CMV, EBV, hepatitis serology
Lumbar puncture
Echocardiogram
Whole-body white cells scan
FDG-PET scan

Inflammatory disorders
RF
ANA, ds-DNA, ENA
ANCA
Iron study
Muscle and/or skin biopsy
Temporal artery biopsy

Malignancy
Serum protein electrophoresis
Serum light chain
Bone marrow aspiration
   and biopsy
Lymph node biopsy
Lesion biopsy
Endoscopy and/or
   colonoscopy
Liver biopsy if abnormal LETs

Others

Establish diagnosis

Yes → Appropriate treatment
No → Empiric treatment if patient is unwell and unstable
No → Watchful waiting, reassessment

Figure 110.1 (a) Positive blood culture; (b) blood culture sensitivity result

(a)   (b)

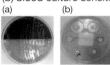

Figure 110.2 (a) CT abdomen shows soft tissue infection in the rectovesical pouch in a man presenting with PUO; (b) CT neck shows bilateral cervical and axillary lymphadenopathy consistent with lymphoma; and (c) CT abdomen shows lymphadenopathy involving bilateral iliac chain consistent with lymphoma

(a)   (c)

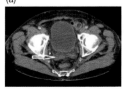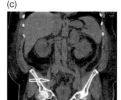

(b)

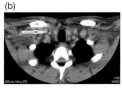

Table 110.2 Suggested further investigations for patients with PUO

Suspected underlying causes	Suggested further investigations
Endocarditis	Echocardiography, trans-oesophageal echocardiography (sensitivity 95–100%, specificity 98% for endocardial vegetations)
Thyroiditis	TFTs and thyroid scan
Abdominal or pelvic abscess	Ultrasound or CT abdomen with contrast
Osteomyelitis	MRI
Tuberculosis	Skin test, interferon-γ release assay, CT chest
Inflammatory disorders	ANA, ENA, dsDNA, ANCA, RF, cryoglobulins
Inflammatory bowel disease	Colonoscopy
Haematological malignancy	Bone marrow biopsy
Viral infection	Serology for EBV, CMV, hepatitis B and C, HIV
Malaria	Thick and thin film, malaria antigen/ICT

Figure 110.3 PET scan shows marked diffuse splenic FDG uptake consistent with lymphoma in a woman presenting with PUO

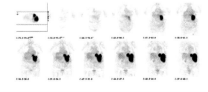

Clinical Investigations at a Glance, First Edition. Jonathan Gleadle, Jordan Li and Tuck Yong. © 2017 John Wiley & Sons, Ltd. Published 2017 by John Wiley & Sons, Ltd.

Pyrexia of unknown origin (PUO) is defined as a fever of 38.3°C (101°F) or more lasting for at least 3 weeks for which no cause can be identified after 1 week of intensive and appropriate investigations.

PUO has a wide differential diagnosis that can be abbreviated as SIM (sepsis, inflammatory disease, malignancy). The commonly encountered underlying causes of the pyrexia are listed in Table 110.1. Worldwide, infectious diseases are still the most likely aetiologies. Local epidemiological trends in the aetiology of PUO should be taken into account.

Initial investigations

Taking and repeating a thorough history and physical examination often leads to a diagnosis. A persistent fever needs to be accurately documented because the pattern of the fever and its relation with the pulse rate (particularly a temperature–pulse disparity) may point to an underlying cause such as typhoid fever, and this will be helpful if there is suspicion of factitious fever. Regular clinical evaluations throughout the course of PUO are important as new signs and symptoms may appear which will change the direction of the investigation plan. While investigating the PUO, two conditions which may warrant urgent treatment should be considered: immunocompromised or neutropenic fever and suspected giant cell arteritis or other vasculitis. These may need empirical treatment with antibiotics or corticosteroids, respectively. Basic laboratory and imaging studies may help to guide further evaluation (see flow diagram on opposite page).

Further investigations

Clues obtained from the history, physical examination and the initial investigation should form the basis for subsequent investigations that are tailored to the individual patient (Table 110.2). In the absence of clues, the following investigations should be considered.

CT of the abdomen and pelvis

Several studies have shown CT of the abdomen and pelvis with contrast to have the highest diagnostic yield in the evaluation of patients with PUO after initial basic work-up, looking specifically for abscesses, lymph nodes or splenomegaly (Figure 110.1).

FDG-PET scan

This may be useful in helping to pinpoint a source of fever. Fluoro-2-deoxy-D-glucose (FDG) is preferentially taken up by tumour cells and inflammatory cells, in which glucose metabolism is high. FDG-PET-localised pathology that directs further tests can lead to a diagnosis in over one-third of patients (Figure 110.2). The diagnostic yield may be increased further by simultaneously using FDG-PET with CT. Several small retrospective studies have shown sensitivities of 56–100%, specificities of 75–81%, and negative predictive values of 100% when a combination of CT and FDG-PET were used. Notably, FDG-PET was of no diagnostic benefit unless patients had an elevated ESR or raised CRP.

Nuclear scintigraphy

Nuclear scan with ^{67}Ga-citrate and ^{111}In-labelled leucocytes is a much cheaper and more widely available imaging technique that may perform a similar role in localising pathology, though it is more time-consuming and has lower sensitivity (75%) and specificity (83%) than FDG-PET. ^{111}In-labelled leucocyte scintigraphy may be helpful in diagnosing inflammatory and infectious conditions but is rarely of use in malignancy.

Bone marrow aspirate with trephine biopsy

This investigation has been found to be diagnostic in nearly 20% of patients with PUO and 'helpful' for diagnosis in nearly one-quarter. This is particularly, though not exclusively, true in the presence of thrombocytopenia or anaemia (haemoglobin <110 g/L). Bone marrow culture has a lower yield in immunocompetent individuals than in those who are immunocompromised.

Biopsy

More invasive tests, such as lymph node or liver biopsy, lumbar puncture and temporal artery biopsy, may be considered when the cause of fever remains unidentified and when clinical suspicion shows that these tests are indicated.

Other considerations

In patients who remain without a diagnosis after an extensive work-up, the prognosis is usually favourable. About 20% of patients with documented PUO never have a confirmed diagnosis. In most of these the fever usually spontaneously resolves in 4 weeks or more. Therefore, a watch-and-wait approach is acceptable in a clinically stable patient. All patients should be monitored until a diagnosis can be made or the fever resolves spontaneously. There is no role for testing tumour markers in the investigation of PUO.

Empirical antibiotics are warranted only for patients who are clinically unstable or neutropenic or immunocompromised. In stable patients, empirical treatment with antibiotics or non-steroidal anti-inflammatory drugs (NSAIDs) or corticosteroids is discouraged.

Key points

- Investigations should be guided by thorough history, physical examination and basic investigation results, with consideration of risk factors and likely causes.
- Initial investigations should include FBC, biochemistry, LFTs, CRP, TFT, urine and blood culture, and CXR.
- If the initial investigation provides no diagnostic clues, further investigations including imaging studies and serological tests for inflammatory disorders may be indicated.

111 Leucopenia and febrile neutropenia

Table 111.1 Common causes of neutropenia

Decreased production
Primary haematological disorders Aplastic anaemia Myelodysplasia Leukaemia *Secondary disorders* Malnutrition Infection Cancers Medication Immunosuppressive drugs, NSAIDs, chemotherapy and radiation therapy

Increased turnover

Acute and overwhelming infections
Drug-related or immune-mediated
  agranulocytosis
Autoimmune neutropenia, SLE and
  rheumatoid arthritis
Hypersplenism

Altered distribution
Severe infections Endotoxaemia Transfusion reactions

Table 111.2 Common causes of lymphopenia

Abnormal production

Primary haematological disorders
Hodgkin's disease
Multiple myeloma
 	
Secondary disorders
Malnutrition
Infection: viral infections, disseminated
  granulomatous infection (mycobacterial,
  fungal)
Radiation and/or chemotherapy
Medication: glucocorticoids, immuno-
  suppressive drugs

Alteration in traffic
Acute bacterial or fungal infection Surgery, trauma Haemorrhage

Destruction or loss
HIV infection Antibody-mediated lymphocyte destruction Protein-losing enteropathy

Table 111.3 Features of systemic compromise in patients with febrile neutropenia

- Hypotension: systolic blood pressure 90 mmHg, or 30 mmHg below patient's baseline blood pressure
- Hypoxia: arterial Po_2 <60 mmHg at room air or oxygen saturation of 90%
- Confusion or altered mental state
- Coagulopathy
- Heart failure or arrhythmia
- Kidney failure
- Liver failure
- Multiorgan failure

Key points

- Neutropenia is suspected in patients with frequent, severe or unusual infections or in patients receiving cytotoxic drugs or radiation therapy. Confirmation is by FBC with differential.
- Blood cultures are the mainstay of investigation. At least two sets of blood cultures should be obtained from all febrile patients; if an indwelling intravenous catheter is present, cultures are drawn from the catheter and from a separate peripheral vein.
- Culture of relevant body fluid and/or radiological investigations are needed to identify a possible source of opportunistic infection in a patient with febrile neutropenia.

Box 111.1 Investigations for febrile and suspected or confirmed neutropenia

- Two sets of blood cultures
- Basic investigations in febrile neutropenia:
  - FBC with differential white cell count
  - Electrolytes, urea, creatinine and LFTs: assessing renal function is important because it can affect the dose of certain antibiotics to be administered
  - Urinalysis and urine culture should also be performed
  - Arterial blood gases and lactate
  - CXR
- Commence intravenous antibiotics within 30 min of presentation. Do not wait for the test results
- Further investigations to locate the source of infection:
  - Mid-stream urine sample for culture
  - Sputum for culture if patient has a productive cough
  - Faeces for culture and *C. difficile* toxin if there is diarrhoea
  - Swab all wounds, recent intravenous catheter site, central venous access sites
  - Chest CT
  - Abdominal ultrasound or CT
  - Lumbar puncture
- Investigations to determine the cause of neutropenia, such as bone marrow biopsy

Leucopenia

Leucopenia is a total WBC count of less than 4.0×10^9/L and neutropenia is an absolute neutrophil count below 1.5×10^9/L. In adults, leucopenia is almost always due to neutropenia and very rarely due to absolute lymphopenia ($<1.0 \times 10^9$/L). Severe neutropenia markedly increases the risk of serious, recurrent and treatment-resistant infections.

Neutropenia may be due to decreased production of neutrophils in the bone marrow, altered distribution of neutrophils in the peripheral blood, or abnormal removal of neutrophils in the extravascular system (Table 111.1). Lymphopenia may be caused by bone marrow failure or increase in destruction (Table 111.2). It also occurs in immunodeficiency syndromes, most importantly with HIV infection.

Acute neutropenia is a relatively frequent finding, is often well tolerated and normalises rapidly, and specialised investigations are often unnecessary. However, neutropenia that persists should be investigated thoroughly. Neutropenia arising as a result of haematological disorders is more significant, with risk of infectious complications.

Laboratory investigations

Initially, review the FBC and differential count to determine if neutropenia, lymphopenia or both are present, and to exclude pancytopenia. Presence of atypical cells in the blood smear may point to an underlying systemic disorder. For example, neutropenia with hypersegmented polymorphs and megaloblastic anaemia suggests folate or vitamin B_{12} deficiency.

In patients with unexplained neutropenia, anaemia or thrombocytopenia, infectious causes, including viruses (EBV, CMV, HIV, measles, hepatitis), bacteria (Gram-positive and Gram-negative, typhoid fever, tuberculosis), parasites (malaria) or fungi, should be considered. Viral PCR and serologic testing for EBV, CMV, hepatitis and HIV may be warranted.

In patients with neutropenia accompanied by splenomegaly, consider cirrhosis, sarcoidosis and lymphoma. In patients with neutropenia but normal levels of other blood cells, consider humoral immune neutropenia. Measure ANA, rheumatoid factor and anti-CCP antibody to further evaluate patients for systemic autoimmune neutropenia and Felty's syndrome.

Patients with severe neutropenia, pancytopenia or severe infection should undergo bone marrow biopsy unless (i) the patient likely has a drug- or toxin-induced neutropenia that promptly resolves after stopping the exposure, or (ii) the patient has a nutritional deficiency (folate or vitamin B_{12}).

Cyclic neutropenia

This is an autosomal dominant disease characterised by severe neutropenia recurring about every 21 days and lasting for 3–6 days, as well as oscillations in other WBC and platelet counts. Skin and respiratory infections are common, but life-threatening infections are not.

Chronic idiopathic neutropenia

Laboratory investigations are normal or near normal, except for monocyte and immunoglobulin levels, which may be increased. Bone-marrow production of neutrophils ranges from normal to a lack of mature polymorphs, but mostly there is ineffective granulocytopoiesis.

Febrile neutropenia

Febrile neutropenia is fever of at least 38.3°C or 38.0°C on two occasions in the setting of an absolute neutrophil count below 0.5×10^9/L. However, patients with neutropenia can present with sepsis without fever, common in elderly patients or patients on corticosteroid therapy.

Febrile neutropenia is a common complication of chemotherapy for cancer and haematological malignancies. Over half of patients with febrile neutropenia have an established or occult infection. Mortality rates for critically ill patients are 10–20%, with rates as high as 40% in Gram-negative bacteraemia.

Initial investigation and risk assessment

All patients presenting with fever following chemotherapy should have the appropriate cultures taken followed by empirical antibiotics without waiting for laboratory confirmation of neutrophil count.

The first step is to determine the presence of systemic compromise (Table 111.3) and whether the patient is at high or low risk for medical complications by performing the basic tests outlined in Box 111.1.

Patients with systemic compromise should receive antibiotics within 30 min of presentation, after the immediate collection of two sets of blood culture. Clinical investigations must never delay prompt administration of antibiotic therapy. The risk of a patient with febrile neutropenia developing medical complications should be assessed using an accepted risk assessment tool, such as the Multinational Association for Supportive Care in Cancer (MASCC) risk index.

Two sets of blood cultures in a 24-hour period will detect more than 90% of cases of bacteraemia in adults with febrile neutropenia. There is no need to wait for fever to exceed 38°C before taking a blood culture. The concurrent collection of blood from vascular catheters in addition to peripheral blood cultures may assist in the diagnosis of catheter-related bloodstream infection (CRBSI) by allowing the time required for blood from the peripheral vein to become positive to be compared with the sample from a central venous catheter. A differential time to positivity of 120 min or more is predictive of CRBSI. For patients with positive blood cultures, repeat peripheral cultures should be performed to document clearance of bacteraemia.

Additional investigations

Respiratory symptoms

A CXR is indicated for patients with febrile neutropenia. In a patient with pulmonary infiltrate, bacterial, viral or fungal pathogens need to be considered. Investigations may include HR CT, sputum culture and/or bronchoscopy with bronchial lavage. Nasal swab (throat swab if thrombocytopenic) for respiratory virus PCR should be performed.

Gastrointestinal symptoms

If the patient has diarrhoea, stool sample should be sent for culture and viral studies. Stool for *Clostridium difficile* toxin assay is needed if there has been recent treatment with antibiotics. In patients with features of abdominal or perineal infection, ultrasound or CT of this region is indicated.

Skin, mouth or vascular catheter site lesions

If there is suspicion of infection, bacterial swab for Gram stain and culture and/or viral swab of vesicular lesions and mouth ulcers for HSV and VZV PCR should be performed.

Central nervous system (CNS) symptoms

CT brain and lumbar puncture (LP) may be indicated if there are new CNS symptoms or signs. Correction of thrombocytopenia and/or coagulopathy must occur prior to LP.

112 Illness in returned travellers

Table 112.1 Incubation periods of common infectious disease

Less than 7 days	7–21 days	Greater than 21 days
Influenza	Malaria	Malaria
Dengue fever	Viral haemorrhagic fevers	Hepatitis A, B, C
Yellow fever	Typhoid fever	Tuberculosis
Paratyphoid fever	Q fever	Schistosomiasis
	Rickettsial diseases	Amoebic liver abscess
	Brucellosis	HIV
		Rabies

Table 112.2 Travel exposure and infectious diseases

Exposure	Infectious disease
Unhygienic, undercooked food	Typhoid fever, salmonellosis
Untreated water	Cholera, typhoid fever, salmonellosis, hepatitis A
Unpasteurised dairy products	Brucellosis, tuberculosis
Animal contact	Brucellosis, Q fever, rabies
Mosquito bite	Dengue fever, malaria
Tick bite	Rickettsial diseases
Close contact	Meningococcal disease, tuberculosis, viral haemorrhagic fevers

Figure 112.1

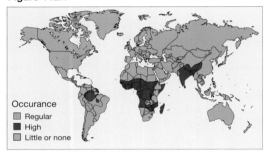

Occurance
- Regular
- High
- Little or none

Table 112.3 Basic investigations for fever in returned travellers

- FBC with differential count and platelet count
- Blood biochemistry and LFTs
- Thick and thin blood smears for malaria (can be supplemented by rapid tests where available)
- Blood culture
- Urinalysis and urine culture
- Stool culture, ova and parasites in diarrhoeal illness
- Store a serum sample for comparison with convalescent-phase sample
- CXR if patient is unwell or has respiratory symptoms or signs

 +

No other symptoms and signs

Typhoid
Dengue
Malaria
Hepatitis
Thick and thin blood film, blood culture, serology tests

 +

Typhoid
Traveller's diarrhoea
Cholera
Dysentery
Stool culture

+

Returned from malaria endemic area, consider malaria first
Thick and thin blood film

 +

Pneumonia
Influenza
Tuberculosis
CXR, viral PCR, sputum smear

 +

Jaundice

Hepatitis A, B, C
EBV
Q fever
Amoebic liver abscess
Hepatitis serology, liver ultrasound

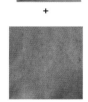 +

Dengue
Rickettsial disease
Viral infection
Serology tests

Figure 112.2 (a) Thick blood film; (b) thin blood film

(a)

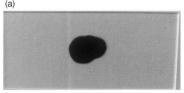

(b)

Figure 112.3 (a, b) Two thin blood smears positive for malaria

(a)   (b)

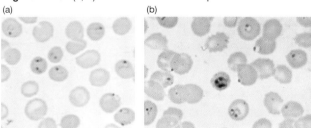

Key points

- Thick and thin blood films for malaria and blood cultures are important initial investigations for febrile returned travellers.
- The diagnosis of dengue fever is made clinically and can be confirmed by a fourfold rise in antibody titre between acute- and convalescent-phase serum samples obtained at least 4 weeks apart.
- Stool microscopy, ova, parasites and culture are important investigations in people with suspected travellers' diarrhoea.

Clinical Investigations at a Glance, First Edition. Jonathan Gleadle, Jordan Li and Tuck Yong. © 2017 John Wiley & Sons, Ltd. Published 2017 by John Wiley & Sons, Ltd.

Fever in returned travellers

Febrile illness (temperature >38°C) occurs in 2–3% of returned travellers. While most travel-related infections present within a few months of return, some infections can present many months or years after exposure, such as strongyloidiasis or schistosomiasis. Infectious causes may be of public health concern, and require specific intervention to prevent spread.

The common causes of travel-related fever include malaria, influenza, dengue fever, rickettsia infections, non-specific viral syndromes and bacterial diarrhoea. However, fever can be caused by common infections such as pneumonia, urinary tract infection, pulmonary emboli, malignancy and autoimmune disorders unrelated to travel.

A detailed travel history is essential and should include all the areas of travel including 'stopovers' and details of the precise areas visited, whether the areas were predominantly urban, rural or both. Time of symptom onset in relation to travel may help eliminate diseases with different incubation periods (Table 112.1). For example, fever beginning over 10 days after departure from an endemic area is unlikely to be dengue, which has a short incubation period. Information about the patient's activities during travel (Table 112.2), pre-travel immunisations and chemoprophylaxis during travel are very helpful.

Initial investigations

The initial investigation should focus on diseases that are life-threatening, most importantly *Plasmodium falciparum* malaria and typhoid fever. Basic investigations are listed in Table 112.3.

FBC can be very helpful. Notably normal or low WBC counts occur in many infections including dengue, malaria, rickettsia and typhoid. Thrombocytopenia is seen in malaria and viral infections, especially viral haemorrhagic fevers including dengue, and in severe sepsis. Neutrophilia usually reflects a bacterial infection, which could include leptospirosis, but more often is due to common pyogenic organisms. Eosinophilia suggests invasive parasitic infection such as schistosomiasis, or the migratory phase of some helminths or strongyloides. It also occurs in drug reactions and some fungal infections. A normal CRP does not rule out serious infection.

Investigations for malaria

The most serious cause of fever in returned travellers from the tropics is *P. falciparum* malaria, which can be rapidly fatal. It generally presents within 6 weeks of return from an endemic area, although onset may be delayed by prophylactic mefloquine. In contrast, malaria caused by *Plasmodium vivax* may present many months after exposure. No signs or symptoms are specific to malaria, although fever is invariable. Malaria should always be considered and investigated if a traveller has returned from an area where transmission occurs, regardless of whether they took chemoprophylaxis or whether they are afebrile now.

Malaria is diagnosed by detecting the parasite in a blood film (Figure 112.1) or circulating malarial antigen. Initial blood films may be negative, and repeat films should be taken every 6–12 hours for 36–48 hours before malaria can be confidently excluded. When malaria smears are ordered, it should be examined by a recognised reference laboratory to minimise the possibility of a false negative. Negative smears can be due to low level of parasitaemia or can occur despite a high load with *P. falciparum* due to sequestration.

Thick and thin blood film microscopy examination remains the gold standard for diagnosis (Figure 112.2); however, simple, sensitive and specific antibody-based rapid diagnostic tests that detect *Pf*HRP2, pan-malaria or species-specific LDH, or aldolase antigens in fingerprick blood are increasingly used.

Investigations for enteric fever

Enteric fever refers to a clinical syndrome caused by *Salmonella typhi* (typhoid fever) or less commonly, *Salmonella paratyphi* (paratyphoid fever). Typhoid fever is common in many developing nations. Diagnosis is achieved by isolation of the organism in cultures of blood, stool, urine, bone marrow, and duodenal aspirates.

Investigations for dengue fever

The diagnosis of dengue fever is made clinically and can be confirmed by a fourfold rise in antibody titre between acute- and convalescent-phase serum samples obtained at least 4 weeks apart. PCR-based tests may offer rapid and specific diagnosis but have a limited window of positivity.

Diarrhoea in returned travellers

Travellers' diarrhoea is defined as three or more unformed or bloody stools within 24 hours passed by a traveller and accompanied by other symptoms (cramps, nausea, vomiting, fever).

The duration of diarrhoea is a useful clue in determining cause. About 50–75% of acute cases of travellers' diarrhoea (duration ≤2 weeks) are caused by bacteria, such as enterotoxic *Escherichia coli* (40–70% of cases), *Campylobacter*, *Salmonella* and *Shigella*. Viruses, most commonly rotaviruses and noroviruses, account for 10–20% of cases, and parasitic agents such as *Giardia*, *Cryptosporidium* and *Cyclospora* for up to 5% of cases. *Vibrio cholerae* is an uncommon cause but should be considered if the patient has travelled in the area of an outbreak. Even with careful laboratory investigation, no pathogen is detected in a substantial proportion of cases. 10–20% of cases are caused by more than one pathogen.

For return travellers with ongoing diarrhoea a good travel and clinical history is paramount. Blood and mucus is characteristic of dysentery, which can be caused by a range of pathogens including *Shigella* and *Entamoeba*. The patient's hydration should be assessed.

Stool testing

Stool microscopy and culture is the key investigation. The stool should be examined for leucocytes, ova, cysts and parasites and cultured for bacteria, as well as viral antigen or PCR tests conducted. Bacterial or viral causes can be identified in 50–70% of travellers who have diarrhoea lasting more than 2 weeks. The triple faeces test (collection of faeces specimens on three consecutive days) has been shown to substantially increase the sensitivity (>80%) of detecting parasites but is often not practical. The stool sample needs to be sent to the laboratory immediately to maximise yield. A *Cryptosporidium* stool antigen test can be performed, and a *Giardia* stool antigen test should be performed for a returning traveller with diarrhoea of 7 days or more. Test stool for *Clostridium difficile* toxin if antibiotics have been used in the past month.

Colonoscopy

Colonoscopy is recommended for persistent diarrhoea to exclude inflammatory bowel disease and pseudomembranous or amoebic colitis.

113 Sepsis

Clinical Investigations at a Glance, First Edition. Jonathan Gleadle, Jordan Li and Tuck Yong. © 2017 John Wiley & Sons, Ltd. Published 2017 by John Wiley & Sons, Ltd.

The aim of investigation in patients with suspected sepsis/bacteraemia/septicaemia is to:
- Establish the presence of septicaemia/bacteraemia and the causative organism
- Identify the main site of infection associated with the septicaemia/bacteraemia
- Assess any organ injury/failure resulting from the septicaemia/bacteraemia

Key points

- Blood culture should be performed in all patients with suspected sepsis regardless of whether the patient is febrile or not.
- A total of 20 mL of blood should be drawn for cultures, and the number of sites is less important than total volume.
- Cultures of relevant body fluids should be collected from an infectious source, including sputum, urine, wound, catheters and CSF.
- CXR should be obtained in every patient suspected of having sepsis, because pneumonia is the most commonly identified infection leading to sepsis.

History and clinical examination

Suspected sepsis or septic shock, commence **treatment**

Non-invasive haemodynamic monitoring, assess airway, breathing, circulation

Basic laboratory and radiographic tests
- FBC with differential, CRP
- Serum biochemistry, creatinine
- Liver function, lactate
- Coagulation studies
- Urine analysis
- CXR

Blood cultures (two peripheral and from each indwelling catheter) before the antibiotics treatment

Body fluids that can be collected for microbiology studies
- Mid-stream urine
- Sputum
- Stool
- Pleural fluid
- Ascitic fluid
- Cerebrospinal fluid (CSF) through lumbar puncture
- Synovial fluid through joint aspiration
- Wound or abscess culture

Consider central venous catheter, mechanical ventilation

Initial fluid resuscitation and consider inotropic support with vasopressor agents

Initial empirical broad-spectrum antibiotic treatment

Further imaging investigations to identify infection source if indicated

Figure 113.1 Blood culture growth of *Pseudomonas aeruginosa*

Figure 113.2 Blood culture growth of *Staphylococcus aureus*

Figure 113.3 Blood culture growth of *Streptococcus pneumoniae* with minimal inhibitory concentration test

Figure 113.4 CSF collection and examination

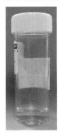

Figure 113.5 CXR shows right middle lobe pneumonia

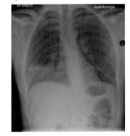

Figure 113.6 USS shows thickened gallbladder wall with tenderness consistent with acute cholecystitis

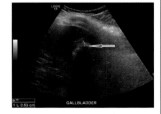

Figure 113.7 CT of the brain shows a round hypodense lesion with surrounding oedema consistent with brain abscess

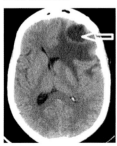

Figure 113.8 CT of the abdomen shows a low-attenuation extraluminal fluid collection with a gas bubble consistent with an intra-abdominal abscess

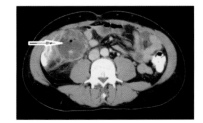

Figure 113.9 MRI of the foot shows osteomyelitis of the heel

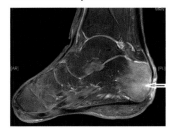

Bacteraemia is the detection of viable bacteria in circulating blood (may be transient) without reference to clinical features. This may not have any clinical significance in people who do not have an underlying illness or immune deficiency or turbulent cardiac blood flow. Harmless, transient bacteraemia can occur following dental work or other minor medical procedures. However, occult bacteraemia can progress to a more severe local or systemic infection if left untreated. Septicaemia is the presence of microorganisms in the bloodstream with a systemic response to infection. Sepsis is the systemic response to the infection, such as fever, hypotension and raised inflammatory markers, but the blood culture result is pending or negative.

Sepsis/bacteraemia/septicaemia can occur in association with many common bacterial infections including pneumonia, pyelonephritis, septic arthritis, osteomyelitis, cellulitis, meningitis, infective endocarditis and intra-abdominal infections. A wide range of bacteria can be involved and risk factors for septicaemia/bacteraemia include splenectomy, neutropenia, intravenous drug use, animal bite, transplant recipients, and hospitalisation with intravenous cannula, indwelling catheter or surgery.

The presentation of sepsis/bacteraemia/septicaemia is often non-specific. Fever and rigors are the most common presenting symptoms. Other clinical features will depend on the main site of infection and these features will usually guide which investigations are needed.

Patients with sepsis may be severely ill or can deteriorate rapidly. It is important to consider the correction of hypotension and hypoxaemia, including the need for intensive care and the administration of broad-spectrum antibiotics. In immunosuppressed patients consider more unusual pathogens and potential sources of infection including sinuses, ears, throat, skin and muscle.

Blood culture

If sepsis/bacteraemia/septicaemia is suspected, blood cultures (Figures 113.1–113.3) must be taken before antibiotics are given. Two sets of venous blood samples should be taken, each into both aerobic and anaerobic culture bottles. For some organisms, an extended period of culture may be needed.

Laboratory investigations

Laboratory studies that may be helpful in the work-up for possible septicaemia/bacteraemia include the following.
• FBC with differentials. Leucocytosis, neutrophilia, toxic changes and left shift are usually observed with clinically significant bacterial infection.
• Biochemistry to determine kidney function, liver function (may affect antibiotic dosing) and any other organ dysfunction as a consequence of the sepsis.
• Arterial blood gases to evaluate gas exchange, lactate and acid–base status.
• CRP does not identify occult bacteraemia but can be useful in monitoring response to treatment.
• Coagulation tests including fibrinogen level can be abnormal in patients with septicaemia, which may be suggestive of disseminated intravascular coagulation.
• Serum lactate above 4 mmol/L may indicate tissue hypoperfusion in severe septicaemia.

Body fluids cluture

Depending on the patient's clinical features, a number of body fluids (see flow diagram on opposite page) can be collected for microscopy, culture (Figure 113.4) and determination of antibiotic susceptibility if an organism is grown.

Radiology

X-ray

CXR is important in the assessment of a patient with septicaemia/ bacteraemia. CXR may reveal pneumonia (Figure 113.5), parapneumonic effusion, empyema or lung abscess. Acute lung injury can develop with severe sepsis. Dental radiological studies may be required for the assessment of occult dental sepsis.

Ultrasound

Ultrasound has many uses in the assessment of septicaemia/ bacteraemia. It can be used to examine the abdomen for evidence of cholecystitis (Figure 113.6), intra-abdominal abscess, renal abscess or ascites. It is also used to guide aspiration of pleural effusion, ascites and joint effusion. Transthoracic and/or transoesophageal echocardiography is indicated if infective endocarditis is suspected as the cause of septicaemia/ bacteraemia.

CT

CT of the head can be used to assess brain abscess (Figure 113.7), paranasal sinus disease, middle ear disease, orbital abscess and mastoid air cells. CT of the chest can help to identify a lung abscess and infective pleural disease. CT of the abdomen and pelvis is useful for identifying any intra-abdominal or pelvic abscess (Figure 113.8) or infective collection related to the liver, spleen, pancreas or kidneys.

MRI

MRI is useful in the assessment of encephalitis and osteomyelitis (Figure 113.9).

Radionuclide scan

Technetium or gallium bone scan is useful for the assessment of osteomyelitis and septic arthritis. Indium (^{111}In)-labelled granulocyte scan can help to localise a deep-seated site of infection or inflammation.

Biopsy

In some cases of osteomyelitis, a biopsy of the bone is required to identify the causative organism and determine the best course of treatment.

Prostheses and devices

Various prostheses (e.g. cardiac valves and joints) and devices or shunts (e.g. venous catheter, urinary catheter or pacemaker leads) can be infected and become a source of septicaemia/ bacteraemia. If the catheter or cannula is removed, this should be sent for culture. In implant-associated infections, for maximum diagnostic yield, deep specimens should be obtained from up to five sites around the implant at debridement.

114 Sepsis: testing for infectious diseases

Table 114.1 Common viral infections and tests

Microorganism	Disease	Test
Rotavirus	Diarrhoea	Stool PCR test
Norwalk virus	Diarrhoea	Stool PCR test
Enteric adenovirus	Diarrhoea	Stool PCR test
Enterovirus (coxsackievirus, echovirus)	Respiratory tract infection; hand, foot and mouth disease; aseptic meningitis; myocarditis; encephalitis	Clinical diagnosis, viral isolation by cell culture-blood or feces CSF PCR
Arboviruses	Encephalitis	Serology test, limited PCR test available
Parvovirus B19	Pure red cell aplastic anaemia, erythema infectiosum	Clinical diagnosis, serology test if needed, positive IgM antibody or fourfold increase in IgG antibody over 4 weeks
Ebola virus	Ebola haemorrhagic fever	Viral PCR, virus isolation/culture, serology test
Human T cell lymphotropic virus (HTLV)-I	T-cell lymphoma, leukaemia	Immunoassay for HTLV-I specific IgG antibodies in serum
HTLV II	Hairy cell leukaemia	Immunoassay for HTLV-II specific IgG antibodies in serum
Human immunodeficiency virus (HIV)	Acquired immunodeficiency syndrome	See Chapter 118
Herpes simplex 1 and 2	Acute herpetic gingivostomatitis or herpetic pharyngotonsillitis, genital herpes, encephalitis	Clinical diagnosis, swab, CSF PCR
Varicella-zoster virus	Shingles or herpes zoster	Clinical diagnosis, vesicular fluid PCR test if needed
Varicella-zoster virus	Chickenpox	Clinical diagnosis, vesicular fluid PCR test
Human herpes virus 6	Roseola subitum	Self-limiting infection, clinical diagnosis, if needed viral PCR
Human herpes virus 8	Kaposi's sarcoma (KS)	Viral PCR in tissues
Hepatitis A virus	Hepatitis A	Anti-HAV IgM and IgG antibody
Hepatitis B virus	Hepatitis B	HBsAg, HBeAg, Anti-HBs, Anti-HBc IgG, Anti-HBc IgM, HBV DNA PCR
Hepatitis C virus	Hepatitis C	Anti-HCV, viral RNA PCR
Hepatitis D virus	Hepatitis D	Anti-HDV, HDV Ag
Hepatitis E virus	Hepatitis E	Anti-HEV
EBV	Infectious mononucleosis	Serology test: viral capsid antigen (VCA)-IgM antibodies, VCA-IgG and D early antigen (EA-D) IgG tests, and Epstein–Barr nuclear antigen (EBNA) antibody test
CMV	Viral illness, pneumonitis, colitis, retinitis	Blood PCR test, histopathology of the biopsy, serology test
Influenza A and B virus	Respiratory tract infection	Nasopharyngeal aspirate for PCR
Parainfluenza virus	Respiratory tract infection	Nasopharyngeal aspirate for PCR
Adenovirus	Respiratory tract infection	Nasopharyngeal aspirate for PCR
Respiratory syncytial virus	Respiratory tract infection	Nasopharyngeal aspirate for PCR
Rhinovirus	Respiratory tract infection	Nasopharyngeal aspirate for PCR
Coronavirus	Respiratory tract infection	Nasopharyngeal aspirate for PCR
Dengue virus	Dengue fever, viral illness, haemorrhagic symptoms, shock	Blood viral PCR, serology test, fourfold increase in antibody over 4 weeks
Measles (morbillivirus)	Measles	Usually clinical diagnosis, nasopharyngeal secretion PCR or serology test
Rubella virus	Rubella	Usually clinical diagnosis, confirmed by serology test
Mumps (paramyxovirus)	Mumps	Clinical diagnosis, serology test if needed, tissue cell culture
Ross river virus	Viral illness and severe joint pain	Serology test: positive for IgM antibody

Infection is caused by the interaction between a microorganism and the human body. The disease and severity depends on the virulence, number and entry of the microorganisms and the immune status of the individual. Some microorganisms cause distinctive patterns of infection which can be diagnosed clinically without the need for extensive investigations. Many microorganisms can cause variable presentations or produce non-diagnostic clinical syndromes. In these contexts, clinical investigations especially cultures, serological tests and PCR tests to identify the microorganisms and antimicrobial sensitivity are essential. The usual investigations for common microorganisms and their infections are listed in Tables 114.1 and 114.2.

Most common infections, such as upper respiratory tract infections and uncomplicated urinary tract infections (UTIs), can be diagnosed clinically and treated empirically and not all infectious diseases need laboratory confirmation or other investigations. Generally speaking, if the patient has severe sepsis, does not respond to empirical treatment or the diagnosis is uncertain, then investigation is indicated. Laboratory microbiological investigations also play an important role in surveillance of infectious diseases and endemic diseases.

It is important to remember that the clinical response should be monitored after the diagnosis and antimicrobial treatment. Superimposed infection, inadequate treatment, development of resistance to antimicrobials, complications of the original infection and immunocompromised patients are the common causes of treatment failure and appropriate investigations should be carried out to identify the causes.

Investigations for infectious diseases are dynamic. New pathogens and new diseases continue to be discovered, such as Ebola and Zika virus and Middle East respiratory syndrome. New diagnostic methods are increasingly available.

Table 114.2 Common bacterial infections and tests

Microorganism	Diseases	Test
Campylobacter jejuni	Diarrhoea, associated with Guillain–Barré syndrome	Stool culture
Salmonella	Diarrhoea	Blood/stool culture
Escherichia coli O157:H7	Diarrhoea, haemolytic–uraemic syndrome	Stool culture serotyping, immunoassay for Shiga toxins
Shigella species	Dysentery	Stool culture
Clostridium difficile	Diarrhoea	Toxin assay
Listeria monocytogenes	Diarrhoea, meningitis	Blood, CSF culture
Streptococcus pneumoniae	Pneumonia, meningitis	Blood, CSF culture
Streptococcus pyogenes	Scarlet fever, pharyngitis	Throat or blood culture, antistreptolysin O titre (ASOT)
Haemophilus influenzae type b	LRTI, pneumonia, meningitis	Blood, CSF culture
Staphylococcus aureus	Cellulitis, osteomyelitis, septic arthritis, endocarditis, sepsis	Blood, fluid, aspirate culture
Klebsiella pneumoniae	Pneumonia, UTIs	Blood or urine culture
Neisseria meningitidis	Meningitis, septicaemia	CSF microscopy examination, blood, CSF culture or PCR
Neisseria gonorrhoeae	See Chapter 116	
Streptococcus agalactiae (Group B)	Postpartum infection, neonatal sepsis, pneumonia, osteomyelitis, septicaemia	Blood culture, vaginal swab
Bordetella pertussis	Whooping cough	Nasopharyngeal aspirate for PCR
Viridans streptococci	Endocarditis	Blood culture
Pasteurella multocida	Cellulitis after dog or cat bite	Wound swab for culture
Clostridium perfringens or C. septicum	Gas gangrene	Clinical diagnosis and confirm by wound swab and blood culture
Enterococcus faecalis	Endocarditis, septicaemia, UTI	Blood and urine culture, collection culture
Proteus species	UTI	Urine and blood culture
Pseudomonas aeruginosa	UTI, septicaemia	Blood and urine culture
Escherichia coli	Diarrhoea, urosepsis, biliary traction, septicaemia	Blood and urine culture, wound swab or abscess culture
Brucellosis	Febrile illness, septicaemia	Blood culture, serology test

Table 114.3 Other common infections and tests

Microorganism	Diseases	Test
Legionella pneumophila	Atypical pneumonia	Legionella urine antigen test Sputum culture for Legionella Serology test: fourfold increase in antibody over 4 weeks
Mycoplasma pneumoniae	Atypical pneumonia	Respiratory secretions PCR Serology test: fourfold increase in antibody over 4 weeks
Chlamydia pneumoniae	Atypical pneumonia	Serology test: fourfold increase in antibody over 4 weeks
Coxiella burnetii (Q fever)	Pneumonia, hepatitis	Serology test, PCR test
Toxoplasma gondii	Asymptomatic in immunocompetent patients, encephalitis in immuno-compromised patients	Serology test IgM and IgG antibody PCR test in body fluid Histological examination
Giardia lamblia	Diarrhoea	Fresh stool specimen or duodenal aspirate examination for cysts or trophozoites
Entamoeba histolytica	Diarrhoea, liver abscess	Direct stool smear and staining and EIA Antigen detection: monoclonal antibody
Cryptosporidium (parasite)	Diarrhoea	Detecting Cryptosporidium in a faecal sample using PCR
Strongyloides stercoralis	Asymptomatic, or diarrhoea, or disseminated infection	Visualisation of larvae on microscopic stool examination ELISA for detecting serum IgG against S. stercoralis is available
Rickettsia species	Rickettsial infections cause febrile illness, lymphadenopathy, rash, eschar	Serology test
Leptospira	Leptospirosis	Culture blood and urine Serology test
Candida species	Septicaemia, UTI, wound infection	Blood and urine culture
Aspergillus species	Pulmonary infection	Blood culture, bronchial lavage culture
Cryptococcus neoformans	CNS infection, UTI, bone, eye infection	Biopsy of cutaneous lesions for fungal stains and culture, blood culture, cryptococcal serology, cryptococcal antigen testing, CSF india ink smear

When considering investigation for infection, the following key points/principles should be observed.

- Specimens should be taken before commencing antimicrobials.
- Collect an adequate quantity of specimen.
- Avoid contamination.
- Collect the appropriate specimen for the suspected microorganism and discuss with the testing laboratory.
- Ask the laboratory for special culture if clinically indicated.
- Place the specimen in the appropriate medium for transport and culture.

115 Osteomyelitis

Figure 115.1 Plain X-ray of the right foot shows periosteal reaction and poor definition of the cortex at the medial aspect of the head of the first metatarsal consistent with osteomyelitis

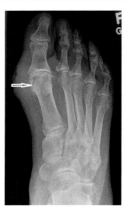

Table 115.1 Sensitivities and specificities of radiological investigation for osteomyelitis

Test	Sensitivity (%)	Specificity (%)
MRI	77–79	53–100
Bone scan	61–100	25–70
WBC scan	80	29
Plain X-ray	60	81

Figure 115.2 MRI of the right foot with contrast shows marrow oedema and enhancement in the posterior aspect of the calcaneum consistent with early osteomyelitis

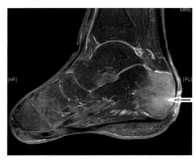

Figure 115.3 Bone scan showing focal hyperaemia centred on the patella suggestive of osteomyelitis

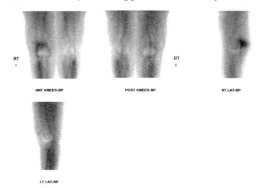

ANT KNEES-BP   POST KNEES-BP   RT LAT-BP

LT LAT-BP

Figure 115.4 USS shows a well-demarcated area of subcutaneous collection over the anteromedial aspect of the left distal tibia

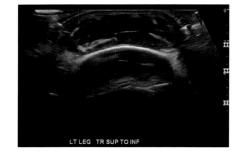

LT LEG   TR SUP TO INF

Figure 115.5 CT-guided aspiration for T12–L1 discitis/osteomyelitis

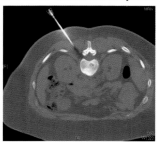

Key points

- Leucocytosis and elevated CRP support the diagnosis of osteomyelitis.
- If radiology is normal but symptoms are suggestive of osteomyelitis, CT or MRI is the imaging of choice to diagnose early osteomyelitis or associated abscesses (e.g. paravertebral or epidural abscess).
- A bone scan can show abnormalities earlier than plain X-ray but does not distinguish between osteomyelitis, fractures and tumours.
- Microbiological diagnosis is essential for guiding therapy of osteomyelitis and should be actively pursued.

Osteomyelitis is infection of bone that can lead to bone destruction and is usually caused by bacteria. The infection can be limited to a single portion of the bone or can involve several regions, such as marrow, cortex and periosteum, and the surrounding soft tissue. Acute osteomyelitis evolves over several days or weeks, as opposed to chronic osteomyelitis, which is arbitrarily defined as infection lasting 6 weeks or more and characterised by the persistence of microorganisms, low-grade inflammation, and the presence of dead bone (sequestrum) and fistulous tracts.

Acute osteomyelitis due to local spread from a contiguous contaminated source of infection usually follows trauma, bone surgery or joint replacement. In this group, identification of patients with a foreign-body implant is important, because of their high susceptibility to infection and treatment challenges. Acute osteomyelitis can be haematogenously acquired and is seen mostly in prepubertal children and in elderly patients. Osteomyelitis secondary to vascular insufficiency occurs predominantly in patients with diabetes and mostly follows a foot soft-tissue infection that spreads to bone. *Staphylococcus aureus* is the most common causative microorganism.

Laboratory investigations

The initial investigations should include FBC, CRP, serum electrolytes, creatinine, urea and LFTs. WBC count is not a reliable indicator and can be normal even when infection is present. The CRP increases usually after 16–24 hours of infection and returns to normal within a week after adequate treatment has begun in most cases. Serum calcium, phosphate and alkaline phosphatase are normal in osteomyelitis, in contrast to metastatic or metabolic bone diseases.

Blood culture

Blood culture should be performed in all patients suspected of osteomyelitis prior to treatment with antibiotics, especially in those with suspected haematogenous spread of infection. A positive culture may preclude the need for more invasive diagnostic procedures. Positive blood cultures are reported in 30–78% of cases of acute osteomyelitis but rarely in chronic osteomyelitis. If osteomyelitis is suspected after imaging is performed and blood cultures do not show growth of microorganisms, a biopsy is usually warranted.

Radiological investigations

Plain X-ray

Plain films can show soft-tissue swelling, narrowing or widening of joint spaces, bone destruction and periosteal reaction (Figure 115.1). However, bone destruction is not apparent on plain films until after 10–21 days of infection. Hence, normal bone X-ray does not exclude osteomyelitis. Plain X-ray can identify other conditions such as fracture, bone neoplasm, avascular necrosis or arthritis. In chronic osteomyelitis, plain X-ray may be diagnostic but cannot demonstrate the extent of marrow infection or soft-tissue abscesses.

CT and MRI scan

Both CT and MRI have excellent resolution and can reveal the destruction of medulla as well as periosteal reaction, cortical destruction, articular damage and soft-tissue involvement, even when plain X-ray is normal (Figure 115.2). CT is prone to image degradation owing to artefacts caused by the presence of bone or metal but is nevertheless useful for guiding needle biopsy. In addition, CT provides excellent definition of cortical bone and a good assessment of the surrounding soft tissues. It is especially useful in identification of sequestrum. MRI, however, is more useful than CT for soft-tissue assessment. MRI also reveals early bone marrow oedema and is therefore most useful for early detection of infection especially in patients with acute vertebral osteomyelitis (90% accuracy). In vertebral osteomyelitis, MRI typically shows high signal intensity within the disc on T2-weighted sequences and loss of the intranuclear cleft. Although MRI is very sensitive, it is not helpful in assessing the response to therapy, given the persistence of bone marrow oedema for many months despite microbiological cure.

Radionuclide bone scan

Bone scan with technetium-99m (^{99m}Tc), which binds to sites of increased bone metabolic activity, is highly sensitive in the early detection of acute osteomyelitis. Leucocyte scanning with WBCs radiolabelled with indium-111 has been used for imaging of osteomyelitis with high sensitivity but lower specificity (Figure 115.3). The limited specificity for radionuclide bone scan is due to diabetic (Charcot) arthropathy, gout, trauma, recent fracture and surgery, which can give false-positive results.

PET scan

PET scan combined with CT appears particularly promising for delineation of lesions and their concomitant inflammatory or infectious activity and when the patient has metallic implants.

Ultrasound

Ultrasound is useful in detecting abscesses in soft tissue or subperiosteal fluid collections. It can be used to guide aspiration of soft-tissue abscesses (Figure 115.4).

Microbiological and histopathological diagnosis

In investigating any kind of osteomyelitis, the most important step is to isolate the offending organisms so that appropriate antimicrobial therapy can be chosen. This can be achieved by blood cultures or by direct biopsy from the involved bone. Biopsy has a higher overall diagnostic yield than blood culture (47–100%). If polymicrobial osteomyelitis is suspected (e.g. from intra-abdominal sepsis), a biopsy should be performed regardless of whether the blood cultures are positive. If the patient has a paravertebral, epidural or psoas abscess, drainage guided by CT (Figure 115.5) with subsequent staining and culture of specimen may make a bone biopsy unnecessary.

Material taken from an open sinus tract by swabbing can give misleading results because the isolates may include non-pathogenic microorganisms that are colonising the site. Whenever bone biopsies are done, the samples should be processed for aerobic and anaerobic cultures. Samples for mycobacterial and fungal cultures should be taken and processed. In implant-associated infections, for maximum diagnostic yield, deep specimens should be obtained from up to five sites around the implant at debridement.

116 Sexually transmitted diseases

Table 116.1 Common STDs

- Genital tract chlamydia infection
- HSV-1 and HSV-2
- Gonorrhoea infection
- Syphilis
- Trichomoniasis
- HPV infection
- HIV infection
- Pelvic inflammatory disease
- Urethritis
- Chancroid

Table 116.2 Patients at higher risk for STDs

- Patients who have multiple sex partners
- Patients who use or have used intravenous drugs
- Patients who have been diagnosed with other STDs
- Men who have sex with men
- Women who have sex with women
- Patients who are sex workers or have unprotected intercourse

Table 116.3 Tests for common STDs

	Test	Specimen	Window period	Indication	Comments
Chlamydia	NAAT	Urine, swab (urethra, cervix)	2–7 days	Screening and diagnosis	NAAT can be performed on self-collected samples
	Culture	Swab, any site			Highly specific, use in legal situations
Herpes	PCR	Lesion	Lesion	Diagnosis	Negative PCR or viral culture does not exclude infection
	Viral cultures	Lesion	Lesion	Diagnosis	
	EIA/ELISA serology test	Blood	3–12 weeks	Screening	Type-specific serology is useful
Gonorrhoea	NAAT	Urine, swab (urethra, cervix)	24 hours	Screening and diagnosis	PCR at high vaginal, throat and rectal sites not validated
	Culture	Swab (urethra, cervix, throat, rectum)		Screening/diagnosis Confirmation of NAAT	Culture allows antibiotic sensitivity testing
Syphilis	Dark-ground microscopy	Lesion	3–30 days, if chancre	Diagnosis early syphilis	
	PCR/LCR	Lesion, tissue, CSF, blood	3–30 days, if chancre	Diagnosis early syphilis	Not widely available
	EIA	Blood	2–12 weeks	Screening	Repeat serology for those with suspected exposure
	RPR/VDRL	Blood, CSF	3–12 weeks	Screening, diagnosis/ staging, treatment response, reinfection	

Table 116.4 Contact tracing for STDs

Infection	How far back to trace
Chlamydia	6 months
Gonorrhoea	2 months
Syphilis	Primary syphilis: 3 months plus duration of symptoms Secondary syphilis: 6 months plus duration of symptoms Early latent syphilis: 12 months
Trichomoniasis	Unknown; important to treat current partner
Mycoplasma genitalium	Unknown; important to treat current partner
Lymphogranuloma venereum	1 month

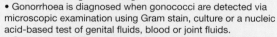
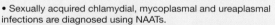

Key points

- Sexually acquired chlamydial, mycoplasmal and ureaplasmal infections are diagnosed using NAATs.
- Gonorrhoea is diagnosed when gonococci are detected via microscopic examination using Gram stain, culture or a nucleic acid-based test of genital fluids, blood or joint fluids.
- Genital warts (HPV infections) are usually diagnosed clinically. HPV testing is available, but its role in HPV management is unclear.
- Genital herpes can be confirmed by PCR on the swab samples.
- Syphilis has three sequential clinical symptomatic stages separated by periods of asymptomatic latent infection. Diagnose using a non-treponemal test (e.g. RPR, VDRL) and confirm positive results using a treponemal antibody test.

Sexually transmitted diseases (STDs) can be caused by bacteria, viruses, fungi and parasites. Early diagnosis can reduce the spread of infections and early treatment can minimise potential complications such as infertility. The individual's age and sexual behaviour and community STD prevalence influence the level of risk, and choice of STD screening tests. The common STDs are listed in Table 116.1.

In pregnant women, the health of both the woman and the fetus are at risk. At the first prenatal visit, the patient should be considered for screening for common STDs, depending on the history and risk level of the patient and the patient's partner.

Chlamydia

Chlamydia trachomatis is the most commonly reported STD in developed countries. It is an important risk factor for pelvic inflammatory disease (PID), ectopic pregnancies and infertility. Patients are usually asymptomatic but can present with an odourless mucoid vaginal discharge. In men, symptoms include a clear to white urethral discharge.

Clinical Investigations at a Glance, First Edition. Jonathan Gleadle, Jordan Li and Tuck Yong. © 2017 John Wiley & Sons, Ltd. Published 2017 by John Wiley & Sons, Ltd.

Nucleic acid amplification test (NAAT) is the investigation of choice, with sensitivity of 85% and specificity of 95%. A negative test performed when clinical suspicion for infection is high should be repeated. NAATs can be done on self-collected (first-pass not mid-stream urine sample or vaginal swab) or clinician-collected samples (vaginal, endocervical or urethral swab). *Chlamydia trachomatis* cultures have the highest specificity and allow for antibiotic sensitivity testing.

Annual screening for chlamydia infection is recommended in sexually active women aged 25 years or less and in women aged over 25 years who are at increased risk for STDs.

Gonorrhoea

Untreated *Neisseria gonorrhoeae* infection can lead to cervicitis, urethritis, proctitis, PID, and adverse outcomes in pregnancy. Infected men frequently present with a urethral discharge; women are often asymptomatic until complications such as PID or ectopic pregnancy occur.

A Gram stain of the discharge has high specificity (98%) and sensitivity (95%). The test is considered highly suggestive for infection with *N. gonorrhoeae* in symptomatic men if the smear contains typical Gram-negative diplococci within polymorphonuclear leucocytes. However, all patients with suspected *N. gonorrhoeae* should have a definitive laboratory test (i.e. culture or NAAT). Culture is highly specific and allows for antibiotic sensitivity testing, but the sensitivity may decrease with lengthy delays between collection and the laboratory. NAAT has high sensitivity (90–95%) and specificity (98–100%) for swab samples. First-void urine samples and self-collected anal swabs are acceptable samples for test; however, in women endocervical swabs are more sensitive than urine samples.

Genital herpes

Both HSV-1 and HSV-2 infections are chronic lifelong viral infections. HSV-2 is the causative agent in the majority of genital herpes cases, but HSV-1 has become more prevalent.

The clinical diagnosis is unreliable and should be confirmed by HSV PCR test. Type-specific PCR is sensitive and specific but can produce false-negative results. Although slow and labour-intensive, viral culture is type specific and has a specificity of nearly 100%.

Human papillomavirus (HPV)

Anogenital HPV is extremely common, with up to 75% of sexually active individuals having evidence of current or past infection. While most infections are subclinical and transient, others may cause genital warts and cervical cancer. Although cervical cancer is a rare outcome of HPV infection, over 99.7% of cervical cancers are positive for HPV DNA. The diagnosis of genital warts is clinical. A biopsy is indicated only if the genital warts appear fixed to underlying structures, are refractory to standard therapy or display ulceration or size over 1 cm.

Syphilis

Syphilis is caused by the bacterium *Treponema pallidum* and transmitted through direct sexual contact with an individual with early syphilis.

Screening for syphilis is performed when the patient presents with symptoms, has had sexual intercourse with a known infected partner, has been diagnosed with other STDs or has engaged in other high-risk behaviours. In pregnant women, screening is typically performed at the first prenatal visit.

Dark-field microscopy of swab from a lesion should be performed to identify *T. pallidum*. In primary syphilis, the sensitivity is 74–86% and specificity 85–100%. Three negative examinations on different days exclude infection. In secondary syphilis, dark-field microscopy may be positive in samples from ulcerative anogenital lesions.

Syphilis serology should be performed in any patient with suspected syphilis even if dark-field microscopy is negative. Screening utilises sensitive and specific treponemal tests, such as enzyme immunoassay, that contain both IgG and IgM components. These are then confirmed by supplementary specific investigations such as *T. pallidum* particle agglutination assay or fluorescent treponemal antibody absorption test. However, these tests do not give an indication of disease activity and usually remain positive regardless of treatment. A non-specific test such as rapid plasma reagin (RPR) or Venereal Disease Research Laboratory (VDRL) test is used to provide a titre to stage the infection, assess treatment response and detect reinfection. Treatment response is monitored using RPR or VDRL titres and a fourfold reduction within 6–12 months is considered a cure.

Neurosyphilis is the most serious complication of syphilis. CSF analysis is required to confirm the diagnosis. The CSF WBC count (usually lymphocytes) is typically raised above $5/mm^3$, protein levels are increased and glucose is normal. CSF VDRL confirms the diagnosis if positive.

All patients with syphilis should be tested for HIV.

Trichomoniasis

Trichomoniasis is caused by the protozoan *Trichomonas vaginalis*. The traditional investigation depends on microscopic observation of motile protozoa from vaginal or cervical samples and from urethral or prostatic secretions, but is only 60–70% sensitive. Many point-of-care tests are available but often result in false positives, particularly in low-prevalence populations. For women, a culture of vaginal secretions is the most sensitive method for diagnosis when microscopy is not conclusive. For men, culture for *T. vaginalis* from urethral swab, urine and semen has the highest sensitivity.

Pelvic inflammatory disease

PID consists of inflammatory disorders of the upper female genital tract, including endometritis, salpingitis, tubo-ovarian abscesses and pelvic peritonitis. Signs and symptoms may be non-specific but early diagnosis can avoid inflammatory sequelae. It is recommended that all women with a diagnosis of acute PID be tested for *N. gonorrhoeae*, *C. trachomatis* and HIV.

Imaging is needed for patients with uncertain clinical diagnosis and those who are severely ill or unresponsive to initial therapy. Transvaginal ultrasound is the primary imaging modality and may be normal in early or uncomplicated cases. It can detect endometritis, salpingitis, oophoritis and abscess. Pelvic CT with both oral and intravenous contrast is indicated in patients with diffuse pelvic pain, peritonitis, or difficult or equivocal ultrasound. Pelvic MRI is considered superior to ultrasound at diagnosing PID when there is a tubo-ovarian abscess, pyosalpinx, fluid-filled tube and/or enlarged polycystic ovaries with free intrapelvic fluid.

Notification and contact tracing

In the case of a notifiable condition, the patient should be informed that case notification to public health authorities will occur. Contact tracing (or 'partner notification') is an essential component of the effective management of STDs as they may be asymptomatic. The aim of contact tracing is to reduce reinfection and complications of disease and to reduce the population burden of STDs (Table 116.4).

117 Tuberculosis

Table 117.1 Patients at increased risk of primary or reactive TB

Elderly patients
Patients from high TB-burden countries, such as sub-Saharan Africa, India, China and other Asian countries
Healthcare workers who have been working in high-burden countries
Immunocompromised states including HIV infection (risk of TB reactivation is 10% per annum, although this is substantially reduced with antiretroviral therapy)
Medication-related, such as chemotherapy and post-transplantation immunosuppressants

```
Always consider TB in symptomatic patients,
in patients from populations at high risk and
in those with undifferentiated illness
                    │
                    ▼
        Is the patient symptomatic?
    ◄─── No                    Yes ───►
        │                            │
        ▼                            ▼
    Latent TB                    Active TB
        │                            │
        ▼                            ▼
  First-line test: IGRA      CXR, three sputum samples
  Second-line test: TST      for smear and culture
        │                            │
   ┌────┴────┐                       │
   ▼         ▼                       ▼
Negative,  Positive, need to   Consider molecular
consider   exclude active TB   PCR assay
alternative                         │
diagnosis                      ┌────┴────┐
                               ▼         ▼
              Positive, consider    Negative, consider
              drug susceptibility   alternative diagnosis
              test
   Consult TB physician  ◄───
   for treatment
```

Figure 117.1 CXR shows a cavity in the right upper lobe and bilateral small infiltrate consistent with active TB

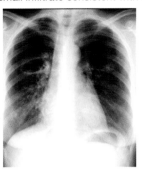

Figure 117.2 CXR shows left apical opacity with left upper lobe collapse and minor right upper lobe scarring consistent with TB

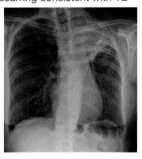

Figure 117.3 CXR shows previous thoracoplasty for surgical treatment of TB and stable scarring in the left upper lobe in keeping with previous TB

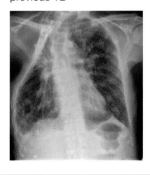

Key points

- IGRA is the investigation of choice for latent TB.
- TST is the second choice in persons at high risk of LTBI or progression to active TB, even if they have received previous BCG vaccination.
- In active TB, patient should have a CXR, sputum smear and culture. The overall sensitivity of three acid-fast smears for identifying active TB is 70%. Sputum culture is the gold standard for the diagnosis of TB.
- Contact tracing and investigation (IGRA testing and CXR) minimises morbidity resulting from transmission of TB and should be guided by the local health authority.

Clinical Investigations at a Glance, First Edition. Jonathan Gleadle, Jordan Li and Tuck Yong. © 2017 John Wiley & Sons, Ltd. Published 2017 by John Wiley & Sons, Ltd.

Tuberculosis (TB) is an infection caused by *Mycobacterium tuberculosis*. TB infection most commonly involves the lungs and is communicable in pulmonary TB, but may affect many other organs (extrapulmonary TB) such as lymph nodes, CNS, bones and kidneys.

TB infects one-third of the world's population, but the diagnosis is often overlooked in developed countries, where the incidence is low. When infection is contained by the immune system it remains latent for many years, termed 'latent tuberculosis infection' (LTBI). It can re-emerge with immunosuppression or advancing age. Overall, LTBI carries a 10% risk of developing active TB during a patient's lifetime, with the greatest risk being within 2 years of infection. Once reactivated, symptoms such as fever, night sweats, weight loss and cough develop.

Tests for suspected active pulmonary TB

A key diagnostic challenge for all clinicians is to 'remember' TB. Patients with symptoms suggestive of active TB, such as night sweats, cough and fever, and household contacts of a confirmed case of TB should undergo the tests described in the following sections. These patients are potentially infectious so precautions should be taken. Table 117.1 lists the groups of patients who are at increased risk of primary TB infection or reactivation of TB and these individuals should carry a low threshold for TB tests.

CXR

Typical changes include air-space consolidation, cavitation and fibrous contraction in one or both upper lobes and superior parts of the lower lobes (Figures 117.1–117.3). In HIV, atypical findings are more common, including a normal CXR despite active disease. Active infection can be difficult to distinguish from LTBI on CXR so further microbiology tests are essential.

Microbiological tests

Sputum smear

Three sputum specimens, preferably early morning, are needed to maximise yield. Nebulised hypertonic saline (3%) may induce sputum production, but occasionally bronchoscopic lavage is necessary. Collection should occur away from other people, and into a jar with a threaded lid. Sputum should be delivered promptly to the laboratory but can be stored in the refrigerator for 1–2 days. Acid-fast microscopy is rapid and inexpensive. Approximately 5000 bacilli per millilitre of sputum are required for a positive smear. Microscopy detects acid-fast bacilli (AFB) in approximately 50% of cases of pulmonary TB. The Ziehl–Neelsen stain is the standard, and utilises the staining properties of the waxy coats of the mycobacterial cell walls. Culture or molecular assays are then required to confirm if AFB are *M. tuberculosis*.

Sputum culture

Culture is the most sensitive and specific test. Automatic liquid cultures are preferred as they are more rapid (1–3 weeks) and sensitive than solid culture media (4–8 weeks) and can also test drug susceptibility. Approximately 80% of pulmonary TB cases in developed countries are sputum culture positive.

Molecular assays

Molecular assays detect DNA specific for *M. tuberculosis*. In smear-positive samples they are highly sensitive (95% sensitivity, 99% specificity), but in smear-negative specimens sensitivity drops to 50% and specificity to 95%. A new rapid PCR test that is not prone to contamination is advocated by some experts.

Sensitivity is equivalent to that of solid culture and simultaneously detects rifampicin resistance.

Drug susceptibility testing

The cultured isolate should be tested against first-line agents. Resistant strains are then tested against second-line drugs. Multiple drug-resistant strains are defined by resistance to both isoniazid and rifampicin. Drug-resistant strains require longer therapy.

Tests for suspected latent tuberculosis

Diagnosis of LTBI depends on tests of immune recognition of *M. tuberculosis* antigens with tuberculin skin testing (TST) or interferon gamma release assay (IGRA). These tests become positive 4–6 weeks after initial infection. Treating LTBI decreases the risk of progression to active TB by 60–90% and eliminates the potential for transmission. The risk of progression to disease is greatest within the first year.

Tuberculin skin test

The TST or Mantoux test evaluates inflammation in the dermis following intradermal injection of tuberculin protein. The test needs to be read 48–72 hours after injection. The diameter of induration gives a semi-quantitative assessment of the likelihood of LTBI. The sensitivity of TST in diagnosing active TB is 75%. False positives can result from previous bacillus Calmette–Guérin (BCG) vaccination and exposure to environmental *Mycobacterium* species. False-negative results occur in 20–25% of patients with active pulmonary TB.

Interferon gamma release assays

IGRAs measure the response of T lymphocytes to TB antigens in order to diagnose prior exposure. If primed by previous TB infection, lymphocytes will produce detectable amounts of gamma interferon. There are two commercially available tests: the Quantiferon Gold In-Tube™ assay (Celestis Australia) and the T-spot™ test (Oxford Immunotech). IGRAs are not affected by previous BCG vaccination. A positive IGRA suggests that the patient's immune system recognises *M. tuberculosis* antigens. This may be due to current infection or a remote past infection. IGRAs do not diagnose active TB; microbiological tests are needed. Similarly a negative test cannot exclude active TB because false-negative results occur in 20–25% of patients with active pulmonary TB.

Neither TST nor IGRA is sufficiently sensitive to rule out TB infection; in particular, those with advanced disease can have normal TST results. In addition, caution is recommended in infants and in immunosuppressed patients.

Tests for extrapulmonary TB

Extrapulmonary TB is diagnosed by sending a tissue sample in normal saline for microscopy and culture. Histopathology may identify typical changes (necrotising granulomas, caseation and AFB). Patients with TB should be screened for HIV infection.

Follow-up tests

Patients diagnosed with active TB should undergo sputum analysis for *M. tuberculosis* weekly until sputum conversion, defined as two consecutive negative cultures. Monitoring for toxicity includes baseline and periodic LFTs, FBC and serum creatinine. Monthly eye examination is recommended for patients on ethambutol, which can cause optic neuritis.

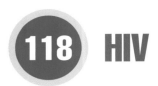

118 HIV

The purpose of investigating patients with newly diagnosed HIV is to:
- Establish the prognosis and the need for highly active antiretroviral therapy (HAART).
- Stage the patient according to WHO or Centers for Disease Control and Prevention (CDC) criteria.
- Monitor the progression of HIV and response to HAART.
- Monitor adverse effects of antiretroviral therapy and resistance genotyping.
- Guide the introduction of prophylactic therapy against opportunistic infections.

Box 118.1 Indications for HIV testing

- Clinical suspicion of HIV infection
- Patients where HIV enters the differential diagnosis
- Diagnosis of a condition with shared transmission route, especially STD
- Sex partners of individual known to be HIV positive
- Unprotected sexual intercourse with a partner whose HIV status is unknown
- Reported reuse of equipment used for skin penetration
- Patients who have used intravenous drugs
- In the setting of contact tracing or in the context of post-exposure prophylaxis
- Patients from countries with high HIV prevalence
- Patient requests an HIV test
- Healthcare workers conducting exposure-prone procedures
- Organ transplant donors and recipients, dialysis patients, blood donors

Table 118.1 Screening and confirmatory tests for HIV

Test	Use	Window period	Sensitivity	Specificity	Comments
HIV antibodies via ELISA	Screening test	21 days after infection	99.3%	99.8%	Gold-standard assays detect antibodies
p24 antigen	Screening test	6 days after infection	79–89%	99.3%	Combined with HIV antibodies improved sensitivity
Western blot	Confirmatory test	21 days after infection	96%	99.7%	Expensive, reserved for investigating equivocal serology results
RNA viral load	Confirmatory test and monitring	10 days after infection	Sensitive to 40 copies/mL	100%	Detects HIV infection before antibodies, decides the need and success of treatment
Proviral DNA	Diagnostic test for baby forn to HIV-infected mother		>99%	98%	Also used in positive serology with undetectable HIV RNA in untreated patients

Table 118.2 Investigation of the adverse effects of HAART

Adverse effects	Investigations
Lactic acidosis	Lactate, LFTs, ABG
Peripheral neuropathy	Vitamin B_{12} level, hepatitis C serology
Hepatotoxicity	LFTs, hepatitis B and C serology, liver ultrasound, liver biopsy if needed
Lipodystrophy	Usually a clinical diagnosis but CT or MRI can be used for assessment
Hyperlipidaemia	Lipid studies
Diabetes mellitus	Fasting glucose, oral glucose tolerance test, glycated haemoglobin, urine albumin/creatinine ratio
Bone disease	Bone densitometry (DEXA scan), calcium, phosphate, 25-hydroxyvitamin D, PTH, testosterone (males), MRI or CT if osteonecrosis is suspected

Table 118.3 Investigations for some of the AIDS-defining illnesses

AIDS-defining illness	Investigations
Cervical cancer	Cervical smear
Cryptococcosis	Histology/cytology in tissue; culture or detection of antigen in fluid or tissue
Cytomegalovirus disease	Histology/cytology in tissue; viral PCR in blood, fluid or tissue
Herpes simplex virus	PCR in fluid or tissue, histology/cytology in tissue
Kaposi's sarcoma	Histology or cytology
Non-Hodgkin's lymphoma	Radiological imaging (CT and PET), excision biopsy of the lesions
Mycobacterium tuberculosis	CXR, CT, AFB in fluid or tissue, culture, tissue histology, bone marrow biopsy
Mycobacterium avium complex	CT, blood culture, tissue histology, bone marrow biopsy
Oesophageal candidiasis	Upper gastrointestinal endoscopy and biopsy
Pneumocystis jiroveci pneumonia	CXR, CT chest, ABG, bronchoscopy
Progressive multifocal leukoencephalopathy	MRI head, lumbar puncture and JC virus PCR
Toxoplasmosis	CT or MRI head, lumbar puncture, histology or cytology

Key points

- Detection of antibodies to HIV is sensitive and specific except during the first few weeks after infection.
- ELISA is rarely false positive. A Western Blot test more specific than ELISA.
- If HIV infection is clinically suspected but antibody tests are negative, the plasma HIV RNA level may be measured. The NAATs used are highly sensitive and specific.
- HIV is monitored by CD4 count and plasma HIV RNA viral loads. Both are useful for determining prognosis, the need for treatment and monitoring treatment.

HIV infection is caused by a retrovirus (HIV types 1 and 2) that infects and replicates in human lymphocytes and macrophages, leading to immune incompetence and a susceptibility to opportunistic and other infections as well as the development of malignancies. It is estimated that over 33 million people worldwide are living with HIV-1 infection.

HIV infection is a chronic disease characterised by three phases: acute primary illness, asymptomatic chronic illness and symptomatic chronic illness. The rate of progression from one phase to another is highly variable. Symptomatic HIV disease is further divided into two phases that are not necessarily contiguous: symptomatic HIV infection and AIDS (acquired immunodeficiency syndrome). The time interval between HIV transmission and the ability to detect the infection in blood using serology tests or PCR viral RNA detection is referred to as the 'window period'.

Initial screening and confirmatory tests

Indications for HIV testing
See Box 118.1.

Which test should be used for initial HIV testing?
The diagnosis of HIV infection is made by detecting circulating antibodies using an enzyme-linked immunosorbent assay (ELISA) and p24 antigen. In some situations, such as pre-seroconversion, measurement of HIV antibodies is unreliable. As a result, direct detection of HIV is done by measuring HIV RNA in blood or tissue culture.

The ELISA test is generally scored as positive (highly reactive), negative (non-reactive) or indeterminate (partially reactive). A positive ELISA is usually observed within 3–6 weeks following infection. False-positive results are rare, with a test specificity of more than 99.8% (causes for false-positive results include antibodies to human leucocyte antigen class II antigens, other autoantibodies, hepatic disease, recent influenza vaccination and acute viral infections). Rapid tests or point-of-care tests are becoming increasingly used. They rely on either serum from fingerprick or saliva from a mouth swab and can give a result in 30 min.

Consent must be obtained prior to a HIV test. Patients should be given the reason why the test is recommended, the benefits of testing and the potential consequences of a positive or negative test. They should be given the details of how the result will be communicated to them and the subsequent healthcare services that are available.

Which confirmatory tests should be used if the screen test is positive?

Serum Western blot test
This is used as a confirmatory test following a positive ELISA or rapid test. During the window period the result may be falsely negative or indeterminate.

HIV RNA quantification
HIV RNA quantification (or viral load) can be achieved by reverse transcriptase polymerase chain reaction (RT-PCR) or branched DNA assay. Both tests can detect 40–50 copies of HIV RNA per millilitre of plasma. Detection of HIV RNA can help diagnose HIV infection where standard serological testing is inappropriate or unclear. Quantification of HIV RNA levels allows prediction of the rate of HIV disease progression and provides a surrogate marker of response to antiretroviral therapy.

HIV proviral DNA PCR
HIV proviral DNA PCR is highly sensitive (>99% detecting one copy of HIV DNA per 10,000–100,000 cells) and specific (98%) but does not replace serology either as a screening test or as a diagnostic test in isolation. The main use is for the qualitative detection of HIV when serological testing is inappropriate, disputed or inconclusive (Table 118.1).

Investigations for newly diagnosed HIV

Baseline investigations
The following laboratory investigations are performed in patients with newly diagnosed HIV.
- Staging of HIV infection: CD4 cell count by flow cytometry (Table 118.1) and HIV viral load.
- Baseline FBC, biochemistry, LFTs, fasting glucose and lipid studies.
- Baseline serology for CMV, *Toxoplasma*, hepatitis A, B and C virus, and syphilis (VDRL).
- Glucose 6-phosphate dehydrogenase in males of African or eastern Mediterranean descent (risk of drug-related haemolysis).

Initial investigations for possible comorbidities
- Testing for STDs (gonorrhoea, *Chlamydia*, syphilis and HSV).
- Cervical cytology in women.
- Routine CXR.
- Mantoux test if at risk of exposure or past exposure to TB.
- Baseline ECG, echocardiogram if cardiovascular risk factors are present.

Follow-up investigations
After the diagnosis of HIV, plasma HIV RNA, CD4 cell count, FBC, electrolytes and LFTs are performed every 3 months, or more frequently if there are clinical indications. Fasting lipids and glucose are monitored every 6 months. Other investigations are undertaken as clinically indicated (see the following sections).

Investigations for drug resistance and antiretroviral therapy adverse effects
The resistance profile of an HIV strain can be tested by examination of the nucleic acid sequence of the target genes for evidence of known resistance mutations (resistance genotyping assay), or directly assessed by tissue culture of HIV (full length or cloned into a common viral backbone) in the presence of a panel of antiretroviral drugs.

Many adverse effects can occur in the setting of combination antiretroviral therapy. Antiretroviral therapy can cause mitochondrial toxicity (lactic acidosis and peripheral neuropathy), hepatotoxicity and metabolic abnormalities (lipodystrophy, hyperlipidaemia, diabetes) and bone disease. Table 118.2 shows some of investigations to diagnose and monitor these adverse effects.

Investigations for diagnosing AIDS-defining illnesses
HIV infection can be complicated by a wide range of opportunistic illnesses leading to substantial morbidity and mortality. Table 118.3 shows some of the commonly encountered AIDS-defining illnesses and their diagnostic investigations.

119 Leucocytosis

Table 119.1 Common causes of neutrophilia

Physiological neutrophilia

Pregnancy
Stress
Exercise

Primary neutrophilia

Acute myeloid leukaemia
Chronic myeloid leukaemia (CML), primary myelofibrosis
  (proliferative phase)
Hereditary neutrophilia

Secondary neutrophilia

Bacterial infections
Inflammation and tissue necrosis
Anaemia
Acute haemorrhage or haemolysis
Solid tumour malignancy
Bone marrow infiltration due to tumour, granulomatous
  disease
Asplenia
Recovering bone marrow function from chemotherapy
Treatment with myeloid growth factors (e.g. G-CSF)

Drug-induced neutrophilia

Corticosteroid therapy
Epinephrine (adrenaline), beta-agonists

Table 119.2 Causes of eosinophilia

Allergic events

Asthma, eczema, food allergy

Infections

Parasitic infections
Other infections: scarlet fever, leprosy, HIV

Drugs

Any drug, especially seen with antibiotics,
  sulphonamides, anticonvulsants

Lung diseases

Löffler's syndrome, Churg–Strauss syndrome,
  allergic bronchopulmonary aspergillosis

Gastrointestinal diseases

Eosinophilic oesophagitis, celiac disease,
  inflammatory bowel disease (IBD)

Autoimmune diseases

Psoriasis, pemphigus and dermatitis,
  rheumatoid arthritis, SLE, adrenal insufficiency

Malignancies

Non-Hodgkin's lymphoma, Hodgkin's disease,
  eosinophilic leukaemia
Myeloproliferative disorders: CML, myelofibrosis

Idiopathic hypereosinophilic syndrome

Table 119.3 Causes of basophilia

- Myeloproliferative disorders: CML, polycythaemia vera, myelofibrosis
- Infections: viral infections (varicella), chronic sinusitis
- Inflammatory conditions: IBD, chronic airway inflammation, chronic
  dermatitis
- Other haematological disorders: chronic haemolytic anaemia,
  Hodgkin's disease, splenectomy

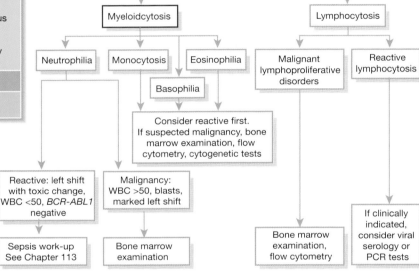

Step 1
Confirm leucocytosis before initiating an intensive investigation
into the cause as it may be due to laboratory artefact

Step 2
Examine the peripheral blood film to confirm the automated blood cell differential

Step 3
Separate the leucocytosis into a myeloid versus a lymphoid process

Step 4
Distinguish malignant from benign leucocytosis, the appropriate response of
normal bone marrow to external stimuli. Bone marrow examination may be required

Myeloidcytosis

Lymphocytosis

Neutrophilia — Monocytosis — Eosinophilia

Basophilia

Malignant
lymphoproliferative
disorders

Reactive
lymphocytosis

Consider reactive first.
If suspected malignancy, bone
marrow examination, flow
cytometry, cytogenetic tests

Reactive: left shift
with toxic change,
WBC <50, *BCR-ABL1*
negative

Malignancy:
WBC >50, blasts,
marked left shift

Sepsis work-up
See Chapter 113

Bone marrow
examination

Bone marrow
examination,
flow cytometry

If clinically
indicated,
consider viral
serology or
PCR tests

Table 119.4 Causes of lymphocytosis

Absolute lymphocytosis

Acute infections: CMV or EBV infection,
  pertussis, hepatitis, toxoplasmosis
Chronic infections: tuberculosis, brucellosis
Lymphoid malignancies: chronic lymphocytic
  leukaemia

Relative lymphocytosis

Acute phase of some viral illnesses
Connective tissue diseases
Thyrotoxicosis
Addison's disease
Splenomegaly with splenic sequestration

Table 119.5 Causes of monocytosis

- Chronic bacterial infections: tuberculosis,
  brucellosis, bacterial endocarditis
- Protozoan infections
- Chronic neutropenia
- Hodgkin's disease
- Myelodysplastic syndrome, CML
- Treatment with myeloid growth factor
  (e.g. GM-CSF)

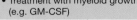

Key points

- The first step in investigating leucocytosis is to manually examine
  the blood smear to confirm the WBC differential count.
- Characteristic features of reactive neutrophilia include a 'shift to the
  left' and presence of cytoplasmic toxic granulation.
- A leukaemoid reaction is a reactive and excessive leucocytosis
  characterised by the presence of immature cells (myeloblasts,
  promyelocytes and myelocytes) in the peripheral blood.
- The first step in the evaluation of lymphocytosis is review of the
  morphology of lymphocytes to see whether it is reactive.

Clinical Investigations at a Glance, First Edition. Jonathan Gleadle, Jordan Li and Tuck Yong. © 2017 John Wiley & Sons, Ltd. Published 2017 by John Wiley & Sons, Ltd.
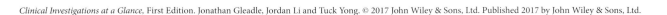

Leucocytosis, a frequently encountered laboratory finding, is a WBC count in excess of 11×10^9/L. It most often results from an increase in neutrophils but other cell types including eosinophils, lymphocytes and monocytes may be responsible, so it is important to check the differential count when interpreting leucocytosis. Leucocytosis typically reflects the response of bone marrow to an infectious or inflammatory process but can be the sign of primary bone marrow disorders such as leukaemia or myeloproliferative disorder.

Diagnostic evaluation

In interpreting leucocytosis on FBC, the patient's clinical features, differential leucocyte count and other counts should be considered. The key steps in evaluation are shown on the page opposite.

Neutrophilia

An increase in circulating neutrophils above 7.5×10^9/L is one of the most frequently encountered FBC changes. The common causes of neutrophilia are shown in Table 119.1. Features often reported with reactive neutrophilia (secondary to bacterial infections, inflammation, neoplasms or acute haemorrhage) include the following.
• 'Shift to the left' in the peripheral blood differential WBC count: an increase in the number of band forms and the occasional presence of more primitive cells.
• 'Toxic changes': the presence of cytoplasmic toxic granulation and Döhle bodies.
Patients taking corticosteroids often have a persistent increase in neutrophils that reflects a number of changes to neutrophil kinetics, including decreased movement into tissues.

The manual differential is key to diagnosis, along with correct enumeration of blasts and blast equivalents, immature granulocytes, basophils and eosinophils, and dysplasia to identify myeloid malignancies. Confirmation and characterisation of myeloid malignancies should be performed with a bone marrow examination. Myeloid leukaemoid reactions can result from infections, show activated neutrophil changes and should prompt evaluation for infection. Imaging studies of chest and abdomen should be performed for possible underlying haematological or non-haematological malignancy.

Eosinophilia

Eosinophilia is defined as an eosinophil count in excess of 0.5×10^9/L. The most common cause of eosinophilia in developed countries is allergic disease, particularly asthma, hay fever and eczema. However, parasitic infection should be considered in at-risk populations. Common causes of eosinophilia are listed in Table 119.2 and can be divided into three categories:
• reactive (or secondary) eosinophilia;
• clonal (or primary) eosinophilia;
• idiopathic hypereosinophilic syndrome.

The investigation of unexplained persistent eosinophilia relies on clinical history (especially allergy, drugs, and travel history) as well as symptoms and signs which may point to a reactive eosinophilia or a specific organ-related eosinophilic syndrome. The following investigations can be considered.
• Tests for allergy: serum total IgE, skin-prick tests and/or allergen-specific IgE tests.
• Tests for parasitic infections: fresh stool specimen for the diagnosis of parasite infections. Duodenal aspirate, sputum, spinal fluid, urine, blood film and tissue biopsy may also be examined if clinically indicated.
• Serological tests for suspected parasitic infections such as schistosomiasis and filariasis.
• Bone marrow aspiration and biopsy.
• Cytogenetic and molecular analysis on bone marrow aspirate.
• Pulmonary function tests and bronchoalveolar lavage if clinically indicated.

Basophilia

Basophilia is an uncommon cause of leucocytosis. Basophils are inflammatory mediators of substances such as histamine. These cells, along with similar tissue-based cells (mast cells), have receptors for IgE and participate in the degranulation of WBCs that occurs during allergic reactions, including anaphylaxis. Underlying myeloproliferative disorders are the most common causes of persistent basophilia (Table 119.3).

Lymphocytosis

Lymphocytes normally represent 20–40% of circulating WBCs. Increased numbers of lymphocytes occur with certain acute and chronic infections (Table 119.4). In EBV infection or glandular fever, the cells may show striking reactive changes, referred to as 'reactive lymphocytes' on the blood film report. Malignancies of the lymphoid system may also cause lymphocytosis. Distinguishing a reactive lymphoid proliferation from a lymphoproliferative disorder requires examination of lymphocyte morphology for pleomorphic lymphocytes versus a monomorphic population, with the latter favouring a lymphoproliferative neoplasm. Samples suspicious for lymphoproliferative disorders can be confirmed and characterised by flow cytometry, although molecular studies and bone marrow examination may be necessary.

Monocytosis

Monocytosis is a monocyte count above 0.8×10^9/L. It is an infrequent finding. Conditions associated with monocytosis are listed in Table 119.5. Mild monocytosis can be seen in chronic infections such as diabetic ulcers, osteomyelitis and tuberculosis or as a bacterial infection is resolving. Blood film assessment is used to exclude dysplastic features.

120 Myelodysplastic syndromes

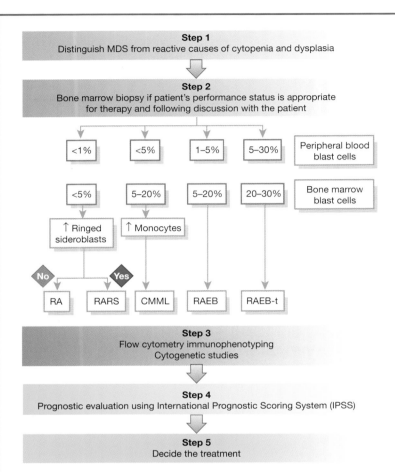

Step 1
Distinguish MDS from reactive causes of cytopenia and dysplasia

Step 2
Bone marrow biopsy if patient's performance status is appropriate for therapy and following discussion with the patient

| <1% | <5% | 1–5% | 5–30% | Peripheral blood blast cells |

| <5% | 5–20% | 5–20% | 20–30% | Bone marrow blast cells |

↑ Ringed sideroblasts   ↑ Monocytes

No   Yes

| RA | RARS | CMML | RAEB | RAEB-t |

Step 3
Flow cytometry immunophenotyping
Cytogenetic studies

Step 4
Prognostic evaluation using International Prognostic Scoring System (IPSS)

Step 5
Decide the treatment

Table 120.1 Initial investigations for suspected MDS

Haematology tests

FBC with differential count, morphologic studies of peripheral blood film, reticulocyte count
RBC indices (mean cell volume), reticulocyte count
RBC folate/serum folic acid, vitamin B12 levels
Iron study
Haptoglobin, direct antiglobulin test (Coombs' test)
β_2-Microglobulin
Serum protein electrophoresis

Biochemistry tests

Electrolytes, creatinine, LFTs, TFTs, LDH

Viral serological tests

HIV
Parvovirus B19 (hypoplastic MDS)
CMV
Hepatitis B and C virus

Other tests

JAK2 mutational testing in patients with myeloproliferative features, e.g. thrombocytosis
Paroxysmal nocturnal haemoglobinuria testing by flow cytometry

Table 120.2 Classification of MDS

- Refractory anemia (RA)
- Refractory anemia with excess blasts (RAEB)
- Refractory anemia with leukemia in transformation RAEB-t)
- Refractory anemia with sideroblasts (RARS)
- Chronic myelomonocytic leukemia (CMML)

Figure 120.1 Peripheral blood film shows hypolobulated neutrophil, anisocytosis and poikilocytosis consistent with MDS

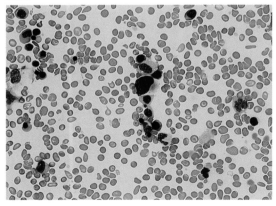

Figure 120.2 Bone marrow smear showing megakaryocytic cells and hypolobulated neutrophil consistent with MDS

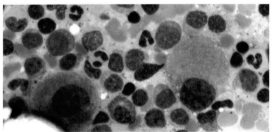

Key points

- Cytopenias secondary to congenital disorders, vitamin deficiencies or drug adverse effects must be ruled out before investigating MDS.
- Diagnosis is by examining peripheral blood and bone marrow and identifying morphological evidence of dysplasia in 10–20% of cells of a particular lineage.
- Cytogenetic abnormalities are detected in about 45–50% of MDS patients, with one or more clonal cytogenetic abnormalities often involving chromosomes 5 or 7.
- Prognosis of patients with MDS should be calculated using the IPSS revised score (IPSS-R).

Myelodysplastic syndromes (MDS) are a group of clonal marrow stem-cell disorders characterised by ineffective haemopoiesis leading to peripheral blood cytopenias, and increased risk of acute myeloid leukaemia (AML) evolution in about one-third of patients. MDS are generally diseases of older people, with a median age at diagnosis of 65–70 years. The cause of MDS is known in only 15% of cases. Hereditary predisposition is uncommon but should be investigated in young adults or in families with other cases of MDS, AML or aplastic anaemia.

Clinical features are non-specific and mainly result from cytopenias, especially anaemia, which is symptomatic in many patients, leading to fatigue and decompensation of underlying cardiovascular disease. Thrombocytopenia is commonly associated with platelet dysfunction, potentially leading to bleeding symptoms. Infections (especially with Gram-negative bacilli, Gram-positive cocci, and fungi) can occur with only moderate neutropenia due to frequent neutrophil function defects. Some patients with MDS also have autoimmune disorders such as vasculitis and seronegative polyarthritis.

Initial clinical investigations

The initial investigation is to distinguish MDS from reactive causes of cytopenia and dysplasia as well as from other malignant cytopenias. The tests that are required in evaluating suspected MDS are listed in Table 120.1.

About 90% of patients with MDS have anaemia that is typically macrocytic and non-regenerative (Figure 120.1). Neutropenia and thrombocytopenia are seen at diagnosis in about 30% of patients. Small numbers of circulating blasts can be found but rarely exceed 5%. If there is no reactive or malignant cause of cytopenia revealed after these initial investigations and MDS is clinically suspected, then bone marrow biopsy is required.

Bone marrow biopsy

The assessment of dysplasia on peripheral blood and bone marrow smears based on the World Health Organization (WHO) 2008 classification of myeloid neoplasms (Table 120.2) is recommended for the diagnosis of MDS.

The bone marrow smear is generally hypercellular and shows dysplastic features in one or several myeloid series (Figure 120.2), differing from those seen in vitamin B_{12} or folate deficiency. The marrow blast percentage (including agranular blasts and myeloblasts, but not promyelocytes) is assessed on at least 500 nucleated cells and is of critical importance for an accurate classification of MDS. Evaluation of bone marrow smears must include iron staining (Prussian blue reaction) to evaluate the presence and number of ring sideroblasts.

A trephine biopsy should be performed in all patients with suspected MDS in which bone marrow examination is indicated. Bone marrow biopsy may aid the exclusion of other diseases presenting with cytopenia and provide information on marrow cellularity, megakaryocyte component, blast compartment, bone marrow fibrosis (present in 15% of cases), and the presence of metastatic cancer cells. However, aspirates are usually sufficient for follow-up including for assessment of treatment efficacy.

Flow cytometry immunophenotyping

Flow cytometry immunophenotyping is able to identify specific aberrations in both the immature and mature compartments of different bone marrow haematopoietic cell lineages. Although no single immunophenotypic parameter has been proven to be diagnostic of MDS, combinations of such parameters in scoring systems have been shown to discriminate MDS from other cytopenias with high sensitivity and acceptable specificity.

Cytogenetic findings

Cytogenetic analysis has a major role in determining clonality and prognosis in patients with suspected MDS. A cytogenetic analysis of bone marrow aspirate should be performed in all patients with suspected MDS in whom bone marrow examination is indicated, and at least 20 metaphases should be analysed whenever possible. Chromosomal abnormalities are observed in 50–60% of patients with MDS; the most frequent single cytogenetic abnormalities include del(5q), monosomy 7 or del(7q), trisomy 8, and del(20q).

Complex cytogenetic findings are common in patients with a major excess of marrow blasts or with therapy-related MDS. Fluorescence *in situ* hybridisation analysis can be useful when fewer than 20 mitoses have been obtained for conventional analysis or when the karyotype is complex in order to identify the chromosomes involved more accurately.

Prognostic evaluation

A high percentage of marrow blasts, increasing number and importance of cytopenias, and abnormal karyotype are the most important independent factors of poor prognosis in MDS; the International Prognostic Scoring System (IPSS) allows classification of patients into four subgroups with largely differing risks of progression to AML and survival.

121 Erythrocytosis

Key points

- If a secondary erythrocytosis related to hypoxia is suspected, arterial blood gas should be performed.
- In patients with suspected primary erythrocytosis, investigation for JAK2 mutation and abdominal ultrasound to evaluate spleen size should be performed.

Erythrocytosis is an increase in the number of RBCs and is defined by a haemoglobin above 18.5 g/dL in a man (>16.5 g/dL in a woman) or haematocrit or packed cell volume (PCV) above 0.52 in a man (>0.48 in a woman). The PCV is a measure of the volume percentage of RBCs in whole blood. Erythrocytosis can be classified as primary or secondary.

Primary erythrocytosis, also known as polycythaemia vera (PV), is a clonal haematopoietic disorder and belongs to the group of Philadelphia chromosome-negative myeloproliferative disorders. It is associated with an increased risk of thrombosis, haemorrhage, myelofibrosis and occasionally progression to acute leukaemia. In primary PV, haematopoietic stem cells acquire genetic mutations that lead to clonal haematopoiesis. A *JAK2* mutation is implicated in 95% of cases of PV.

The common conditions that underlie secondary erythrocytosis include hypoxia from respiratory disease (the most common secondary causes), cardiac disease, high altitude habitat, renal cell carcinoma and exogenous administration of erythropoietin. Factors associated with apparent erythrocytosis are obesity, alcohol excess, smoking and hypertension.

Patients with erythrocytosis can be asymptomatic or present with myalgia, generalised weakness, fatigue, pruritus, headache and facial redness.

Initial investigations (Box 121.1)

If erythrocytosis is suspected, FBC and blood smear should be performed. If the FBC is suggestive of erythrocytosis, it should be repeated (minimum of 1-week interval) to see whether the rise is transient. It is useful to determine if FBC has been done in the past and whether the raised PCV is a new finding. If present for some time, this suggests a true erythrocytosis. One-off borderline increases in PCV often return to the normal range.

Blood film should be reviewed to look for features of myeloproliferative disease. Urinalysis, pulse oximetry or arterial blood gas (for hypoxia), serum ferritin (because iron deficiency can mask the degree of erythrocytosis), and renal and liver function should be checked to look for undiagnosed underlying diseases which can cause erythrocytosis.

Second-line investigations (Box 121.1)

If PV is suspected, blood test for the *JAK2* mutation should be performed. An abdominal ultrasound is performed in all patients with suspected PV and those with confirmed disease to assess for splenomegaly. An enlarged spleen is seen radiographically in two-thirds of patients with PV, although this may not be clinically palpable.

If *JAK2* testing is negative, measurement of serum erythropoietin can be helpful. A low value suggests a primary bone marrow disease and should prompt testing for the rarer exon 12 mutation of *JAK2*. Bone marrow aspiration and trephine biopsy should also be considered. If erythropoietin is raised, a cause of exogenous production of erythropoietin should be sought (see Other investigations). For patients without a *JAK2* mutation and normal erythropoietin, the next step is to measure red cell mass, which is the definitive way to determine whether a true erythrocytosis exists. The measurements of red cell mass and plasma volume can be performed using ^{51}Cr-labelled RBCs and ^{125}I-labelled albumin, respectively.

Other investigations

In patients with erythrocytosis secondary to hypoxic conditions, the following investigations should be considered:
- CXR;
- pulmonary function test and arterial blood gas;
- sleep study;
- echocardiogram;
- renal tract ultrasound.

Clinical Investigations at a Glance, First Edition. Jonathan Gleadle, Jordan Li and Tuck Yong. © 2017 John Wiley & Sons, Ltd. Published 2017 by John Wiley & Sons, Ltd.

122 Haemolytic anaemia

Table 122.1 Common causes of haemolytic anaemia

Type	Aetiology	Association	Diagnostic tests
Acquired haemolytic anaemia			
Immune-mediated	Antibodies to RBC surface antigens	Idiopathic, malignancy, drugs, autoimmune disorders, infections, transfusions	Spherocytes and positive DAT
Microangiopathic	Mechanical disruption of RBCs in circulation	TTP, HUS, DIC, pre-eclampsia, eclampsia, malignant hypertension, prosthetic valve	Schistocytes
Infection	Malaria (Figure 122.6), *Clostridium* infections		Cultures, thick and thin blood smears, serology tests
Congenital haemolytic anaemia			
Enzymopathies	G6PD deficiency	Infections, drugs, ingestion of fava beans	Measurement of low G6PD activity
Membranopathies	Hereditary spherocytosis		Spherocytes, family history, negative DAT
Haemo-globinopathies	Thalassaemia and sickle cell disease		Haemoglobin electrophoresis, genetic studies

Table 122.2 Investigations for haemolytic transfusion reactions

- Repeat the group on pre- and post-transfusion samples and on the donor blood, and repeat the cross-match
- DAT on the post-transfusion sample
- Plasma haemoglobinaemia
- Tests for DIC
- Blood cultures of donor sample
- Post-transfusion urine sample should be examined for haemoglobinuria

Key points

- If haemolysis is suspected, peripheral blood film should be examined and serum bilirubin, LDH and haptoglobin measured.
- Abnormalities of RBC morphology are seldom diagnostic but often suggest the presence and cause of haemolysis.
- Laboratory tests that can help determine the causes of haemolysis include quantitative haemoglobin electrophoresis, RBC enzyme assays, flow cytometry and cold agglutinins test.
- The pattern of the direct antiglobulin reaction can help distinguish warm antibody haemolytic anaemia from cold agglutinin disease.

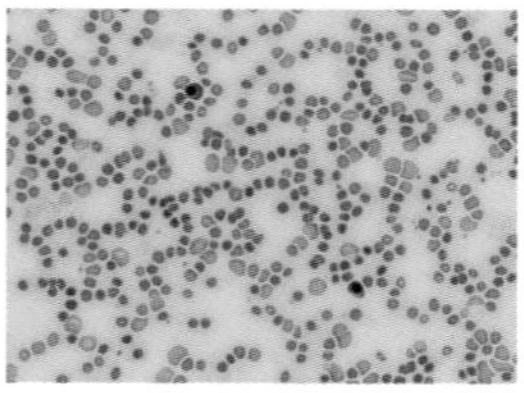

Patients with suspected haemolytic anaemia

Laboratory investigations to confirm haemolysis

	Extravascular	Intravascular
Haematological investigations		
FBC and peripheral blood film	Normocytic anaemia, spherocytosis	Normocytic anaemia, RBC fragmentation
Reticulocyte count	↑	↑
Serum biochemistry and other tests		
Bilirubin	Unconjugated	Unconjugated
LDH	↑	↑↑
Haptoglobin	↓	↓↓
Plasma haemoglobin	Normal/↑	↑↑
Urine tests		
Bilirubin	0	0
Haemosiderin	0	+
Haemoglobin	0	0/+

Figure 122.1 Blood smear shows autoimmune haemolytic anaemia

Positive, confirmed haemolytic anaemia, investigate underlying causes

Negative, consider alternative diagnosis, other causes of anaemia

| Spherocytes, positive DAT | Spherocytes, negative DAT, family history | RBC fragments | Hypochromic, microcytic anaemia, ethnic background | Sickle cell | Drug exposure | Fever, travel to malaria endemic area |

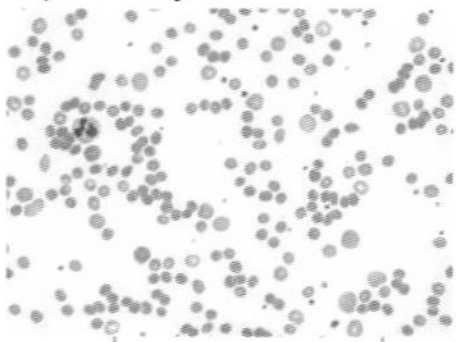

Figure 122.2 Blood smear shows spherocytes

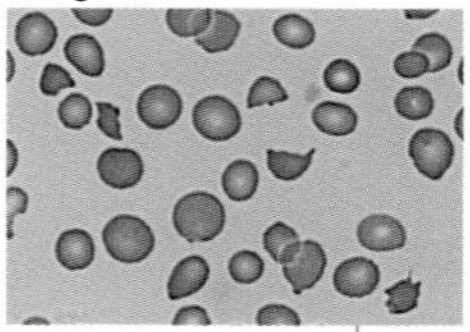

Figure 122.3 Blood smear shows RBC fragments

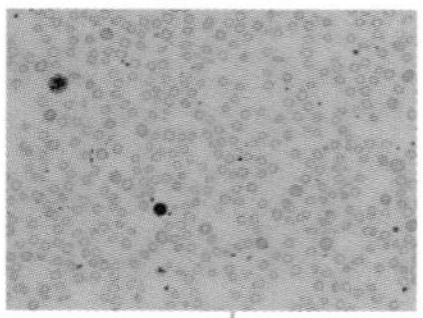

Figure 122.4 Blood smear shows hypochromic microcytic anaemia due to thalassaemia

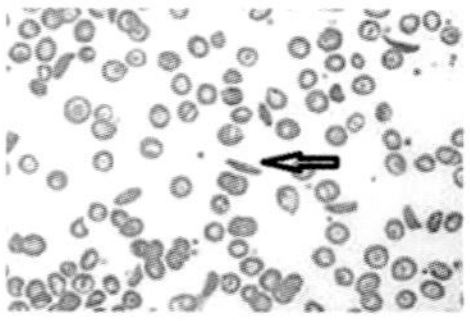

Figure 122.5 Blood smear shows sickle cell anaemia

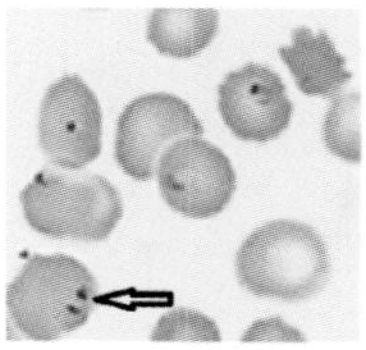

G6PD activity

G6PD deficiency

Thick and thin blood film, blood culture

Figure 122.6 Blood film shows malaria

AIHA, further investigations to exclude secondary causes: CLL, drugs,infection, transfusion NHL, SLE

Hereditary spherocytosis

MAHA, check blood pressure, coagulation study, renal function, LFTs

Thalassaemia

Haemoglobin electrophoresis

Sickle cell anaemia

Haemoglobin electrophoresis

Further investigations for possible TTP, HUS, DIC, malignant hypertension, pre-eclampsia

Clinical Investigations at a Glance, First Edition. Jonathan Gleadle, Jordan Li and Tuck Yong. © 2017 John Wiley & Sons, Ltd. Published 2017 by John Wiley & Sons, Ltd.

Haemolysis is the destruction or removal of RBCs from the circulation before their normal lifespan of 120 days. There are two mechanisms of haemolysis: extravascular and intravascular.

Investigations to confirm haemolysis

Haematological tests

The characteristic feature of haemolysis is reticulocytosis, which is expressed either as a percentage of the total number of RBCs (>3%) or as an absolute number (>100×10^9/L). In the absence of concomitant bone marrow disease, reticulocytosis should be observed within 5 days after a drop in haemoglobin. The anaemia of haemolysis is usually normocytic but a marked reticulocytosis can lead to an elevated mean corpuscular volume (MCV); the average MCV of a reticulocyte is 150 fL. Review of the peripheral blood film is a critical step. Extravascular haemolysis is associated with spherocytosis (Figures 122.1 and 122.2) and intravascular haemolysis with RBC fragmentation (Figure 122.3).

Biochemical tests

Bilirubin, LDH and haptoglobin levels should be measured. LDH is present in RBCs. LDH and haemoglobin are released into the circulation when RBCs are haemolysed. Liberated haemoglobin is converted into unconjugated bilirubin in the spleen or bound by haptoglobin in the plasma. The haemoglobin–haptoglobin complex is cleared quickly by the liver, leading to low or undetectable haptoglobin levels.

Urinary tests

In cases of severe intravascular haemolysis, the binding capacity of haptoglobin is exceeded rapidly, and free haemoglobin is filtered by the glomeruli. The renal tubule cells may absorb the haemoglobin and store the iron as haemosiderin; haemosiderinuria is detected by Prussian blue staining of sloughed tubular cells in the urinary sediment approximately 1 week after the onset of haemolysis. Haemoglobinuria, which causes red-brown urine, is indicated by a positive urine dipstick reaction for haem in the absence of RBCs.

Investigating the cause of haemolytic anaemia

It is essential to investigate the aetiology of haemolysis. The clinical presentation, age of onset, evidence of intravascular versus extravascular haemolysis, and coexisting medical problems can help to classify haemolytic anaemia into either an acquired or hereditary cause (Table 122.1).

Autoimmune haemolytic anaemia (AIHA)

AIHA is mediated by autoantibodies and subdivided into: (i) warm haemolysis, where IgG autoantibodies maximally bind RBCs at body temperature (37°C); and (ii) cold haemolysis, where IgM autoantibodies (cold agglutinins) bind RBCs at lower temperatures (0–4°C). When warm autoantibodies attach to RBC surface antigens, these IgG-coated RBCs are partially ingested by the macrophages of the spleen, leaving microspherocytes, the characteristic cells of AIHA (Figure 122.1).

The direct antiglobulin test (DAT), or Coombs' test, demonstrates the presence of antibodies or complement on the surface of RBCs and is the hallmark of AIHA. The patient's RBCs are mixed with rabbit or mouse antibodies against human IgG or C3. Agglutination of the patient's antibody- or complement-coated RBCs by anti-IgG or anti-C3 serum constitutes a positive test. RBC agglutination with anti-IgG serum reflects warm AIHA, while a positive anti-C3 DAT occurs in cold AIHA. Although most cases of AIHA are idiopathic, potential causes such as CLL, NHL and SLE should always be sought. Cold AIHA may occur following infections, particularly infectious mononucleosis and *Mycoplasma pneumoniae* infection.

Drug-induced haemolytic anaemia

Drug-induced immune haemolysis is classified according to three mechanisms of action: drug absorption (hapten-induced), immune complex, or autoantibody. These IgG- and IgM-mediated disorders produce a positive DAT and are clinically and serologically indistinct from AIHA.

Alloimmune (transfusion) haemolytic anaemia

Haemolytic transfusion reactions may be immediate or delayed. Immediate life-threatening reactions associated with massive intravascular haemolysis are the result of complement-activating antibodies of IgM or IgG classes (e.g. ABO antibodies). If a patient develops a severe transfusion reaction, the transfusion should be stopped and investigations for blood group incompatibility and bacterial contamination of the blood must be initiated (Table 122.2). Further samples of blood should be taken at 6 and/or 24 hours after transfusion for blood count and bilirubin, free haemoglobin and methaemalbumin estimations. In the absence of positive findings, the patient's serum should be examined 5–10 days later for RBC or WBC antibodies.

Microangiopathic haemolytic anaemia (MAHA)

MAHA is caused by mechanical disruption of the membrane of circulating RBCs, leading to intravascular haemolysis and the appearance of fragmented RBCs (Figure 122.3), the defining peripheral smear finding of MAHA. MAHA occurs in a diverse group of disorders, including thrombotic thrombocytopenic purpura (TTP), haemolytic–uraemic syndrome (HUS), disseminated intravascular coagulation (DIC), pre-eclampsia, eclampsia, malignant hypertension, scleroderma renal crisis and, intravascular devices such as prosthetic cardiac valves.

Hereditary haemolytic anaemia

Defects in any RBC component – enzymes, membrane or haemoglobin – can lead to haemolysis (Table 122.1).

Enzymopathies

The most common enzymopathy causing haemolysis is glucose 6-phosphate dehydrogenase (G6PD) deficiency, which is due to various point mutations in the *G6PD* gene on the X chromosome.

There are several tests for detecting G6PD deficiency, based on assessing the production of NADPH by RBCs in the presence of an excess of glucose 6-phosphate. If there is decreased G6PD level, then the patient is more likely to experience haemolysis when exposed to an oxidative stress. If a *G6PD* genetic mutation is detected, the patient will likely have some degree of G6PD deficiency. G6PD levels may be normal during an acute episode, because only non-haemolysed younger cells are assayed. The assay should be repeated in 3 months, when cells of all ages are again present. Pyruvate kinase deficiency can also cause haemolysis.

Membranopathies

Hereditary spherocytosis is an autosomal dominant disorder caused by mutations in the RBC membrane skeleton protein genes. Although there is marked variability in phenotype, hereditary spherocytosis is typically a chronically compensated, mild to moderate haemolytic anaemia. The diagnosis is based on the combination of spherocytosis noted on peripheral smear, a family history (in 75% of cases), and a negative DAT. Hereditary elliptocytosis is relatively common and can be recognised by the very characteristic RBC shape.

Haemoglobinopathies

Chronic haemolysis can be a characteristic of disorders of haemoglobin synthesis, including sickle cell anaemia and thalassaemias. The thalassaemias are a heterogeneous group of inherited anaemias characterised by defects in the synthesis of the α or β subunit of the haemoglobin tetramer ($\alpha_2\beta_2$). Beta-thalassaemia can be diagnosed by haemoglobin electrophoresis, which shows elevated levels of haemoglobins A_2 and F, while the diagnosis of alpha-thalassaemia requires genetic studies. Thalassaemias are characterised by hypochromia and microcytosis; target cells are frequently seen on the peripheral smear (Figure 122.4).

Sickle cell anaemia is an inherited disorder caused by a point mutation leading to substitution of valine for glutamic acid in the sixth position of the β-chain of haemoglobin. Haemoglobin electrophoresis reveals a predominance of haemoglobin S. Sickle cells are observed on the peripheral smear (Figure 122.5).

123 Leukaemia

Table 123.1 Classification and features of leukaemias

Types of leukaemia	Clinical features
Acute leukaemias: proliferation of immature blast cells	
Acute lymphoblastic leukaemia	Short history of feeling unwell
Acute myeloid leukaemia	Often present with fever or bleeding
	Organ infiltration may occur: skin, gums, testes, meninges
	Peripheral blood shows leucocytosis with circulating blasts and cytopenias
Chronic leukaemias: proliferation of mature cells	
Chronic lymphocytic leukaemia	Often diagnosed incidentally
Chronic myeloid leukaemia	Often present with non-specific symptoms
Less common chronic leukaemias: large granular lymphocytic leukaemia, hairy cell leukaemia	Splenomegaly is common
	Lymphadenopathy is common in CLL
	Peripheral blood usually shows leucocytosis with circulating mature lymphocytes or myeloid cells, blasts are rare

Table 123.2 Examples of common immunophenotypic patterns seen in leukaemia

Leukaemia	Immunophenotypic patterns
T-ALL	cCD3, CD7, TdT positive
B-ALL	CD10, CD19, surface Ig positive
AML	CD13+, CD33+, ± CD34, ± CD14 positive
CLL	CD5, CD19, CD23, weak surface Ig positive

Table 123.3 Examples of karyotypic abnormalities in leukaemia

Leukaemia	Karyotypic abnormalities	
ALL	t(9;22)	Philadelphia chromosome, poor prognosis
	t(4;11)	Poor prognosis
	Hyperdiploidy	Increase in total chromosome number, good prognosis
AML	Hypodiploidy	Decrease in total chromosome number, poor prognosis
CML	t(8;21)	AML M2, has better prognosis
	t(15;17)	AML M3, has better prognosis
	t(9;22)	Philadelphia chromosome translocation creates BCR-ABL chimeric gene

Table 123.4 Baseline investigations in the management of leukaemia

- FBC, full coagulation screen including fibrinogen and D-dimer
- Blood group and antibody screen
- Serum electrolyte, creatinine, urea, LFTs, calcium, albumin, phosphate, urate, LDH
- If patient is a possible candidate for bone marrow transplantation, HLA typing at tissue typing laboratory
- Viral studies: HIV, CMV, HSV, VZV, measles, hepatitis B and C, Toxoplasma serology
- Microbiological screening-blood cultures, MSU, nose and throat swab, culture of potential infected areas, if there is concern for infection
- CXR, ECG
- Lumbar puncture for those with clinical suspicion of CNS involvement
- Serum gamma-globulin level especially in CLL
- Echocardiography or multiple gated acquisition (MUGA) scanning is needed because many of the chemotherapeutic agents are cardiotoxic

Figure 123.1 Blood film shows ALL

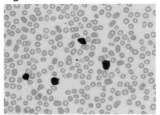

Figure 123.2 Blood film shows AML

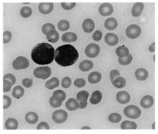

Figure 123.3 Blood film shows CML

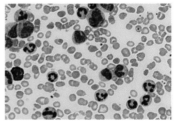

Figure 123.4 Bone marrow examination (trephine) shows CLL

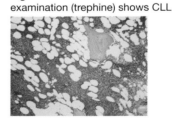

Figure 123.5 Blood film shows CLL

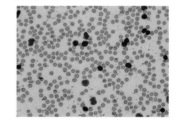

Key points

- FBC usually reveals leucocytosis or other abnormally elevated or depressed cell lines.
- Examination of peripheral blood film and bone marrow is essential to confirm diagnosis and classify the subtype.
- Acute myelogenous leukaemia is characterised by the presence of Auer rods on a peripheral smear. However, Auer rods are not commonly detected and flow cytometry and cytogenetic testing are required to distinguish between AML and ALL and subtypes.
- Peripheral blood flow cytometry is the most valuable test for confirming a diagnosis of CLL.

Clinical Investigations at a Glance, First Edition. Jonathan Gleadle, Jordan Li and Tuck Yong. © 2017 John Wiley & Sons, Ltd. Published 2017 by John Wiley & Sons, Ltd.

Leukaemia can be divided into acute and chronic types according to the degree of cell differentiation. When immature WBCs or blasts proliferate, presentation is usually acute, whereas leukaemia arising from mature cells tends to be chronic. Leukaemia can be further classified as myelogenous or lymphocytic and into several subtypes according to the predominant type of cell involved (Table 123.1).

Patients with acute leukaemia usually present with symptoms and signs of bone marrow failure: recurrent infections, spontaneous bruising, abnormal bleeding or symptoms of anaemia (Table 123.1). In chronic leukaemia, non-specific symptoms such as fatigue, low-grade fevers, night sweats and unexplained weight loss are common. Of cases of chronic lymphocytic leukaemia (CLL), the commonest form of adult leukaemia, 75% are diagnosed incidentally in asymptomatic patients after FBC is performed.

Initial investigations to establish the diagnosis of acute or chronic leukaemia

Step 1: Recognition of abnormal blood count in FBC

Leucocytosis is typically present in leukaemia, which may be accompanied by one or more cytopenias. Aggressive leukaemias may present with only a mild increase in the WBC count, whereas some indolent forms are often accompanied by dramatic leucocytosis. Therefore, unlike cytopenia, the degree of leucocytosis is a poor indicator of disease severity. The absence of leucocytosis does not exclude a diagnosis of leukaemia. These 'aleukaemic' leukaemias can have a normal or low WBC count but are usually accompanied by cytopenias. Leukaemia is very unlikely in the presence of a normal FBC.

Step 2: Review the blood film in patients with an abnormal blood count

This helps to decide whether the leucocytosis is likely to be caused by malignancy or inflammation (Figures 123.1–123.3). Most laboratories perform a blood film automatically when blood count abnormalities are found, but this practice is not universal, and clinicians should request a film after review of blood count results.

Step 3: Bone marrow biopsy

Bone marrow samples are obtained by bone marrow aspiration and biopsy. Although it is often possible to establish a diagnosis of acute leukaemia from peripheral blood examination, bone marrow aspiration should nevertheless be carried out (Figures 123.4–123.5). This is both because the likelihood of successful cytogenetic analysis is higher if bone marrow cells are used and because a baseline is needed for comparison with bone marrow aspirates performed during treatment.

In chronic myeloid leukaemia (CML), a bone marrow aspirate is indicated for cytogenetic analysis. Furthermore, if the accelerated phase of the disease or blast transformation is suspected, bone marrow aspiration and trephine biopsy are both important. The diagnosis of CLL can usually be made from the peripheral blood features and the immunophenotyping. A bone marrow aspirate is therefore not essential in patients with early-stage disease, particularly in elderly patients in whom treatment may never become necessary. Bone marrow assessment is indicated before treatment is undertaken. This should always include a trephine biopsy, which permits accurate assessment of the extent of infiltration and gives information of prognostic importance.

Specialised investigations

The specialised investigations include (i) characterisation of cell surface antigens by flow cytometry/immunophenotyping, (ii) cytogenetics and (iii) molecular cytogenetic analysis. These tests should be performed in a haemato-oncology diagnostic unit. The clinical, morphological, immunophenotypic and genetic data are often integrated at a multidisciplinary team meeting and the leukaemia is assigned to a WHO category.

Immunophenotyping

Immunophenotyping (flow cytometry and immunohisto-chemistry) describes the identification and quantification of cell types using monoclonal antibodies specific for cell surface proteins. These proteins are denoted according to their cluster of differentiation (CD) markers. Most cells express many different proteins and the pattern of expression allows cellular characterisation. Immunophenotyping is used in conjunction with standard morphological analysis of blood and marrow cells and enables:
- diagnosis and classification of leukaemias and lymphomas (Table 123.2);
- assessment of clonality;
- evaluation of prognosis;
- monitoring of minimal residual disease (the lowest level of malignancy that can be detected using standard techniques).

Cytogenetic analysis

Cytogenetic analysis examines the number of chromosomes in each cell and detects structural abnormalities between chromosomal pairs (Table 123.3). In haematological malignancies, cytogenetic analysis can be used to:
- diagnose and classify haematological disorders;
- assess clonality;
- evaluate prognosis;
- monitor response to therapy;
- determine engraftment and chimerism after allogeneic transplantation.

Molecular cytogenetics analysis is the identification of specific genetic abnormalities associated with haematological disorders. For example, *BCR-ABL* probes are used in diagnosis and monitoring of treatment response to CML. Specific probes may be used in diagnosis and monitoring of subtypes of acute leukaemia.

Other baseline investigations in the management of leukaemia

See Table 123.4.

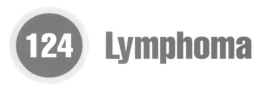

124 Lymphoma

Table 124.1 Simple classification of lymphoma

Hodgkin's lymphoma
Nodular sclerosis Lymphocyte predominance Mixed cellularity Lymphocyte depletion
Non-Hodgkin's lymphoma
Follicular lymphoma Diffuse large B-cell lymphoma Mantle cell lymphoma
Immunodeficiency-associated lymphoma
Lymphoproliferative diseases associated with primary immune disorders HIV-related lymphomas Post-transplant lympho-proliferative disorders Methotrexate-associated lymphoproliferative disorders

Table 124.2 Indications for flow cytometry test

Cytopenias, especially bicytopenia and pancytopenia
Unexplained leucocytosis
Atypical cells or blasts in blood, marrow or body fluids
Plasmacytosis or monoclonal gammopathy
Unexplained organomegaly and tissue masses
Staging a previously diagnosed haematolymphoid neoplasm
Monitoring response to treatment

Table 124.3 Ann Arbor staging system for lymphoma

I	Involvement of one lymph node region or one extranodal organ or site
II	Involvement of two or more lymph node regions on the same side of diaphragm
III	Involvement of lymph node regions on both sides of the diaphragm
IV	Diffuse or disseminated involvement of one or more distant extranodal organs with or without associated lymph node involvement
Modifiers	
A	No symptoms
B	Presence of fever (>38°C), night sweats, weight loss (>10% of body weight) in the 6 months preceding presentation

Table 124.5 Late effects and their specific investigations

Late effects	Tests	Frequency
Hypothyroidism	TFTs	Yearly in patients having radiotherapy to the neck
Thyroid cancer	Physical examination, ultrasound	Yearly
Leukaemia and myelodysplastia	FBC	Yearly
Breast cancer	Mammography	Yearly screening from 10 years after treatment or >40 years of age
Heart failure	ECG, echo	When suspected
Lung cancer	CXR	When suspected

Step 1
Baseline investigations in patient with suspected lymphoma: FBC, biochemistry, creatinine, LFTs, LDH, β2-microglobulin, viral serology, CXR

Figure 124.1 CXR shows right mediastinal mass

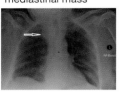

Figure 124.2 (a) Flow cytometry report

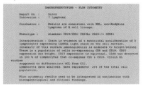

Step 2
Confirm the diagnosis with excisional biopsy, aided by flow cytometry

Figure 124.2 (b) flow cytometry shows typical mantle cell lymphoma

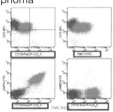

Figure 124.3 Lymph node biopsy shows typical NHL

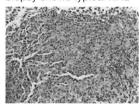

Step 3
Staging

Figure 124.4 (a) CT abdomen shows extensive para-aortic lymph node involvement in a patient with NHL. (b) CT of abdomen shows spleen involvement in a patient with NHL

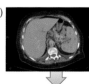
(a)   (b)

Figure 124.5 PET scan shows a splenic lymphoma

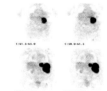

Step 4
Other pretreatment investigations

Figure 124.6 Radionuclide cardiac scan to assess cardiac function before treatment of lymphoma

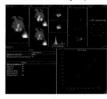

Step 5
Investigations for recurrent disease and monitoring the late effects of treatment

Key points

- The diagnosis of lymphoma should be established by excisional biopsy.
- Molecular genetic tests and flow cytometry are important.
- Imaging tests are important in defining the extent of a tumour mass and possible extension into extranodal sites.
- PET scan can assist in distinguishing residual non-neoplastic masses from persistent lymphoma.

Clinical Investigations at a Glance, First Edition. Jonathan Gleadle, Jordan Li and Tuck Yong. © 2017 John Wiley & Sons, Ltd. Published 2017 by John Wiley & Sons, Ltd.

Lymphoma is a heterogeneous disease and can be divided into Hodgkin's lymphoma (HL), non-Hodgkin's lymphoma (NHL) and immunodeficiency-associated lymphoma (Table 124.1). HL is distinguished by the histopathological presence of Reed–Sternberg cells and accounts for 10% of all lymphomas. While over 30 specific subtypes of NHL exist, B-cell lymphomas represent more than 85% of all NHLs and T-cell and natural killer (NK)-cell lymphomas less than 15% of all NHLs. About 70–80% of lymphomas arise from the lymph nodes; the remainder are extranodal.

Clinical presentation is dependent on the site of involvement, natural history of the lymphoma subtype, and the presence or absence of 'B' symptoms (weight loss >10%, night sweats, body temperature >38°C). Two-thirds of patients present with painless lymphadenopathy. Any organ can be the primary site of NHL. The gastrointestinal tract is the most frequent extranodal site, with the stomach most commonly involved.

Confirm the diagnosis

In patients with suspected lymphoma the following investigations should be performed.

FBC

FBC will often reveal a normochromic normocytic anaemia and occasionally autoimmune haemolytic anaemia in lymphoma. In advanced disease with bone marrow involvement, neutropenia, thrombocytopenia or leuco-erythroblastic features may be detected. Eosinophilia is frequently present in HL. Lymphoma cells with variable nuclear abnormalities may be found in the peripheral blood in some patients.

Biochemistry

LDH and β_2-microglobulin are raised in aggressive and extensive lymphoma and are used as prognostic indicators. Increased creatinine may occur with kidney involvement. Hypercalcaemia may occur. Abnormal LFTs may suggest disseminated disease. Viral serology should be performed (hepatitis B and C and HIV).

CXR

A CXR is performed in the initial evaluation and lymphoma may present as mediastinal masses (Figure 124.1), lung parenchymal involvement, pleural effusion or infective complications such as pneumonia.

Flow cytometry

The indications for flow cytometric immunophenotyping are listed in Table 124.2. In these clinical situations, flow cytometry can provide a sensitive screen for the presence of lymphoma and assist in demonstrating the absence of disease (Figure 124.2).

Lymph node biopsy

Excised lymph nodes, extranodal tumour samples or adequate core biopsy is required for the diagnosis of lymphoma (Figure 124.3). Fine-needle aspiration or fine-gauge needle biopsies have a much lesser accuracy of diagnosis. Histological examination enables definition of the subtype and tumour grade. Immunological markers, chromosome findings and gene rearrangement are analysed for molecular profiling.

Bone marrow biopsy

In NHL, bone marrow biopsy may show focal involvement. Bone marrow involvement is observed in 5–8% of patients with HL and in less than 1% with early-stage disease. Therefore in those with early-stage disease, a routine bone marrow biopsy is not recommended.

Staging and preparation for treatment

NHL is staged using the Ann Arbor classification system (Table 124.3).

CT is the standard approach for evaluating the lymphoma stage above and below the diaphragm (Figure 124.4).

MRI is better than CT in detecting central nervous system and bone diseases.

PET scan Different subtypes of NHL have varied avidity for 2-[^{18}F]fluoro-2-deoxy-D-glucose (FDG). The more common subtypes (diffuse large B-cell, follicular and mantle-cell lymphomas) are usually FDG avid (Figure 124.5). In subgroups that are usually FDG avid, PET detects disease with a sensitivity of 80% and specificity of 90%. In combination with CT, PET is used for staging, end-of-treatment and interim assessment and follow-up surveillance.

PET is more accurate than CT in the reassessment of patients after completion of treatment because it can differentiate between residual active disease and necrosis or fibrosis. The negative predictive value of PET is high (85–96%) but the positive predictive value is not as reliable (85% in NHL). False positives occur because of infection, inflammation, increased uptake in brown fat and reactive changes after treatment. Therefore to ascertain relapse, histological evidence is preferred to PET alone.

Cardiac and other investigations

Baseline ECG and radionuclide cardiac scan (Figure 124.6) or echocardiogram are performed prior to treatment with anthracycline-containing chemotherapy regimens or targeted therapy which can affect cardiac function or radiotherapy to the mediastinal region. Gastric lymphoma should be investigated with upper gastrointestinal endoscopy. Lumbar puncture and CSF analyses may be indicated with meningeal involvement.

Prognosis

The International Prognostic Index (IPI) is the most widely used prognostic model in aggressive NHL (predominantly diffuse large B-cell lymphoma). Clinical findings associated independently with survival are age (≤60 vs. >60 years), LDH (normal vs. abnormal), Eastern Cooperative Oncology Group performance status (<2 vs. ≥2), Ann Arbor stage (I/II vs. III/IV) and number of extranodal sites implicated (1 or >1). From this, four risk groups are developed.

Monitoring late effects of treatment

One of the late effects of treatment for lymphoma is the development of secondary malignancies, which can involve solid organs (most commonly lung, skin, breast and gastrointestinal) or be of haematological origin (leukaemia, myelodysplasia). The risk of secondary malignancies is highest after treatment in childhood. The most common secondary malignancy in female patients is breast cancer and the guidelines recommend yearly screening from 10 years after treatment or at 40 years of age (whichever is earlier). Fertility issues should also be considered before commencing treatment of lymphoma. The other late effects and specific investigations are listed in Table 124.4.

125 Multiple myeloma

Table 125.1 International Myeloma Working Group diagnostic criteria

Symptomatic myeloma
All three criteria needed for diagnosis
- Monoclonal plasma cells in marrow ≥10%
- Monoclonal protein in serum or urine (unless non-secretory; if so, need ≥30% monoclonal plasma cells in bone marrow)
- Evidence of myeloma-related organ or tissue impairment:
  - Hypercalcaemia: >2.6 mmol/L (10.5 mg/dL) or upper limit of normal
  - Renal insufficiency: serum creatinine >176.8 µmol/L (2 mg/dL)
  - Anaemia: haemoglobin <10.0 g/dL or 2.0 g/dL below normal range
  - Lytic bone lesions, osteoporosis, or pathological fractures

Asymptomatic (smouldering) myeloma
Both criteria needed for diagnosis
- Monoclonal protein ≥30 g/L or monoclonal plasma cells in marrow ≥10%
- Absence of myeloma-related organ or tissue impairment

Monoclonal gammopathy of unknown significance
All three criteria needed for diagnosis
- Monoclonal protein <30 g/L
- Monoclonal plasma cells in bone marrow <10%
- Absence of myeloma-related organ or tissue impairment

Table 125.2 Initial investigations for suspected MM

- FBC and blood film
- Serum electrolyte, urea, creatinine, urate, calcium, LDH and LFTs
- Erythrocyte sedimentation rate (ESR)
- Serum electrophoresis and immunofixation, FLC analysis and quantification of isotypic and non-isotypic immunoglobulins
- Concentrated urine electrophoresis studies (measurement of urinary Bence Jones protein)
- Skeletal survey

Table 125.3 Tests performed to estimate tumour burden and prognosis

- Cytogenetics or fluorescence *in situ* hybridisation (FISH) analysis of bone marrow aspirate
- Serum β_2-microglobulin concentration
- Serum albumin concentration
- Quantification of monoclonal proteins in serum and urine

Table 125.4 International staging system for multiple myeloma

Stage I: median survival 62 months
Serum β_2-microglobulin <3.5 mg/L and albumin ≥35 g/L
Stage II: median survival 44 months
Does not fit criteria for stage I or III
Stage III: median survival 29 months
Serum β_2-microglobulin ≥5.5 mg/L (regardless of albumin level)

Key points

- Serum electrophoresis identifies paraprotein in about 80% of patients while FLCs are usually found in the remaining 20%.
- Serum level of β_2-microglobulin is measured if diagnosis is confirmed as it is used to stage patients as part of the international staging system.
- Bone marrow involvement can be patchy: some samples from patients with MM may show <10% plasma cells but the number of plasma cells in bone marrow is always abnormal. Plasma cell phenotyping by flow cytometry and/or immunohistochemistry on trephine biopsy sections is recommended.
- Skeletal radiograph survey is the recommended initial imaging work-up for MM. Nuclear bone scans and dual energy X-ray absorptiometry have no role in the diagnosis of MM.

Figure 125.1 Electrophoresis shows paraprotein

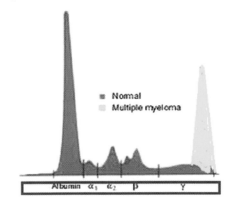

■ Normal
□ Multiple myeloma

Albumin α₁ α₂ β γ

Figure 125.2 Skeletal survey shows (a) multiple lytic lesions in the skull; (b) multiple lytic lesions in the left femoral shaft
(a)   (b)

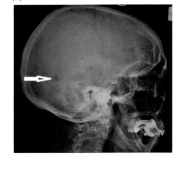
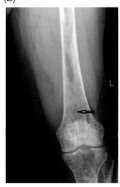

Figure 125.3 (a) Bone marrow aspirate shows multiple myeloma; (b) bone marrow trephine shows multiple myeloma
(a)   (b)

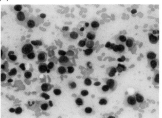
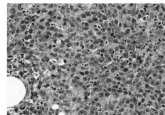

Figure 125.4 Kidney biopsy shows cast nephropathy

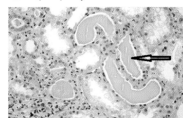

Clinical Investigations at a Glance, First Edition. Jonathan Gleadle, Jordan Li and Tuck Yong. © 2017 John Wiley & Sons, Ltd. Published 2017 by John Wiley & Sons, Ltd.

Multiple myeloma (MM) is a plasma cell malignancy characterised by a clonal population of bone marrow plasma cells that usually secrete a monoclonal paraprotein or an immunoglobulin free light chain (FLC). The majority of cases present *de novo* but it is now recognised that myeloma is preceded by an asymptomatic monoclonal gammopathy of undetermined significance (MGUS) phase in most patients. Distinguishing symptomatic MM, which typically requires treatment, from MGUS or smouldering MM can be challenging. Other plasma cell disorders include Waldenström's macroglobulinaemia and primary amyloidosis. Monoclonal gammopathy is characterised by a rearrangement of immunoglobulin genes resulting in the production of a monoclonal protein. Secondary monoclonal gammopathy can occur in patients with AIDS, hepatitis C and rheumatoid arthritis.

The classical manifestations of MM are often abbreviated into the acronym CRAB: hyper*c*alcaemia (30% at diagnosis), *r*enal impairment (25%), *a*naemia (75%) and *b*ony lesions (70%). The diagnostic suspicion for MM should be heightened by the presence of any of these symptoms. Less common presentations include recurrent bacterial infections (more than two episodes per year) due to hypogammaglobulinaemia, or symptomatic hyperviscosity resulting in confusion, visual changes and headaches. MM can be classified into three categories (Table 125.1).

Initial investigations

If MM is clinically suspected, the recommended tests are listed in Table 125.2. Serum electrophoresis (Figure 125.1) establishes the presence of a monoclonal band, while immunofixation increases diagnostic sensitivity to 93% and determines the precise nature of the paraprotein (e.g. IgA, IgG) and whether kappa or lambda FLCs are present. IgM myeloma is extremely rare and the presence of IgM paraprotein should raise suspicion of Waldenström's macroglobulinaemia or lymphoplasmacytic lymphoma. A serum FLC analysis must always be included because a small proportion of patients do not have measurable disease on serum electrophoresis and immunofixation. The combination of these three tests (electrophoresis, immunofixation and FLC) has a diagnostic sensitivity of 97–98%. About 2% of patients have true non-secretory disease that is undetectable by any of these methods.

FBC, blood film and electrolytes should be performed to detect evidence of MM-related organ involvement. If hypercalcaemia is present, parathyroid hormone and vitamin D are measured.

A skeletal survey (whole-body X-ray) is performed to detect osteolytic lesions (Figure 125.2). Those with more advanced disease may present with a pathological fracture from minimal trauma. MRI short-tau inversion recovery (STIR) is more sensitive and can identify lytic lesions in suspicious cases when the skeletal survey does not yield a diagnosis. Nuclear bone scintigraphy has no role in MM because skeletal uptake of technetium relies on the osteoblastic reaction, which is reduced or absent in MM. PET-CT scan may have a role in screening for, and monitoring of, extramedullary sites of disease, especially in non-secretory myeloma.

Non-secretory myeloma poses particular diagnostic difficulties as there is no serum paraprotein and no urinary Bence Jones protein excretion. The serum FLC assay is informative in about two-thirds of patients. While the clinical presentation is essentially similar to that of standard myeloma, anaemia and lytic lesions may be seen more frequently while renal failure is uncommon.

Investigations to confirm the diagnosis

Bone marrow aspirate and trephine biopsy (Figure 125.3) with plasma cell phenotyping by flow cytometry and/or immunohistochemistry are required to confirm the diagnosis and for prognostic purposes. In MM, plasma cell infiltration in the bone marrow is greater than 10%. This helps to differentiate MM from MGUS and solitary plasmacytoma.

Investigations to estimate myeloma burden and prognosis (Table 125.3)

Prognosis is commonly evaluated using the IPI, which is divided into three stages (Table 125.4). Specific genetic lesions or gene signatures are associated with worse outcomes. IgH translocations involving chromosomes 4 and 16 are associated with a worse prognosis. The tumour suppressor gene *TP53* is located on the short or p arm of chromosome 17, at 17p13, and deletion of this region, del(17p), is associated with a worse outcome.

In MGUS, the type and quantity of paraprotein and the presence of abnormal serum FLCs can assist in ascertaining the risk of transformation to overt MM. These parameters can also guide the frequency of monitoring.

Investigations of myeloma-related organ involvement

Kidney

FLCs are filtered in the glomeruli and reabsorbed in the proximal tubules. When the FLC load exceeds this reabsorptive capacity, FLCs precipitate out as casts in the distal tubule (Figure 125.4), causing tubular obstruction and tubulo-interstitial inflammation, leading to AKI. Other causes of kidney injury include amyloid deposition, dehydration, hypercalcaemia and hyperviscosity. Kidney biopsy can help to define the type of kidney injury and determine the degree of pathological activity and chronicity, which can guide treatment and predict outcome.

Spinal cord compression

Spinal cord compression due to retropulsion of pathological vertebral fractures or extramedullary soft tissue plasmacytomas occurs in 5% of patients with MM. If cord compression is suspected, dexamethasone should be started immediately, followed by urgent MRI or CT of the spine if MRI is unavailable.

Neuropathy

Paraproteinaemia is associated with neuropathies. Infiltration of peripheral nerves by amyloid can be a cause of carpal tunnel syndrome and other sensorimotor mononeuropathies and polyneuropathies. Nerve conduction and electromyographic studies can be performed to assess neuropathies.

Bone lesions and hypercalcaemia

Lytic lesions or osteoporosis with compression fractures can be confirmed by MRI or CT. Corrected serum calcium above 2.75 mmol/L is defined as hypercalcaemia.

Hyperviscosity syndrome

Hyperviscosity syndrome may develop in patients with high serum paraprotein levels, particularly those of IgA and IgG3 type. Symptoms including blurred vision, headaches and mucosal bleeding commonly appear when plasma viscosity exceeds 4 or 5 mPa·s and urgent plasma exchange may be indicated. This usually corresponds to a serum IgM level of at least 30 g/L, an IgA level of 40 g/L and an IgG level of 60 g/L. All patients with high paraprotein levels should undergo fundoscopy, which may demonstrate retinal vein distension, haemorrhages and papilloedema.

126 Platelet disorders

Table 126.1 Common causes of thrombocytosis

Reactive thrombocytosis
Infections
Inflammation
Acute blood loss
Haemolysis
Metastatic cancer
Post splenectomy
Drugs
Iron deficiency anaemia

Primary thrombocytosis
Myeloproliferative disorders
Myelodysplastic syndromes
Other myeloid malignancies

Congenital thrombocytosis

Figure 126.1 Normal platelet morphology and numbers in blood smear

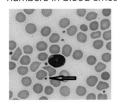

Figure 126.2 Platelet clumping

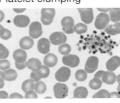

Figure 126.3 Blood smear showing RBC fragmentation in patient with TTP

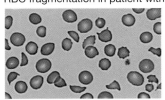

Table 126.2 Findings that help to distinguish between primary and reactive thrombocytosis

Finding	Primary thrombocytosis	Secondary (reactive) thrombocytosis
Underlying systemic disease	No	Often clinically apparent
Digital or cerebrovascular ischaemia	Characteristic	No
Large-vessel arterial or venous thrombosis	Increased risk	No
Bleeding complications	Increased risk	No
Splenomegaly	Yes (40% of patients)	No
Peripheral blood film	Giant platelets	Normal platelets
Platelet function	May be abnormal	Normal
Bone marrow megakaryocytes	Increased	Normal
Quantity	Increased	Increased
Features	Giant, dysplastic with increased ploidy; associated with large masses of platelet debris	Normal

Table 126.3 Causes of thrombocytopenia

Decreased platelet production
• Viral infections
• Drugs especially cytotoxic drugs
• Radiotherapy
• Megaloblastic anaemia and aplastic anaemia
• Leukaemia
• Lymphoma
• Myelodysplastic syndromes
• Multiple myeloma
• Marrow infiltration by cancer

Dilutional loss
• Massive transfusion
• Pregnancy
  Gestational thrombocytopenia
  Pre-eclampsia

Increased platelet consumption
• Immune-related
  Autoimmune (idiopathic)
  Drug-induced including heparin
• SLE
  CLL and lymphoma
  Infections: HIV, viruses, malaria
  Post-transfusional purpure
• Disseminated intravascular coagulation
• Thrombotic thrombocytopenic purpura

Abnormal platelet distribution
• Splenomegaly

Platelet count <150 × 10⁹/L

Repeat platelet count by collecting blood in both an EDTA tube and a citrated tube

Platelet count >150 × 10⁹/L, pseudothrombocytopenia ← → Platelet count <150 × 10⁹/L

Any suspected medications including heparin

Yes → Drug-induced thrombocytopenia or HIT

No → Blood smear

Drug-induced thrombocytopenia or HIT → HIT suspected

Blood smear → RBC fragment / WBC and RBC abnormality / Normal

HIT suspected → Discontinue heparin, start alternative anticoagulant

RBC fragment → HUS/TTP

WBC and RBC abnormality → Bone marrow disorders, MDS, leukaemia

Normal → Exclude secondary ITP → ITP

Discontinue heparin, start alternative anticoagulant → Anti-PF4/heparin antibody, ELISA

Anti-PF4/heparin antibody, ELISA → Positive / Weak positive / Negative

Positive → Functional assay → HIT

Weak positive → High clinical probability / Low clinical probability

High clinical probability → Functional assay

Low clinical probability → HIT unlikely

Negative → HIT unlikely

Key points

• Pseudothrombocytopenia due to platelets clumping in the presence of EDTA should be excluded first.
• Persistent isolated thrombocytopenia with normal RBC morphology and larger-than-usual platelets but without any immature WBCs are typical of ITP.
• Serological tests for HIV, hepatitis and B and C, EBV, and autoantibody screen for SLE and, when appropriate, a pregnancy test should be performed to exclude secondary ITP. If the smear shows abnormalities other than thrombocytopenia, such as nucleated RBCs or abnormal or immature WBCs, bone marrow biopsy is indicated.
• If suspected TTP–HUS, investigations should be performed promptly including FBC, peripheral blood smear, reticulocyte count, serum LDH, and creatinine. Fragmented RBCs on the blood smear are indicative of microangiopathic thrombocytopenia.

Clinical Investigations at a Glance, First Edition. Jonathan Gleadle, Jordan Li and Tuck Yong. © 2017 John Wiley & Sons, Ltd. Published 2017 by John Wiley & Sons, Ltd.

Thrombocytosis

Thrombocytosis is a platelet count in excess of 400×10^9/L. The common causes are listed in Table 126.1. Congenital thrombocytosis is extremely rare and sometimes associated with mutations of thrombopoietin or its receptor.

The first step is to distinguish reactive from primary thrombocytosis (Table 126.2). The presence of a history of infection, a connective tissue disorder, vasculitis, haemolysis, active bleeding, recent surgery, history of splenectomy, or cancer favours reactive thrombocytosis. The presence of chronic thrombocytosis, thrombohaemorrhagic complications, microvascular symptoms or splenomegaly favours primary thrombocytosis.

FBC and blood smear examination

FBC and peripheral blood film can provide clues for reactive thrombocytosis such as Howell–Jolly bodies due to surgical or functional hyposplenism. An increase in haematocrit or leucocyte count suggests myeloproliferative disorders, whereas the presence of abnormal platelet morphology is consistent with essential thrombocytosis.

CRP and iron study

Increased CRP suggests but does not establish a diagnosis of reactive thrombocytosis associated with an occult inflammatory or malignant condition. A normal iron study excludes iron deficiency anaemia-associated reactive thrombocytosis.

JAK mutation testing

*JAK*2V617F mutation testing is now part of the diagnostic work-up for thrombocytosis, according to the WHO diagnostic criteria for essential thrombocytosis and polycythaemia vera (PV). However, peripheral blood mutation screening for *JAK*2V617F cannot substitute for bone marrow examination, since the mutational frequency is estimated at 60% in patients with essential thrombocytosis.

Bone marrow biopsy

Bone marrow morphology appears normal in reactive thrombocytosis. In essential thrombocytosis, bone marrow findings include increased numbers of megakaryocytes and other myeloid cells, abnormality in cell morphology, and presence of megakaryocyte clusters.

Essential thrombocytosis

Essential thrombocytosis is a persistent platelet count of 450×10^9/L or greater that is neither reactive nor associated with a defined myeloid malignancy including PV, primary myelofibrosis, CML and MDS. Therefore, before making a diagnosis of essential thrombocytosis one must exclude CML by conventional cytogenetics and by testing for *BCR-ABL*. Bone marrow histology should be carefully examined for both trilineage dysplasia, which would suggest MDS, and intense marrow cellularity accompanied by atypical megakaryocytic hyperplasia, which would suggest pre-fibrotic primary myelofibrosis, associated with elevated levels of LDH, increased peripheral blood CD34 cell count and a leucoerythroblastic peripheral blood smear. It is important to distinguish essential thrombocytosis from pre-fibrotic primary myelofibrosis, as the latter is associated with significantly worse overall and leukaemia-free survival.

Thrombocytopenia

Thrombocytopenia is a platelet count below 150×10^9/L. However, platelet counts between 100 and 150×10^9/L do not necessarily indicate disease if they have been stable for more than 6 months. Clinically significant spontaneous bleeding does not usually occur until the platelet count is less than $10–20 \times 10^9$/L. However, the presence of thrombocytopenia can aggravate surgical or traumatic bleeding or prevent the administration of chemotherapy. There are many causes of thrombocytopenia (Table 126.3) and these may be related to reduced platelet production, increased platelet consumption, abnormal platelet distribution, or dilutional loss as seen in massive transfusion.

FBC and blood smear examination

Examination of the peripheral blood smear is essential. Spurious thrombocytopenia due to platelet clumping (Figures 126.1 and 126.2) or platelets adhering to neutrophils (platelet satellitism) can be seen on a smear.

Giant platelets are often seen in patients with hereditary thrombocytopenia. In thrombotic thrombocytopenic purpura (TTP) RBC fragmentation (Figure 126.3) is seen in addition to thrombocytopenia, elevated LDH level and brisk reticulocytosis. Examination of the blood film is essential to exclude rare instances of acute leukaemia presenting as thrombocytopenia.

Bone marrow biopsy

Bone marrow biopsy is not necessary in most cases of thrombocytopenia. Bone marrow biopsy is indicated in patients with an atypical course such as those who have splenomegaly, protracted fever, bone or joint pain, unexplained macrocytosis, neutropenia or will undergo splenectomy and in patients aged over 60 years, as thrombocytopenia may be the initial manifestation of MDS. Bone marrow biopsy in patients with ITP shows megakaryocytic hyperplasia. Quantifying the megakaryocytes in the bone marrow is technically difficult. Usually, two to three megakaryocytes are present in each spicule in typical marrow.

Heparin-induced thrombocytopenia (HIT)

When HIT is suspected, testing for heparin-dependent antibodies is indicated with either immunological or functional assays. Immunological assays that detect circulating antibodies against heparin–PF4 complexes via ELISA are the first-line tests. However the main disadvantage of the immunological assays is limited specificity and false positives are common. Therefore, those with a positive ELISA are tested further with a functional assay. The functional assay uses platelets and serum from the patient, which are incubated with heparin and then tested for the release of serotonin, a marker of platelet activation.

Immune thrombocytopenic purpura (ITP)

The diagnosis of ITP remains one of exclusion. The following investigations are essential for patients with suspected ITP:

- FBC, reticulocyte count including peripheral blood film;
- quantitative immunoglobulin measurement;
- bone marrow biopsy only in patients with atypical features or older than 60 years;
- blood group (Rh);
- direct antiglobulin test;
- HIV and hepatitis C serology.

127 Bleeding disorders

Table 127.1 Causes of bleeding disorders

Platelet defects
Disorders of platelet numbers (thrombocytopenia)
Disorders of platelet function
Congenital
Acquired
Pharmacological platelet inhibitors
Severe renal failure
Vascular disorders
Hereditary
Hereditary haemorrhagic telangiectasia
Ehlers–Danlos syndrome
Marfan's syndrome
Acquired
Scurvy (vitamin C deficiency)
Henoch–Schönlein purpura
Corticosteroid-induced
Senile purpura
Coagulation disorders
Congenital
Haemophilia A (FVIII deficiency)
Haemophilia B (Christmas disease or FIX deficiency)
von Willebrand disease
Other factor deficiencies
Acquired
Anticoagulant drugs
Vitamin K deficiency
Liver disease
Disseminated intravascular coagulation
Acquired coagulation factor inhibitors

Table 127.4 Laboratory findings in bleeding disorders

Bleeding disorder	PT	APTT	TT	Fibrinogen	Platelet count
FVIII, FIX, FXI deficiency	N	↑	N	N	N
FVII deficiency	↑	N	N	N	N
FII, FV and FX deficiency	↑	↑	N	N	N
Acquired or congenital haemophilia, with an inhibitor	N	↑	N	N	N
VWD	N	N or ↑	N	N	N
Fibrinogen deficiency (hypofibrinogen-aemia) or dysfunction	N or ↑	N or ↑	↑	↓	N
Vitamin K deficiency (or warfarin therapy)	↑	N or ↑	N	N	N
Unfractionated heparin: therapy or sample contamination	N	↑	↑	N	N
Low-molecular-weight heparin therapy	N	N	N or ↑	N	N
Direct thrombin inhibitors	N	N	↑	N	N
Direct inhibitors of FXa	N or ↑	N or ↑	N	N	N
Fibrinolytic therapy	↑	↑	↑	↓	N
Lupus anticoagulant	N or ↑	N or ↑	N	N	N
Liver disease	N or ↑	N or ↑	N or ↑	↓ or N	↓
DIC	↑	↑	↑	↓	↓
Massive transfusion	↑	↑	↑	↓	↓

Table 127.2 Symptoms suggestive of bleeding disorders

Bruises >2 cm in size with minimal or no trauma
Bleeding from trivial wounds lasting >15 min
Heavy, prolonged or recurrent bleeding after surgical procedures
Spontaneous and recurrent epistaxis (>1 episode/month) lasting >10 min
Anaemia that required a blood transfusion
Heavy menses characterised by large clots, changing a pad or tampon more than hourly
A family history of bleeding disorder

Table 127.3 Coagulation studies used in bleeding disorders

Investigations	Factors measured	Common causes of prolongation
PT or INR	Deficiency or inhibition of one or more of the following factors: VII, X, V, II, fibrinogen	Chronic liver disease Warfarin therapy Disseminated intravascular coagulation (DIC)
APTT	Deficiency or inhibition of one or more of the following factors: XII, XI, IX, VIII, X, V, II, fibrinogen	Haemophilia A Haemophilia B Chronic liver disease Heparin therapy DIC

Table 127.5 Main clinical and laboratory findings in haemophilia and VWD

	Haemophilia A	Haemophilia A	VWD
Inheritance	Sex-linked	Sex-linked	Autosomal dominant (variable penetrance)
Main sites of haemorrhage	Muscle, joints, post trauma or operation	Muscle, joints, post trauma or operation	Mucous membranes, skin, post trauma or operation
Platelet count	N	N	N
Bleeding time	N	N	↑
PT	N	N	N

Key points

- PT detects abnormalities in the extrinsic and common pathways of coagulation.
- APTT detects abnormalities in factors of the intrinsic and common pathways.
- Patients with isolated prolonged APTT or with normal APTT, PT, platelet count and fibrinogen level in the presence of bleeding signs or symptoms should have VWF antigen, VWF:RCo and factor VIII assays to test for VWD.
- A mixing study determines if there is a clotting factor deficiency or an inhibitor to a factor.

Bleeding disorders are a group of acquired or inherited disorders characterised by extended bleeding after injury, surgery, trauma, menstruation and sometimes spontaneously. Numerous disorders can cause abnormal bleeding (Table 127.1). A bleeding disorder may be suggested by the symptoms listed in Table 127.2.

Approach to investigation for bleeding disorders

Laboratory tests are essential for the diagnosis of bleeding disorders. Pre-test probabilities should be taken into consideration. Patients seen in preoperative clinics for assessment of bleeding disorders have low pre-test probability for a bleeding disorder. On the other hand, patients with anaemia and family history of bleeding disorder are much more likely to have a bleeding disorder. Population/social factors such as consanguinity also affect the prevalence of bleeding disorder.

All bleeding disorder investigations should start with screening tests and, when necessary, more specific tests such as coagulation factor assays should be undertaken. Specimen collection, storage, temperature, transport and handling should adhere to local protocols and depends on the assays.

Initial investigations

FBC and peripheral blood film

Thrombocytopenia can be detected on FBC. A peripheral blood film can help to exclude pseudothrombocytopenia and to look for abnormally shaped platelets. Haemoglobin needs to be determined and monitored when bleeding is massive or difficult to control. ABO blood group should be determined.

Renal function and liver function tests

Tests to determine renal and liver function should be performed.

Coagulation studies

Prothrombin time (PT) measures the factors involved in the extrinsic and common pathways. Deficiencies of these factors (most notably factor VII) will prolong the PT (Table 127.3). The international normalised ratio (INR) is used to standardise the reporting of PT. Thrombin time (TT) and fibrinogen concentration should be measured.

Activated partial thromboplastin time (APTT) measures the factors involved in the intrinsic and common pathways. Deficiencies of these factors, including factor VIII (haemophilia A) and factor IX (haemophilia B), will prolong the APTT. Factor VIII levels may be low in patients with von Willebrand disease (VWD) and therefore these patients could present with a prolonged APTT.

Inhibitors – autoantibodies that bind to a factor and inhibit clot formation – can also prolong the APTT. The most common inhibitors are the factor VIII inhibitors and the lupus anticoagulant. A factor VIII inhibitor should be suspected in anyone who has no history of bleeding but develops significant bleeding and has a prolonged APTT (Table 127.4).

Second-line investigations

If the initial coagulation screen is normal but history is suggestive of bleeding disorders, repeat tests should be performed and the following tests should be considered.

- Von Willebrand's screen: FVIII, von Willebrand factor (VWF) antigen plus activity.
- Platelet function activity test with PFA-100.
- Perform relevant factor assays if prolonged PT/APTT, with inhibitor assays if indicated:
  - If isolated prolonged PT: FVII activity.
  - If isolated prolonged APTT: FVIII, FIX, FXI activity.
  - If prolonged PT and APTT but normal fibrinogen/TT: FII, FV, FX initially.
- A lupus inhibitor test should be performed in the face of isolated prolongation of the APTT.
- Consider mixing tests with pooled normal plasma if indicated.

Platelet function activity

Bleeding time is now not used in the evaluation of platelet function. The Platelet Function Analyzer (PFA-100) has been shown to be superior to bleeding time in detecting platelet dysfunction. The sensitivity of the PFA-100 for diagnosing VWD and other platelet function disorders is 88–90% with a specificity of 86–94%. Although the PFA-100 is more sensitive than bleeding time, it is reasonable to use normal platelet function activity results to rule out a significant platelet defect in patients who have low clinical suspicion of such a defect. However, if clinical suspicion of a platelet defect is high, then a normal result should not be used to rule out this possibility and further testing for VWD or other platelet function disorders are indicated.

Classical light transmission aggregometry assesses platelet function. Despite its widespread use, the test is poorly standardised and there are wide variations in laboratory practice. It can be used to detect the effects of aspirin and clopidogrel in preoperative patients scheduled for major elective surgery.

Mixing studies, inhibitor and factor assays

A mixing study determines if the patient has a clotting factor deficiency or an inhibitor to a factor. When one part of the patient's blood is mixed with one part of normal blood, the inhibitor in the patient's blood disables the factor in the normal blood. The APTT stays prolonged and does not 'correct'. Inhibitor assays are then performed to identify which inhibitor is present. When the blood from a patient with a factor deficiency is mixed with normal blood, the APTT should normalise. Factor assays are then performed to identify which factor is deficient (Table 127.5).

Investigations for VWD

VWF mediates blood platelet adhesion and accumulation at sites of blood vessel injury, and also carries factor VIII that is important for generating procoagulant activity. VWD, the most common inherited bleeding disorder, affects males and females and reflects deficiency or defects of VWF that may also cause decreased factor VIII. It may also occur less commonly as an acquired disorder (acquired VWD).

The bleeding score is determined by scoring the worst episode for each symptom and then summing all scores. For more information, see www.path.queensu.ca/labs/james/bq.htm. For VWD, a bleeding score of 4 or above has a sensitivity of 100%, specificity 87%, positive predictive value 0.20 and negative predictive value 1.00. The higher the bleeding score, the greater the likelihood of a bleeding disorder, including possible VWD. The initial VWD assays include VWF antigen, VWF:RCo and factor VIII.

128 Thrombophilia

Aims of investigation:
- To determine the underlying causes for thrombophilia
- To develop strategies to prevent the occurrence of thrombosis
- To assist with decisions about effective antithrombotic treatment and duration
- To identify family members at risk

Table 128.1 Laboratory investigations for thrombophilia

FBC
Serum biochemistry, creatinine, LFTs
Urine analysis for proteinuria and haematuria
Coagulation study: INR, APTT
Factor V Leiden (APC resistance)
Plasma homocysteine
Prothrombin G20210A mutation
Anticardiolipin antibodies
Lupus anticoagulant
Antithrombin III
Factor VIII activity
Protein C, protein S

Key points

- Investigations for thrombophilic disorders should be considered only if the results would influence management decisions.
- Routine testing for hereditary thrombophilias in elderly patients (>65 years old) with a first VTE is not helpful in predicting risk of recurrence or altering initial therapy.
- Patients with VTE at atypical sites, such as the hepatic, mesenteric or cerebral veins, and those with arterial thrombosis should be evaluated for haematological disorders or malignancy.
- Extensive screening for occult malignancy in patients with VTE is not cost-effective and does not reduce mortality or improve survival.

Box 128.1 Indications for investigation

If there is a clear predisposing factor (e.g. recent surgery or trauma, prolonged immobilisation, cancer, generalised atherosclerosis), further investigation is not indicated; if no predisposing factor is readily apparent, further evaluation should be conducted in patients with:

- Family history of venous thrombosis (VTE)
- More than one episode of VTE
- Venous or arterial thrombosis before age 50
- Unusual sites of venous thrombosis (e.g. cavernous sinus, mesenteric veins)
- No identifiable provoking risk factors
- Recurrent pregnancy loss
- VTE with oral contraceptive pill or hormone-replacement therapy

Table 128.2 Frequency and relative risk of venous thrombosis for the thrombophilia factors

Thrombophilia factors	Patients with deep venous thrombosis	General population	Relative risk of thrombosis
Factor V Leiden	50%	4%	Eightfold
Prothrombin gene mutation	15%	3%	Fourfold
Antithrombin III, protein C and S deficiency	10%	1%	Up to 20-fold
Hyperhomocysteinaemia	15%	5%	Threefold
Antiphospholipid antibodies	Common	1%	Eightfold

Clinical Investigations at a Glance, First Edition. Jonathan Gleadle, Jordan Li and Tuck Yong. © 2017 John Wiley & Sons, Ltd. Published 2017 by John Wiley & Sons, Ltd.

Thrombophilia, an increased tendency to venous or arterial thrombosis, can be recurrent or familial or presents at an unusual site or at a young age. The thrombosis can be catastrophic leading to death, permanent disability, prolonged hospitalisation or chronic venous insufficiency. Over 80% of patients with thrombophilia have an abnormality of the natural anticoagulant system. Thrombophilia has both acquired and inherited causes. The clinical history, physical examination and some directed investigations may be used to assess acquired thrombophilia. The risk factors for acquired thrombophilia include age older than 50 years, previous thrombosis, exogenous estrogens, prolonged immobilisation, orthopaedic surgery (especially knee and hip replacement), chronic inflammation and malignancy. This chapter focuses on the investigation of inherited thrombophilia.

Accurate clinical assessment is important to establish the site and severity of thrombosis and whether it occurred spontaneously or in association with a well-identified precipitating factor such as estrogen therapy, an operation or plane travel. A previously undiagnosed malignancy (particularly a mucin-secreting adenocarcinoma) or a myeloproliferative disorder may present with a similar picture of unusual thrombosis. These conditions should be considered before testing for thrombophilia.

Why investigate thrombophilia?

Although the acute management of thrombosis is not dependent on the results of thrombophilia investigation, testing may influence decisions relating to the prevention of recurrent thrombosis (secondary prophylaxis) and the duration and intensity of anticoagulant treatment. Testing may also be beneficial for those family members of the proband who are carriers of the defect but are still asymptomatic. These individuals may be offered primary prophylaxis when exposed to risk situations.

Who should be investigated?

Any patient with spontaneous, unusual, recurrent or strong family history of venous thromboembolism (VTE) or evidence of premature arterial occlusion should be investigated (Box 128.1). It is reasonable to test first-degree relatives of individuals with demonstrated heritable causes. Finding the abnormality will provide an opportunity to modify other risk factors and ensure appropriate prophylaxis against VTE in high-risk situations.

When is the best time to investigate thrombophilia?

Acute thromboembolic events with or without concomitant therapy may influence laboratory investigations (except DNA analysis) or make the interpretation of results difficult. Hence, tests on thrombophilia should be performed either at the presentation of thrombosis or 6 months after the acute thrombotic episode. Furthermore, oral anticoagulants, given for treatment of VTE after the acute event, affect the results of testing for protein C, protein S and activated protein C (APC) resistance. Therefore, the laboratory investigation should be performed at least 2 weeks after discontinuation of oral anticoagulant treatment. Testing a patient during the acute thrombotic event is practical as long as the results are interpreted appropriately and tests with abnormal results are repeated 3 months later.

What are the appropriate tests for thrombophilia?

Whenever possible, testing should be performed by means of functional assays. DNA analysis is required for the prothrombin gene mutation G20210A. The recommended thrombophilia tests are summarised in Table 128.1. Abnormal results should be confirmed by repeat testing. This is because the levels of the natural anticoagulant factors may be altered by consumption in the clotting process, blood collection artefacts, and standardisation and reproducibility problems inherent in most of the clotting-based laboratory techniques. The frequency and relative risk of VTE for positive thrombophilia factors are listed in Table 128.2.

Protein C and protein S are vitamin K-dependent anticoagulant factors and so deficiency cannot be diagnosed while the patient is on warfarin. However, all the thrombophilia factors can be tested while the patient is on therapeutic heparin or low-molecular-weight heparin.

Thrombophilia and arterial thrombosis

There is no solid evidence that congenital deficiencies of the main anticoagulant pathways of blood coagulation increase the risk of arterial thrombosis. Although studies have shown that factor V Leiden, APC resistance or the prothrombin G20210A gene mutation may be contributory risk factors for myocardial infarction or stroke in selected groups of patients, the most comprehensive prospective study, carried out on American physicians, showed that factor V Leiden does not increase the risk of myocardial infarction or stroke. Hence, laboratory screening for thrombophilia in patients who present with arterial thrombosis is of little value. However, these patients should be considered for investigation for antiphospholipid antibodies and hyperhomocysteinaemia, which are frequently associated with arterial thrombosis.

129 Breast cancer

The purpose of investigation in breast cancer is to:
- Screen asymptomatic patients
- Establish the diagnosis for a patient with breast symptoms
- Assess regional lymph nodes and stage the disease if cancer is diagnosed
- Assess patient's general health status

Table 129.1 Current recommendation for breast cancer screening

Age group	Risk factors	Screen method	Reduction of mortality
50–74	None	Biennial screening mammography	14–32%
40–49	None	Controversial due to the lower breast cancer risk, lower mammographic sensitivity and higher false positive results	Not available
≥75	None	Not recommended due to lack of data, consider patient's life expectancy, functional status before screen	Not available
>30	Familial breast cancer with or without proven BRCA mutations	Annual screening with MRI of the breast in combination with mammography	Unknown

Table 129.2 Risks associated with mammographic screen

False positive result leading to recall, with or without biopsy
False negative result leading to false reassurance and feeling of security among patients and doctors
Overdiagnosis (Breast cancers will be detected that will never be clinically important) and overtreatment
Radiation-induced breast cancer

Table 129.3 Risk factors for *BRCA1* or *BRCA2* gene mutation

Breast cancer diagnosed before age 50
Two breast cancers, either bilateral or ipsilateral
Family history of breast cancer before age 50
Male breast cancer
Personal or family history of ovarian cancer
Previously identified *BRCA* mutation in the family
Eastern European Jewish heritage

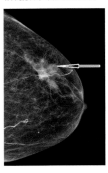

Figure 129.1 Mammogram shows a stellate mass in the upper-outer quadrant of left breast consistent with invasive carcinoma

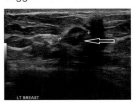

Figure 129.2 USS of the left breast shows an irregular hypoechoic round lesion suggestive of breast cancer

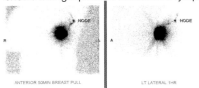

Figure 129.3 Breast lymphoscintigraphy shows a single positive left sentinel lymph node

Key points

- Initial complete evaluation for suspected breast cancer includes clinical examination, radiological imaging and biopsy.
- Histopathological examination should provide a diagnosis, confirm the removal of the lesion and provide extra information such as tumour markers and oestrogen receptor status.
- Additional investigations for staging such as chest CT, abdominal CT scan and bone scan should be considered for patients with clinically positive axillary nodes, large tumours (e.g. ≥5 cm) or clinical signs, symptoms or laboratory results suggesting the presence of metastases.
- Mammography is the only screening test shown to reduce breast cancer–related mortality. Screening is offered biennially to women 50 to 74 years of age.

Clinical Investigations at a Glance, First Edition. Jonathan Gleadle, Jordan Li and Tuck Yong. © 2017 John Wiley & Sons, Ltd. Published 2017 by John Wiley & Sons, Ltd.

Breast cancer is the most common cancer diagnosed in women and the leading cause of deaths from cancer among women worldwide. In mammographic screening, more than 60% of cancers detected are impalpable by clinical examination.

Screening for breast cancer

The purpose of population-based mammographic screening is to detect breast cancers at a preclinical stage to improve survival (Table 129.1). Screening mammography should only be performed in patients with a life expectancy of 5 years or more. Digital and film mammography in asymptomatic women aged over 50 years has equivalent sensitivity and specificity. Mammographic screening is associated with risks (Table 129.2). The estimated risk of radiation-induced breast cancer is 86 cancers and 11 deaths per 100,000 women screened annually aged 40–55 years and biennially thereafter; ratio of benefit to risk is 4.5 : 1 for lives saved and 9.5 : 1 for life-years saved.

Initial diagnostic investigations

Complete clinical evaluation for suspected breast cancer includes clinical examination, radiological imaging and biopsy. The initial investigation should focus on assessment of primary tumour and regional lymph nodes.

Mammography

A diagnostic mammography can confirm clinical suspicion of malignancy and typically shows a spiculated opacity or microcalcification (Figure 129.1). In patients with palpable breast cancer, the combined use of clinical examination and mammography can provide the best assessment of disease extent. However, mammography does not show evidence of malignancy in 10% of patients with breast cancer.

Breast and axillary ultrasound

Ultrasound is reliable for evaluation of tumour size especially in dense breast parenchyma where mammography may be limited in demonstrating tumour margins (Figure 129.2). It is also useful in detecting small cancers in patients with dense breast tissue. Some types of breast cancer such as invasive lobular carcinoma may not be detectable by either mammography or ultrasound.

Metastatic involvement of axillary lymph nodes (commonly termed 'node-positive' cancer) is an important prognostic determinant. The majority of patients with early breast cancer will have no palpable malignant nodes at diagnosis and will be investigated with sentinel lymph node biopsy (SLNB). Preoperative ultrasound of the axilla is part of the routine evaluation of women with invasive breast cancer. Sensitivity of ultrasound for detection of lymph node metastases is modest (60%) and specificity is 82%. SLNB can be performed by lymphoscintigraphy and gamma probe detection. Lymphoscintigraphy defines the pattern of lymph flow and may reduce failure or false-negative biopsies (Figure 129.3).

Biopsy

Fine-needle aspiration (FNA)

Cytological examination of FNA can establish a preoperative diagnosis in palpable breast cancer. FNA cytology has a sensitivity and specificity for malignancy of 85% and 100%, respectively. When a diagnostic sample of malignant cells is obtained, it may be possible to proceed directly to definitive surgery without a preliminary open biopsy. If the FNA is non-diagnostic, it should be repeated or another technique used.

Core biopsy

Core biopsy uses a wide-bore needle (14 or 16 gauge) to obtain a tissue sample. Core biopsy may be performed on palpable lesions, or with mammographic or hand-held ultrasound guidance on impalpable tumours. Core biopsy allows testing for hormone receptor and human epidermal growth factor receptor (HER)-2 status.

Open excision biopsy

When a cytological or histological diagnosis has not been obtained prior to surgery and there is a strong suspicion of malignancy, an open biopsy can be used. Impalpable lesions may require needle localisation under mammographic or ultrasound control.

Pathological examination and genetic testing for BRCA

Pathological examination should provide a diagnosis, confirm the removal of the lesion and provide extra information such as tumour markers and estrogen receptor status. It should provide information on tumour size, type, histological grade, tumour margins, presence or absence of multifocality, the presence or absence of Ductal carcinoma in situ (DCIS), the presence or absence of vascular invasion in the main tumour, status of axillary node removed, estrogen receptor, progesterone receptor and HER-2 status. If two or more risk factors for BRCA are established (Table 129.3), genetic testing is recommended.

Investigations for breast cancer staging

In early breast cancer, routine staging investigations are directed at locoregional disease, as asymptomatic distant metastases are very rare and patients do not benefit from comprehensive laboratory (including tumour markers) and radiological staging. Additional investigations such as chest CT, abdominal ultrasound or CT scan and bone scan should be considered for patients with clinically positive axillary nodes, large tumours (≥5 cm) or clinical signs, symptoms or laboratory values suggesting metastases. FDG-PET/CT scan may be useful when conventional methods are inconclusive.

Investigations for general health status

FBC and liver, bone and renal function tests should be performed. Assessing menopausal status is imperative, if in doubt by measuring serum estradiol and follicle-stimulating hormone levels. Test for cancer antigen (CA)15-3 is non-specific and unreliable.

Follow-up investigations

In the first year after treatment with curative intent, history and examination is undertaken every 3 months and mammography at 6–12 months after radiotherapy for conserved breast. After the first year, mammography is indicated every year. Heart failure is associated with anthracycline chemotherapy, requiring investigation with ECG and echocardiography.

130 Spinal cord compression

Table 130.1 Common causes of spinal cord compression

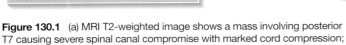

Metastasis
Primary vertebral tumour
Intervertebral disc protrusion
Infections
Osteomyelitis
Epidural abscess
Trauma: vertebral fracture
Degenerative anterolisthesis: spondylosis
Rheumatoid arthritis

Key points

• MRI is the gold standard in the assessment of suspected spinal cord or cauda equina compression.
• If MRI is contraindicated or not available, CT with contrast may be of use if there is a well-defined clinical level of compression. The sensitivity and specificity of CT compared with MRI for the detection of MSCC is 89% and 92%, respectively.
• MRI can identify intramedullary metastases and leptomeningeal disease.

Figure 130.1 (a) MRI T2-weighted image shows a mass involving posterior T7 causing severe spinal canal compromise with marked cord compression; (b) normal MRI T2-weighted image of the spine for comparison

(a)   (b)

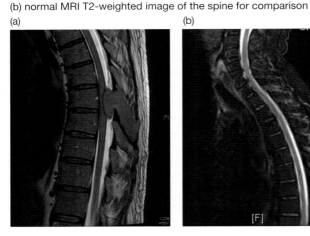
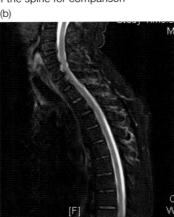

Figure 130.2 Whole bone scan shows multiple metastatic disease

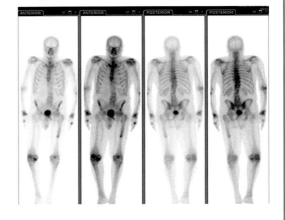

Spinal cord compression is a medical emergency. Early recognition, investigation and treatment are essential to prevent permanent neurological impairment. Once paraplegia develops it is commonly irreversible. There are many causes of cord compression (Table 130.1).

Metastatic spinal cord compression (MSCC) is a well-recognised complication of cancer that occurs in 4% of all patients with cancer. Breast, prostate and lung cancer each account for 20% of cases, while non-Hodgkin lymphoma, myeloma and renal cell carcinoma each account for 5–10% of cases; 60% of metastases are thoracic, 30% lumbosacral and 10% cervical. About 30% of people with metastasis to the spine will have metastases in more than one area of the spine. Commonly, breast and lung cancers cause thoracic lesions, while colon and pelvic carcinomas affect the lumbosacral spine.

Spinal cord compression can be the initial presentation of a cancer. Back pain is the most common symptom of spinal cord compression. A detailed history and thorough clinical examination is required prior to imaging. If spinal cord compression is suspected, administration of systemic glucocorticoid therapy should not be delayed while awaiting investigations to establish the diagnosis.

Radiological investigations

MRI

MRI is the key investigation and gold standard in detecting spinal cord compression (sensitivity 93%, specificity 97%, overall accuracy 95%) (Figure 130.1). Diagnosis of spinal cord compression depends on the demonstration of a neoplastic mass or bone fragment compressing the thecal sac. In the case of back pain suggestive of spinal metastases and neurological symptoms or signs suggestive of MSCC, MRI reveals metastatic lesions and finding unsuspected lesions is common. An MRI of the entire spine is therefore required, including T1-weighted sagittal images with T1- or T2-weighted axial images in areas of interest, and/or short T1 inversion recovery (STIR) sequences.

CT and myelogram

If MRI is unavailable, CT with or without myelogram may be an alternative. Although myelography and CT myelography can demonstrate extrinsic cord compression, vertebrae which are infiltrated with tumour that has not yet compressed the cord may not be demonstrated. MRI is able to demonstrate bone disease which is not yet compressing the cord. MRI of the entire spinal axis for the exclusion of cord compression takes about 20 min while myelography and post-myelogram CT can take up to 2 hours and can involve considerable discomfort for the patient. Plain spinal X-ray may show lytic bone lesions but have inadequate sensitivity for spinal cord compression.

Radionuclide whole-body bone scan

Bone scan is required to establish the extent of bone involvement in some patients in whom the diagnosis has not been made prior to presentation (Figure 130.2).

Laboratory investigations

Laboratory studies may help direct tests to detect a primary tumour, rule out other possible diagnoses (e.g. infection, multiple myeloma) and assess for complications such as hypercalcaemia. Anaemia and thrombocytopenia are common in patients with extensive metastatic bone disease because tumour cells are displacing the bone marrow. The evaluation should include serum immunoelectrophoresis, serum free light chains, FBC, creatinine, calcium, ALP and, for men, PSA.

Laboratory investigations are seldom diagnostic for metastatic disease except positive immunoelectrophoresis suggestive of myeloma, and PSA for prostate carcinoma. Because of their lack of specificity, tumour serum markers generally provide little information about the location and nature of an undetected primary tumour.

131 Cancer of unknown primary

Table 131.1 Cytokeratin pattern and the anatomical origin of adenocarcinomas

CK7+ and CK20+	CK7+ and CK20–	CK7– and CK20+	CK7– and CK20–
Pancreatic adenocarcinoma	Lung adenocarcinoma	Colorectal carcinoma	Hepatocellular carcinoma
Ovarian adenocarcinoma	Breast adenocarcinoma	Merkel cell carcinoma	Renal cell carcinoma
Cholangiocarcinoma	Thyroid carcinoma		Prostate carcinoma
	Cervical carcinoma		Squamous cell and small cell lung cancer
			Head and neck carcinoma

Table 131.2 Immunochemistry of CUP biopsy and the tumour primary site

Marker	Primary site
CDX2	Colon
CK7	Lung, pancreas, breast, ovarian
CK20	Colon, oesophageal
Mesothelin	Ovarian, mesothelioma
TTF-1	Lung

Table 131.3 Specific immunohistochemistry tests for CUP

Cancers	Markers
Breast cancer	GCDFP-15, ER, PR, HER-2
Cholangiocarcinoma	CK19
Colorectal cancer	CEA, CK7, CK20, CDX-2
Germ cell carcinoma	β-hCG, AFP
Lung cancer	TTF-1, surfactant A and B, CK7
Medullary thyroid carcinoma	TTF-1, calcitonin
Mesothelioma	Calretinin
Prostate cancer	PSA, PAP
Urothelial carcinoma	Uroplakin III, THR, HMWCK, CK7, CK20

The aim of investigation in cancer of unknown primary origin:
- Confirm histologically the metastatic lesions and identify the cell lineage
- Identify primary cancer
- Identify cancer with favourable prognosis, which may derive benefit from appropriate treatment

Step 1: Initial evaluation
- History and clinical examination
- Electrolytes, LFTs, FOBT
- CXR
- CT chest, abdomen and pelvis
- Basic immunohistochemistry study on biopsy samples
- Identify cancers with specific cell lineages

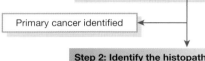

Primary cancer identified

Step 2: Identify the histopathology subtype of CUP and further investigation
- Serum tumour marker
- Consider appropriate endoscopy
- Mammography
- Testicular ultrasound
- PET/CT scan
- Specific immunohistochemistry tests

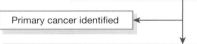

Primary cancer identified

Step 3: Focused immunohistochemistry or gene profiling
- Molecular study: *in situ* hybridisation, RT-PCR, cDNA microarray
- Specific immunohistochemistry tests (Table 131.3)

Key points

- Immunohistochemical panels and the use of emerging molecular markers can help to identify the primary cancer.
- In considering imaging tests, the focus should be on finding the primary site cancer and the appropriate site for tissue biopsy.

Figure 131.1 (a) Histopathology study of the biopsy sample shows features of squamous cell carcinoma; (b) USS-guided FNA for a parotid mass

Figure 131.2 MRI of the head and neck in patients with CUP shows a locally invasive mass within the deep parotid

Figure 131.3 PET scan shows occult lung cancer

(a)

(b)

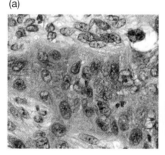

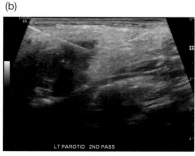

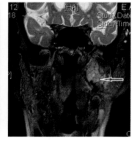

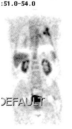

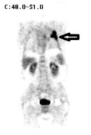

Clinical Investigations at a Glance, First Edition. Jonathan Gleadle, Jordan Li and Tuck Yong. © 2017 John Wiley & Sons, Ltd. Published 2017 by John Wiley & Sons, Ltd.

Cancer of unknown primary (CUP) refers to histologically confirmed metastatic cancer for which clinicians are unable to identify a primary tumour after medical history, physical examination and standardised diagnostic work-up. CUP accounts for 3–5% of all malignancies. The fundamental characteristics of CUP are:

- clinical absence of primary site at presentation;
- early dissemination;
- generally aggressive cancer;
- unpredictable metastatic pattern.

The most common histological type of CUP is adenocarcinoma, with well-differentiated to moderately differentiated adenocarcinomas accounting for 50% of cases of CUP, and poorly or undifferentiated adenocarcinomas accounting for a further 35%. Squamous cell carcinomas account for 10% of CUP cases, while undifferentiated neoplasms, including neuroendocrine tumours, lymphomas, germ cell tumours, melanomas, sarcomas and embryonic malignances, account for 5%.

Comprehensive history and physical examination, including breast, nodal areas, skin, genital, rectal and pelvic examination, are vital to guide further investigation. Available data show that the antemortem frequency of detection of primary site by imaging, endoscopy or immunohistochemistry studies remains around 30%. At autopsy, the primary site is found in 73% of cases, with the most common primary sites being lung (27%) and pancreas (24%).

Initial laboratory investigations

FBC, biochemistry, calcium, LDH, liver function and renal function should be performed in all patients with CUP.

Tumour markers

Routine evaluation of commonly used tumour markers is not very helpful in the diagnostic process. Non-specific multiple overexpression of adenocarcinoma tumour markers (CEA, CA125, CA15-3, CA19-9) occurs in most CUP patients. Around 70% of CUP patients will have high serum levels of more than one tumour marker. However, the following tests are worthwhile considering:

- AFP in patients with hepatic tumours;
- β-hCG and AFP in men with undifferentiated tumours (especially with midline distribution);
- CA125 in women with papillary adenocarcinoma of the peritoneal cavity;
- CA15-3/CA27-29 in women with adenocarcinoma involving only axillary lymph nodes;
- PSA in men with bone metastatic adenocarcinoma.

Histopathology study

Histopathology, especially immunohistochemical examination of biopsy samples, is the first step in the investigation of CUP (Figure 131.1).

In immunochemistry studies, the pattern of cytokeratins (CK7 and CK20 positivity) is widely used to predict the anatomical origin of adenocarcinomas (Table 131.1). The immunochemistry of a CUP biopsy can help to establish whether the cancer is carcinoma, melanoma, lymphoma or sarcoma; whether the subtype is adenocarcinoma, germ-cell tumour, hepatocellular, renal, thyroid, neuroendocrine or squamous carcinoma; and the primary site of adenocarcinoma, i.e. prostate, lung, breast, colon, pancreas, biliary or ovarian (Table 131.2).

Molecular genetic testing

Molecular testing will become an important method in tissue-of-origin identification to lend support to a suspected diagnosis. Such methods could allow appropriate specific treatment including targeted therapy. However, this approach is evolving and the current role of molecular testing in CUP remains uncertain.

Radiological investigations

A CXR is a prerequisite before any further imaging. CT scans of the neck, chest, abdomen and pelvis or targeted MRI scan (Figure 131.2) are useful, with a detection rate of 40% for an occult primary site, and can provide useful guidance for biopsy. Mammography can be performed in all women with adenocarcinoma involving the axillary lymph nodes or skeletal CUP, but it has very low sensitivity whereas breast MRI enables detection of occult primary breast cancers in as many as 70% of cases. Testicular ultrasound should be performed in men when germ cell tumours are suspected. FDG-PET scan can be helpful, especially in patients with occult head and neck cancers or lung cancer (Figure 131.3).

Endoscopy

The detection accuracy, sensitivity and specificity of endoscopic procedures in CUP are very low. Therefore endoscopic procedures should be used only in patients presenting with relevant symptoms or signs, or in the presence of specific histopathological changes:

- ENT pan-endoscopy for patients with cervical node involvement;
- bronchoscopy for patients who have a positive CXR or CT scan with a cough;
- colonoscopy is useful in patients with relevant symptoms or signs, such as a positive faecal occult blood test (FOBT);
- proctoscopy and colposcopy for patients with inguinal node involvement.

132 Tumour markers

- Screening high-risk individuals
- Confirming diagnosis together with other tests; the presence of a tumour marker alone is usually insufficient to diagnose cancer
- Staging disease
- Predicting prognosis
- Assisting in making treatment decisions
- Monitoring treatment response
- Monitoring for recurrence

- An elevated tumour marker level may be caused by disease other than cancer
- Tumour marker levels may be elevated in people without cancer
- Tumour marker levels may vary over time
- The level of a tumour marker may not rise until a person's cancer is advanced, which is not helpful for early detection, screening or monitoring for recurrence

Table 132.1 Recommendations for tumour marker testing in common malignancies

Tumour marker	Relevant cancer	Screening	Diagnosis	Staging / planning treatment / prognosis	Monitoring treatment	Detecting recurrence	Non-malignant conditions that can cause increased levels
AFP	Germ cell / testicular tumour	No	Yes	Yes	Yes	Yes	Pregnancy
AFP	HCC	Yes, in selected patients	Yes	Yes	Yes	Yes	Liver regenerative disease, chronic hepatitis
Calcitonin	Medullary thyroid carcinoma	No	Yes	No	Yes	Yes	
CA125	Ovarian cancer	No	Yes	Yes	Yes	Yes	Cirrhosis, CKD, CCF, non-malignant ascites, pancreatitis
CA15-3	Breast cancer	No	No	No	Yes	Yes	Acute hepatitis
Estrogen receptor (ER) and progesterone receptor (PR)	Breast cancer	No	No	Yes, decide the need for hormone treatment	No	No	
HER-2	Breast cancer	No	No	Suitability of anti-HER2 treatments	No	No	
CA19-9	Pancreatic cancer	No	Yes	No	Yes	Yes	Cholangitis, pancreatitis, cholestasis, cirrhosis
CEA	Colorectal cancer	No	No	Yes	Yes	Yes	Cirrhosis, colitis, diverticulitis, CCF
β-hCG	Germ cell and testicular cancers; trophoblastic neoplasia	No	Yes	Yes	Yes	Yes	Pregnancy
PSA	Prostate cancer	No	Yes	Yes	Yes	Yes	UTI, prostatitis, acute urinary retention
Thyroglobulin	Thyroid cancer	No	No	No	Yes	Yes	

Clinical Investigations at a Glance, First Edition. Jonathan Gleadle, Jordan Li and Tuck Yong. © 2017 John Wiley & Sons, Ltd. Published 2017 by John Wiley & Sons, Ltd.

Tumour markers are substances, usually proteins, that are produced by the body in response to cancer growth or by the cancer itself. These markers can be found in blood, urine, stool, other body fluids, or tissues. Most tumour markers are made by normal cells as well as cancer cells; but at much higher levels in cancerous conditions. The roles of tumour markers are listed in Box 132.1.

The ideal marker would be a 'blood test' for cancer whereby a positive result would occur only in patients with malignancy, it would correlate with stage, response to treatment and recurrence, and be easily and reproducibly measured. No tumour marker currently meets this ideal. The limitations of current tumour markers are shown in Box 132.2.

Screening asymptomatic populations

Although a screening test to detect early cancer has long been the goal, screening for cancer with tumour markers has very limited application. When the likelihood of cancer in the population is low, tumour markers should not be used for screening due to low sensitivity and specificity. Currently, there is no evidence to support any serum tumour marker-based screening programme in a general healthy population and even PSA has significant limitations and is controversial (see Chapter 134).

Clinically useful tumour markers in diagnosis and monitoring (Table 132.1)

AFP: hepatocellular carcinoma (HCC)

AFP is elevated in 80% of patients with HCC and exceeds 1000 ng/mL in 40% of patients with HCC. Annual AFP and ultrasound screening in patients with well-compensated non-alcohol-induced cirrhosis is recommended. AFP above 200 µg/L is regarded as virtually diagnostic of HCC in patients with hypervascular lesions.

β-hCG: non-seminomatous germ cell tumours

The AFP or β-hCG level is elevated in 85% of patients with non-seminomatous germ cell tumours (NSGCT) but in only 20% of patients with stage I disease. Hence, these markers have no role in screening. AFP levels above 10,000 ng/mL or β-hCG levels over 50,000 mIU/mL at initial diagnosis indicates poor prognosis (50% survival rate at 5 years). Following AFP and β-hCG levels is important in monitoring response to treatment in patients with NSGCT.

CEA: colorectal cancer

CEA is overexpressed in colorectal cancer and levels above 10 ng/mL are rarely due to benign disease. Sensitivity and levels increase with advancing tumour stage, with 50% of patients with lymph node involvement and 75% of those with distant metastasis having elevated CEA levels; however, fewer than 25% of patients with disease restricted to the colon have an elevated CEA level. CEA has no role in screening for or diagnosis of colorectal cancer. A CEA level should be ordered only after malignancy has been confirmed. CEA levels return to normal within 4–6 weeks after successful surgical resection. The major role for CEA is in following patients for relapse after intended curative treatment. In patients who underwent CEA monitoring there was a 9% improvement in survival after 5 years. CEA levels should be monitored every 3 months for 2 years in patients with stage II or III disease who are surgical candidates. When an abnormal level is found, the test should be repeated; if CEA elevation is confirmed, patients should undergo imaging of potential recurrence sites.

CA27-29: breast cancer

CA27-29 is highly associated with breast cancer; CA27-29 levels above 100 U/mL are rare in benign conditions. Because of superior sensitivity and specificity, CA27-29 has supplanted CA15-3 as the preferred tumour marker in breast cancer. The CA27-29 level is elevated in approximately one-third of women with early-stage breast cancer (stage I or II) and in two-thirds of women with late-stage disease (stage III or IV). CA27-29 has no role in screening for or diagnosing breast cancer. CA27-29 may detect asymptomatic recurrence or metastasis.

CA19-9: pancreatic cancer

CA 19-9 has a sensitivity and specificity of 80–90% for pancreatic cancer and a sensitivity of 60–70% for biliary tract cancer. CA19-9 has no value in screening because its positive predictive value is less than 1%, but the positive predictive value of levels above 1000 U/mL is 97% when CA19-9 testing is used in clinical situations that are consistent with pancreatic cancer.

CA125: ovarian cancer

CA125 levels are elevated in 85% of women with ovarian cancer, but in only 50% of those with stage I disease. Higher levels are associated with increasing bulk of disease. Insensitivity in early-stage disease and low disease prevalence limit the usefulness of CA125 in ovarian cancer screening.

Molecular tumour markers

A number of molecular genetic markers are used in predicting response to targeted therapy. The most commonly used are mutations in the *KRAS* gene, which are indicative of lack of response to anti-epidermal growth factor receptor (EGFR) antibodies. Other useful molecular tumour markers are described in the following sections.

Breast cancer

Mutations of *BRCA1* and *BRCA2* genes account for 75% of hereditary breast cancers (which comprise 5–10% of all breast cancers) and confer a lifetime risk of 85% by age 70 years. These mutations are uncommon in sporadic breast cancers. Other predictive molecular markers in breast cancer are estrogen receptor, progesterone receptor and HER-2 receptor. The use of adjuvant systemic therapies is decided by the patients' receptor status.

Lung cancer

Testing for EGFR mutations in non-small cell lung cancer is essential prior to the treatment with EGFR tyrosine kinase inhibitors such as gefitinib or erlotinib. Importantly, high response rates to gefitinib and erlotinib can be achieved based on EGFR gene mutation status.

Key points

- Annual AFP and ultrasound screening in patients with well-compensated non-alcohol-induced cirrhosis is recommended.
- Insensitivity in early-stage disease and low disease prevalence limit the usefulness of CA125 in ovarian cancer screening.
- Mutations of *BRCA1* and *BRCA2* genes should be tested for in suspected hereditary breast cancers.

133 Ovarian cancer

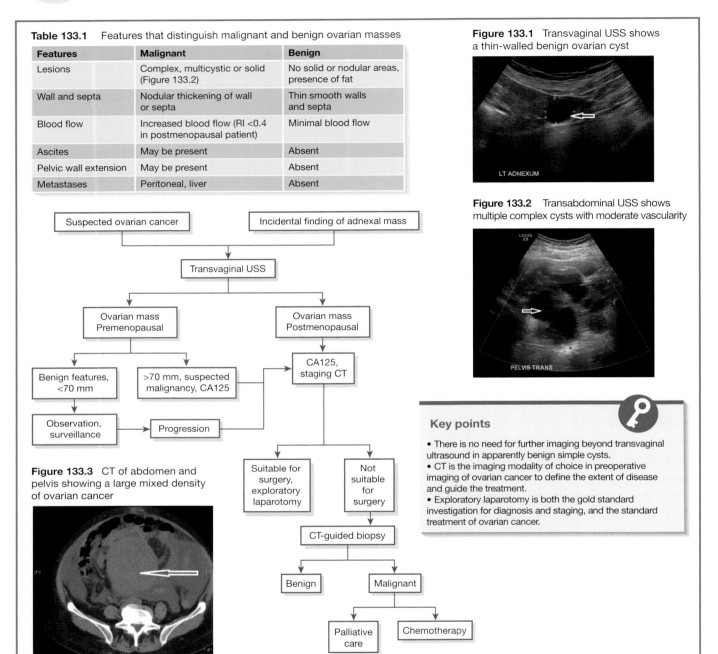

Table 133.1 Features that distinguish malignant and benign ovarian masses

Features	Malignant	Benign
Lesions	Complex, multicystic or solid (Figure 133.2)	No solid or nodular areas, presence of fat
Wall and septa	Nodular thickening of wall or septa	Thin smooth walls and septa
Blood flow	Increased blood flow (RI <0.4 in postmenopausal patient)	Minimal blood flow
Ascites	May be present	Absent
Pelvic wall extension	May be present	Absent
Metastases	Peritoneal, liver	Absent

Figure 133.1 Transvaginal USS shows a thin-walled benign ovarian cyst

LT ADNEXUM

Figure 133.2 Transabdominal USS shows multiple complex cysts with moderate vascularity

LOGIQ E9

PELVIS TRANS

Suspected ovarian cancer / Incidental finding of adnexal mass

Transvaginal USS

Ovarian mass Premenopausal / Ovarian mass Postmenopausal

Benign features, <70 mm / >70 mm, suspected malignancy, CA125

CA125, staging CT

Observation, surveillance / Progression

Suitable for surgery, exploratory laparotomy / Not suitable for surgery

Figure 133.3 CT of abdomen and pelvis showing a large mixed density of ovarian cancer

CT-guided biopsy

Benign / Malignant

Palliative care / Chemotherapy

Key points

• There is no need for further imaging beyond transvaginal ultrasound in apparently benign simple cysts.
• CT is the imaging modality of choice in preoperative imaging of ovarian cancer to define the extent of disease and guide the treatment.
• Exploratory laparotomy is both the gold standard investigation for diagnosis and staging, and the standard treatment of ovarian cancer.

Ovarian cancer is the fourth commonest cause of female cancer death in the developed world. The high mortality is partially due to the delay in investigation and diagnosis (60% present with stage III or IV) because of non-specific presenting symptoms. Subtypes of ovarian cancer include epithelial, germ cell and sex-cord stromal tumours. Women with a genetic predisposition to ovarian cancer are diagnosed about 10 years earlier than the median age of diagnosis. Women with germline *BRCA1* or *BRCA2* mutations have a 40–60% lifetime risk of epithelial ovarian cancer. A high index of suspicion and subsequent investigation of ovarian cancer is essential due to the non-specific nature of the symptoms, and lack of awareness of ovarian cancer.

Initial investigation

Transvaginal ultrasound

Transvaginal ultrasound is the first investigation of choice in the initial investigation of suspected ovarian cancer, with a specificity of 92% (Figures 133.1 and 133.2). However, its sensitivity in symptomatic women remains low, so a negative test cannot completely rule out cancer. Features distinguishing malignant and benign lesions are described in Table 133.1.

Serum CA125

Serum CA125 is a blood test which can be helpful in the diagnosis of ovarian cancer.
- In 80% of patients with advanced-stage disease, CA125 levels are elevated.
- In a postmenopausal patient, CA125 of 65 U/mL or greater is almost diagnostic of malignancy, with 98% specificity; an elevated CA125 level in this group requires further investigation.
- In premenopausal patients, elevations between 35 and 65 U/mL are associated with a 50–60% risk of cancer.
- CA125 can be elevated in many non-malignant conditions (e.g. endometriosis, uterine fibroids, pregnancy, ascites due to other causes and ovarian cysts) and in malignant conditions (e.g. pancreatic, breast, lung, gastric and colon cancers).
- Normal CA125 levels cannot exclude ovarian cancer, as 50% of patients with early-stage ovarian cancers have a normal CA125.
- CA125 levels alone cannot diagnose ovarian cancer; surgery and histopathology are ultimately necessary for diagnosis.
- CA125 levels are most useful after a histological diagnosis of ovarian cancer. It can be followed to assess disease recurrence as well as response to treatment. However, the use of CA125 for surveillance and detection of relapse has not been demonstrated to improve patient survival.
- LDH, AFP and hCG should be measured in all women aged under 40 years with a complex ovarian mass because of the possibility of germ cell tumours.

The combination of CA125 and transvaginal pelvic ultrasound is more sensitive and specific than either alone in distinguishing benign lesion from malignant adnexal masses.

Radiological investigation

CT of the abdomen and pelvis is the modality of choice in preoperative imaging of ovarian cancer. It can estimate the extent and sites of tumour involvement (Figure 133.3). MRI might be helpful in further assessment of the pelvic tumour. Sometimes the tumour arises in the peritoneum producing widespread low-volume cancer, without a discrete ovarian tumour, in which case the tumour is referred to as a primary peritoneal cancer, which is almost always of serous type. CT has good sensitivity and specificity for detecting peritoneal disease (92% and 82%, respectively). This is similar to MRI and superior to ultrasound. For lymph node and hepatic parenchymal disease, CT has low sensitivity (40–43%) but good specificity (89–96%). PET or integrated PET-CT can help distinguish between benign and malignant tumours based on standardised uptake values.

Tissue diagnosis

Exploratory laparotomy is both the gold standard investigation for diagnosis and staging and the standard treatment of ovarian cancer. The diagnosis of ovarian cancer is based on histopathology. When an ovarian mass is detected, biopsy is *not* recommended as this can disseminate tumour cells in the peritoneal cavity. Surgical extirpation of the affected ovary is necessary for definitive diagnosis. However, in patients for whom initial radical cytoreductive surgery is considered inappropriate because of widespread bulky disease or poor clinical state, a tissue sample can be taken using image-guided core biopsy. This allows for an immunohistological diagnosis of the tumour and may guide further management. In patients presenting with ascites, a sample of fluid should be obtained and cytological analysis and measurement of CA125 levels performed.

Screening

Screening for ovarian cancer in the general population is not recommended

Attempts to screen the general population using measurement of serum CA125 level, transvaginal ultrasound, or both have not yet provided convincing evidence that early-stage, curable ovarian cancer can be detected in sufficient numbers, without an excessive number of non-malignant lesions leading to unnecessary surgery. Unlike cervical cancer, ovarian cancer does not have a detectable pre-invasive phase.

High-risk screening

- Women with a strong family history of breast and/or ovarian cancer should be tested for *BRCA1* and *BRCA2* mutations as well as for mutations associated with hereditary non-polyposis colorectal cancer (HNPCC).
- A woman with germline *BRCA* mutations has a lifetime risk of developing ovarian cancer of 55–60%.
- There is limited evidence to support the effectiveness of screening these high-risk women; most practice guidelines recommend pelvic ultrasound with concomitant CA125 levels every 6 months.
- Currently, prophylactic bilateral salpingo-oophorectomy and oral contraceptives remain the only means of risk reduction in this population.

134 Prostate cancer

The purpose of investigations is to:
- Establish the diagnosis of prostate cancer
- Stage the disease (TNM system, Gleason score) prior to treatment
- Monitor response to treatment and detect early cancer recurrence

Table 134.1 Conditions that can cause elevation of PSA

Benign prostatic hyperplasia (BPH)
Prostatitis
Urinary tract infection
Post-prostate biopsy
DRE
Ejaculation
Strenuous physical exercise or bicycle riding
Acute urinary retention and catheterisation

Table 134.2 Age-specific PSA ranges

Age (years)	PSA, upper limit of the reference intervals (ng/mL)
40–49	≤2.5
50–59	≤3.5
60–69	≤4.5
70–79	≤6.5

Table 134.3 Active surveillance for low-risk prostate cancer

Timing	Investigations
At time of diagnosis	Multiparametric MRI
Year 1	PSA 3-monthly, monitor PSA kinetics, DRE 6-monthly
Years 2–4	PSA 6-monthly, monitor PSA kinetics, DRE 6-monthly
Year 5 and every year thereafter	PSA 6-monthly, monitor PSA kinetics, DRE yearly

Table 134.4 Key points regarding the prostate cancer screen

- PSA test is inaccurate: two of three men who have a high PSA will not have prostate cancer
- A raised PSA blood test initiates a cascade of diagnostic and treatment events that have significant harms and these should be considered before testing (Table 134.5)
- Up to 25% of men with normal PSA actually have prostate cancer
- Most men diagnosed with prostate cancer will have slow-growing cancer and will not benefit from invasive testing
- Finding prostate cancer, especially in older men, may not increase lifespan and treatment may lead to a poorer quality of life
- Overdiagnosis: the major harms of PSA screening relate to treatment of detected cancers. About half of those detected would never cause clinical problems in a man's lifetime, even in the absence of treatment. Treatment complications include long-term erectile, urinary and bowel dysfunction
- Overtreatment: about 30% of patients aged over 60 years have prostate cancer that is unlikely to cause harm during their lifetime. This greatly exceeds the 3% lifetime risk of dying of prostate cancer even if untreated

Table 134.5 Benefits and harms of screening for prostate cancer

Benefits of screening	Every 1000 men screened
Number of men who die from prostate cancer with no screening	5
Number of men who die from prostate cancer with screening	4.5
Number of men who avoid death from prostate cancer because of screening	0.1
Harms of screening	
Number of men who experience a false-positive PSA test	120
Number who develop serious treatment-related cardiovascular events	2
Number who develop treatment-related venous thromboembolism	1
Number who develop erectile dysfunction	29
Number who develop urinary incontinence	18

Fig 134.1 (a) Transrectal USS-guided prostate biopsy; (b) USS-guided prostate biopsy; (c) biopsy gun

(a)
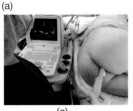
(b)
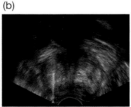
(c)
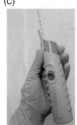

Figure 134.2 Staging CT in a patient with prostate cancer shows liver metastases and right obstructive uropathy

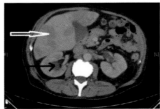

Figure 134.3 Whole-body bone scan shows extensive bony metastatic prostate cancer

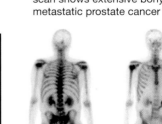
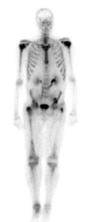

Clinical Investigations at a Glance, First Edition. Jonathan Gleadle, Jordan Li and Tuck Yong. © 2017 John Wiley & Sons, Ltd. Published 2017 by John Wiley & Sons, Ltd.

Prostate cancer is the most frequently diagnosed cancer other than skin cancer in men and the second leading cause of death from cancer. Prostate cancer is predominantly a disease of older men but 25% of cases occur in men younger than 65. Established risk factors for prostate cancer include increasing age (>50 years), black ethnic origin, and a family history of prostate cancer in a close male relative. There are no specific symptoms of early-stage prostate cancer. Currently, the majority of prostate cancers are identified in patients who are asymptomatic. Diagnosis in such cases is based on abnormalities in a screening PSA level or findings on digital rectal examination (DRE).

Initial investigations

Prostate-specific antigen (PSA)

PSA is a glycoprotein produced solely by the prostate and is elevated in prostate cancer. However, PSA is tissue-specific but not cancer-specific, as PSA can be elevated in other conditions (Table 134.1).

PSA is not a diagnostic test; a patient should receive explanation that invasive investigations (prostate biopsy) may be needed if PSA level is elevated and that PSA within the reference interval does not exclude cancer. Age-specific PSA ranges are used to interpret elevated PSA (Table 134.2).

Free-to-total PSA ratios are used to discriminate patients with benign prostatic hyperplasia (BPH) and those with prostate cancer because levels of bound PSA are higher in prostate cancer. Ratios below 15% are more suspicious of cancer. PSA velocity is a measure of annual increase in PSA levels and an increase of more than 0.75 ng/mL within 2 years is suspicious of cancer.

Transrectal ultrasound-guided biopsy

Transrectal ultrasound-guided prostate biopsy (Figure 134.1) is undertaken for tissue diagnosis in patients with elevated PSA levels or abnormal DRE findings. A 12-core systematic biopsy incorporating apical and far-lateral cores in a template distribution allows maximal cancer detection, avoidance of repeat biopsy, and adequate information for planning therapy while minimising the detection of occult, indolent prostate cancers. Indolent disease can be detected and clinically important cancers missed. These errors can lead to poor risk attribution; for example, a man with low-risk cancer on ultrasound-guided biopsy has a one in three chance of harbouring higher-grade disease. Consider multiparametric MRI (using T2- and diffusion-weighted imaging) for men with a negative transrectal ultrasound 10–12 core biopsy to determine whether another biopsy is needed. If the MRI is negative, repeat biopsy is not required.

Other investigations

FBC, serum electrolytes including calcium, creatinine and LFTs should be checked. If hormone therapy is considered, bone densitometry should be performed.

Staging investigations

MRI and CT have equivalent accuracy for staging (Figure 134.2). Consider MRI or CT for men with histologically proven prostate cancer if knowledge of the T or N stage could affect management. Do not offer imaging to men who are not candidates for radical treatment. For metastasis staging, bone scan with technetium-99m (^{99m}Tc) is typically used (Figure 134.3). It is not indicated in asymptomatic patients with PSA below 10 ng/mL.

Surveillance

Active surveillance (Table 134.3) is an option for patients with low-risk localised prostate cancer for whom radical prostatectomy or radical radiotherapy is suitable.

Monitoring recurrent disease

Radical prostatectomy should stop PSA production and levels should fall to zero. Persistence of PSA level or rising level after radical surgery indicates failure to remove the gland completely, cancer recurrence or metastases. Regular PSA every 6 months can help monitor the outcome of treatments such as brachytherapy and radiation or hormone treatment. A positive response can see PSA return to near zero levels. Serial measurements showing a rise in PSA may mean disease is recurring or progressing.

Screening for early prostate cancer

Use of the PSA test for prostate cancer screening is controversial. No study has reported that PSA screening for prostate cancer leads to a reduction in overall mortality. Currently, universal screening is not recommended but, if undertaken, the combination of DRE and PSA may improve the predictive value of both as early detection tests. PSA screening is done on a 'case-by-case' basis. The best evidence of possible benefits of PSA screening is in men aged 55–69 years or men with a family history of prostate cancer. The key issues that impact the decision to test are listed in Tables 134.4 and 134.5.

135 Stroke

Table 135.1 Classification and common causes of stroke

Haemorrhagic stroke (15%)
Intracerebral (66%)
Subarachnoid (34%)
Ischaemic stroke (85%)
Atherosclerotic thromboembolism (20%)
Lacunar (25%)
Cardiogenic emboli (20%)
Cryptogenic (30%)
Others (5%)

Table 135.2 Sensitivity and specificity of investigations

Investigation	Sensitivity (%)	Specificity (%)
Carotid ultrasound	87	75
CTA	95	85
MRA	92	75
Combined MRA and USS	96	80
Digital subtraction angiography (DSA)	Gold standard	

Table 135.3 Investigation of complications in the recovery phase

Complication	Investigation
Aspiration or hospital-acquired pneumonia	CXR
Venous thromboembolism (VTE)	CTPA and/or duplex USS of lower limbs
Urinary tract infection (UTI)	Urine culture
Urine retention	Post-void ultrasound scan
Dysphagia	Barium swallow test
Vision disturbance	Formal visual field test

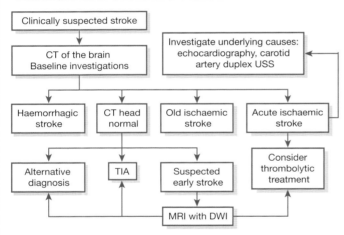

Clinically suspected stroke → CT of the brain, Baseline investigations → Haemorrhagic stroke / CT head normal / Old ischaemic stroke / Acute ischaemic stroke

Investigate underlying causes: echocardiography, carotid artery duplex USS

Alternative diagnosis / TIA / Suspected early stroke / Consider thrombolytic treatment

MRI with DWI

Figure 135.3 MRI T2 FLAIR image shows acute occipital infarct

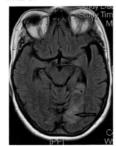

Figure 135.4 CT angiogram shows a 90% stenosis in the proximal left internal carotid artery

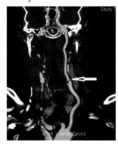

Figure 135.1 CT of the brain shows left basal ganglia haemorrhage consistent with hypertensive bleed

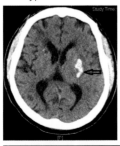

Figure 135.2 CT of the brain shows hypodensity involving grey and white matter in the left occipital lobe consistent with early infarct

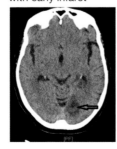

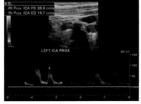

Figure 135.5 Carotid duplex USS shows left proximal internal carotid artery 70% stenosis

Key points

- Initial brain imaging with CT is intended to distinguish between ischaemic and haemorrhagic stroke and localise the area of pathology.
- Urgent imaging and baseline laboratory investigations are required in patients considered suitable for thrombolytic therapy.
- MRI is more sensitive than CT for acute ischaemic stroke.
- If an ischaemic stroke is confirmed, additional investigations such as ECG, echocardiography and carotid artery duplex ultrasound may be warranted depending on the clinical presentation.

A stroke is a clinical syndrome characterised by rapid development of focal or global loss of brain function, lasting more than 24 hours. Transient ischaemic attack (TIA) is characterised by a transient episode of neurological dysfunction caused by focal brain, spinal cord or retinal ischaemia, without acute infarction, usually lasting less than 24 hours. TIA is a warning sign of stroke, with 20% of patients having a subsequent stroke within 90 days. Half of these will have a stroke within 48 hours of the TIA. Approximately 85% of strokes are ischaemic, caused by a transient or permanent critical reduction in cerebral blood flow due to arterial occlusion or stenosis.

The classification and causes of stroke are summarised in Table 135.1. Uncommon causes should be considered, especially if patients are young (<50 years) and have no cardiovascular risk factors. In patients with neck trauma, carotid artery dissection should be considered; fever and new onset of a cardiac murmur raises the possibility of infective endocarditis; headache and an elevated CRP in patients older than 50 years of age suggest giant cell arteritis. Cryptogenic stroke has no identifiable cause despite extensive investigation.

Acute stroke is suspected by the sudden onset or rapid progression of a focal neurological deficit such as dysphasia, dysarthria, hemianopia, weakness, ataxia, sensory loss, and neglect. Symptoms and signs are often unilateral, and consciousness is generally normal or slightly impaired, except in the case of some infarcts in the posterior circulation. Loss of neurological function can be documented by the National Institutes of Health (NIH) Stroke Scale. Acute ischaemic stroke is a clinical emergency, and timely investigation, diagnosis and intervention can improve outcome.

Initial investigations

Brain imaging

In all patients with suspected stroke, CT or MRI of brain must be performed as soon as possible, ideally within 30 min of arrival in the emergency department. Brain imaging is used to determine:

- if the patient has had a stroke;
- the vascular territory of the stroke;
- the aetiology of the stroke.

Ischaemic stroke cannot be distinguished with certainty from intracerebral haemorrhage on the basis of symptoms and signs alone. The decision to perform thrombolysis should be based on CT or MRI of the head. Non-contrast CT is the first choice and can exclude intracerebral haemorrhage (Figure 135.1). Compared with MRI, CT head is more widely available, faster, less susceptible to motion artefacts and less expensive. Non-contrast CT will show an abnormality within 6 hours of the ischaemic event in 50% of patients with cortical infarcts (Figure 135.2).

MRI has a much higher sensitivity than CT for acute ischaemic changes, especially in the posterior fossa, lacunar infarcts and in the first hours after an ischaemic stroke (Figure 135.3). Oedema is detectable within minutes after the onset of ischaemia, with reduced apparent diffusion coefficient on diffusion-weighted (DWI) and gradient-echo sequences imaging.

For patients in whom acute invasive treatment such as intra-arterial thrombolysis or mechanical clot retrieval are considered, urgent CT angiography (CTA) or magnetic resonance angiography (MRA) is useful for identifying the site of arterial occlusion (Figure 135.4). If arterial dissection is suspected, CTA or MRA should be performed (Table 135.2). CTA is faster than MRA and provides higher resolution for imaging extracranial and intracranial arteries to demonstrate the presence and location of persistent arterial occlusions, stenosis or dissections.

Laboratory investigations and CXR

Laboratory tests that should be performed at presentation are listed in Box 135.2. Blood culture should be performed if there is a suspicion of infective endocarditis. A baseline CXR should be obtained to identify cardiac or pulmonary abnormalities and for later comparison.

Ultrasound

Carotid duplex ultrasound (Figure 135.5) and transcranial Doppler ultrasound can be used in the subacute stage to detect carotid artery occlusion or critical stenosis.

ECG and echocardiography

An ECG should be performed, which may reveal atrial fibrillation or an acute or previous myocardial infarction as potential causes of thromboembolism. Urgent echocardiography is indicated if infective endocarditis is suspected. When the patient is stable, transthoracic or transoesophageal echocardiography may be indicated to rule out cardioembolism. Contrast echocardiography can detect cardiovascular shunts. Persistent patent foramen ovale is associated with stroke especially in young patients with cryptogenic stroke and other disorders related to paradoxical embolism.

Investigations of vascular risk factors

Patients with difficult-to-control blood pressure may require investigation for secondary causes of hypertension. Fasting blood glucose or HbA$_{1c}$ for patients with suspected or established diabetes mellitus and lipid profile should be determined.

Investigations for thrombophilia (protein C, protein S, antithrombin III, factor V Leiden, prothrombin G20210A mutation and fasting homocysteine level), antiphospholipid antibodies (anticardiolipin antibody, lupus anticoagulant), syphilis serology, HIV serology and autoimmune antibodies should be performed in selected patients.

Investigations of complications in the recovery phase

See Table 135.3.

Investigations for TIA

All patients should have a CT brain scan to exclude haemorrhage and other space-occupying lesions and carotid duplex ultrasound (if symptoms are within the carotid artery territory and the patient would be potentially suitable for carotid revascularisation) within 48–72 hours. If CT brain is normal and clinical features are suggestive of stroke, MRI with DWI should be performed. Other routine investigations should include FBC, electrolytes, renal function, lipid studies, blood glucose level, CRP and ECG.

136 Haemorrhagic stroke

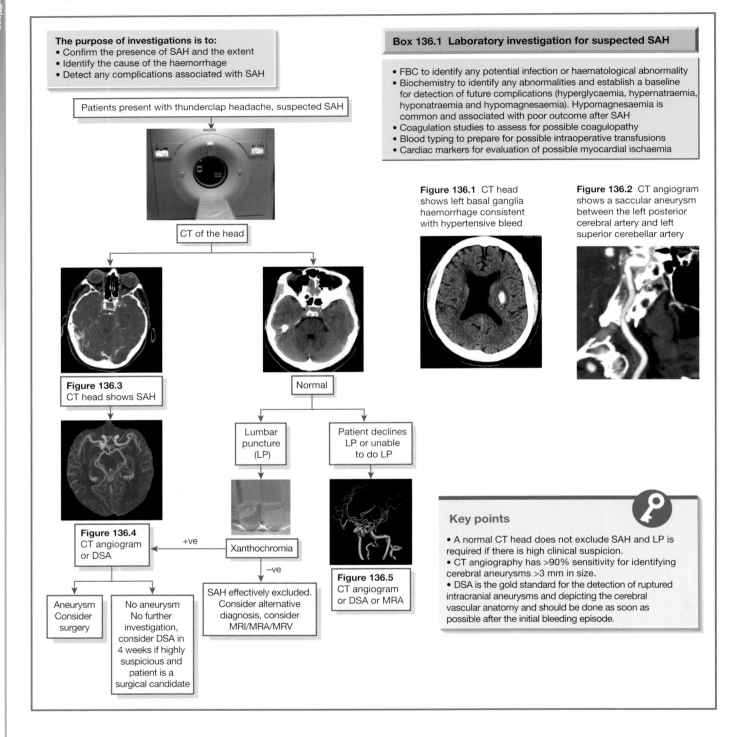

The purpose of investigations is to:
- Confirm the presence of SAH and the extent
- Identify the cause of the haemorrhage
- Detect any complications associated with SAH

Box 136.1 Laboratory investigation for suspected SAH

- FBC to identify any potential infection or haematological abnormality
- Biochemistry to identify any abnormalities and establish a baseline for detection of future complications (hyperglycaemia, hypernatraemia, hyponatraemia and hypomagnesaemia). Hypomagnesaemia is common and associated with poor outcome after SAH
- Coagulation studies to assess for possible coagulopathy
- Blood typing to prepare for possible intraoperative transfusions
- Cardiac markers for evaluation of possible myocardial ischaemia

Patients present with thunderclap headache, suspected SAH

CT of the head

Figure 136.1 CT head shows left basal ganglia haemorrhage consistent with hypertensive bleed

Figure 136.2 CT angiogram shows a saccular aneurysm between the left posterior cerebral artery and left superior cerebellar artery

Figure 136.3 CT head shows SAH

Normal

Figure 136.4 CT angiogram or DSA

Lumbar puncture (LP)

Patient declines LP or unable to do LP

+ve

Xanthochromia

−ve

Figure 136.5 CT angiogram or DSA or MRA

Aneurysm Consider surgery

No aneurysm No further investigation, consider DSA in 4 weeks if highly suspicious and patient is a surgical candidate

SAH effectively excluded. Consider alternative diagnosis, consider MRI/MRA/MRV

Key points

- A normal CT head does not exclude SAH and LP is required if there is high clinical suspicion.
- CT angiography has >90% sensitivity for identifying cerebral aneurysms >3 mm in size.
- DSA is the gold standard for the detection of ruptured intracranial aneurysms and depicting the cerebral vascular anatomy and should be done as soon as possible after the initial bleeding episode.

Intracranial haemorrhage

Stroke is divided into ischaemic and haemorrhagic stroke. Haemorrhagic stroke is caused by the rupture of a cerebrospinal artery resulting in bleeding into brain parenchyma that may extend into the intraventricular and subarachnoid space. Haemorrhagic stroke accounts for 10–15% of cases of stroke and is associated with the highest mortality rate (25–58%) within the first 6 months after the bleeding episode.

Primary intracerebral haemorrhage (80% of cases) originates from the spontaneous rupture of small vessels damaged by chronic hypertension or amyloid angiopathy. Secondary intracerebral haemorrhage occurs in patients with vascular malformations, tumours or impaired coagulation. Hypertension is the most important risk factor for primary haemorrhagic stroke.

The presenting symptoms of haemorrhagic stroke are highly variable depending on the mechanism, volume and location of stroke. Patients with a large intracerebral haemorrhage usually have a decreased level of consciousness.

Brain imaging

CT of the head is essential for diagnosing haemorrhagic stroke. It can distinguish between ischaemic stroke and intracerebral haemorrhage (Figure 136.1) and exclude other neurological conditions that mimic stroke. MRI with gadolinium enhancement and MRA can be used to identify secondary causes of intracerebral haemorrhage, such as arteriovenous malformation (AVM), intracranial aneurysm, dural venous sinus thrombosis and neoplasm.

Conventional angiography should be performed in all patients with no clear cause of haemorrhage who are candidates for surgery, particularly young patients without hypertension whose condition is clinically stable. Patients with lobar haemorrhage or suspected vasculitis, aneurysm or AVM should also be considered for angiography. CT angiography (CTA) is the first choice (Figure 136.2) as it has high spatial resolution and is non-invasive.

Angiography should also be considered in patients who have subarachnoid blood associated with a parenchymal haemorrhage and in patients with recurrent haemorrhages. In patients who have initially negative findings on imaging but who have a high likelihood of secondary intracerebral haemorrhage, angiography can be repeated 2–4 weeks after the resolution of haematoma when vascular anomalies may become visible. Angiography is not required for older hypertensive patients who have a haemorrhage in the basal ganglia, thalamus, cerebellum or brainstem and in whom CT findings do not suggest a structural lesion.

Laboratory investigations

These should include FBC, biochemistry and coagulation studies, especially for patients who are on anticoagulants. Serology and measurement of autoantibodies, such as ANA and ANCA, should be performed in patients with suspected underlying vasculitis. CXR and ECG should be routinely performed.

Subarachnoid haemorrhage

Non-traumatic subarachnoid haemorrhage (SAH) accounts for 5% of strokes but tends to affect younger patients. Ruptured aneurysms account for 85% of patients with non-traumatic SAH, whereas 10% are related to non-aneurysmal perimesencephalic haemorrhage and the remaining 5% are caused by rare aetiologies such as mycotic aneurysms, vasculitis, vascular malformations and cocaine abuse.

Sudden severe headache, often described as the worst headache ever, is the most characteristic symptom of SAH and is present in about 75% of patients, but may be the only manifestation in 30% of cases. It can be associated with nausea, vomiting and photophobia. Confusion, seizures, reduced consciousness level and coma are among the other possible presenting symptoms.

A high index of suspicion of SAH is essential and must be excluded in anyone presenting with sudden severe headache that is maximal within minutes. SAH can be a diagnostic challenge and prompt investigation is mandatory as no clinical feature is sufficiently reliable to make the diagnosis.

Initial investigations

CT of the brain

Non-contrast CT of the head is the first-line investigation for patients with suspected SAH and should be performed as soon as possible. The ability of CT to detect SAH is dependent on the interval after symptom onset, the amount of subarachnoid blood and the resolution of the scanner. CT performed within 48–72 hours of the onset of symptoms will usually demonstrate the presence of high-attenuation blood in the subarachnoid space (Figure 136.3) and may indicate the site of the aneurysm if focal clot is present. A negative CT does not exclude the diagnosis of SAH because the sensitivity of the procedure declines within hours of symptom onset. Third-generation CT scanners miss about 2% of cases of SAH within 12 hours and about 7% of cases by 24 hours. SAH blood is almost completely reabsorbed within 10 days.

Repeat CT scan may be needed to diagnose or rule out hydrocephalus. Patients with intraventricular blood or with extensive haemorrhage in the perimesencephalic cisterns are predisposed to developing acute hydrocephalus.

MRI of the brain

In the first 5 days after haemorrhage, MRI with proton density and FLAIR images is as sensitive as CT. After that, MRI is more sensitive than CT in detecting subacute haemorrhage.

Angiography

Angiography is the investigation of choice for determining the cause of SAH. If CT is positive or lumbar puncture (LP) reveals xanthochromia or fresh blood in the CSF in a patient with clinical acute SAH, catheter DSA is performed in order to establish the source of the haemorrhage. However, catheter angiography is associated with some risk, namely transient or permanent ischaemic neurological complications (about 1.8%) and aneurysm rupture (1–2%). With conventional angiography as the gold standard, CTA has a sensitivity of about 95% for detecting ruptured aneurysms (Figures 136.4 and 136.5). MRA has similar test characteristics to CTA. MRA is not feasible for patients who are restless or need mechanical ventilation.

Laboratory and other investigations

Laboratory studies for patients with suspected SAH are listed in Box 136.1. Troponin measurement is important in patients with SAH, even in those without underlying cardiac conditions because there is an association between troponin levels and neurological complications and outcome.

ECG abnormalities that can be detected in some patients with SAH include non-specific ST and T wave changes, decreased PR intervals, increased QRS intervals, increased QT intervals, and presence of U waves or dysrhythmias.

All patients with SAH should have a CXR to serve as a reference point for evaluation of possible pulmonary complications.

Second-line investigation: lumbar puncture

Patients with suspected SAH and a normal CT require LP. A small number of patients with sudden headache caused by SAH will have a normal CT head initially. In this setting, LP may help clarify the diagnosis by detecting xanthochromia. It may be necessary to wait until at least 6 hours and preferably 12 hours have elapsed after the onset of headache to perform the LP so that bilirubin has been formed in the interval from the breakdown of erythrocytes in the CSF.

The opening pressure of CSF must be recorded. The CSF should be protected from light to prevent degradation of bilirubin and analysed for protein, cells and glucose (paired with a serum sample) routinely. If the CSF is bloodstained, it should be centrifuged immediately. If the supernatant is yellow, the diagnosis of SAH is practically certain but formally the presence of bilirubin should be established. Spectrophotometry can be used to confirm the presence of bilirubin and also to exclude it. The estimation of erythrocyte counts in three consecutive samples of CSF does not reliably distinguish SAH from a traumatic tap.

If CT and CSF (including spectrophotometry) are normal within 2 weeks of a sudden severe headache, then SAH is excluded and an alternative diagnosis must be considered. CTA or MRA should be considered for patients who present 2 weeks or more after a highly suspected SAH.

Screening for new aneurysms after SAH

Although patients who have survived a sporadic episode of SAH are at increased risk of a new episode from a new aneurysm or from recurrence of the treated aneurysm, screening of these patients in general cannot be recommended because of reduced quality of life and increased cost. However, some exceptions to this recommendation include patients with an initial episode at a very young age and the presence of multiple aneurysms at the initial haemorrhage.

Screening for aneurysms in relatives of patients with SAH

Screening should be considered in individuals with two or more affected first-degree relatives and in patients with autosomal dominant polycystic kidney disease, at least after age 20 years, and provided the life expectancy is not too short. If a first screen is negative, repeat screening every 5 years should be discussed because the rate of finding an aneurysm at 5 years after the initial screening is about 7%. However, in individuals with only a single affected first-degree relative, screening is not effective or efficient.

137 Brain abscess

Figure 137.1 CT head shows a hypodense area due to brain abscess

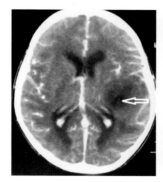

Figure 137.2 CT head shows a ring-enhancing lesion due to brain abscess

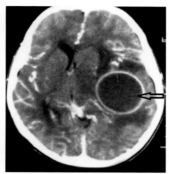

Key points

- Contrast-enhanced MRI or, if unavailable, contrast-enhanced CT is required to diagnose brain abscess.
- If it is difficult to distinguish from a tumour or infarction, CT-guided aspiration with biopsy and culture is the next investigation.
- Aspirate culture, including aerobic, anaerobic and acid-fast organisms and fungi, confirms the diagnosis and helps direct antibiotic therapy.

Brain abscess can be caused by bacteria, mycobacteria, fungi or parasites (protozoa and helminths). In most patients with brain abscess, there is an identifiable predisposing factor, such as taking immunosuppressants, head trauma, operative procedures, mastoiditis, sinusitis, or a systemic source of infection such as endocarditis or bacteraemia. Bacteria enter the brain through contiguous spread in about 50% of cases and through haematogenous dissemination in about 30% of cases, with unknown mechanisms accounting for the remaining cases. The common clinical features of brain abscess are headache, fever and altered level of consciousness. Neurological signs depend on the site of the abscess and can be subtle for days to weeks.

Neuroimaging

CT of the brain with contrast is required in all patients with suspected brain abscess. It can detect the size, number and location of abscesses (Figures 137.1 and 137.2). MRI, combined with DWI and apparent diffusion coefficient (ADC) images, can differentiate brain abscess from primary, cystic or necrotic tumours. DWI MRI has 96% sensitivity and 96% specificity for the differentiation of brain abscesses from primary or metastatic cancers (positive predictive value, 98%; negative predictive value, 92%).

For patients with a decline in consciousness, immediate brain imaging is indicated to detect impending brain herniation or hydrocephalus. Abscess rupture into the ventricular system results in ventriculitis, often leading to hydrocephalus, and is associated with high mortality (27–85%). In patients with rupture, placement of an external ventricular catheter provides a way of sampling, draining CSF and monitoring intracranial pressure, as well as providing a direct route for the administration of intraventricular antibiotics. Hydrocephalus is common in patients with abscesses in the posterior fossa. A decline in consciousness may also be caused by seizures or status epilepticus.

Microbiology investigations

Cultures of blood and CSF identify the causative pathogen in about 25% of patients. Culture of CSF is valuable in patients with coexisting meningitis. However, LP should only be performed when there is clinical suspicion of meningitis or abscess rupture into the ventricular system and there are no contraindications for LP, such as brain shift on head CT or coagulation disorders. Underlying dental, paranasal sinus, ear and skin foci of infection should be cultured; surgical removal of these foci may be required.

Stereotactic aspiration should be performed for the purposes of diagnosis and decompression unless it is contraindicated because of the patient's poor health status or multiple comorbidities. If brain imaging does not show a central cavity in the abscess, careful consideration should be given to the choice between performing a stereotactic biopsy of the area of presumed cerebritis and empirically administering antimicrobial treatment with follow-up neuroimaging. In HIV-infected patients with probable toxoplasmosis, presumptive therapy may be justified in the absence of a tissue-based diagnosis when tests for anti-*Toxoplasma* IgG antibodies are positive. Diagnostic aspiration should be aimed at achieving maximal drainage of the abscess. Continuous drainage can be achieved by placing a catheter into the abscess cavity, which may decrease reoperation rates.

Microbiological study of CSF, blood or aspirate from the abscess should include Gram stain and aerobic and anaerobic cultures. In immunocompromised patients and those with risk factors for tuberculosis or opportunistic infection, smears and cultures should include mycobacteria, *Nocardia* species, and fungi. If a bacterial brain abscess is strongly suspected but the culture results are negative, PCR-based 16S ribosomal DNA sequencing may provide a definitive aetiological diagnosis, allowing for targeted antimicrobial therapy.

In immunocompromised patients, investigations are also required to assess the severity and aetiology (see Chapter 43). If infective endocarditis is suspected, transoesophageal echocardiography is indicated.

Clinical Investigations at a Glance, First Edition. Jonathan Gleadle, Jordan Li and Tuck Yong. © 2017 John Wiley & Sons, Ltd. Published 2017 by John Wiley & Sons, Ltd.

138 Encephalitis

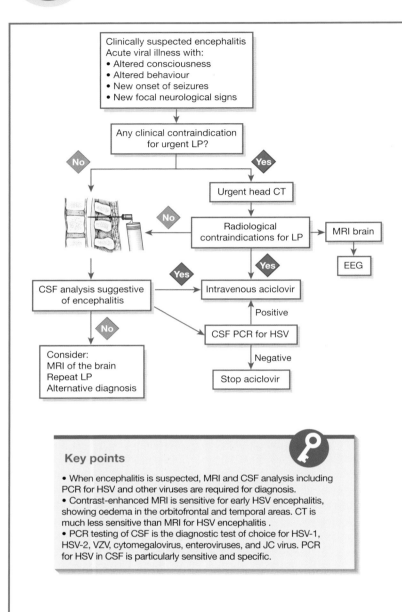

Clinically suspected encephalitis
Acute viral illness with:
• Altered consciousness
• Altered behaviour
• New onset of seizures
• New focal neurological signs

Any clinical contraindication for urgent LP?

No — Yes

Urgent head CT

No — Radiological contraindications for LP → MRI brain → EEG

Yes

Yes — Intravenous aciclovir

Positive

CSF analysis suggestive of encephalitis

CSF PCR for HSV

No

Negative

Consider:
MRI of the brain
Repeat LP
Alternative diagnosis

Stop aciclovir

Key points

• When encephalitis is suspected, MRI and CSF analysis including PCR for HSV and other viruses are required for diagnosis.
• Contrast-enhanced MRI is sensitive for early HSV encephalitis, showing oedema in the orbitofrontal and temporal areas. CT is much less sensitive than MRI for HSV encephalitis .
• PCR testing of CSF is the diagnostic test of choice for HSV-1, HSV-2, VZV, cytomegalovirus, enteroviruses, and JC virus. PCR for HSV in CSF is particularly sensitive and specific.

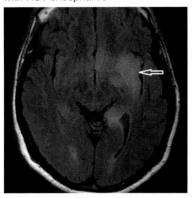

Figure 138.1 MRI of the head shows oedema in the left temporal area consistent with HSV encephalitis

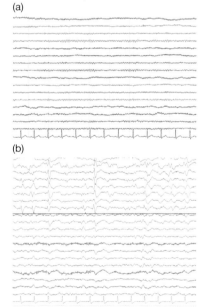

Figure 138.2 (a) Normal EEG; (b) EEG shows characteristic PLEDs consistent with HSV encephalitis
(a)

(b)

Encephalitis is inflammation of the brain parenchyma but the meninges can also be involved (meningo-encephalitis). The clinical presentation and course can be varied but the classic presentation is altered state of consciousness and/or diffuse or focal neurological symptoms and signs such as personality changes, seizures, cranial nerve palsies, speech problems, and motor and sensory deficits. Encephalitis may be associated with a number of complications, including seizures, syndrome of inappropriate antidiuretic hormone secretion (SIADH), increased intracranial pressure and coma.

Encephalitis is caused by a variety of infectious and non-infectious diseases that directly involve brain tissue. However, an aetiological agent is not identified in up to 60% of cases. Although bacterial, fungal and autoimmune disorders can cause encephalitis, most cases are caused by viruses such as herpes simplex virus (HSV) types 1 and 2, varicella zoster virus (VZV), Epstein–Barr virus (EBV), arboviruses, measles, mumps and rubella virus. It is difficult to estimate the frequency and prevalence of encephalitis because of the myriad causes with different prevalence rates in different countries. There is increasing recognition of autoimmune antibody-mediated encephalitis.

Neuroimaging

CT of the head with contrast should be performed in all patients with suspected encephalitis. This should be done prior to LP if there are focal neurological symptoms and signs to suggest elevated intracranial pressure, obstructive hydrocephalus, or mass effect due to focal brain infection. Head CT scan also helps to exclude brain haemorrhage or infarction as a cause of an encephalopathic state. MRI is more sensitive than CT in demonstrating brain abnormalities earlier in the disease course.

In HSV encephalitis, MRI may show several foci of increased T2 signal intensity in medial temporal lobes and inferior frontal grey matter (Figure 138.1). Head CT commonly shows areas of oedema or petechial haemorrhage in the same areas. In toxoplasmosis, contrast-enhanced CT of the head typically reveals several nodular or ring-enhancing lesions. Because lesions may be missed without contrast, MRI should be performed in patients for whom use of contrast material is contraindicated.

Lumbar puncture and CSF analyses

LP should be performed on all patients suspected of having viral encephalitis. A platelet count and coagulation profile should be checked before LP. The most important diagnostic test in LP is to rule out bacterial meningitis by prompt Gram staining and bacterial culture. PCR for HSV in the CSF should be done in all patients with suspected encephalitis. PCR for HSV DNA is 100% specific and 75–98% sensitive within the first 24–48 hours. Types 1 and 2 HSV cross-react, but no cross-reactivity with other herpesviruses occurs. PCR for other viruses should be performed depending on the clinical context.

Electroencephalography (EEG)

In HSV encephalitis, EEG often shows characteristic paroxysmal lateral epileptiform discharges (PLEDs), even before neuroradiographic changes (Figure 138.2). PLEDs are present in 80% of cases but the presence of PLEDs is not pathognomonic for HSV encephalitis.

Brain biopsy

In situations where the diagnosis remains unclear after the above-mentioned investigations, brain biopsy can be performed.

Other laboratory investigations

Basic laboratory tests should be performed first in any patient with suspected encephalitis. The blood glucose level should be determined immediately to rule out confusion due to simply treatable hypoglycaemia and to compare with the CSF glucose level. FBC with differential should be performed, although findings are often within the normal range. Serum electrolyte levels are usually normal unless dehydration is present; SIADH can occur in patients with encephalitis. Urea and creatinine levels and liver function tests are helpful for assessing organ dysfunction or the need to adjust the dose of antimicrobial therapy. Urine or serum toxicology screening may be indicated in selected patients presenting with delirium or confusional state.

The diagnosis of paraneoplastic limbic encephalitis can be established with the detection of paraneoplastic antibodies such as anti-Hu, anti-Yo, anti-CV2 and anti-Ma2 in serum or CSF. These antibodies can be found in patients who have cancer without encephalitis; conversely, approximately 40% of patients who have encephalitis do not have detectable antibodies.

139 Brain tumours

Figure 139.1a MRI T1-weighted imaging with contrast shows a glioblastoma multiforme

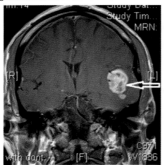

Figure 139.1b T2-weighted imaging with contrast shows a glioblastoma multiforme

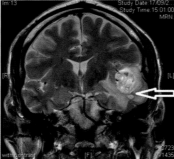

Figure 139.1c DWI imaging shows a glioblastoma multiforme

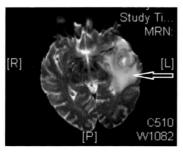

Figure 139.1d ADC imaging shows a heterogeneously contrast-enhancing left frontal lesion consistent with glioblastoma multiforme

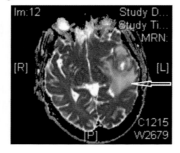

Figure 139.1e Magnetic resonance spectroscopy showing elevated choline to N-acetyl-aspartate ratio of >4 within the lesion consistent with glioblastoma multiforme

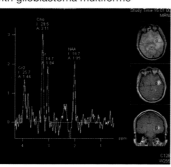

Figure 139.2 CT head with contrast shows a solitary contrast-enhancing lesion in the left frontal region with surrounding vasogenic oedema consistent with meningioma.

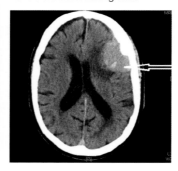

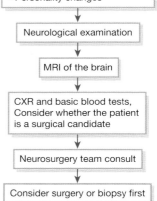

Symptoms that might be produced by a brain tumour:
- Persistent headache
- Seizures
- Nausea, vomiting
- Neurocognitive symptoms
- Personality changes

↓

Neurological examination

↓

MRI of the brain

↓

CXR and basic blood tests, Consider whether the patient is a surgical candidate

↓

Neurosurgery team consult

↓

Consider surgery or biopsy first

Key points

- MRI is the preferred initial imaging study in the evaluation of neoplastic brain lesions. It is superior to CT because it can produce better images and more precise assessment of lesions in the posterior fossa and spine.
- Primary brain tumours rarely metastasise outside the CNS and there is no need for extracranial staging.
- Round, peripherally enhancing mass lesions on MRI are typical of metastases, but gliomas can have the same appearance. Multiple enhancing lesions do not exclude multifocal glioma.
- Definitive diagnosis of brain tumours requires stereotactic biopsy for morphological, immunohisto-chemical and possibly molecular genetic studies.

Clinical Investigations at a Glance, First Edition. Jonathan Gleadle, Jordan Li and Tuck Yong. © 2017 John Wiley & Sons, Ltd. Published 2017 by John Wiley & Sons, Ltd.

A brain tumour can occur from any tissue within the cranium including the brain, cranial nerves, meninges, skull, pituitary gland and pineal gland. Tumours may be benign or malignant and can be divided into primary tumours (originate from within the cranium) or metastatic tumours. Gliomas are the most frequent primary brain tumours in adults, accounting for 70% of adult malignant primary brain tumours. Primary central nervous system (CNS) lymphomas, meningiomas and pituitary adenomas are also common in adults. Patients commonly present with symptoms of increased intracranial pressure such as headache, nausea and/or vomiting, altered mental status, seizures, and focal neurological signs. There are many types of brain tumours which can be classified according to 2007 WHO criteria.

When a brain tumour is suspected, confirmatory imaging with MRI or CT of the head should be done. It can be very difficult to distinguish between different types of brain tumours clinically and radiologically. Therefore, biopsy is required for pathological confirmation.

MRI of the head

In the absence of contraindications, standard MRI with T1-weighted spin-echo sequence, T2 fluid-attenuated inversion recovery (FLAIR), and gadolinium contrast is the imaging modality of choice in diagnosing brain tumours. A poorly marginated hypo-iso-signal T1-weighted and hypersignal T2-weighted sequence or FLAIR lesion is characteristic of a brain tumour (Figures 139.1a–d). MRI can show the integrity of the blood–brain barrier. Additionally, multimodal MRI can now be used to provide information about cellularity, metabolism and angiogenesis.

• Diffusion-weighted imaging (DWI): assesses tumour-cell density and can differentiate a cystic brain tumour from a brain abscess.

• Proton magnetic resonance spectroscopy (Figure 139.1e): can estimate the proliferation rate of tumour cells (choline to N-acetyl-aspartate ratio) and necrosis (lipids or lactates).

• Dynamic contrast-enhanced and perfusion MRI: can assess angiogenesis, which provides information about the malignancy of the lesion.

Neuroimaging remains non-specific, and histological examination of the tumour is mandatory to diagnose the type of brain tumour, especially gliomas. The differential diagnosis with brain metastasis is usually difficult, particularly when the brain lesion is solitary and in the absence of known systemic cancer. A biopsy or resection of the brain lesion may be needed. A thorough history and clinical examination including skin and breast, whole-body CT scan or PET can be performed to detect a primary neoplastic lesion.

In CNS lymphoma, MRI often shows unique or multiple periventricular, homogeneously enhancing lesions. However, primary CNS lymphomas can also manifest a large spectrum of radiological presentations, including non-enhancing infiltrating lesions, and can simulate inflammatory (sarcoidosis and multiple sclerosis) or infectious diseases, or other brain tumours such as meningiomas and malignant gliomas.

CT of the head

When MRI is not available, CT with intravenous contrast can assist in identifying the presence of brain tumours which usually demonstrate contrast enhancement. Brain tumours may appear hypodense, isodense or hyperdense, or may have mixed density (Figure 139.2). Metastases to the brain tend to be multiple, but certain tumours, such as renal cell carcinomas, often produce solitary metastatic brain lesions.

Cerebral biopsy

Definitive diagnosis of brain tumours requires stereotactic biopsy performed by the neurosurgical team. The tissue samples require morphological, immunohistochemical and possibly molecular genetic studies. Efforts should be made to avoid corticosteroid therapy prior to biopsy.

Laboratory investigations

In patients with suspected primary or metastatic brain tumours, laboratory studies should include FBC, coagulation studies, electrolytes, renal function, liver function and bone profile. Patients with cancer are predisposed to medical complications such as hyponatraemia due to SIADH and hypercalcaemia. Blood film review and other investigations (see Chapter 124) should be done if CNS lymphoma is suspected.

Lumbar puncture

In patients with suspected primary CNS lymphoma, LP should be performed unless features of raised intracranial pressure are present. It will usually reveal the presence of abnormal cells, low glucose, high protein and high pressure. Cerebral biopsy can be avoided if lymphoma cells are discovered in the CSF (10–30%). Because identification of a systemic site of lymphoma has important implications in the treatment strategy, CT scan, bone marrow biopsy and PET in the staging are usually required.

140 Multiple sclerosis

The purpose of investigation for suspected MS is to supplement clinical evidence to:
- Establish the diagnosis of MS
- Define disease activity and classification
- Determine the anatomical dissemination of lesions in time and space (imaging, CSF analysis for intrathecal inflammation)

Laboratory investigations
FBC
Biochemistry
TFTs, vitamin B12
Autoimmune serology
Antibody against aquaporin 4
Syphilis (if applicable)

Clinically suspected MS

Brain and spinal cord MRI

Atypical or negative | Typical, MS confirmed

Lumbar puncture
Cell count
Glucose
Protein
Oligoclonal band
IgG

Evoked potentials and CSF

Normal VEPs — Latency 108 msec
Multiple sclerosis VEPs — Latency 136 msec

Typical, MS confirmed | Normal, consider alternative diagnosis | Single lesion on MRI and evoked potenials, follow-up 3 months and consider alternative diagnosis

Table 140.1 Revised (2010) McDonald Criteria for the diagnosis of multiple sclerosis

Clinical presentation	Additional data needed for MS diagnosis
Two or more attacks Objective clinical evidence of two or more lesions with reasonable historical evidence of a prior attack	None; clinical evidence will suffice. Additional evidence (e.g. brain MRI) desirable, but must be consistent with MS
Two or more attacks Objective clinical evidence of one lesion	Dissemination in space demonstrated by MRI or await further clinical attack implicating a different site
One attack Objective clinical evidence of two or more lesions	Dissemination in time demonstrated by MRI or second clinical attack
One attack Objective clinical evidence of one lesion (clinically isolated syndrome)	Dissemination in space demonstrated by MRI or await a second clinical attack implicating a different CNS site and dissemination in time, demonstrated by MRI or second clinical attack
Insidious neurological progression suggestive of MS	One year of disease progression and dissemination in space, demonstrated by two of the following: One or more T2 lesions in brain, in regions characteristic of MS Two or more T2 focal lesions in spinal cord Positive CSF

Note: An attack is defined as a neurological disturbance of the kind seen in MS. It can be documented by subjective report or by objective observation, but it must last for at least 24 hours. To be considered separate attacks, at least 30 days must elapse between onset of one event and onset of another event.

Key points

- Brain MRI is abnormal in the majority of patients with MS.
- MRI with gadolinium during the first attack can provide evidence of lesions in the brain and spinal cord and exclude other disease that may mimic MS.
- Sensory evoked potential testing is useful in demonstrating the presence of subclinical lesions in sensory pathways or in providing objective evidence of lesions suspected on the basis of subjective complaints.
- In 90% of patient with MS, the CSF IgG level is elevated.

Figure 140.1 MRI FLAIR axial image: high-signal foci of demyelination in the periventricular white matter consistent with MS

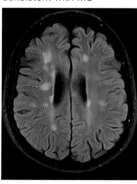

Figure 140.2 MRI T2 sagittal image: high-signal foci of demyelination extending from the corpus callosum into the pericallosal white matter consistent with MS

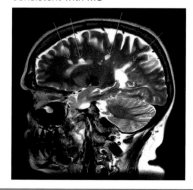

Figure 140.3 MRI T2 cervical spine sagittal image; high T2 foci of demyelination in the cervical cord consistent with MS

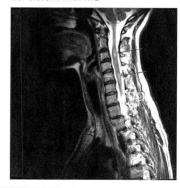

Multiple sclerosis (MS) is an inflammatory disorder of the brain and spinal cord in which focal lymphocytic infiltration leads to damage of myelin and axons. MS is often a disabling disease primarily affecting young female adults that exhibits marked clinical, radiological and pathological heterogeneity. The cause and pathogenesis of MS is unclear and affects about 0.1% of the population worldwide.

MS is classified into four clinical forms. About 85% of patients with MS present with the relapsing–remitting form (RRMS), comprising episodic relapses and remissions that may be partial or complete. A first attack is categorised as a clinically isolated syndrome. After many years most of these patients will enter a phase of progression with or without attacks, called secondary progressive MS (SPMS). About 15% of patients present with a slowly progressive pattern called primary progressive MS (PPMS). A few of them may later relapse, called progressive-relapsing MS (PRMS). Of patients with RRMS, 15% have a mild course with minimal disability after 15 years, called benign MS.

In most patients, clinical manifestations indicate the involvement of motor, sensory, visual and autonomic systems but few of the clinical features are disease-specific. MS is a clinical diagnosis. The most frequent error is making a diagnosis of MS in patients with progressive disease at a single site (usually spinal) where a structural lesion has not been excluded. The current diagnostic criteria for MS are the Revised McDonald Criteria (Table 140.1).

Laboratory investigations

Results of blood tests are usually normal. However, laboratory investigations are performed to exclude other conditions such as vasculitis, rheumatologic conditions, syphilis infection, thyroid disease, vitamin B_{12} deficiency and sarcoidosis. Neuromyelitis optica (Devic's disease) can be confirmed by the presence of serum antibodies against aquaporin 4, a water channel expressed at major fluid–tissue barriers in the CNS.

MRI

All patients with suspected MS should undergo MRI of brain and spinal cord with gadolinium contrast, which has a sensitivity of 95% for patients with clinically definite MS. More than 95% of patients with MS have T2-weighted white matter abnormalities on MRI (Figures 140.1 and 140.2), but these are not diagnostic. Typical sites of lesions seen on MRI include periventricular white matter (if at right angles to the corpus collosum, these are referred to as 'Dawson fingers'), juxtacortical white matter,

corpus collosum, optic nerve (with gadolinium enhancement in acute neuritis), infratentorial structures (pons, cerebellar peduncles and cerebellum) and spinal cord (Figure 140.3).

The main practical use of MRI is in the investigation of individuals with clinically isolated lesions or progressive disease at a single site. However, the presence of white matter lesions alone on MRI do not confirm the diagnosis of MS because these lesions can appear in people without clinical evidence of disease and because many individuals aged over 50 years have non-specific white matter cerebral lesions which should not be misinterpreted. Nonetheless, at any age, lesions detected in the spinal cord are abnormal.

Lumbar puncture

Lumbar puncture with CSF analysis is no longer routine in the investigation of MS, but may be of use when MRI is unavailable or MRI findings are non-diagnostic. CSF is evaluated for oligoclonal bands and intrathecal IgG production, as well as for signs of infection. Oligoclonal bands are found in 90–95% of patients with MS, and intrathecal IgG production in 70–90% of patients.

Neurophysiological studies

Evoked potentials (i.e. recording of the timing of CNS responses to specific stimuli) can be useful neurophysiological studies for evaluation of MS. Visual evoked potentials (VEPs), somatosensory evoked potentials (SSEPs) and brainstem auditory evoked potentials (BAEPs) are used to identify subclinical lesions but are non-specific for MS. VEPs are performed by having a patient focus on a reversing black-and-white checkerboard pattern. Delays in latencies indicate demyelination in the anterior visual pathways (see page opposite). VEPs are not necessary for patients with clear clinical evidence of optic neuritis. SSEPs evaluate the posterior column of the spinal cord, the brainstem and the cerebral cortex. BAEPs are performed to evaluate ipsilateral asymptomatic MS lesions in the auditory pathways but are less sensitive than VEPs and SSEPs.

Pretreatment investigations

If treatment with a targeted immunomodulator is required, patients should be tested for evidence of latent tuberculosis (see Chapter 117). Testing for JC virus antibodies is also performed when targeted therapy such as natalizumab is being considered because of the potential risk of progressive multifocal leukoencephalopathy.

141 Spinal cord disorders

Table 141.1 Common causes of myelopathy

Compressive
Degenerative
Traumatic: spinal cord injuries (motor vehicle accident, sports injuries)
Bone lesion
Disc herniation
Epidural haemorrhage
Infectious (abscess)
Tumours
Extradural: benign and malignant
Intradural: intramedullary and extramedullary
Vascular
Arteriovenous malformation
Syringomyelia

Non-compressive
Infectious transverse myelitis
Viral, HIV, polio
Bacterial, TB
Acute disseminated encephalomyelitis
Demyelinating diseases
Multiple sclerosis
Vascular
Spinal arterial thrombosis
CNS vasculitis (lupus, sarcoidosis)
Degenerative
Motor neuron disease
Hereditary
Familial spastic paraparesis
Spinocerebellar ataxia
Friedreich's ataxia
Metabolic
Vitamin B_{12} deficiency
Paraneoplastic

Table 141.2 Common CSF results in spinal cord disorders

CSF analysis	Results and spinal cord disorders
CSF cell count, cell differential, protein level, IgG index, oligoclonal bands	Increased cell count (>5 WBCs/mm³) and increased protein level suggest transverse myelitis; <50 WBCs/mm³ with lymphocytic differential and presence of increased IgG index or oligoclonal bands suggest MS
CSF Gram stain, cultures (bacterial, tubercular, fungal), and India ink smear	Positive in specific infectious myelitis
CSF PCR for HSV-1, HSV-2, VZV, CMV, EBV	Positive in specific viral infection
CSF VDRL	Positive CSF VDRL is 100% specific for syphilis, but a negative result does not exclude the diagnosis
CSF cytology	Positive in malignancy
CSF myelin basic protein level	Elevated in acute disseminated encephalomyelitis

Neurological dysfunction consistent with spinal cord lesion
↓
Contrast MRI of whole spinal cord
↓
Compression | Non-compression

Compression:
Degenerative spine
Trauma
Tumour
Infection (abscess)

Non-compression:
Lumbar puncture to determine any evidence of spinal cord inflammation
MRI head
Evoked potential studies
↓
Site of demyelination
↓

Brain, optic tract and spinal cord
Multiple sclerosis
Acute disseminated encephalomyelitis

Spinal cord
Transverse myelitis

Optic tract and spinal cord
Neuromyelitis optica

Figure 141.1 (a) MRI T2 sagittal image showing diffuse high-T2 signal and expansion of the cord centrally with enhancement post contrast which is suggestive of myelitis; (b) MRI T1 fat saturation post contrast imaging of the same patient

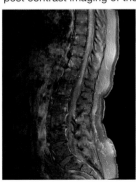
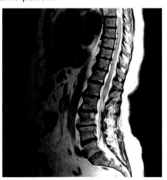

Key points

- The history, neurological examination, CSF analysis and MRI are useful in the diagnosis and classification of non-compressive spinal cord disorders.
- If a patient is suspected of a spinal cord lesion or compression, MRI is the investigation of choice.
- Contrast media can help to differentiate ischaemic spinal cord disorders from inflammatory, tumour or infectious causes.

Spinal cord disorders can have devastating consequences, ranging from quadriplegia and paraplegia to severe sensory deficits. Myelopathy is a broad term that refers to spinal cord disorders of multiple aetiologies. Spinal cord disorders are critical neurological emergencies, as prognosis depends on an early and accurate diagnosis. Therefore, the early recognition of signs and symptoms of spinal cord disorders and prompt investigation, especially with MRI, are paramount. The common causes of myelopathy can be grouped into compressive and non-compressive (Table 141.1). About 40% of acute non-compressive myelopathies are secondary to multiple sclerosis (MS), 16% are due to a systemic disease, 14% to a spinal cord infarct, 6% to an infectious disease, 4% are secondary to radiation, and the remainder are idiopathic.

Spinal cord syndromes are classified as follows.
- Complete spinal cord: involvement of all the tracts (trauma, compression or acute transverse myelitis).
- Brown-Séquard or hemi-spinal cord syndrome: ipsilateral corticospinal tract, posterior columns and contralateral spinothalamic tract (MS and compression).
- Anterior spinal cord syndrome: anterior horns, corticospinal, spinothalamic and autonomic tracts (anterior spinal artery infarct and MS).
- Posterior spinal cord syndrome: posterior columns (vitamin B_{12} or copper deficiency).
- Central syndrome: spinothalamic crossing, corticospinal and autonomic tracts (syringomyelia, neuromyelitis optica).
- Medullary cone: sacral emerging fibres (post-viral myelitis).
- Cauda equina: cauda equina nerves (acute cytomegalovirus infection, polyradiculits and compression).

The imaging strategy in patients with suspected myelopathy depends on the clinical setting. In patients without a history of trauma, MRI is the first-choice investigation. In cases following trauma, investigations include plain X-ray, CT and MRI (see Chapter 46).

Radiographic investigation

Plain X-ray

Cervical spine X-ray is the first radiological investigation in patients following spinal trauma with neurological signs in order to delineate fractures and/or dislocation (see Chapter 46).

MRI of the spine

If a patient is suspected of a spinal cord lesion or compression, MRI is the investigation of choice. MRI is useful for the following reasons:
- to identify intrinsic cord lesions such as tumour, demyelination or syrinx;
- to localise the lesion affecting the spinal cord and determine its nature;
- to demonstrate bony disease which has not yet compressed the cord;
- to demonstrate leptomeningeal disease, for example inflammatory, infective or neoplastic disease.

Once compression is excluded as the cause of myelopathy, an inflammatory cause such as transverse myelitis should be considered. The diagnosis of an inflammatory myelopathy requires evidence of spinal cord inflammation, which can be confirmed by MRI and CSF analysis. MRI with gadolinium will show increased T2-weighted signal within the spinal cord, usually with gadolinium enhancement of the lesion (Figure 141.1). If a disseminated demyelinating process is suspected, MRI of the brain should be undertaken.

In some cases of acute myelopathy, the image on MRI is normal. There are several explanations for this.
- The syndrome is not a myelopathy (Guillain–Barré syndrome, inflammatory radiculopathy).
- The picture may not be acute but rather a decompensated existing myelopathy (Friedreich's ataxia, motor neuron disease, vitamin B_{12} deficiency, HIV myelopathy).

Lumbar puncture and CSF fluid analysis

If inflammatory, MS, rupture of a vascular malformation or infective myelitis is suspected. Lumbar puncture and CSF fluid analysis should be performed (Table 141.2).

Other investigations

Depending on the clinical scenario, additional investigations are for evaluating systemic conditions such as vitamin B_{12} deficiency, infections, vasculitis, sarcoidosis, systemic lupus erythematosus and malignancies. Electromyography (EMG) may show decreased spinal cord conduction and can be used to monitor changes in cord function and determine the prognosis. Urodynamic studies may be required for proper assessment of sphincter dysfunction.

142 Peripheral neuropathy

Box 142.1 Common causes of peripheral neuropathy

- Autoimmunity: inflammatory demyelinating polyradiculoneuropathies
- Vasculitis: connective tissue diseases
- Systemic illness: diabetes, uraemia, sarcoidosis, myxoedema, acromegaly
- Cancer: paraneoplastic neuropathy
- Infections: diphtheria, leprosy, Lyme disease, AIDS, herpes zoster
- Dysproteinaemia: myeloma, cryoglobulinaemia
- Nutritional deficiencies and alcoholism
- Compression and trauma
- Toxic industrial agents and drugs
- Inherited neuropathies

Key points

- Electrodiagnostic studies are recommended if the diagnosis remains unclear after initial history and physical examination.
- If GBS suspected, patients should be admitted to a hospital for electrodiagnostic testing, CSF analysis, and monitoring of forced vital capacity (FVC) every 8 hours. Normal initial electrodiagnostic studies do not exclude the diagnosis and should not delay treatment.
- If clinical findings and electrodiagnostic test results are inconclusive, a biopsy may be required (nerve biopsy for suspected large-fibre neuropathy or skin punch biopsy for suspected small-fibre neuropathy).
- Genetic testing is indicated if a hereditary neuropathy is suspected.

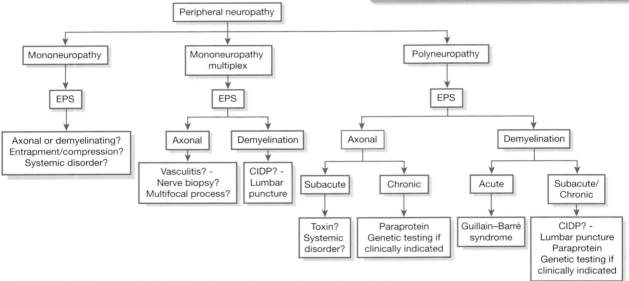

Table 142.1 Nerve conduction findings in axonal degeneration or demyelination

	Axonal degeneration	Demyelination
Sensory or motor amplitudes	Small or absent	Normal or slightly reduced
Distal latencies	Normal	Prolonged
Conduction velocities	Normal or slightly reduced	Significantly reduced
F wave latencies	Normal or slightly prolonged	Significantly prolonged or absent
H reflex latencies	Normal or slightly prolonged	Significantly prolonged or absent
Conduction block/temporal dispersion	Not present	Present

Peripheral neuropathy refers to any disorder of the peripheral nervous system including the cranial nerves, the spinal nerve roots, the dorsal root ganglia, the peripheral nerve trunks and their terminal branches, and the peripheral autonomic nervous system. The mechanisms of peripheral neuropathy include axonal degeneration, demyelination and vascular nerve damage.

Classification of neuropathy into the subtypes of mononeuropathy, mononeuropathy multiplex or polyneuropathy is helpful in guiding further investigations. The term 'mononeuropathy' implies a focal lesion of a single peripheral nerve. Mononeuropathy multiplex describes the involvement of multiple separate non-contiguous peripheral nerves either simultaneously or serially.

The common causes of mononeuropathy are trauma, focal compression, and entrapment. The most common mononeuropathy is carpal tunnel syndrome caused by entrapment of the median nerve in the carpal tunnel. In the developed world, the most common cause of peripheral polyneuropathy is diabetes mellitus. In global terms, leprosy remains an important cause of neuropathy. Other common causes of peripheral neuropathy include alcohol, nutrition, Guillain–Barré syndrome (GBS), hereditary, toxins and drugs, vasculitis, amyloid, paraneoplastic and infection (Box 142.1).

Clinical investigation

There are four steps in the investigation of peripheral neuropathy: (i) determining the presence of a peripheral neuropathy; (ii) confirming the type of peripheral neuropathy; (iii) confirming the pattern of peripheral neuropathy; and (iv) investigating the underlying cause of the peripheral neuropathy.

Is this a peripheral neuropathy?

This is usually answered by a careful history and neurological examination. Presenting features of peripheral neuropathy include combinations of altered sensation, pain, muscle weakness or atrophy, and autonomic symptoms. The earliest symptoms are usually sensory abnormalities such as numbness or burning in the toes or feet.

Confirm the type of peripheral neuropathy

The most important step in investigating peripheral neuropathy is to determine the type (demyelinating vs. axonal vs. mixed type), the duration and the course of the neuropathy. Electrodiagnostic tests include nerve conduction study (NCS) and needle electromyography (EMG) examination and are essential in determining whether the primary pathophysiology is demyelinating or axonal (Figure 142.1).

Sensory, motor or mixed nerves can be studied in an NCS. Pairs of electrodes are used: one to initiate the impulse and the other to record the response further along the path (distally within the innervated muscle for motor nerves or proximally along sensory nerves). The parameters obtained include the following.
- Amplitude: from baseline to peak, reflecting the number of conducting fibres; reduced in axonal loss.
- Latency (ms): from stimulus to onset of evoked response.
- Duration of response (ms).
- Conduction velocity (m/s): reflects integrity of the myelin sheath and is reduced in demyelinating processes.

The key differences in NCS results between axonal loss and demyelination are summarised in Table 142.1. The most common abnormality with axonal loss is reduction in compound amplitude, reflecting fewer functional axons. In demyelination, reduction in conduction velocities and temporal dispersion (increase in duration) are typical.

One of the limitations of NCS is that it mainly tests large myelinated fibres corresponding to modalities of fine touch, vibration and proprioception. Small-fibre neuropathies may have normal sensory studies and early disease changes can be subtle and overlooked.

EMG can detect active axonal damage, as evidenced by the presence of spontaneous muscle fibre activity at rest resulting from denervation. EMG is also used to diagnose myopathies, to distinguish between radiculopathy and peripheral nerve lesions, to localise the level of peripheral nerve or root lesions, and to detect widespread denervation in motor neuron disease.

Confirm the pattern of peripheral neuropathy

Mononeuropathy
The electrodiagnostic tests can localise the site of injury and determine the severity of the lesion. Focal mononeuropathy, especially carpal tunnel syndrome and ulnar neuropathy at the elbow, can be associated with more generalised metabolic or toxic neuropathies such as diabetic polyneuropathy.

Mononeuropathy multiplex
Electrodiagnostic studies can confirm mononeuropathy multiplex. Assessment of patients with mononeuropathy multiplex is important because serious underlying disorders such as vasculitis or other systemic diseases (e.g. sarcoidosis, lymphoma, amyloidosis, leprosy, HIV infection) may be responsible. Up to one-third of patients with the picture of mononeuropathy multiplex have electrodiagnostic findings of multifocal demyelination, usually secondary to chronic inflammatory demyelinating polyneuropathy (CIDP) or a variant such as multifocal motor neuropathy.

Acute polyneuropathy
Acute symmetrical polyneuropathy presenting as rapidly progressive paralysis with areflexia and variable sensory involvement is usually one of the variants of GBS. The recognition of this pattern is important since it can progress rapidly to respiratory failure (25% of cases).

Chronic polyneuropathy
This is the most common type of polyneuropathy and usually evolves over months or years. The focus of the investigation is to determine whether the neuropathy is primarily demyelinating or primarily axonal by electrodiagnostic studies. This distinction provides a branch point in evaluating polyneuropathy since each subtype (demyelinating vs. axonal) has different causes, treatments and prognosis.

Chronic demyelinating polyneuropathy
Chronic demyelinating polyneuropathies can be genetic or acquired (Table 142.2). Electrodiagnostic features are helpful because uniform symmetrical slowing of nerve conduction usually indicates a genetically determined neuropathy, whereas multifocal slowing and conduction block are indicative of acquired demyelinating neuropathies. Most genetically determined demyelinating polyneuropathies are variants of Charcot–Marie–Tooth (CMT) disease, and 70–80% of patients have a duplication of the *PMP22* gene.

Box 142.2 Basic laboratory tests in investigating peripheral neuropathy

- FBC, CRP, vitamin B_{12}, folate
- Comprehensive biochemistry panel, fasting blood glucose, renal and liver function, thyroid function
- Serum protein electrophoresis with immunofixation, serum light chains
- Glycosylated haemoglobin or glucose tolerance test
- Urinalysis, urine protein, urine Bence Jones protein and light chains

Table 142.2 Common causes of chronic demyelinating polyneuropathy

Genetic
Charcot–Marie–Tooth disease types 1, 4 and X1
Hereditary liability to pressure palsies
Metachromatic leukodystrophy
Globoid cell leukodystrophy
Refsum disease

Acquired
Chronic inflammatory demyelinating polyradiculoneuropathy
Multifocal motor neuropathy
Paraproteinaemic demyelinating polyneuropathy
Associated with antibodies to myelin-associated glycoprotein (MAG)
Associated with monoclonal gammopathy of unknown significance or myeloma

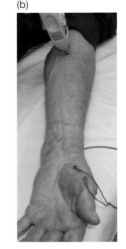

Figure 142.1 (a) Nerve conduction test equipment; (b) nerve conduction test; (c) nerve conduction test report

The acquired demyelinating neuropathies represent a heterogeneous group of mostly immunologically mediated neuropathies. Electrodiagnostic tests can refine the classification by determining the pattern of demyelination and the spectrum of fibre involvement. CIDP is the most common type, with either a relapsing or gradually progressive course. In CIDP, CSF examination can be helpful in confirming the diagnosis since the protein in the CSF is almost always raised.

Chronic axonal polyneuropathy

The commonest cause is diabetes mellitus. However, other causes include a range of systemic diseases and metabolic disorders, such as nutritional deficiencies, CKD, malignancy and alcohol abuse. Several varieties of hereditary neuropathy, especially the axonal forms of CMT2 disease, can present with this pattern of neuropathy. Even after thorough evaluation of chronic polyneuropathy, no cause is found in 25% of patients.

Investigate the underlying cause of peripheral neuropathy

All patients with peripheral neuropathy should have the following basic laboratory tests (Box 142.2).

Tests for infectious causes

Since infection with *Campylobacter jejuni* or cytomegalovirus might precede GBS, antibody testing for these agents is useful in supporting the diagnosis of GBS. Hepatitis B and C virus, HIV, Lyme disease and syphilis serology tests should be carried out if there is clinical suspicion.

Tests for suspected connective tissue diseases and vasculitis

Tests for ANA, RF, anti-Ro, anti-La, ANCA, serum angiotensin-converting enzyme (ACE) and cryoglobulins should be performed. Tests for anti-myelin associated glycoprotein (MAG) antibodies and anti-ganglioside antibody profile (GM1, GD1a, GD1b, GD3, GQ1b, GT1b) may help in the investigation of other immune-mediated neuropathies.

Tests for malignant causes (cancer, myeloma, lymphoma)

Skeletal radiographic survey, mammography, ultrasound of abdomen and pelvis, and CT of chest, abdomen and pelvis should be performed. CSF analysis for cytology can be considered. Serum antibodies to anti-nerve and anti-ganglioside antigens may be found in paraneoplastic and other immune-mediated neuropathies. Commercially available tests for anti-Hu (ANNA-1), anti-Ri (ANNA-2), anti-CV2/CRMP5 and anti-Yo (PCA-1) antibodies are used to investigate paraneoplastic neuropathies.

Genetic tests

Molecular genetic tests are available for an increasing number of hereditary neuropathies, such as CMT disease, hereditary neuropathy with liability to pressure palsies, and hereditary amyloidosis.

CSF tests

If there is suspicion of an infectious, immune-mediated or neoplastic cause of neuropathy, CSF should be analysed. Neurotropic infectious agents and malignant diseases often cause CSF pleocytosis. Immune-mediated neuropathies such as GBS and CIDP usually show an increased protein level with a normal cell count in the CSF (i.e. albuminocytological dissociation).

Tests for toxins and heavy metals

Although analysis of blood and urine for heavy metals is often performed in patients with neuropathies, the yield is very low unless there is strong suspicion of heavy metal exposure. In idiopathic chronic polyneuropathies, a 24-hour urine collection for heavy metals is almost always unproductive. A particular caution applies to finding elevated total levels of arsenic in urine collections since this can occur after eating certain seafood. Arsenic found in seafood is in the form of arsenobetaine, which has low toxicity and is not associated with neuropathy. If, in a particular chronic axonal polyneuropathy, heavy metal intoxication is suspected, analysis of hair or nail samples is indicated. In patients with suspected porphyria, blood, urine and stool porphyrins should be tested.

Nerve biopsy

Nerve biopsy is most useful in investigation of inflammatory disorders such as vasculitis, sarcoidosis and CIDP, infectious diseases such as leprosy, and infiltrative disorders such as amyloidosis or tumour and is valuable in mononeuropathy multiplex. The procedure is best reserved for patients in whom the diagnosis cannot be obtained by other means or in rapidly progressive and asymmetric polyneuropathies. For the rare cases of storage disease (e.g. Fabry disease) or other unusual hereditary neuropathies (e.g. giant axonal neuropathy) nerve biopsy can confirm the diagnosis. Most common hereditary neuropathies, especially the variants of CMT disease, can be confirmed by a combination of electrodiagnostic tests and molecular genetic testing.

The usual site of nerve biopsy is the sural nerve. In suspected vasculitis the diagnostic yield is higher if muscle is also examined, and some recommend combined nerve and muscle biopsy. This can be achieved through a single incision for the superficial peroneal sensory nerve and peroneus brevis muscle or for the sural nerve and gastrocnemius muscle.

143 Movement disorders

Table 143.1 Classification of common causes of tremor

Postural tremor
Physiological tremor
Essential tremor
Tremor with basal ganglia disease
Dystonia
Wilson's disease
Cerebellar postural tremor
Tremor with peripheral neuropathy
Hereditary peripheral neuropathy
Acquired neuropathy
Post-traumatic tremor
Alcoholic tremor
Resting tremor
Parkinson's disease
Kinetic tremor
Cerebellar intention tremor
Task-specific tremor
Primary writing tremor
Vocal tremor
Orthostatic tremor
Drug and metabolic induced tremor
Psychogenic tremor

Table 143.2 Other Parkinson-plus syndromes

Multisystem atrophy
Progressive supranuclear palsy
Corticobasal degeneration
Vascular Parkinsonism
Lewy body dementia

Table 143.3 Investigations in common movement disorders

Condition	Investigations
Essential tremor	Clinical diagnosis
Drug-induced tremor	Clinical diagnosis
Enhanced physiological tremor	TFTs, LFTs, creatinine, glucose, blood alcohol
Parkinson's disease	Clinical diagnosis, PET or SPECT for atypical presentation
Atypical Parkinsonism, or Parkinson-plus syndromes	MRI or CT head
Wilson's disease	Serum caeruloplasmin and copper levels, LFTs, 24-hour urine copper excretion, and liver biopsy if necessary
Huntington's disease	Genetic testing (CAG repeat number for each allele)
Tic disorders	Clinical diagnosis
Dystonias	None for typical adult-onset primary focal dystonia. Genetic testing for the DYT1 mutation in patient <30 years old. MRI of the brain for suspected secondary dystonia
Psychogenic tremor	Clinical diagnosis

Key points

- The diagnosis of most movement disorders is based on history and physical examination.
- Many peripheral neuropathies are associated with tremors, which are predominantly postural and kinetic.
- There is no consistently reliable test that can distinguish Parkinson's disease from other conditions that have similar clinical presentations. The diagnosis is primarily clinical.
- For particularly difficult cases, SPECT to visualise the integrity of the dopaminergic pathways may be useful for diagnosing Parkinson's disease.
- Structural MRI may be considered for the differential diagnosis of Parkinsonian syndromes.

Movement disorders are neurological motor disorders that can be divided into hyperkinetic disorders, characterised by excessive and abnormal involuntary movements, and hypokinetic disorders, manifested by paucity or slowness (bradykinesia) of movement.

Movement disorders can be primary (idiopathic or genetic disease) or secondary to a wide range of neurological or systemic diseases. Cerebrovascular disease causes about 20–25% of secondary movement disorders. When investigating movement disorders, the first step is to define the movement disorder class based on the clinical features and video documentation is very useful.

The investigation of movement disorders depends on the clinical presentation; if features are typical of a primary movement disorder, such as essential tremor, further investigation is unnecessary.

Investigation of tremor

Tremor is an involuntary movement characterised by rhythmic oscillations of one or more parts of the body. Tremor is the most common movement disorder and a useful classification scheme is shown in Table 143.1. The diagnosis of tremor is clinical but can be supported and further characterised by electrophysiological studies using surface electromyography (EMG) and accelerometers if needed.

If the family history and examination findings are indicative of essential tremor, no laboratory or imaging studies are required; however, if there are atypical features, the following investigations should be considered.

Laboratory investigations
- Serum electrolytes panel, liver and thyroid function tests.
- Serum caeruloplasmin for suspected Wilson's disease.
- Vitamin B_{12}, serum and red cell folate levels for suspected Lewy body dementia.

Imaging of the head
Findings on CT and MRI of the head are usually normal in essential tremor. MRI helps to exclude structural and inflammatory lesions (including multiple sclerosis) and Wilson's disease. Therefore MRI should be performed if the tremor has an acute onset or a stepwise progression.

Although the classic resting tremor of Parkinson's disease is different in many aspects from that of essential tremor, it can be difficult to distinguish variants. Single-photon emission CT (SPECT) using ioflupane (^{123}I) can be used to support a diagnosis of Parkinsonism, so decreasing the misdiagnosis of essential tremor as Parkinson's disease. SPECT can visualise the integrity of the dopaminergic pathways in the brain.

Investigation for Parkinsonism

Parkinson's disease is a clinical diagnosis. No laboratory biomarkers exist, and findings on MRI and CT of the head are unremarkable. However, patients with atypical features (e.g. atypical course, dementia, significant imbalance in early disease, autonomic dysfunction, gaze abnormalities, or atypical abnormalities on neurological examination) should be considered for MRI to exclude brain lesions such as stroke, tumour or demyelination. In patients considered for deep-brain stimulation therapy, detailed CT or MRI is performed to decide the target for electrode implantation.

PET and SPECT can detect abnormalities of the dopaminergic system that may help distinguish Parkinsonism from essential tremor. These PET and SPECT tracers typically bind to the dopamine transporter or vesicular monoamine transporter.

Atypical Parkinsonism, or Parkinson-plus syndromes, are neurodegenerative disorders that have Parkinsonian features (Table 143.2). Investigations in such patients may include serum caeruloplasmin for Wilson's disease or sphincter EMG for multisystem atrophy.

Investigation for Huntington's disease

Huntington's disease (HD) is a progressive, adult-onset, autosomal dominant inherited disorder associated with cell loss within a specific subset of neurons in the basal ganglia and cortex. Characteristic features include involuntary movements, dementia and behavioural changes.

Genetic testing for HD is commercially available, with results being reported as the CAG repeat number for each allele of the *HTT* (or Huntingtin) gene. Genetic testing may not be necessary in a patient with a typical clinical picture and a genetically proven family history of HD. In the absence of a family history of HD, patients with a suggestive clinical presentation should undergo genetic testing. If the genetic test is negative for HD, then tests for systemic lupus erythematosus, antiphospholipid antibody syndrome, thyroid disease, syphilis, Wilson's disease and other less common causes of chorea should be carried out. No single imaging technique is accurate for diagnosis of HD. Measurement of the bicaudate diameter (the distance between the heads of the two caudate nuclei) by CT or MRI is a reasonable marker of HD.

The diagnosis of HD has significant impact on a patient's life, employment, insurance and family. Therefore, informed consent should be obtained before testing. This may include informing patients of the potential insurance and familial implications of a diagnosis. Genetic testing can be deferred until a time of the patient's choosing and this may help them decide how they wish to manage ongoing life, financial and work issues. Persons at risk of HD who request presymptomatic testing should undergo extensive genetic counselling and neurological and psychiatric evaluation, given the implications of receiving a positive (or negative) result for an untreatable, familial and progressive neurodegenerative disease.

Investigation for Wilson's disease

It is important to exclude Wilson's disease while investigating movement disorders. The investigation should include slit-lamp examination for Kayser–Fleischer rings, serum ceruloplasmin and copper levels, liver function tests, 24-hour urine copper excretion, and liver biopsy if necessary (Table 143.3).

144 Septic and crystal arthropathies

The goal of investigation in septic arthritis is to confirm the diagnosis by:
- Isolation of a pathogenic organism from an affected joint, *or*
- Isolation of a pathogenic organism from another source (e.g. blood) in the context of a hot, red joint suspicious of sepsis, *or*
- Typical clinical features and culture-negative turbid joint fluid in the presence of previous antibiotic treatment

Table 144.1 Summary of the characteristics of synovial fluid in different arthritis

	Appearance	WBC count (×10⁹/L)	Crystals	Culture
Septic arthritis	Turbid	50–200 neutrophils	Nil	Positive
Gout	Clear, low viscosity	0.5–200 neutrophils	Needle-shaped and negatively birefringent	Negative
Pseudogout	Clear, low viscosity	0.5–10 neutrophils	Block-shaped and positively birefringent	Negative
Inflammatory arthritis	Turbid, yellowish -green	2–100 neutrophils	Nil	Negative
Osteoarthritis	Clear, large volume	0–2 mononuclear	Nil	Negative

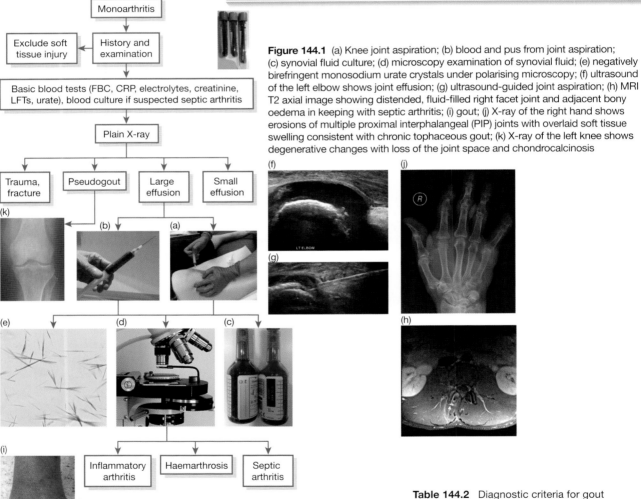

Figure 144.1 (a) Knee joint aspiration; (b) blood and pus from joint aspiration; (c) synovial fluid culture; (d) microscopy examination of synovial fluid; (e) negatively birefringent monosodium urate crystals under polarising microscopy; (f) ultrasound of the left elbow shows joint effusion; (g) ultrasound-guided joint aspiration; (h) MRI T2 axial image showing distended, fluid-filled right facet joint and adjacent bony oedema in keeping with septic arthritis; (i) gout; (j) X-ray of the right hand shows erosions of multiple proximal interphalangeal (PIP) joints with overlaid soft tissue swelling consistent with chronic tophaceous gout; (k) X-ray of the left knee shows degenerative changes with loss of the joint space and chondrocalcinosis

Key points
- Arthrocentesis is required in most patients with monoarthritis and is mandatory if infection is suspected.
- When an infection is suspected, synovial fluid should be sent for WBC count with differential, crystal analysis, Gram stain, and culture. Synovial fluid tests for lipid panels, rheumatoid factor or uric acid are not useful.
- Light microscopy may be useful to identify gout crystals, but polarised microscopy is preferred.

Table 144.2 Diagnostic criteria for gout (American College of Rheumatology)

More than one attack of acute arthritis
Maximum inflammation developed within 1 day
Monoarthritis attack, redness observed over joints
First metatarsophalangeal joint painful or swollen
Unilateral first metatarsophalangeal joint attack
Unilateral tarsal joint attack
Tophus (confirmed or suspected)
Hyperuricaemia
Asymmetric swelling within a joint on X-ray film
Subcortical cyst without erosions on X-ray film
Joint culture negative for organism during attack

Clinical Investigations at a Glance, First Edition. Jonathan Gleadle, Jordan Li and Tuck Yong. © 2017 John Wiley & Sons, Ltd. Published 2017 by John Wiley & Sons, Ltd.

The presentation of a patient with an acute, hot and swollen joint is a common and important medical presentation. The two commonest causes are septic arthritis and crystal arthropathy. The most serious cause is septic arthritis and delayed investigation and treatment can lead to irreversible joint destruction. All acute cases of monoarthritis should be considered septic arthritis until proven otherwise. The diagnosis of septic or crystal arthritis depends on the integration of history, examination and the results of laboratory investigations showing evidence of acute inflammation; however, investigations to detect bacteria and/or crystals in synovial fluid are essential.

Septic arthritis

The most frequent causative organisms are *Staphylococcus aureus* followed by streptococci. The frequency of Gram-negative organisms is increased in the elderly. In young adults, gonococcal infection is an important cause of septic arthritis.

Basic laboratory investigations

FBC, measurement of CRP, urate, serum electrolytes, and renal and liver function tests should be performed. However, blood tests alone cannot confirm a diagnosis in monoarthritis. CRP and WBC count are usually raised in septic or crystal arthropathy but normal values for these variables at presentation do not exclude septic or crystal arthropathy. WBC count and CRP level might not distinguish septic arthritis from other forms of acute arthritis. Rheumatoid factor (RF) and other autoantibodies should be measured if inflammatory arthritis is suspected.

Blood culture

Blood culture should always be performed in patients with suspected septic arthritis before starting antibiotic treatment to increase the chances of obtaining causative organisms. Blood cultures are positive in about 25% of cases where organisms are identified in the synovial fluid; in a further 9% of patients, blood cultures are the only source of a positive microbiological diagnosis.

Synovial fluid aspiration

In all cases of suspected native joint sepsis or assessment of a hot swollen joint, the joint should be aspirated (Figures 144.1a,b) and sent for immediate Gram stain and culture (Figure 144.1c). Gram staining of synovial fluid can identify the causative organism in 50% of cases and this rises to 67% after culture. For suspected sepsis of a prosthetic joint, it should always be aspirated with full aseptic precautions in an operating theatre. Neither overlying cellulitis nor anticoagulation is an absolute contraindication to native joint aspiration. The absence of organisms on Gram stain, or a subsequently negative synovial fluid culture, does not exclude the diagnosis, although it does make it less likely.

To diagnose crystal arthritis, samples of synovial fluid should be examined by polarising-light microscopy (Figures 144.1d,e). Samples should be processed immediately or stored at room temperature before analysis because artificial crystals can form on refrigeration. Quantification of the synovial WBC count may be helpful in distinguishing between crystal and septic arthritis; a WBC count in excess of 50×10^9/L is suggestive of septic arthritis (Table 144.1).

Radiological investigations

Plain X-ray of the joint should be done as a baseline investigation. It may not help the diagnosis but can reveal underlying joint disease. Ultrasound may show the presence of an effusion to guide aspiration (Figures 144.1f,g). Plain X-ray, technetium bone scans, CT and MRI can be used to assess the presence and extent of inflammation, destruction and tissue response; they cannot accurately distinguish between infective and other causes of acute inflammatory arthritis. However, MRI can assess both coexistent osteomyelitis and deep joints (such as the hip or facet joint; Figure 144.1h) in patients with septicaemia with localised musculoskeletal pain. Furthermore, MRI will also indicate any tracking of purulent material into surrounding soft tissues from a primary joint infection.

Infection associated with prosthetic joints

Infection of prosthetic joints occurs in 0.8–1.9% of knee replacements and 0.3–1.7% of hip replacements. Staphylococci (*S. aureus* and coagulase-negative *Staphylococcus* species) account for over half of prosthetic joint infections. Identification of the involved organisms and their antimicrobial susceptibility is important to guide antimicrobial therapy. In patients with suspected prosthetic joint infection, the following tests should be performed

CRP

In the absence of coexisting inflammatory conditions, CRP is a useful test for detecting prosthetic joint infection. Raised CRP (>10 mg/L) has a sensitivity of 73–91% and a specificity of 62–80% for the diagnosis of prosthetic-knee or prosthetic-hip infection. A normal CRP generally indicates the absence of prosthetic joint infection but false negatives may occur in patients who have been treated with antibiotics or who have an infection caused by a low-virulence organism such as *Propionibacterium acnes*.

Radiological investigations

Plain X-ray has low sensitivity and specificity for detecting prosthetic joint infection. CT and MRI are hampered by artefacts produced by prostheses. Bone scans are non-specific for detecting infection and these scans will be abnormal for more than 12 months after implantation. PET scan has a sensitivity of 82% and a specificity of 87% for the detection of prosthetic-knee or prosthetic-hip infection but is not widely available.

Synovial fluid aspiration

When there is uncertainty about the diagnosis, the most useful preoperative test is aseptic aspiration of joint synovial fluid for culture. However, aspiration should not be performed through overlying cellulitis. Synovial fluid culture has a sensitivity of 56–75% and a specificity of 95–100%. To achieve optimal sensitivity and specificity, the fluid should be inoculated into a blood culture bottle. If an organism of questionable clinical significance is isolated, repeat synovial fluid aspiration should be considered.

Intraoperative microbiological testing

Specimens should be collected for microbiology at the time of surgery. Antimicrobial therapy should be discontinued at least 2 weeks before surgery if possible and perioperative antimicrobial coverage should be deferred until culture specimens have been collected. Cultures of sinus tract exudates should be avoided; these are often positive because of microbial skin colonisation and correlate poorly with cultures of surgical specimens. Multiple specimens should be collected from periprosthetic tissue for aerobic and anaerobic bacterial culture because of the poor sensitivity of a single culture and to distinguish contaminants from pathogens. A sample should be obtained from the surface of the prosthesis if it is removed as microorganisms form a biofilm on the prosthesis surface.

Gout

Gout is an inflammatory arthritis caused by the deposition of monosodium urate crystals in synovial fluid and other tissues. It is often associated with hyperuricaemia. Gout has two clinical phases. The first is characterised by intermittent acute attacks with asymptomatic periods between attacks. The second phase is chronic tophaceous gout, which often involves polyarticular attacks, symptoms between attacks and crystal deposition (tophi) in soft tissues or joints. The diagnostic investigations include the following.

Arthrocentesis

The gold standard for diagnosing gout remains synovial fluid or tophus aspiration with identification of negatively birefringent monosodium urate crystals under polarising microscopy (Figures 144.1e,i). The joint aspiration will also help to exclude septic arthritis or other crystal-induced arthropathies. Joint aspiration with Gram stain and culture must be performed routinely even if monosodium urate crystals are identified because gout and septic arthritis can coexist.

Urate levels and basic laboratory investigations

Urate should be measured 2 weeks after the attack as hyperuricaemia may not be present during acute gout attacks. Gout can develop with normal levels of urate.

FBC, renal function, liver function and urinary uric acid (to determine over- or under-excretion of urinary uric acid relative to serum urate levels) should be performed to determine the contributing factors to hyperuricaemia.

Plain X-ray of the joints

This has no role in the investigation of an acute attack of gout. In chronic gout, X-rays may show erosions, overlaid by soft tissue swelling and often containing secondary calcific deposits (Figure 144.1j).

Clinical diagnosis

Alternatively, diagnosis of gout can be made based on fulfilment of six or more of the criteria from the American College of Rheumatology (Table 144.2) without arthrocentesis.

Pseudogout

Pseudogout, known as calcium pyrophosphate deposition disease (CPPD), occurs almost exclusively in articular tissues, most commonly fibrocartilage and hyaline cartilage, and is the most common cause of chondrocalcinosis. CPPD is the third most common inflammatory arthritis. The affected joints are more likely to be the knee, wrist or shoulder. Attacks are commonly precipitated by surgery, medical illnesses and trauma. CPPD is associated with a large number of diseases such as osteoarthritis, previous joint trauma/injury, and metabolic disease. About 20% of patients with hyperparathyroidism have CPPD, while 40–45% of patients with haemochromatosis have this condition.

Arthrocentesis can confirm the diagnosis by revealing intracellular or extracellular birefringent rhomboid-shaped crystals under polarised light.

Laboratory investigations

Serum electrolytes including calcium and magnesium levels, which can be normal or decreased, should be checked. Parathyroid hormone and iron studies are useful to exclude hyperparathyroidism or haemochromatosis as the underlying cause of CPPD.

Plain X-ray

One of the main features of CPPD is chondrocalcinosis, the calcification of hyaline cartilage that produces a fine line parallel to the joint surface (Figure 144.1k). Chondrocalcinosis is most likely to be seen in the knee, symphysis pubis and wrist.

145 Osteoarthritis

The purpose of investigations is to:
- Establish the diagnosis by excluding other causes of joint pain such as septic arthritis or crystal arthropathy
- Identify any associated injuries to cartilage or meniscus
- Assist in the planning of surgical interventions in applicable situations

Key points
- Confirm the diagnosis of osteoarthritis with X-ray findings such as:
  - marginal osteophytes
  - narrowing of the joint space
  - increased density of the subchondral bone
  - sometimes subchondral cyst formation and joint effusion.
- Laboratory studies are normal in osteoarthritis but may be required to rule out other disorders such as rheumatoid arthritis or to diagnose an underlying disorder causing secondary osteoarthritis.
- If osteoarthritis causes joint effusions, synovial fluid analysis can help differentiate it from inflammatory arthritides; in osteoarthritis, synovial fluid is usually clear and viscous and has a WBC count of 2×10^9/L or less.
- Conditions associated with osteoarthritis, haemochromatosis and acromegaly, may warrant additional investigations.

Figure 145.1 X-ray of the right hip shows severe osteoarthritis with joint space loss, marginal osteophytes, subchondral sclerosis and cyst formation

Figure 145.2 MRI of the left knee shows central radial tear of the posterior horn and posterior body of the medial meniscus

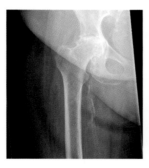

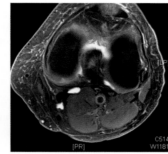

Osteoarthritis is a degenerative joint disorder that involves the entire joint, including the articular cartilage, subchondral bone, capsule and synovium. The condition leads to loss of cartilage, sclerosis and eburnation of the subchondral bone, osteophytes and subchondral cysts. Osteoarthritis is the most common joint disorder and is the leading cause of disability in older adults. There is a pronounced female preponderance for severe grades of osteoarthritis as well as osteoarthritis of the hand and knee. Joints commonly affected by osteoarthritis include the spine, hip, knee, hands and feet.

Risk factors for primary osteoarthritis include old age, high bone mass, genetic predisposition, obesity, joint injury, developmental deformities, participation in weight-bearing sports and occupations requiring prolonged standing or lifting of heavy objects. Systemic causes of osteoarthritis include haemochromatosis, osteonecrosis and rheumatoid or septic arthritis, hyperparathyroidism, hypothyroidism, acromegaly, Paget's disease, gout and chondrocalcinosis.

The main clinical features of osteoarthritis are pain, deformity, instability and restricted movement, as well as functional impairment.

Radiological investigations

Plain X-ray of affected joints

Typical X-ray findings of osteoarthritis include loss of joint space, osteophyte formation, subchondral sclerosis and cysts (Figure 145.1). However, the radiological findings correlate poorly with the severity of pain and a normal X-ray does not exclude osteoarthritis.

Ultrasound

Currently, ultrasonography has no role in the routine clinical assessment of the patient with osteoarthritis. However, it is being investigated as a tool for monitoring cartilage degeneration, and it can be used to guide injections of joints.

CT

CT is rarely used in the diagnosis of primary osteoarthritis but may be used in the diagnosis of malalignment of the patellofemoral joint or of the foot and ankle joints.

MRI

MRI is not used in the investigation of osteoarthritis unless additional pathology amenable to surgical repair is suspected. Pathology that can be seen on MRI includes joint narrowing, subchondral osseous changes, and osteophytes. Unlike plain X-ray, MRI can directly visualise articular cartilage and other joint tissues such as meniscus, tendon, muscle or effusion (Figure 145.2).

Laboratory investigations

No blood tests are routinely required in the assessment of a patient with typical osteoarthritis unless there are clinical features to suggest inflammatory or septic arthritis.

CRP is typically within the reference range in patients with osteoarthritis but it may be elevated in inflammatory or septic arthritis or in gout. No single biomarker has proved reliable for diagnosis and monitoring.

Other laboratory investigations such as serum calcium concentration, parathyroid hormone, iron studies, haemochromatosis gene studies, urate, RF and anti-CCP antibody should be performed if clinically indicated.

Synovial fluid aspiration

Examination of synovial fluid is indicated if inflammatory arthritis or crystal arthropathy is suspected or if septic arthritis is a concern. A WBC count below 1×10^9/L in the synovial fluid is consistent with osteoarthritis, whereas higher WBC counts suggest inflammatory arthritis.

Clinical Investigations at a Glance, First Edition. Jonathan Gleadle, Jordan Li and Tuck Yong. © 2017 John Wiley & Sons, Ltd. Published 2017 by John Wiley & Sons, Ltd.

146 Spondyloarthropathies

Table 146.1 Techniques for imaging sacroiliac joints

	Advantages	Disadvantages
Plain X-ray	Quick and cheap	Changes are detected late
CT	Able to detect early changes. May clarify diagnosis when plain X-rays are equivocal	Higher ionising radiation exposure
MRI	Able to detect early changes	Expensive and limited accessibility
Radionuclide studies	May detect early changes	Of uncertain value in adolescent skeleton

Key points

- Plain X-ray is of little use in AS diagnosis within the first 5 years of symptoms, because it takes on average 8–10 years before radiographic changes of sacroiliitis occur.
- In patients with less than 5 years of symptoms, or where pelvic X-rays do not confirm the suspected diagnosis of AS, MRI including both the sacroiliac joints and lumbar spine is indicated.
- X-ray findings common in psoriatic arthritis include DIP joint involvement, resorption of terminal phalanges, arthritis mutilans and extensive destruction.

Table 146.2 Clinical features of different spondyloarthropathies

Features	Ankylosing spondylitis	Reactive arthritis	Psoriatic arthritis	IBD-associated spondyloarthropathy
HLA-B27	90–95%	80%	40%	30%
Sacroiliitis	Sacroiliitis	Sacroiliitis	Sacroiliitis	Sacroiliitis
Frequency	100%	40–60%	40%	20%
Distribution	Symmetric	Asymmetric	Asymmetric	Symmetric
Peripheral arthritis	Peripheral arthritis	Peripheral arthritis	Peripheral arthritis	Peripheral arthritis
Frequency	Occasional	Common	Common	Common
Distribution	Asymmetric, lower limbs	Asymmetric, lower limbs	Asymmetric, any joint	Asymmetric, lower limbs
Ethesitis	Common	Common	Common	Occasional
Dactylitis	Uncommon	Common	Common	Uncommon
Skin lesions	None	Circinate balanitis, keratoderma blenorrhagicum	Psoriasis	Erythema nodosum, pyoderma gangrenosum
Nail changes	None	Onycholysis	Pitting, onycholysis	Clubbing
Ocular complications	Acute anterior uveitis (40%)	Acute anterior uveitis, conjunctivitis	Chronic uveitis	Chronic uveitis
Oral complications	Ulcers	Ulcers	Ulcers	Ulcers
Cardiac complications	Aortic regurgitation (10%), conduction defects	Aortic regurgitation, conduction defects	Aortic regurgitation, conduction defects	Aortic regurgitation
Respiratory complications	Upper lobe fibrosis (15%)	None	None	None
Gastrointestinal complications	IBD (10%)	Diarrhoea	None	Crohn's disease, ulcerative colitis
Renal complications	Amyloidosis, IgA nephropathy	Amyloidosis	Amyloidosis	Nephrolithiasis
Genitourinary complications	Prostatitis	Urethritis, cervicitis	None	None

Figure 146.2 X-ray of the cervical spine shows marginal syndesmophytes and osteophyte formation consistent with ankylosing spondylitis

Figure 146.3 CT bony windows axial image shows bilateral sacroiliac joint sclerosis and fusion in keeping with advanced sacroiliitis

Figure 146.1 X-ray of the pelvis shows bilateral sacroiliitis

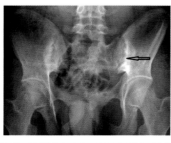

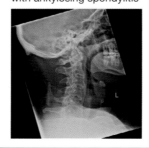

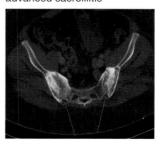

Clinical Investigations at a Glance, First Edition. Jonathan Gleadle, Jordan Li and Tuck Yong. © 2017 John Wiley & Sons, Ltd. Published 2017 by John Wiley & Sons, Ltd.

Spondyloarthropathies are inflammatory arthritides that characteristically affect the spine and entheses (insertions of tendons and ligaments) and are often associated with the HLA-B27 gene. The spondyloarthropathies include ankylosing spondylitis (AS), reactive arthritis and Reiter's syndrome, psoriatic arthritis and inflammatory bowel disease (IBD)-associated spondyloarthropathy.

Ankylosing spondylitis

AS is the commonest spondyloarthropathy. It usually presents as insidious onset of inflammatory back pain. Enthesitis is common at the Achilles tendon and plantar fascia calcaneal insertions and is typically worse with rest and improves with activity. A high index of suspicion, early investigation and diagnosis is essential in AS because it can lead to severe spinal restriction and disability; effective treatment with anti-tumour necrosis factor (TNF) therapies can improve symptoms and function and prevent structural damage.

Laboratory investigations

There is no single laboratory test for diagnosing AS.
• HLA-B27 assay: a positive HLA-B27 is non-specific for AS. Only 1–2% of HLA-B27-positive people develop AS but can be found in 90% of white AS patients. Patients with suspected AS and positive for HLA-B27 should have MRI.
• FBC may show anaemia of chronic disease.
• CRP is elevated in 50–70% of patients but correlates poorly with disease activity.
• Alkaline phosphatase (ALP) is elevated in 50% of patients; this indicates active ossification but does not correlate with disease activity.

Radiological investigations

X-ray of the spine and sacroiliac joints is the first line of imaging for identifying the features of AS, which include bilateral symmetric sacroiliitis (Figure 146.1) and ossification of the annulus fibrosus in the lumbar spine resulting in the formation of marginal syndesmophytes in a gradually ascending pattern ('bamboo spine') (Figure 146.2).

MRI or CT of the sacroiliac joints, spine and peripheral joints can reveal early sacroiliitis, erosions and enthesitis that are not apparent on plain X-ray (Figure 146.3). MRI using fat-saturating techniques such as short tau inversion recovery (STIR) or MRI with gadolinium is sensitive for inflammatory lesions of enthesitis (Table 146.1). Patients who develop bowel or bladder dysfunction should be evaluated immediately with MRI to assess for cauda equina syndrome secondary to spinal stenosis.

Extra-articular features are frequently present and should be investigated (Table 146.2). Patients suspected of pulmonary fibrosis should be investigated with CXR, pulmonary function tests and HRCT of the chest. If associated cardiac conditions are suspected, ECG and echocardiography should be performed.

Reactive arthritis and Reiter's syndrome

Reactive arthritis is an aseptic arthritis that occurs after exposure to certain gastrointestinal and genitourinary infections, particularly *Chlamydia*, *Campylobacter jejuni*, *Salmonella enteritidis*, *Shigella*, and *Yersinia* species. Reiter's syndrome is a reactive arthritis with a clinical triad of urethritis, conjunctivitis and arthritis. Reactive arthritis usually begins 1–4 weeks after a genitourinary or gastrointestinal infection. The arthritis tends to be oligoarticular and preferentially affects the lower limbs. There is no specific test for diagnosing reactive arthritis. Rather, a group of the following tests are used to confirm reactive arthritis.

Laboratory investigations

• CRP is usually elevated.
• FBC may reveal normocytic normochromic anaemia, mild leucocytosis and thrombocytosis.
• Autoimmune screen for RF and ANA are usually negative.
• HLA-B27 is positive in 65–96% of cases of reactive arthritis. HLA-B27 testing is not diagnostic of reactive arthritis and thus not required but is helpful for supporting the diagnosis in patients with joint-restricted symptoms. The HLA-B27 test is moderately expensive, and sensitivity and specificity for reactive arthritis are low.
• Urogenital and stool cultures may reveal inciting infections (e.g. *Chlamydia*, *Salmonella*, *Shigella*) though test results may be negative if obtained weeks after the onset of symptoms. *Chlamydia* should be sought in every case of reactive arthritis via serology test or PCR assay.
• HIV test: the incidence of reactive arthritis is high among patients with AIDS, and HIV testing is recommended in patients in whom reactive arthritis is newly diagnosed, even if they do not have risk factors.

Arthrocentesis and fluid analysis

These may be needed to exclude septic or crystal arthritis especially in monoarticular arthritis with constitutional symptoms. Synovial fluid analysis in reactive arthritis usually reveals a high WBC count ($10–40 \times 10^9$/L) with polymorphonuclear leucocytes predominating.

Radiological investigation

On plain radiology of the affected joints and axial skeleton, the features of reactive arthritis include enthesitis with periosteal reaction, asymmetrical sacroiliitis (<10%) and discontinuous spondylitis with non-marginal syndesmophytes. However, these occur late and sensitivity and specificity of imaging are low.

MRI of the sacroiliac joints can detect disease earlier than plain X-ray. MRI is more sensitive than CT or radionuclide studies in detecting sacroiliitis and enthesitis. Ultrasound may reveal enthesitis (as periosteal reaction and tendinosis) more accurately than physical examination.

Psoriatic arthritis

Psoriatic arthritis occurs in up to 20% of patients with psoriasis. Skin manifestations usually precede arthritis. Psoriatic arthritis is usually asymmetric and distal joints are often affected. Psoriatic arthritis exhibits five patterns: (i) oligoarticular (≤4 joints; >70% of cases), (ii) polyarticular (≥5 joints), (iii) predominant distal interphalangeal (DIP) joint involvement, (iv) arthritis mutilans and (v) psoriatic spondylitis. Psoriatic arthritis is diagnosed clinically and laboratory and radiological investigations are used to exclude other diagnoses and assess the severity of the disease.

Radiological investigations

Plain X-ray of the hands and feet in patients with psoriatic arthritis may reveal an erosive arthritis, with frequent DIP joint involvement and pencil-in-cup changes because of marked resorption of bone. Erosion of the tuft of the distal phalanx, and even of the metacarpals or metatarsals, can progress to complete dissolution of the bone. This form of acro-osteolysis is not diagnostic but highly suggestive of psoriatic arthritis. Other findings include periosteal reaction, sacroiliitis and spondylitis.

CT and MRI may be useful for detecting early joint synovitis. MRI with gadolinium is sensitive for detecting sacroiliitic synovitis, enthesitis and erosions. MRI may show inflammation in the small joints of the hands, involving the collateral ligaments and soft tissues around the joint capsule, a finding not found in persons with rheumatoid arthritis.

Laboratory investigations

An elevated CRP is found in approximately 40% of patients with psoriatic arthritis. Patients with psoriatic arthritis are typically seronegative for RF and anti-CCP antibody. Because of the increased risk of metabolic syndrome in psoriatic disease, patients should have the appropriate metabolic screening, including a lipid profile, fasting blood glucose and uric acid levels.

Arthrocentesis and fluid analysis

Synovial fluid is inflammatory in psoriatic arthritis, with WBC counts ranging from 5 to 15×10^9/L, with more than 50% of cells being polymorphonuclear leucocytes.

Spondyloarthropathy associated with IBD

Spondyloarthropathy occurs in up to 20% of patients with IBD. The association is more frequent in Crohn's disease than in ulcerative colitis. Radiology of the pelvis or the sacroiliac joints may detect bilateral symmetrical sacroiliitis. The spine may show syndesmophytes and apophyseal joint involvement. Erosive disease is uncommon in the peripheral joints, but bony spurs at the heel (enthesitis) may be observed. Ultrasonography may be useful in identifying early soft-tissue pathology, such as tenosynovitis. MRI is useful for early detection of spinal and sacroiliac lesions characteristic of the spondyloarthropathies.

147 Scleroderma and Raynaud's phenomenon

Table 147.1 Characteristics in subsets of scleroderma

Disease characteristic	Limited cutaneous systemic sclerosis	Diffuse scleroderma
Frequency	70% of scleroderma cases	30% of scleroderma cases
Disease course	Slow onset and progression, better prognosis except in the subset with PAH	Rapid onset and progression, internal organ involvement common
Skin involvement	Limited to face, forearms, below knee lower limbs	Distal and proximal extremities, face and trunk
Raynaud's phenomenon	May precede skin changes by many years	May occur simultaneously or a year or two prior to/after the onset of skin disease
Internal organ involvement	Gastrointestinal, PAH	ILD, renal, gastrointestinal, cardiac
Nailfold capillaries	Dilatation without dropouts	Dilatation with dropout
Antinuclear antibodies	Anti-centromere	Anti-topoisomerase I

Table 147.2 Autoantibodies in scleroderma

Antibodies	Prevalence (%)	Clinical association
Anti-centromere	20–30	Limited scleroderma, CREST syndrome, PAH
Anti-topoisomerase (anti-Scl-70)	15–20	Diffuse scleroderma, ILD
Anti-PM-Scl	2–3	Polymyositis/scleroderma overlap
Anti-To/Th	2–5	Limited scleroderma
Anti-RNA polymerase	20	Diffuse scleroderma
Anti-fibrillarin	4	Diffuse scleroderma, myositis, PAH, renal disease
Anti-Ku, anti-Sm, anti-U1-RNP	Rare	Overlap syndromes with features of scleroderma
Anticardiolipin antibodies	20–25	Limited/diffuse subsets, features of secondary antiphospholipid antibody syndrome rare

Table 147.3 Clinical features of primary and secondary Raynaud's phenomenon

Primary Raynaud's phenomenon	Secondary Raynaud's phenomenon
Age at onset <30 years	Age at onset >30 years
Symmetrical involvement of both hands	Episodes are intense, painful, asymmetric
Vasospasm attacks triggered by cold or emotional stressors	Associated with ischaemic skin lesions
Absence of tissue necrosis or gangrene	Clinical features suggestive of connective tissue disease
Normal nailfold capillaries	Microvascular disease on microscopy of nailfold capillaries
Normal CRP	Raised CRP
Negative ANA and other autoantibodies	Positive ANA and specific autoantibodies

The purpose of investigation in scleroderma is:
- To confirm the diagnosis
- To classify the scleroderma into 'limited' and 'diffuse' variants
- To assess the extent of organ involvement
- To monitor disease progression

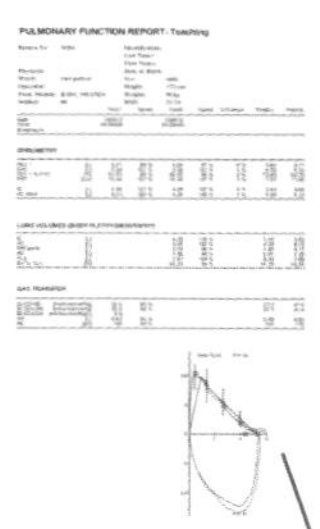

Figure 147.3 PFTs are essential in patients with scleroderma

Figure 147.4 CXR shows bibasal pulmonary fibrosis

Figure 147.5 CT chest shows bilateral pulmonary fibrosis

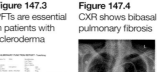
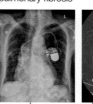
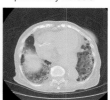
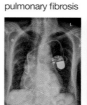

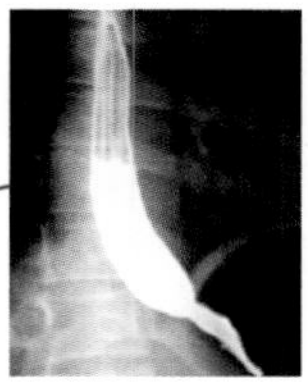

Figure 147.1 Barium swallow study shows hypomotility and fibrotic strictures of the oesophagus

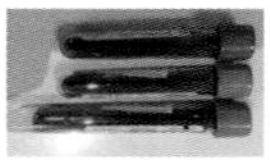

Figure 147.7 Echocardiogram shows pulmonary hypertension

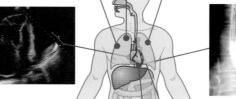

Basic investigations
- FBC
- Electrolytes, creatinine
- LFTs
- CRP
- Autoantibodies

Figure 147.2 Endoscopy shows reflux oesophagitis

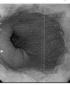

Figure 147.8 Urinalysis and urine protein

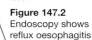
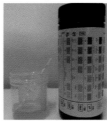

Figure 147.6 Cardiac perfusion scan can be used to assess fibrosis of the myocardium

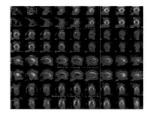

Clinical Investigations at a Glance, First Edition. Jonathan Gleadle, Jordan Li and Tuck Yong. © 2017 John Wiley & Sons, Ltd. Published 2017 by John Wiley & Sons, Ltd.

Scleroderma

Scleroderma is characterised by a triad of fibrosis, vasculopathy and autoimmunity. Scleroderma can be classified into two main types according to the extent of skin involvement (Table 147.1). Patients with limited cutaneous scleroderma (LcSSc) may have Raynaud's phenomenon for years before the appearance of the characteristic features: calcinosis, oesophageal dysmotility and reflux, sclerodactyly and telangiectasia (CREST syndrome). In later stages pulmonary arterial hypertension (PAH) and interstitial lung disease (ILD) may occur. Patients with diffuse cutaneous scleroderma (DcSSc) often have an abrupt onset of Raynaud's phenomenon, and arthritis and myositis are common. Rapid progression of skin disease is accompanied by an increased risk of hypertensive renal crisis, ILD and cardiac and gastrointestinal disease.

The diagnosis of scleroderma is based on typical features of skin thickening, Raynaud's phenomenon and visceral organ involvement, and supported serologically by distinct autoantibodies.

Laboratory investigation

- FBC may reveal anaemia due to chronic disease, iron deficiency due to gastrointestinal blood loss, vitamin B_{12} or folate deficiency secondary to bacterial overgrowth due to intestinal hypomotility, or microangiopathic haemolytic anaemia secondary to scleroderma renal crisis.
- CRP is usually not elevated.
- Serum electrolytes and renal and liver function tests should be performed.
- Urine analysis and urine protein/creatinine ratio.

Autoantibodies in scleroderma

Antinuclear antibodies (ANA)

ANA is positive in 90–95% of patients with scleroderma. ANA specificities include distinct antibody subsets with different clinical associations (Table 147.2).

Anti-centromere antibody (ACA)

The frequency of ACA in patients with LcSSc is as high as 50%, but is below 5% in patients with DcSSc. When found in patients with Raynaud's phenomenon, it predicts the development of scleroderma. ACA is strongly associated with CREST syndrome.

Anti-topoisomerase-I antibody (anti-Scl-70 antibody)

This is found in up to 40% of patients with DcSSc but less than 10% of patients with LcSSc. When present in patients with Raynaud's phenomenon, it predicts the risk of developing scleroderma. ACA and anti-Scl-70 exist in isolation and are rarely found together. Anti-Scl-70 antibody is associated with ILD.

Anti-fibrillarin antibody (anti-U3RNP antibody)

This is found in 4% of patients with scleroderma. It is associated with DcSSc with myositis, PAH and renal disease.

Anti-PM-Scl antibody

This is found in 50% of the patients with polymyositis/scleroderma overlap syndrome and as many as 80% of patients with these antibodies will have this disease. It is found in 3% of patients with scleroderma and 8% of patients with myositis.

Anti-U1-RNP antibody

This is seen in association with overlap syndromes, specifically with Raynaud's phenomenon, joint involvement, myositis, LcSSc and a more favourable outcome.

Anti-Th/To antibodies

These are directed against the ribonuclease mitochondrial RNA processing complex (MRP) and ribonuclease P complexes. They are present in 2–5% of patients with scleroderma, and are also seen in patients with SLE and polymyositis.

Anti-RNA polymerase group (I and III) antibodies

These are found in 20% of patients with scleroderma, associated with DcSSc and are correlated with right heart failure secondary to PAH and higher mortality.

Other autoantibodies

Anti-Ku antibody is found in patients with overlap syndrome with features of scleroderma and SLE. Anti-Ro antibody is identified in scleroderma patients with Sjögren's syndrome. Anti-Sm antibody is seen rarely in patients with scleroderma but if present predicts a poor prognosis with frequent renal involvement. Anticardiolipin antibodies are seen in 20–25% of patients with scleroderma, although secondary antiphospholipid antibody syndrome is rare. Of patients with clinical scleroderma, 40% do not have a known scleroderma-specific autoantibody.

Wide-field microscopy of the nailfold capillary bed

This can reveal characteristic architectural abnormalities of the microvasculature in scleroderma. The changes include enlargement and tortuosity of individual capillary loops interspersed with areas of capillary loop dropout. At later stages of disease, punctate telangiectasia develop with typical locations including fingers, face, lips and oral mucosa.

Skin biopsy

In most cases, skin biopsy is not indicated as the diagnosis is clinical, but may be helpful in atypical presentations of disease.

Investigations for organ involvement

Gastrointestinal involvement

Oesophageal hypomotility is common and can be revealed by manometry or barium swallow (Figure 147.1). Endoscopy can detect oesophagitis, stricture and telangiectases (Figure 147.2). Scleroderma can cause malabsorption and bacterial overgrowth and should be investigated if there is clinical suspicion (see Chapter 71).

Pulmonary involvement

All patients should undergo PFTs (Figure 147.3) to measure forced vital capacity and diffusing capacity for carbon monoxide (D_{LCO}). In ILD these two parameters tend to decline in parallel, whereas in isolated PAH the D_{LCO} shows a disproportionate decline.

CXR is an insensitive screening test but at advanced stages reveals increased interstitial markings, most prominently at the bases, or the changes of PAH (Figure 147.4). HRCT is more sensitive than CXR, and should be used for screening. ILD is usually associated with ground-glass opacification (Figure 147.5).

Table 147.4 Common causes of secondary Raynaud's phenomenon

Mechanical vascular disease	Normal small artery, abnormal vasoconstriction
Thoracic outlet syndrome (cervical rib)	Drug-induced (beta-blockers, ergots)
Crutch pressure	Phaeochromocytoma
Small artery disease	Carcinoid syndrome
Scleroderma, SLE, dermatomyositis,	Migraine
overlap syndromes	**Normal artery, blood disorders**
Cold injury	Cryoglobulinaemia
Vibration disease	Paraproteinaemia
Arteriosclerosis	Cold agglutinin disease
Chemotherapy with vinblastine	Polycythaemias

Key points

• ANA and extractable nuclear antigens (ENA) are useful investigations to support the diagnosis of scleroderma.
• Echocardiography, PFT, CXR and HRCT of the chest should be performed at diagnosis of systemic sclerosis and considered at regular intervals thereafter.

PAH can be screened and diagnosed by echocardiography, which estimates pulmonary artery pressure.

Cardiac involvement

Patchy fibrosis of the myocardium is present at autopsy in 80% of patients, but is rarely clinically significant. Myocardial perfusion scintigraphy is the most sensitive technique for diagnosis (Figure 147.6). Echocardiography is abnormal in 50% of patients and includes pericardial thickening and right ventricular or biventricular heart failure (Figure 147.7). ECG abnormalities include atrial and ventricular arrhythmias and conduction system disturbances.

Renal involvement

The syndrome of scleroderma renal crisis is defined as sudden onset of accelerated hypertension, rapidly progressive renal insufficiency (defined as a fall in eGFR >20 mL/min/1.73 m^2 from baseline within 1 week), microangiopathic haemolysis, consumptive thrombocytopenia and hyperreninaemia. Renal involvement is uncommon in limited scleroderma. Urinalysis typically reveals protein and red cells although casts are unusual (Figure 147.8).

Raynaud's phenomenon

Raynaud's phenomenon is episodic vasospasm that causes digits to change colour to white (pallor) from lack of blood flow, usually brought on by cold temperatures. Affected areas subsequently turn blue (due to deoxygenation) or red (due to reperfusion) or both. It can be painful and can lead to complications.

The diagnosis of Raynaud's phenomenon is made clinically. Laboratory investigations help to distinguish primary and secondary Raynaud's phenomenon (Table 147.3) and discover the underlying causes (Table 147.4).

The following investigations should be performed in patients with Raynaud's phenomenon to test for an underlying connective tissue disease:
- FBC and CRP;
- biochemistry including kidney and liver function tests;
- total immunoglobulin and protein electrophoresis;
- ANA, ENA, ANCA and dsDNA;
- nailfold capillaroscopy;
- urinalysis;
- hand X-ray;
- CXR.

148 Rheumatoid arthritis

The goal of the investigations in RA is to:
- Confirm the diagnosis of RA when it is clinically suspected
- Identify and assess the severity of any extra-articular manifestations
- Assess disease activity, severity, response to treatment and prognosis
- Monitor any adverse effects of therapy
- Diagnose complications related to RA and its treatment such as osteoporosis

Table 148.1 American College of Rheumatology and European League Against Rheumatism 2010 diagnostic criteria for RA

Joint involvement (0–5)
One medium-to-large joint (0)
2–10 medium-to-large joints (1)
1–3 small joints (large joints not counted) (2)
4–10 small joints (large joints not counted) (3)
>10 joints (at least one small joint) (5)
Serology (0–3)
Negative RF and negative antibodies against citrullinated antigens (ACPA) (0)
Low positive RF or low positive ACPA (1)
High positive RF or high positive ACPA (2)
Acute-phase reactants (0–1)
Normal CRP and normal (ESR) (0)
Abnormal CRP or abnormal ESR (1)
Duration of symptoms (0–1)
<6 weeks (0)
≥6 weeks (1)

Points are shown in parentheses. Cut-off point for RA is 6 points. Patients can also be classified as having RA if they have (i) typical erosions or (ii) long-standing disease previously satisfying the classification criteria.

Figure 148.1 Plain X-ray shows (a) a normal right hand; (b) bilateral erosive arthritis in PIP and MCP joints consistent with RA

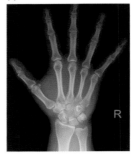

(a)   (b)

Figure 148.2 Plain X-ray shows extensive distruction and deformity of the mid-foot intertarsal and tarsometatarsal joints due to advanced RA

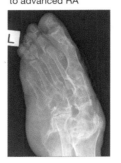

Figure 148.3 MRI of the spine shows C1–C2 subluxation in a patient with RA

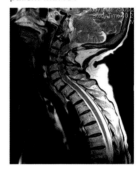

Table 148.2 Investigation of extra-articular disease in RA

Extra-articular disease	Investigations
Pulmonary Pulmonary nodules, pleural effusion, pulmonary fibrosis	Arterial blood gas (ABG), pulmonary function test (PFT), CXR, HRCT chest, echocardiography, pleural fluid analysis, lung biopsy
Ocular Keratoconjunctivitis sicca (Sjögren's syndrome), episcleritis, scleritis	Investigations for Sjögren's: Schirmer's test, ENA, salivary gland biopsy
Systemic vasculitis	Tissue biopsy, urine microscopy, kidney ultrasound and biopsy (if renal involvement suspected)
Cardiac Pericarditis, pericardial effusion, valvular heart disease, conduction defects	ECG, CXR, echocardiography
Neurological Nerve entrapment, cervical myelopathy, peripheral neuropathy, mononeuritis multiplex	MRI neck (cervical myelopathy), nerve conduction test, nerve biopsy
Cutaneous Pyoderma gangrenosum, vasculitic rashes, leg ulceration	Skin biopsy
Amyloidosis	Serum and urine protein, electrophoresis, radionuclide studies, tissue biopsy

Key points

- For patients presenting with painful and swollen joints and suspected RA, investigations should include CRP, RF and anti-CCP antibody levels.
- Anti-CCP antibody testing is the standard evaluation of early inflammatory polyarthritis to achieve early accurate diagnosis of RA and support early treatment with disease-modifying anti-rheumatic drugs.
- All patients with suspected RA should have plain X-ray for hands and feet. It can also be used as a prognostic indicator and for monitoring disease progression.
- All patients with RA needing general anaesthesia should have cervical spine X-ray to evaluate the risk of atlantoaxial subluxation.

Clinical Investigations at a Glance, First Edition. Jonathan Gleadle, Jordan Li and Tuck Yong. © 2017 John Wiley & Sons, Ltd. Published 2017 by John Wiley & Sons, Ltd.

Rheumatoid arthritis (RA) is a systemic inflammatory disorder that affects the synovial joints, especially the small joints of the hands. RA affects 0.5–1.0% of adults in developed countries and is three times more common in women than men. Prevalence increases with age. RA can cause severe pain and destruction of the joints can be very disabling. Furthermore, RA is a systemic disease that can affect many other organs causing, for example, pulmonary fibrosis and premature coronary artery disease.

The key to early diagnosis of RA is the clinical identification of synovitis and then appropriate investigations. The early diagnosis and initiation of disease-modifying anti-rheumatic drugs within 3 months of disease onset makes a significant difference to long-term outcomes as the joint destruction from synovitis can occur rapidly and early.

The diagnostic criteria are listed in Table 148.1. There is no single diagnostic test for RA which accurately differentiates it from normality or from other types of arthritis. The diagnosis is first made clinically, then the tests described in the following sections help to confirm the most likely diagnosis. However, laboratory results and radiology may all be normal in the early stages, even in patients with definite RA, particularly if this is just affecting small joints. Useful initial investigations of patients with suspected RA include basic laboratory tests and X-ray of the hands, wrists and feet.

Laboratory investigations

• FBC may reveal normocytic normochromic anaemia with normal WBC count and mild to moderate thrombocytosis. The severity of haematological changes generally reflects the severity of the RA. Leucopenia and thrombocytopenia may occur in Felty's syndrome.

• CRP is generally elevated in active RA, which indicates an inflammatory process, but has low specificity for RA. It can be useful in monitoring disease activity and response to treatment.

• Rheumatoid factor (RF) is elevated in the early phases of the disease in 60–70% of patients. RF is usually associated with more severe disease and is frequently present in patients with rheumatoid nodules, Sjögren's syndrome, vasculitis, respiratory involvement and peripheral neuritis.

• Anti-CCP antibodies are more specific for the diagnosis of RA than RF but sensitivity is similar. The sensitivity and specificity of anti-CCP for diagnosis of RA are 66.0% and 90.4%, respectively. In comparison, the sensitivity and specificity of RF for diagnosis of RA are 71.6% and 80.3%, respectively. Positivity for anti-CCP antibodies is associated with progression to erosive disease and low remission rate.

• ANA is positive in 20–40% of patients with RA with a homogeneous pattern, particularly in those with Sjögren's syndrome.

• Serum biochemistry and liver function tests: evaluation of kidney and liver function is necessary because many therapies used in RA can cause toxicity to these organs and may be contraindicated if impairment is present. Lipid profile and glucose status should be checked periodically as patients with RA have increased risk of cardiovascular disease.

Radiological investigations

Plain X-ray

X-ray of the hands and feet is indicated. The earliest erosions are often seen in the metacarpophalangeal (MCP) or metatarsophalangeal joint (low sensitivity, 23–30%; high specificity, 85–88%; negative predictive value, 66%; positive predictive value, 50%). Although plain X-ray is a blunt instrument for detecting joint inflammation, there are occasions when erosive damage will be detected when other tests are normal, and it acts as a baseline for future determinations of disease progression. Juxta-articular erosions characterise progressive established RA and are usually irreversible (Figure 148.1). Extensive damage on X-ray (Figure 148.2) suggests the disease is inadequately controlled and rapid progression of joint damage needs intensive treatment.

Ultrasound and MRI

Ultrasound and MRI are superior to clinical examination in the detection of synovitis, and MRI is more sensitive in detecting the presence of erosions and other early inflammatory changes than conventional X-ray. Negative ultrasound findings have useful negative predictive value in patients with suspected RA or with development of RA. If clinically suspected or as part of the preoperative assessment for RA patients with cervical spine involvement, particularly when general anaesthesia is planned, MRI of the neck should be performed to investigate the presence or absence of atlantoaxial subluxation (Figure 148.3). The mortality rate of patients with atlantoaxial subluxation is eight times higher than that of unaffected patients.

Aspiration of synovial fluid

If a large joint is swollen, it may be possible to aspirate synovial fluid for analysis. An increased WBC count (predominantly polymorphonuclear cells) will confirm the inflammatory nature of the fluid and counts between 5 and 50×10^9/L are usually seen in RA.

Investigations for disease monitoring

RF titre and anti-CCP positivity are good predictors of prognosis. In addition to clinical assessment, FBC, CRP and RF are usually evaluated every 3 months to monitor the patient's progress and response to treatment. In general, progressive decline in CRP and RF is evidence that the patient is responding to treatment. Serial X-ray, at yearly intervals, can provide a useful index of disease activity and response to treatment.

Investigations of extra-articular disease

A range of extra-articular features can complicate RA in up to 30% of patients. Table 148.2 shows extra-articular diseases that occur in RA and the diagnostic investigations that should be performed.

149 Systemic lupus erythematosus

The purpose of investigation in SLE is to:
- Confirm the diagnosis
- Assess SLE activity and severity
- Assess other organ involvement
- Monitor treatment toxicities

Table 149.1 Systemic Lupus Erythematosus International Collaborating Clinics classification criteria

Clinical criteria	Immunological criteria
Acute cutaneous lupus or subcutaneous lupus	ANA
Chronic cutaneous lupus	Anti-dsDNA
Oral ulcers or nasal ulcers	Anti-Sm
Non-scarring alopecia	Low complement
Synovitis involving two or more joints	Direct Coombs' test
Serositis	Antiphospholipid antibodies
Renal	Persistent proteinuria >0.5 g/day or >3+ or cellular casts: may be red cell, haemoglobin, granular tubular, or mixed
Neurological	Seizures: in the absence of offending drugs or known metabolic derangements Psychosis: in the absence of offending drugs or known metabolic derangements
Haematological disorder	Haemolytic anaemia with reticulocytosis, or leucopenia $<4 \times 10^9$/L, or lymphopenia $<1.5 \times 10^9$/L, or thrombocytopenia $<100 \times 10^9$/L in the absence of offending drugs

Table 149.3 Autoantibody tests for SLE

Test	Description
ANA	Screening test; sensitivity 95%; not diagnostic without clinical features
Anti-dsDNA	High specificity; sensitivity only 70%; level is variable based on disease activity
Anti-Sm	Most specific antibody for SLE; only 30–40% sensitivity
Anti-SSA (Ro) or Anti-SSB (La)	Present in 15% of patients with SLE and other connective-tissue diseases such as Sjögren's syndrome; associated with neonatal lupus
Anti-ribosomal P	Uncommon antibodies that may correlate with risk for CNS lupus
Anti-RNP	May indicate mixed connective-tissue disease with overlap SLE, scleroderma, and myositis
Anticardiolipin	IgG/IgM variants measured with ELISA are among the anti-phospholipid antibodies used to screen for APS in patients with SLE
Lupus anticoagulant	Multiple tests (e.g. direct Russell viper venom test) to screen for inhibitors in the clotting cascade in APS
Direct Coombs' test	Positive Coombs' test suggests anaemia may be due to haemolysis
Anti-histone	Drug-induced lupus ANA antibodies are often of this antibody (e.g. with procainamide or hydralazine)

Table 149.2 Conditions other than SLE associated with positive ANA

Systemic autoimmune diseases
Scleroderma (sensitivity 85%)
Sjögren's syndrome (sensitivity 48–73%)
Polymyositis or dermatomyositis (sensitivity 61%)
Rheumatoid arthritis (sensitivity 41%)
Mixed connective tissue disease
Organ-specific autoimmune disease
Autoimmune hepatitis
Primary biliary cirrhosis
Graves' disease
Hashimoto's thyroiditis
Idiopathic pulmonary fibrosis
Non-autoimmune associations
Viral infections, e.g. infectious mononucleosis, hepatitis C, HIV
Bacterial infections, e.g. infective endocarditis, tuberculosis
Malignancy

Table 149.4 Classification of lupus nephritis (LN)

Class I	Minimal mesangial LN
Class II	Mesangial proliferative LN
Class III	Focal LN
Class IV	Diffuse LN
Class V	Membranous LN
Class VI	Advanced sclerosing LN

Key points

- Antibody testing should not be used alone to diagnose SLE. A positive ANA test alone is not sufficient to establish the diagnosis.
- Anti-dsDNA and anti-Sm, particularly in high titres, have high specificity for SLE but their sensitivity is low. Therefore, a positive result helps to establish the diagnosis of SLE, but a negative result does not rule it out.
- ANA test is commonly used for screening SLE. The presence of anti-DNA, anti-Sm and antiphospholipid antibodies is more specific for diagnosing SLE.

Clinical Investigations at a Glance, First Edition. Jonathan Gleadle, Jordan Li and Tuck Yong. © 2017 John Wiley & Sons, Ltd. Published 2017 by John Wiley & Sons, Ltd.

Systemic lupus erythematosus (SLE) is a chronic multisystem autoimmune disorder. Approximately 85% of patients with SLE are women, with onset usually in the reproductive years. Patients with SLE can have persistently active disease or a relapsing and remitting pattern. Appropriate investigations can lead to earlier diagnosis and better management that may result in a lower rate of life-threatening complications and slow progression to end-stage organ failure.

The clinical presentation of SLE can be diverse because the disease can affect nearly every organ system and symptoms may accumulate over time. The Systemic Lupus Erythematosus International Collaborating Clinics (SLICC) group has proposed revised classification criteria to improve the sensitivity and specificity of diagnosis (Table 149.1). Diagnosis of definitive SLE requires four or more criteria with at least one clinical and one laboratory criterion, with the exception of biopsy-proven lupus nephritis. Criteria are cumulative and need not be present concurrently.

Immunological investigations

Antinuclear antibodies

The presence of ANA is the serological hallmark of SLE. Up to 98% of patients with SLE are positive for ANA, making it a highly sensitive test. Positive ANA is diagnostic of SLE when it occurs together with the other criteria for the classification of SLE. A positive ANA in the absence of clinical features of SLE may be irrelevant. A negative ANA makes SLE very unlikely and other diagnoses should be sought. ANA is generally non-specific; Table 149.2 shows other causes that can be associated with positive ANA.

It is important to consider both titre and pattern of ANA. A titre above 1 : 320 is considered clinically significant. Low-titre ANA can be found in healthy individuals (titre 1 : 40 in 25–30%; 1 : 80 in 10–15% and 1 : 160 in 5%). The more common patterns observed in SLE are homogeneous and speckled.

Other autoantibodies (Table 149.3)

Antibodies to double-stranded DNA (dsDNA) are specific for SLE. An increase in anti-dsDNA titre may signify onset of disease flare. Other autoantibodies which can be tested on the extractable nuclear antigen panel can also be associated with SLE. For example, anti-Smith (anti-Sm) is highly specific in SLE.

Complement

Tissue deposition of immune complexes can lead to a reduction in serum complement levels (especially C3 and C4). Sequential measurements can be used to gauge disease activity and follow response to treatment.

CRP

Patients with SLE have systemic inflammation. ESR and CRP may be elevated but they are non-specific markers.

Investigations for specific organ/system involvement in SLE

Cutaneous investigations

The spectrum of cutaneous manifestations of SLE is broad but the classical forms are acute malar and chronic discoid lupus erythematous rash. Skin biopsy can help in diagnosing SLE (Figure 149.1). Lupus skin rash often demonstrates inflammatory infiltrates at the dermoepidermal junction and vacuolar change in the basal columnar cells. Discoid lesions demonstrate more significant skin inflammation, with hyperkeratosis, follicular plugging, oedema and mononuclear cell infiltration at the dermoepidermal junction. In many SLE rashes, immunofluorescent stains demonstrate immunoglobulin and complement deposits at the dermoepidermal basement.

Haematological investigations

Anaemia is a common feature. This is usually due to chronic inflammation and sometimes autoimmune haemolytic anaemia. Leucopenia is usually due to lymphopenia rather than neutropenia. Thrombocytopenia is another potential manifestation. A Coombs' test should be requested if initial blood count shows anaemia and features of haemolysis, such as elevated reticulocyte count.

Coagulation studies should be performed. Measurement of antiphospholipid antibodies, anticardiolipin antibodies, lupus anticoagulant and anti-β_2-glycoprotein 1 should be requested in patients with features which are suggestive of antiphospholipid syndrome (APS), such as a history of venous or arterial thromboses, recurrent miscarriages, or in patients with prolonged activated partial thromboplastin time (APTT).

Musculoskeletal investigations

Up to 95% of patients with SLE have intermittent arthritis and X-rays can detect erosive changes. Myalgia is a common manifestation but myositis is rare but can be detected with the measurement of creatine kinase in the blood. The prevalence of avascular necrosis or osteonecrosis is increased in patients with SLE because of heavy steroid use. MRI is the investigation of choice (Figure 149.2). Baseline bone density should be performed (Figure 149.3).

Renal investigations

Lupus nephritis is one of the more serious complications of SLE that is associated with higher mortality. It occurs in over half of SLE patients during the course of disease.

To evaluate renal involvement, urinalysis and urine sediment microscopy should be performed. Protein/creatinine ratio or 24-hour urine protein measurement can be used to quantify proteinuria (Figure 149.4). Serum creatinine and electrolytes should be checked. A renal ultrasound should be performed to exclude other causes of renal impairment.

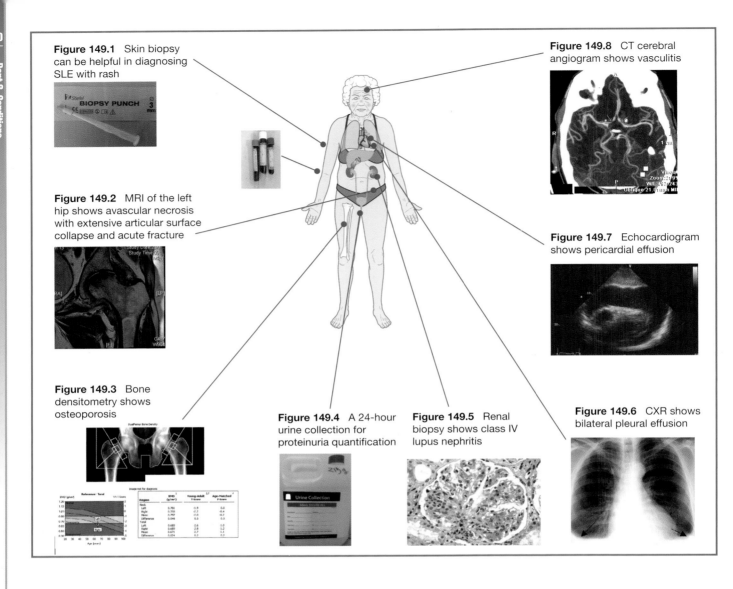

Figure 149.1 Skin biopsy can be helpful in diagnosing SLE with rash

Figure 149.2 MRI of the left hip shows avascular necrosis with extensive articular surface collapse and acute fracture

Figure 149.3 Bone densitometry shows osteoporosis

Figure 149.4 A 24-hour urine collection for proteinuria quantification

Figure 149.5 Renal biopsy shows class IV lupus nephritis

Figure 149.6 CXR shows bilateral pleural effusion

Figure 149.7 Echocardiogram shows pericardial effusion

Figure 149.8 CT cerebral angiogram shows vasculitis

Renal biopsy is the most sensitive and specific test for confirming the diagnosis and classification of lupus nephritis based on the International Society of Nephrology/Renal Pathology Society (ISN/RPS) classification (Table 149.4 and Figure 149.5). The indications for renal biopsy include:
- increasing serum creatinine in the absence of evidence for another aetiology;
- proteinuria of more than 1.0 g in 24 hours;
- proteinuria of 0.5 g or more in 24 hours, with active urine sediment defined as (i) haematuria ($\geq$5 RBCs/hpf) or (ii) cellular casts.

Cardiopulmonary investigations

Pleural and pericardial inflammation and effusion can occur during active SLE (Figures 149.6 and 149.7). Other cardiopulmonary manifestations include interstitial lung disease (ILD) and pulmonary hypertension. CXR and CT of the chest can be used to detect ILD and to assess for pneumonitis and pulmonary emboli. PFT and ABG are useful in evaluating ILD.

Echocardiography is used to assess for pericardial effusion and pulmonary hypertension.

Neuropsychiatric investigations

Brain MRI or magnetic resonance angiography (MRA) is the modality of choice for evaluating central nervous system (CNS) lupus white-matter changes, vasculitis (Figure 149.8) or stroke, although findings are often non-specific and may be absent in as many as 42% of cases with neuropsychiatric symptoms.

Lumbar puncture is performed to exclude CNS infection or other conditions. Non-specific elevations in cell count and protein level and decrease in glucose level may be found in the CSF of patients with CNS lupus.

Evaluation of associated comorbidities

Patients with SLE are at significantly increased risk of premature atherosclerosis so measurement of lipid profiles and fasting glucose are recommended at regular intervals. Measurement of bone mineral density is also recommended, especially for those on long-term glucocorticoid therapy.

150 Sjögren's syndrome

The purpose of investigations in a patient with suspected Sjögren's syndrome is to:
- Establish the diagnosis of Sjögren's syndrome
- Identify the primary condition associated with secondary Sjögren's syndrome
- Identify any extraglandular manifestations of Sjögren's syndrome

Table 150.1 Extraglandular manifestations of Sjögren's syndrome

Extraglandular manifestations	Frequency (%)	Investigations
Skin Purpura/cutaneous vasculitis (usually with cryoglobulinaemia) Annular erythema	10–15 5–10	Cryoglobulin, skin biopsy
Joints Non-erosive symmetrical arthritis	15–30	X-ray of the joint, joint aspiration
Lungs COPD/bronchiectasis Interstitial lung disease Bronchiolitis obliterans	8–10 5 <5	ABG, CXR, HRCT of chest, PFT
Cardiovascular Raynaud's phenomenon Pericarditis	18–37 <5	ECG, CXR, echocardiography
Renal Renal tubular acidosis Glomerulonephritis Interstitial nephritis Recurrent renal calculi	11 <5 <5 <5	FBC, biochemistry, urinalysis, urine protein, microscopy and culture, ultrasound, kidney biopsy (glomerular disease suspected)
Liver/pancreas Primary biliary cirrhosis Autoimmune hepatitis Recurrent pancreatitis	3–8 <5 <5	LFTs, autoimmune markers, ultrasound, liver biopsy Lipase
Peripheral nervous system Mixed polyneuropathy Pure sensory neuropathy Mononeuritis multiplex Autonomic dysfunction	5–10 5 5 55	Nerve conduction test
Central nervous system White matter lesions Cranial nerve involvement Myelitis	50–55 7 <5	MRI, CSF analysis
Thyroid Autoimmune thyroiditis	14–33	Thyroid function test, thyroid autoantibodies
Haematological Anaemia of chronic disease Autoimmune haemolytic anaemia Severe thrombocytopenia B-cell lymphoma	25 <5 <5 5	FBC, biochemistry including calcium, LDH and LFT, serum electrophoresis, CT from head to pelvis and PET (if lymphoma suspected), bone marrow biopsy

Key points

- Schirmer's test or the Rose Bengal test can be used in patients with eye symptoms.
- Non-stimulated whole saliva flow collection (<1.5 mL in 15 min) can be used in patient with oral symptoms.
- Anti-SSA and anti-SSB antigens are not specific to Sjögren's syndrome; they may be present in persons with other diseases such as SLE and in healthy persons.
- Minor salivary gland biopsy from the lip is the gold standard for diagnosis of Sjögren's syndrome, but is not always necessary in typical cases.

Figure 150.1 Labial biopsy of minor salivary glands shows infiltrations of lymphocytes and plasma cells, and the lumen of the salivary duct has an eosinophilic deposit of the thickened secretion consistent with Sjögren's syndrome

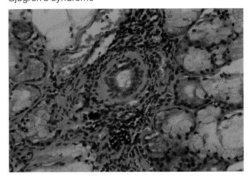

Figure 150.2 Schirmer's test

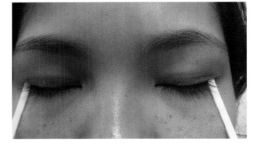

Clinical Investigations at a Glance, First Edition. Jonathan Gleadle, Jordan Li and Tuck Yong. © 2017 John Wiley & Sons, Ltd. Published 2017 by John Wiley & Sons, Ltd.

Sjögren's syndrome is an autoimmune disorder characterised by diminished lacrimal and salivary gland secretion causing dry eyes and mouth, but it can also affect other organs. Sjögren's syndrome is more common in women than men, with a ratio of 9 : 1. Sjögren's syndrome can be classified as primary or as secondary (60% of cases) when it is associated with another autoimmune disease such as rheumatoid arthritis, scleroderma or SLE.

Sjögren's syndrome must be differentiated from non-autoimmune sicca syndrome (dry mouth and eyes), which is not a systemic disease and does not have extraglandular complications. Sicca syndrome occurs in about 25% of those aged over 65 years and may be related to age-related atrophy of exocrine glands and/or drug side effects.

The clinical presentation of primary Sjögren's syndrome is variable and the onset can be insidious. A low threshold for investigation and early diagnosis of Sjögren's syndrome may prevent complications such as dental caries, corneal ulceration and sialadenitis, and allows clinical surveillance for the development of serious extraglandular systemic manifestations.

An American–European Consensus Group (AECG) has established criteria for the investigation and diagnosis of Sjögren's syndrome. These criteria require objective evidence of autoimmunity for a definite diagnosis of Sjögren's syndrome, either anti-Ro or anti-La antibodies or a labial biopsy demonstrating focal sialadenitis. The sensitivity and specificity of the AECG criteria for the diagnosis of primary Sjögren's syndrome are 85% and 97%, respectively.

Diagnostic investigations

Salivary gland biopsy

Characteristic histopathology on salivary gland biopsy (Figure 150.1) is the gold standard for confirming the diagnosis and is necessary in patients who are negative for anti-Ro and anti-La antibodies. It is best performed by labial biopsy of the minor salivary glands. Histopathology is characterised by lymphocytic infiltration, defined as at least one focus of dense inflammatory infiltrate containing at least 50 lymphocytes per 4 mm^2 in labial salivary gland biopsy.

Tests for autoantibodies

The presence of autoantibodies is a hallmark of primary Sjögren's syndrome. About 80% of patients are positive for ANA, 70% are positive for anti-Ro (or SSA) antibodies and 50% for anti-La (or SSB) antibodies. The presence of both anti-Ro and anti-La antibodies together occurs in 90–100% of patients with Sjögren's syndrome and is associated with younger age at disease onset, increased glandular dysfunction and extraglandular manifestations. In pregnant women, these antibodies predispose the developing fetus to neonatal lupus and congenital heart block, which complicate 1–2% of anti-Ro or anti-La positive pregnancies. Up to 60% of patients with primary Sjögren's syndrome are positive for RF but the clinical relevance is uncertain.

Patients with secondary Sjögren's syndrome typically have serum autoantibodies specific to their primary disorder rather than anti-Ro and anti-La antibodies; these include anti-CCP antibody in rheumatoid arthritis, anti-dsDNA antibody in SLE and anti-centromere or topoisomerase antibodies in scleroderma.

Schirmer's test

Ocular gland testing can be done by Schirmer's test, which involves positioning a strip of sterile filter paper overhanging the lateral third of the lower eyelid of each eye and left in place for 5 min (Figure 150.2). The test is positive if less than 5 mm of paper is wetted after 5 min. Alternative tests to show objective ocular dryness include the Rose Bengal test, lissamine green test and tear break-up time, which require a slit lamp and are usually performed by an ophthalmologist.

Investigation and monitoring for extraglandular manifestations

Extraglandular manifestations of primary Sjögren's syndrome include constitutional symptoms such as fatigue, low-grade fever, myalgias and arthralgias, as well as organ-specific complications (Table 150.1). Patients with Sjögren's syndrome have a 44-fold relative risk of developing lymphoma compared to the general population.

Laboratory tests including FBC, biochemistry and CRP should be performed at the time of diagnosis, and then every 6–12 months to monitor for extraglandular complications. About 25% of patients with primary Sjögren's syndrome have anaemia of chronic disease, and often have an elevated CRP.

Raised GGT or AST/ALT may indicate primary biliary cirrhosis or autoimmune hepatitis, respectively. Abnormal thyroid function (frequently hypothyroidism), together with positive thyroid autoantibodies, are found with autoimmune thyroiditis. In patients who develop dyspnoea, CXR, HRCT of the chest and PFTs are useful for evaluation.

The presence of abnormal RBCs and casts suggests glomerular disease. Patients with low plasma bicarbonate and potassium levels should be investigated for possible distal renal tubular acidosis; these patients have normal anion gap metabolic acidosis with a urine pH above 5.5 caused by a defect in distal urinary acidification.

151 Vasculitis

The goal of investigation in vasculitis is to:
- Confirm the diagnosis
- Differentiate primary and secondary vasculitis
- Determine whether this is a specific type of vasculitis
- Assess the extent of vasculitis

Table 151.2 Tests to exclude secondary causes of vasculitis

Secondary causes of vasculitis	Tests
Hepatitis B and C infection	Hepatitis B and C serology
HIV infection	HIV antibody
Rheumatoid arthritis	RF and anti-CCP antibodies
SLE	ANA, dsDNA
Endocarditis	Blood culture, echocardiogram
Cryoglobulinaemia	Cryoglobulin

Table 134.3 Investigation of a patient with cutaneous vasculitis

Laboratory
FBC
Biochemistry, liver and kidney function
CRP
Blood cultures
Hepatitis B and C serology
Anti-CCP antibodies, RF, ANA, anti-dsDNA, ENA, ANCA, C3, C4, cryoglobulin
Anticardiolipin antibodies, lupus anticoagulant
CXR
Electromyography
Skin lesion biopsy

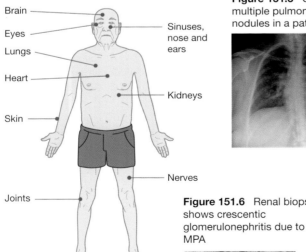

Brain
Eyes
Lungs
Heart
Skin
Joints
Sinuses, nose and ears
Kidneys
Nerves

Table 151.1 Classification of systemic vasculitis

Dominant vessels involved	Primary	Secondary
Large vessels	Giant cell arteritis Takayasu's arteritis Isolated aortitis Primary angiitis of central nervous system	Aortitis associated with RA or AS
Medium vessels	Classical polyarteritis nodosa (PAN) Kawasaki's disease	Hepatitis B-associated PAN
Small vessels	ANCA-associated vasculitis Granulomatosis with polyangiitis Microscopic polyangiitis Churg–Strauss syndrome Henoch–Schönlein purpura Cryoglobulinaemic vasculitis Cutaneous leucocytoclastic angiitis	Vasculitis secondary to RA, SLE, Sjögren's syndrome Drug-induced vasculitis HIV-associated vasculitis Hepatitis C-associated vasculitis

Figure 151.1 Biopsy shows (a) normal small artery; (b) small-artery vasculitis

(a)　　　　　(b)

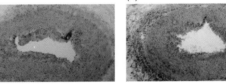

Figure 151.2 Renal biopsy shows polyarteritis nodosa with aneurysm formation

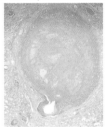

Figure 151.3 CXR shows multiple pulmonary nodules in a patient with GPA

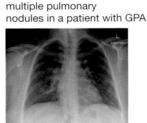

Figure 151.4 Chest CT shows consolidation and patchy ground-glass opacities in a patient with GPA

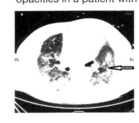

Figure 151.5 CT sinus shows sinus involvement in a patient with GPA

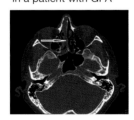

Figure 151.6 Renal biopsy shows crescentic glomerulonephritis due to MPA

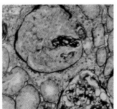

Key points

- Biopsy is the gold standard for establishing the diagnosis of vasculitis but may be misleading due to sampling error or immunosuppressive therapy prior to biopsy.
- Urinary analysis/microscopy and quantification of proteinuria are important investigations for renal vasculitis involvement.
- Immunological tests such as ANCA are important in considering vasculitis.

Clinical Investigations at a Glance, First Edition. Jonathan Gleadle, Jordan Li and Tuck Yong. © 2017 John Wiley & Sons, Ltd. Published 2017 by John Wiley & Sons, Ltd.

Vasculitis is the inflammation of blood vessels and can affect any organ system; many of these diseases have typical recognisable patterns. Systemic vasculitis can be classified as primary or secondary, i.e. associated with infection, drugs or systemic autoimmune diseases such as SLE (Table 151.1). The possibility of vasculitis should be considered in patients with unexplained fever, weight loss, myalgia, rash, renal impairment, respiratory symptoms or neuropathy.

Basic investigations

Laboratory investigations

- Urinary analysis/microscopy and quantification of proteinuria: the finding of haematuria, RBC casts and proteinuria in combination is suggestive of renal involvement in vasculitis and kidney biopsy is indicated.
- FBC: anaemia is common in vasculitis; FBC is needed in monitoring treatment toxicity.
- Serum electrolytes, creatinine and LFTs: systemic vasculitis can cause different forms of glomerulonephritis leading to AKI or CKD and abnormal LFTs.
- CRP is a non-specific marker of inflammation; it is usually raised in active systemic vasculitis.
- Other tests to exclude secondary causes of vasculitis (Table 151.2).

Antineutrophil cytoplasmic autoantibodies

The presence of antineutrophil cytoplasmic antibody (ANCA) is strongly correlated with certain forms of vasculitis, but it cannot establish a diagnosis of vasculitis alone. In general, a cytoplasmic ANCA (c-ANCA) is associated with antibodies against proteinase-3 (PR3-ANCA) and is characteristic of granulomatosis with polyangiitis (GPA or Wegener's granulomatosis). A perinuclear ANCA (p-ANCA) is associated with antibodies against myeloperoxidase (MPO-ANCA) and is characteristic of microscopic polyangiitis (MPA).

There are two types of ANCA assay currently in use:
- indirect immunofluorescence assay (IIF) using alcohol-fixed buffy coat leucocytes;
- enzyme-linked immunosorbent assay (ELISA) using purified specific antigens.

Of these two techniques, the IIF is more sensitive and the ELISA is more specific. Therefore, the clinical approach is to screen with IIF first, and then confirm all positive results with ELISAs directed against the vasculitis-specific target antigens PR3 and MPO. Both positive IIF and ELISA tests have a positive predictive value of 88% and a negative predictive value in excess of 97%.

ANCA is a useful quantitative marker for vasculitis, and the level reflects the degree of inflammation. ANCA levels increase during recurrence and are useful in monitoring response to treatment and relapse. Approximately 10% of patients with granulomatosis with polyangiitis or MPA have negative ANCAs; a negative result does not therefore completely exclude vasculitis. In addition, ANCAs have been reported in other conditions, such as infections, inflammatory bowel disease and drug-induced vasculitis.

Biopsy of affected tissue

Biopsy is the gold standard for establishing the diagnosis of vasculitis but may be misleading due to sampling error or immunosuppressive therapy prior to biopsy. All biopsies should be examined by direct immunofluorescence, as the pattern of immunoglobulin deposition may provide additional clues to the underlying aetiology. Biopsy sites usually include lung, kidney, sinus and skin. The pathognomonic features on biopsy for vasculitis include (Figure 151.1):

- presence of immune-mediated blood vessel wall injury;
- fibrinoid necrosis of the vessel wall;
- red cell extravasation.

Radiological investigations

CXR can show pulmonary infiltrates, nodules, patchy consolidation and pleural effusion (Figure 151.3). Organ-specific CT or MRI should be guided by clinical symptoms (Figures 151.4 and 151.5).

CT angiography or MRA can be helpful in diagnosing medium- and large-vessel vasculitis but does not have a role in the investigation of a small-vessel vasculitis. Beading, aneurysms, and smooth tapering vessel stenosis are consistent with medium- or large-vessel vasculitis.

Nerve conduction study

Motor and sensory neuropathy can occur in systemic vasculitis. Nerve conduction studies should be performed if suspected.

Specific types of vasculitis

Takayasu's arteritis

Takayasu's arteritis is a granulomatous inflammation of the aorta and its main branches that most commonly affects women aged under 40 years. Its clinical manifestations can vary from general inflammatory features to those due to ischaemia. The critical diagnostic investigation is digital subtraction arteriography, which provides extensive evaluation of the arterial tree. MRI and ultrasound can be useful.

Classical polyarteritis nodosa (PAN)

PAN is a necrotising inflammation of medium or small arteries without glomerulonephritis or vasculitis in arterioles, capillaries or venules (Figure 151.2). The dominant clinical features are associated with organ infarction. Angiography of abdominal arteries is the gold standard for diagnosis. All patients with PAN should have hepatitis B serology checked and ANCA by definition should be negative.

ANCA-associated vasculitides

Granulomatosis with polyangiitis

- CRP is elevated in 90% of patients with active GPA; it may decrease in response to treatment.
- ANCA: PR3-ANCA is seen in 70–80% and MPO-ANCA in 10% of patients with GPA. The sensitivity for ANCA by IIF and/or ELISA is as high as 90% in active generalised GPA but as low as 60% in limited disease.

Microscopic polyangiitis

- ANCA testing: about 60% of MPA patients are MPO positive and 30% are PR3 positive.
- Tissue biopsy, usually of the kidney, lung and/or skin, is performed (Figure 151.6).

Churg–Strauss syndrome

Churg–Strauss syndrome is characterised by asthma, hypereosinophilia and transient pulmonary infiltrates, and myocardial vasculitis can occur.

ANCA is present in 40% of patients with Churg–Strauss syndrome. Most of these patients are MPO-ANCA positive.

Cutaneous leucocytoclastic vasculitis

In addition to history and examination, the evaluation of patients with suspected cutaneous vasculitis is summarised in Table 151.3. Diagnosis is made by clinical appearance and biopsy.

152 Polymyalgia rheumatica and giant-cell arteritis

The goals of investigation include:
- Providing laboratory investigation evidence to support the clinical diagnosis
- Confirmation of diagnosis
- Assessment of severity
- Monitoring of relapse and steroid side effects

Figure 152.3 T1 MRI (a) before and (b) after intravenous gadolinium shows mural thickening and enhancement in the right occipital artery consistent with GCA

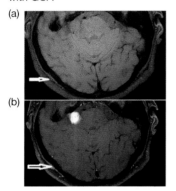

(a)

(b)

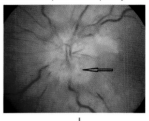

Clinical suspicion: new-onset headache with constitutional symptoms such as fatigue, anorexia and weight loss in a patient older than 50 years, jaw claudication

Figure 152.1 Fundi examination of a patient with GCA showing arterial ischaemic optic neuropathy

Figure 152.2 Biopsy of temporal artery shows marked fibrous thickening of the intimal layer complicated by thrombosis and presence of multinucleate giant cells

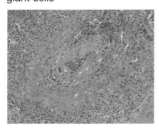

Table 152.2 Laboratory investigations for suspected PMR/GCA

Test	Result
ESR	>50 mm/hour
CRP	Raised; more sensitive indicator of disease activity
FBC	May be normocytic anaemia, leucocytosis
LFTs	Mildly elevated transaminases and ALP

Table 152.1 Criteria for diagnosis of PMR

Age ≥65 years
ESR >50 mm/hour or raised CRP
Stiffness in the morning >1 hour in the neck, shoulder and pelvic girdles
Bilateral upper arm tenderness
Symptom duration >2 weeks
Associated with depression and/or weight loss

Table 152.3 American College of Rheumatology classification criteria for GCA

Age at disease onset ≥50 years
New headache
Temporal artery abnormality
ESR >50 mm/hour
Abnormal artery biopsy: biopsy specimen showing vasculitis characterised by a predominance of mononuclear cell infiltration or granulomatous inflammation, usually with multinucleated giant cells

Key points

- If the ESR or CRP is normal, active PMR and/or GCA is unlikely.
- If clinically suspected GCA, a temporal artery biopsy should be performed to diagnose GCA. The biopsy is positive in 60–80% of patients with GCA and only 15–20% of patients with PMR.
- A negative temporal artery biopsy result does not rule out GCA because other arteries can be involved, or the artery with inflammation may not have been biopsied.

Clinical Investigations at a Glance, First Edition. Jonathan Gleadle, Jordan Li and Tuck Yong. © 2017 John Wiley & Sons, Ltd. Published 2017 by John Wiley & Sons, Ltd.

Polymyalgia rheumatica (PMR) and giant-cell arteritis (GCA) or temporal arteritis are closely related disorders of unknown cause that affect people of middle age and older. Its incidence increases with advancing age. Women are affected two to three times more commonly than men. Population-based studies have shown that 16–21% of patients with PMR have GCA and PMR is present in 40–60% of patients with GCA. PMR might begin before, simultaneously or after clinical manifestations of GCA. In GCA, inflammation mainly affects the large-sized and medium-sized muscular arteries, especially the proximal aorta and its branches. GCA is the most common of all the vasculitides.

Polymyalgia rheumatica

PMR has a wide range of clinical manifestations resulting in a challenging diagnosis. Criteria for diagnosis are shown in Table 152.1. The diagnosis of PMR can be made if a patient has at least three of these six criteria.

As PMR has a non-specific clinical presentation and few significant sequelae, it should be diagnosed with caution. Investigations to rule out other illnesses, such as cancers or insidious-onset rheumatoid arthritis, are the priority. Always specifically enquire about symptoms that may suggest GCA, such as unilateral temporal headaches, scalp tenderness, jaw claudication or visual symptoms. If there is suspicion, the patient should be investigated for GCA (see below).

Laboratory investigations

Laboratory investigations for suspected PMR are listed in Table 152.2. Autoantibodies including RF and anti-CCP antibody are usually negative; if positive, a diagnosis of late-onset rheumatoid arthritis should be considered. Raised creatine kinase (CK) or persistent elevation of transaminases in the setting of muscle weakness is not a feature of PMR and should prompt investigation for myopathies or thyroid disorders.

Radiological investigations

Imaging studies are not required to establish a diagnosis of PMR. Ultrasound can reveal bicipital tenosynovitis, subacromial bursitis, subdeltoid bursitis and trochanteric bursitis. X-ray of other joints may be required to distinguish PMR from arthropathy such as rheumatoid arthritis, spondyloarthropathies and osteoarthritis.

Giant-cell arteritis

A patient with suspected GCA is a medical emergency. Visual loss can occur in up to one-fifth of patients, which may be prevented by prompt recognition (Figure 152.1), investigation and treatment. Criteria for diagnosis are shown in Table 152.3. The diagnosis of GCA can be made if a patient has at least three of these five criteria.

Laboratory investigations

ESR

A raised ESR is considered a hallmark for the diagnosis of GCA. ESR above 50 mm/hour is one of the diagnostic criteria (Table 152.3). A normal ESR makes GCA less likely but 1% of all cases of GCA have a normal ESR.

CRP

CRP is a more sensitive indicator of disease activity than ESR in patients with GCA. Unlike ESR, CRP is unaffected by age and gender and quantitation is precise and reproducible. Histopathological studies have shown that over 40% of patients thought to be in clinical remission with normal CRP have active arteritis.

Other laboratory investigations

FBC may show normochromic normocytic anaemia and thrombocytosis. One-third of the patients have mildly abnormal liver function tests, particularly ALP. Levels of CK and other muscle enzymes are normal.

Temporal artery biopsy

Temporal artery biopsy (Figure 152.2) is the gold standard for diagnosis of GCA.
• A negative biopsy does not exclude GCA. The false-negative rate is 5–13% depending on the length of the specimen, the presence of skip lesions, and the duration of preceding corticosteroid treatment.
• Biopsy specimen length should be 1.5–3.0 cm to keep false-negative results to a minimum as a result of skip inflammatory lesions.
• A negative unilateral biopsy is associated with a very low frequency (1–3%) of subsequent positive contralateral biopsy.
• When possible, biopsy should be done before treatment but biopsy might still show arteritis after 2 weeks of corticosteroid therapy. The commencement of corticosteroids should not be delayed pending biopsy results.

Radiological investigations

CXR

Thoracic aortic aneurysms are 17 times more frequent in patients with GCA than in non-affected people. A CXR every year is adequate to screen for thoracic aortic aneurysm.

Duplex ultrasound

Colour duplex ultrasound is an adjunctive method in the diagnosis of GCA. It can reveal stenoses or occlusion of large vessels, or both, and also inflammatory oedema of the vessel wall (halo sign), which has a high specificity for GCA. However, ultrasound alone lacks diagnostic sensitivity but can serve to target biopsy site.

CT angiography

CT angiography can be used to evaluate large-vessel involvement in GCA. CT is often required to further evaluate the presence of a thoracic aortic aneurysm identified on CXR.

MRI

MRI can show inflammatory changes in temporal arteries or other affected extracranial arteries (Figure 152.3). Bright enhancement, which is a sign of mural inflammation of the temporal artery on high-resolution contrast-enhanced MRI, is highly specific for GCA. Vessel wall oedema on MRI is useful for indicating disease activity.

Arteriography

Rarely, arteriography can be used to outline bilateral stenoses or occlusions of the subclavian, axillary and proximal brachial arteries. Arteries in the legs are less frequently involved.

PET scan

FDG-PET can detect occult involvement of the aorta and large vessels in patients with GCA, especially those presenting with fever of unknown origin. The sensitivity is 80% and specificity 79%.

153 Osteoporosis

The aim of investigations is to:
- Assess the severity and predict fracture risk
- Exclude other bone diseases that mimic osteoporosis, such as myeloma and metastasis
- Identify the causes and predisposing factors of osteoporosis
- Guide treatment and monitor progression

Table 153.1 WHO diagnostic criteria of bone mineral density

Diagnostic category	Criterion based on BMD or BMC value
Normal	Within 1.0 SD of the reference mean for young adults
Low bone mass (osteopenia)	More than 1.0 SD but less than 2.5 SD below the mean for young adults
Osteoporosis	2.5 SD or more below the mean for young adults
Severe osteoporosis (established osteoporosis)	2.5 SD or more below the mean for young adults in combination with one or more fragility (low-trauma) fractures

Table 153.2 Indications for bone density testing

Women aged 65 years and older
Postmenopausal women under age 65 years with risk factors for osteoporosis
Men aged 70 years and older
Adults with fragility fracture
Adults with a disease or condition associated with low bone mass or bone loss
Patients receiving glucocorticoid therapy for 3 months or more
Adults taking medications associated with low bone mass or bone loss
Anyone being considered for pharmacological osteoporosis therapy
Anyone being treated for low bone mass to monitor treatment effect
Anyone not receiving therapy in whom evidence of bone loss would lead to treatment
Women discontinuing estrogen should be considered for testing according to the above indications

Figure 153.1 (a) DEXA scan at the hips; (b) DEXA scan showing the lowest T-score of −2.7 at lumbar spine (L1–L3), which is in the osteoporotic range

(a)

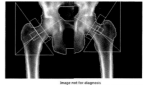

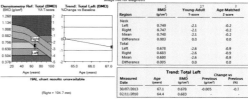

(b)

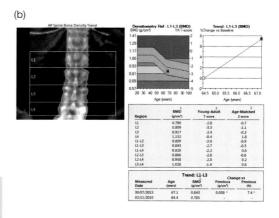

Table 153.3 Bone turnover markers

Bone turnover markers	Specimen
Bone resorption	
C-terminal telopeptide of type 1 collagen	Serum/plasma
N-terminal telopeptide of type 1 collagen	Urine, serum
Pyridinium cross-links: deoxypyridionoline, pyridinoline	Urine
Bone formation	
Alkaline phosphatase (total)	Serum/plasma
Alkaline phosphatase (bone specific)	Serum/plasma
Procollagen type 1 N propeptide	Serum/plasma
Osteocalcin	Serum

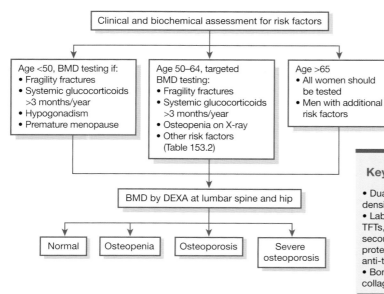

Clinical and biochemical assessment for risk factors

Age <50, BMD testing if:
- Fragility fractures
- Systemic glucocorticoids >3 months/year
- Hypogonadism
- Premature menopause

Age 50–64, targeted BMD testing:
- Fragility fractures
- Systemic glucocorticoids >3 months/year
- Osteopenia on X-ray
- Other risk factors (Table 153.2)

Age >65
- All women should be tested
- Men with additional risk factors

BMD by DEXA at lumbar spine and hip

Normal | Osteopenia | Osteoporosis | Severe osteoporosis

Key points

- Dual-energy X-ray absorptiometry is the gold standard for bone density measurement.
- Laboratory investigations (FBC, serum calcium, creatinine, ALP, TFTs, PTH and 25-hydroxyvitamin D) are indicated to evaluate secondary causes of osteoporosis. If clinically indicated, serum protein electrophoresis and light chains, 24-urine calcium and anti-tissue transglutaminase antibodies should be performed.
- Bone turnover markers (e.g. C-terminal telopeptide of type 1 collagen) can be used to monitor the effects of treatment.

Osteoporosis is the most common bone disease and is characterised by compromised bone strength with increased susceptibility to fractures. Bone strength reflects the integration of bone density and bone quality. Bone density is expressed as grams of mineral per area or volume and in any given individual is determined by peak bone mass and amount of bone loss. Bone quality refers to architecture, turnover, damage accumulation (e.g. microfractures) and mineralisation. Osteoporosis is a major risk factor for fracture, particularly in postmenopausal women and older persons in general.

Bone densitometry

Currently there is no accurate measure of overall bone strength. Bone mineral density (BMD) is used as a proxy measure and accounts for approximately 70% of bone strength. The World Health Organization (WHO) defines osteoporosis as a BMD 2.5 standard deviations (SD) below the mean for young white adult women.

Dual-energy X-ray absorptiometry (DEXA) is the investigation of choice for diagnosing osteoporosis or low BMD, for estimating the future risk of fracture and for monitoring changes in BMD over time (Figure 153.1). DEXA measures bone mineral content (BMC, grams) and bone area (cm^2), then calculates BMD by dividing BMC by bone area. T-score is the parameter used for diagnosis of osteoporosis, which is calculated by subtracting the mean BMD of a young-adult reference population from the patient's BMD and dividing by the SD of young-adult population. The Z-score is used to compare the patient's BMD to a population of peers. It is calculated by subtracting the mean BMD of an age-, ethnicity- and sex-matched reference population from the patient's BMD and dividing by the SD of the reference population.

The diagnosis of osteoporosis can be made by DEXA using the lowest T-score of the lumbar spine (L1–L4), total proximal femur or femoral neck (Table 153.1). BMD measurement may not be valid in patients with skeletal structural abnormalities such as severe osteoarthritis or scoliosis. BMD measurements do not help predict fracture risk in other bone disorders (e.g. renal bone disease).

BMD can also be measured by quantitative CT. This tool can evaluate cortical and trabecular bone separately and is a sensitive measure of early bone loss in the vertebrae. However, this technique is more costly and results in greater exposure to radiation than DEXA.

Indications for bone densitometry test

The value of bone density in predicting fracture risk is established, and there is general consensus that bone density measurement is indicated in the conditions listed in Table 153.2.

Laboratory investigations

Laboratory investigations are indicated to rule out secondary causes of osteoporosis. These investigations should include FBC, measurements of serum calcium and creatinine, liver function tests (including ALP), TFTs, parathyroid hormone and 25-hydroxyvitamin D. If clinically indicated, serum protein electrophoresis and light chains, 24-urine calcium and anti-tissue transglutaminase antibodies should be performed. In men, osteoporosis often has secondary causes and the most frequent include excessive alcohol intake, hypogonadism and corticosteroid use. Therefore measurement of total testosterone is recommended in men with osteoporosis.

Vitamin D is critical for bone mineralisation. Vitamin D deficiency in adults can precipitate or exacerbate osteopenia and osteoporosis, cause osteomalacia and muscle weakness, and increase the risk of fracture. The serum 25-hydroxyvitamin D level is the best indicator of overall vitamin D status because this measurement reflects total vitamin D from dietary intake and sunlight exposure. 25-Hydroxyvitamin D levels change with the seasons, exposure to sunlight and dietary intake. Levels of vitamin D that fall below the 'target' range are very prevalent in many populations but there is no strong evidence to support the health benefits of vitamin D supplementation for those with mild insufficiency (40–60 nmol/L) on routine testing and might even be harmful.

Bone turnover markers

Bone turnover markers are classified as markers of bone resorption or bone formation (Table 153.3). ALP was the earliest marker of bone turnover and is useful in detecting conditions with gross elevations in turnover. A bone-specific ALP can also be measured and is more specific than ALP but there is up to 20% cross reactivity with the liver isoform.

Very high levels of bone turnover markers (>1.5 times upper reference limit) are suggestive of a cause other than postmenopausal osteoporosis. Other causes of increased bone turnover include acute fracture (elevated for up to 6 months), hyperparathyroidism, hyperthyroidism, Paget's disease, malignancy including myeloma or advanced-stage CKD.

Bone turnover markers can be used to monitor the effects of treatment. Bone resorption markers typically fall by over 40% within 3 months of starting bisphosphonate. Most bone turnover markers are renally excreted and increase in renal insufficiency, except for ALP.

154 Dementia

Table 154.1 Types of dementia

Type of dementia	Frequency	Features
Alzheimer's disease	70%	Poor judgement, disorientation, confusion, behaviour change and difficulty speaking, swallowing. Deposits of the protein fragment β-amyloid and protein tau in the brain
Vascular dementia	17%	Impaired judgement or ability to make decisions, plan or organise. Caused by multiple small or large strokes in the brain
Dementia with Lewy bodies	10%	Well-formed visual hallucinations, muscle rigidity or other Parkinsonian movement features. Lewy bodies present in the cortex
Frontotemporal lobar dementia	3%	Changes in personality and behaviour and difficulty with language. Neurons in the frontal and temporal regions are affected but no distinguishing microscopic pathology
Alcohol-related dementia	1%	Also called Korsakoff's syndrome, profound memory impairment. Caused by severe deficiency of thiamine
Mixed dementia		Characterised by the hallmark abnormalities of more than one type of dementia, most commonly Alzheimer's and vascular dementia

Table 154.2 Differences between dementia and delirium

Features	Dementia	Delirium
Onset	Slow, gradual	Acute
Causes	Alzheimer's disease	Infection, AMI, CCF, medications, pain
Reversible	No, progressive process	Yes
Attention impaired	No, until late stage	Yes
Consciousness	No	Impaired
Investigation	See below	See Chapter 155

Table 154.3 Other causes of cognitive impairment/dementia and key findings

Causes	Key findings
Vitamin B$_{12}$ deficiency	Ascending paraesthesiae, tongue soreness, limb weakness, weight loss
Normal-pressure hydrocephalus	Broad-based shuffling gait, urinary incontinence
Adverse effects from medication	Current use of psychoactive drugs, such as benzodiazepines or anticholinergics
Hypothyroidism	Fatigue, cold intolerance, constipation, weight gain, reduced body hair
Subdural haematoma	Head trauma within the previous 3 months, headache, seizures, hemiparesis, papilloedema
Wernicke–Korsakoff syndrome	History of alcoholism, nystagmus or extraocular muscle weakness, broad-based gait and stance
HIV-associated dementia	History of high-risk sexual behaviour or drug use, hyperreflexia, incoordination, peripheral neuropathy
Neurosyphilis	History of high-risk sexual behaviour or drug use, hyporeflexia, papillary abnormalities, decreased proprioception

Figure 154.4 Brain SPECT shows symmetrical reduced perfusion to both temporal, parietal and posterior frontal lobes consistent with Alzheimer's disease

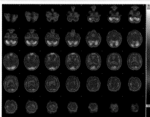

The goals of investigation in dementia are to:
- Confirm the diagnosis of dementia
- Identify treatable conditions which cause the dementia
- Determine the type of dementia

Table 154.4 Recommended basic investigations for patients with suspected dementia

Laboratory tests	Tests to consider in patients with specific risk factors
• Full blood count (FBC) • Biochemistry, calcium level • Urea, creatinine • Fasting blood glucose level • Liver function test • Folate and vitamin B$_{12}$ • Thyroid function tests • Urinalysis	• Lipid study • Chest X-ray (CXR) • Urine culture • Cerebrospinal fluid (CSF) analysis • HIV test • Syphilis serology • Apolipoprotein E

Figure 154.1 CT of the brain shows bilateral chronic subdural haematoma

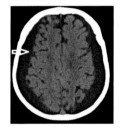

Figure 154.2 MRI of the head shows dilatation of the lateral and third ventricles out of keeping with cerebral atrophy suggestive of hydrocephalus

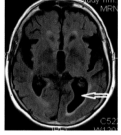

Figure 154.3 CT of the brain shows extensive periventricular white matter hypodensity consistent with chronic small-vessel ischaemic changes and cerebral atrophy

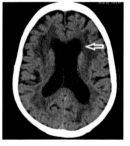

Key points

- FBC, biochemistry, creatinine, liver and thyroid function tests, vitamin B$_{12}$ and folate should be performed in patients with suspected dementia.
- Although brain imaging is neither diagnostic for dementia nor accurate in differentiating different subtypes of the condition, findings can identify pathologies that may mimic dementia.
- Genetic testing should only be considered in early-onset dementia.

Dementia affects 10% of those aged 65 years and older, with 20% of those aged 80 years and older suffering from severe dementia. The transition between normal cognition and dementia is cognitive impairment, which is defined as memory impairment without meeting criteria for dementia. Each year, 10–15% of patients with mild cognitive impairment develop Alzheimer's disease (AD). Types of dementia are listed in Table 154.1.

Risk factors for dementia include age, family history of dementia, apolipoprotein E4 genotype, cardiovascular comorbidities, chronic anticholinergic use, and lower educational level. The greatest risk factor for dementia is increasing age.

Initial clinical evaluation

Dementia can be diagnosed if cognitive or behavioural symptoms interfere with the patient's ability to function at work or socially, if there is a decline from previous functioning, and if cognitive or behavioural impairments are detected. The cognitive or behavioural impairments must be present in at least two of the following domains:

- ability to recall new information
- reasoning
- visuospatial ability
- language
- personality.

Mild cognitive impairment is defined as (i) impairment in at least one of these domains; (ii) concern about cognition as expressed by the patient, a caregiver or the clinician; and (iii) preservation of independence and the ability to work. When dementia is suspected, a history from the patient and especially from a family member or caregiver should be obtained because patients with dementia may not have insight into their deficits.

At first presentation, the three D's should be considered in the differential diagnosis of a patient with cognitive impairment: Dementia, Delirium and Depression. Dementia and depression share many similar features in older persons, including apathy, the inability to concentrate, societal withdrawal, and dramatic changes in mood and affect. Therefore depression should be assessed as part of the assessment for dementia. The Geriatric Depression Scale (GDS-15) (Yesavage, 1988) is a series of 15 yes/no questions; a score of 5 or greater is considered positive. The GDS-15 has a sensitivity of 72–93% and a specificity of 65–78% for detection of depression. A positive GDS-15 can help differentiate between dementia and depression. The differences between dementia and delirium are listed in Table 154.2. Other common causes of dementia which may be treatable are summarised in Table 154.3.

Testing for cognitive impairment

Mini-mental state examination (MMSE)

The MMSE is a 30-item questionnaire that assesses orientation, attention, concentration, memory, language, and construction abilities. It has good sensitivity (71–92%) and specificity (56–96%) for cognitive impairment. Lower educational levels can affect MMSE scores, and information on literacy and educational status should be gathered before scoring.

Clock drawing test

The clock drawing test is a quick cognitive assessment tool that evaluates organisation and planning. The patient is given a blank sheet of paper and told to draw the face of a clock with all the numbers, and then set the time to 10 minutes past 11. The clock drawing test can be graded as normal (time correctly shown with short hour hand and long minute hand, and numbers in the appropriate location) or abnormal (any other result) when it is used as part of a cognitive assessment.

Basic laboratory investigations

Table 154.4 lists the recommended basic investigations in any patient with suspected dementia. These tests help to rule out other causes, especially reversible causes of cognitive impairment.
- If the patient has a history of risk factors for sexually transmitted diseases, testing for syphilis and HIV infection is necessary.
- Lumbar puncture with CSF analysis may be indicated if there is suspicion of neurosyphilis, HIV infection, cerebral Lyme disease, or vasculitis.
- EEG can be considered in suspected delirium, frontotemporal dementia or Creutzfeldt–Jakob disease and associated seizure disorder.

Radiological investigations

The yield for neuroimaging in the investigation of dementia is low (approximately 5%); however, it is important to exclude alternative causes of dementia such as brain tumour, subdural haematoma (Figure 154.1) and normal-pressure hydrocephalus (Figure 154.2) that would otherwise be missed. If imaging studies are indicated, CT is the first choice; however, if there is a high degree of suspicion of alternative causes of dementia, MRI is the preferred study.

Neuroimaging should be considered in patients with:
- newly diagnosed dementia but no previous neuroimaging;
- onset of symptoms before 65 years;
- abrupt onset or rapid cognitive decline within weeks to months;
- focal neurological symptoms/signs;
- predisposing conditions such as malignancy, HIV infection, or receiving anticoagulation;
- patients with suspected subacute stroke, normal-pressure hydrocephalus, infection or subdural haematoma.

Cerebral atrophy, visualised on CT or MRI as enlarged ventricles and cortical sulci (Figure 154.3), is a feature that overlaps with normal ageing and other dementias, resulting in limited diagnostic value in AD. Neuroimaging can be useful for identifying cerebrovascular disease such as cerebral infarcts and white-matter lesions, which is important in identifying vascular dementia (Figure 154.3).

PET scan has good diagnostic sensitivity: hypometabolism in the temporal, parietal and posterior cingulate cortex can be used to differentiate patients with AD from cognitively normal elderly patients. PET can help differentiate among types of dementia, including frontotemporal dementia. PET may be considered as part of the evaluation of patients with dementia when presenting symptoms are unusual or there are diagnostic uncertainties between AD and frontotemporal dementia. Single photon emission computed tomography (SPECT) (Figure 154.4) can provide information similar to that obtained with PET.

155 Delirium

The main purpose of investigations in delirium is to:
- Identify factors that are contributing to the delirium
- Exclude potentially life-threatening disorders such as hypoxaemia, hypercapnia, hypoglycaemia, severe hyperglycaemia, acute myocardial infarction and sepsis

Is the patient at risk of delirium?

↓

Conduct or obtain baseline cognitive function assessment

↓

Determine any changes in cognitive function

↓

Assess for delirium with screen tool CAM

↓

Confirm the diagnosis of delirium

↓

Investigate for potentially reversible precipitating factors:

- Has hypoxia been excluded?
- Has hypotension been excluded?
- Has hypoglycaemia been excluded?
- Has electrolyte disturbance been excluded?
- Has a medication review been performed?
- Has an infection been excluded?
- Has urinary retention been excluded?
- Has constipation and faecal impaction been excluded?
- If person agitated/distressed, have pain, thirst and hunger been excluded?
- Is an alcohol withdrawal syndrome possible?

Table 155.1 Risk factors for delirium

Predisposing factors	Precipitating factors
• Dementia • Cognitive impairment • Previous history of delirium • Visual impairment • Hearing impairment • Severe medical illness • Depression • History of stroke or transient ischaemic attack (TIA) • Parkinson's disease • Alcohol misuse • Older age (>70 years) • Residential care residents	• Drugs: polypharmacy (see Table 155.2) • Renal failure • Hypoglycaemia • Hypovolaemia • Hypercarbia or hypoxaemia • Electrolyte disturbance: hyponatraemia, metabolic acidosis • Sepsis • Acute stroke • Surgery and anaesthesia • Trauma • Untreated pain • Sleep deprivation • Acute myocardial infarction (AMI) • Change of environment • Urinary retention • Constipation • Use of indwelling catheter • Use of physical restraints

Table 155.2 Common medications that can cause delirium

Antidepressants: amitriptyline, selective serotonin reuptake inhibitors (SSRIs)
Antipsychotics: haloperidol, olanzapine
Opioid analgesics: morphine, oxycodone
Anticonvulsants: levetiracetam
Beta-blockers: metoprolol, atenolol
Benzodiazepines: diazepam, nitrazepam
Digitalis: digoxin
Dopaminergic agents: levodopa, bromocriptine, pergolide
Steroids: prednisolone
NSAIDs: ibuprofen

Table 155.3 Basic laboratory investigations for delirium

Medical conditions	Suggested investigations
Baseline investigations	FBC, electrolytes, calcium, creatinine, glucose, liver and thyroid function
Sepsis	Urinalysis, blood and urine culture, CXR, CRP
AMI	ECG and troponin
Respiratory failure	Arterial blood gases (ABG)
Malnutrition	Vitamin B12, folate levels
Drug toxicity	Measurement of drug levels

Key points

- FBC, biochemistry including serum glucose, calcium, liver and thyroid function tests should be performed in the initial evaluation of delirium.
- Relevant culture of body fluids should be performed if a focus of infection is suspected to be the cause of delirium.
- ABG should be performed if hypoxia or hypercapnia is suspected to contribute to the delirium.
- Brain imaging is indicated if there are new-onset focal neurological abnormalities associated with the delirium.

Delirium is a complex syndrome characterised by fluctuating disturbances of consciousness, attention, memory, perception and thought. The highest incidence of delirium is noted in postoperative, palliative-care and intensive-care settings. The prevalence of delirium in general medical and aged care wards is 18–35% but low in the community (1–2%). The mean duration of delirium is 7 days. Delirium is associated with increased mortality, decline in physical function and increased rates of cognitive decline. There are three subtypes of delirium.

• Hyperactive delirium: restless, agitated, delusional, risk of harm.
• Hypoactive delirium: lethargic, monosyllabic, often overlooked.
• Mixed type.

The cause of delirium is usually multifactorial in elderly people but can have a single factor. The common risk factors and precipitating factors for delirium are listed in Table 155.1.

Delirium is a clinical diagnosis, which is often unrecognised and easily overlooked. Key diagnostic features are an acute onset and fluctuating course of symptoms, impaired consciousness, inattention, and diffuse cognitive impairment (e.g. disorientation, memory impairment, language changes). Supportive features include disturbance in sleep–wake cycle, hallucinations, delusions, psychomotor disturbance (hypoactive or hyperactive), inappropriate behaviour and emotional lability.

The most important step in diagnosing delirium is to obtain a history from the patient and a collateral history from family member, caregiver or staff member. The most widely used instrument for identification of delirium is the Confusion Assessment Method (CAM), which is specifically designed for use with the hospitalised older person to improve delirium identification and recognition and has been validated in high-quality studies. Instruments that are used to measure the severity of delirium include the Delirium Rating Scale (DRS) and Memorial Delirium Assessment Scale.

Review medications

Table 155.2 lists common medications that can cause delirium. Reviewing medications that may cause delirium is the first step in the investigation of delirium, focusing particularly on those which have been commenced recently.

Laboratory investigations

Basic laboratory investigations for delirium are listed in Table 155.3. Beware of blaming common mildly abnormal findings such as bacteriuria or mild hyponatraemia as the sole cause of delirium and look for other contributors.

Lumbar puncture

Lumbar puncture should be considered when meningitis, encephalitis or subarachnoid haemorrhage is suspected, and might be indicated when delirium is persistent or no cause can be identified.

EEG

EEG has little sensitivity and specificity in the diagnosis of delirium and should not be used routinely. However, delirium has a characteristic pattern of diffuse slowing with increased theta and delta activity and poor organisation of background rhythm and this correlates with severity of delirium. EEG can be useful in distinguishing organic causes from functional or psychiatric disorders in difficult-to-assess patients with dementia, and in the identification of occult seizures such as non-convulsive status epilepticus or atypical complex partial seizures.

Radiological investigations

Neuroimaging, including non-contrast head CT and MRI, has a low yield in unselected patients. It is recommended in the assessment of patients with focal neurological findings, because stroke or intracranial haemorrhage can present with delirium, and in patients with a history or signs of recent fall, unexplained decreased consciousness level or fever associated with encephalopathy.

156 Falls

Key points

- FBC, electrolytes, urea, creatinine, LFT and calcium should be evaluated to identify any reversible contributing factors to the fall.
- ECG, echocardiography and occasionally Holter monitor are indicated if a cardiac-related condition is suspected to be contributing to the fall.
- X-ray of the relevant region and CT head may be indicated if an injury is suspected to be sustained as a result of the fall.
- Risk of osteoporosis and secondary causes of bone loss should be investigated as clinically indicated.

Box 156.2 Basic laboratory investigations

- FBC
- Electrolytes
- Urea, creatinine
- Glucose
- Calcium
- Albumin
- Vitamin B$_{12}$, folate
- TFTs

Figure 156.2 CT head shows a moderate subdural haematoma extending around the left hemisphere

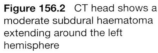
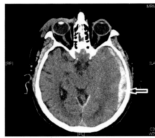

Figure 156.3 Anterior–posterior X-ray of the pelvis shows transcervical fracture through the left neck of femur

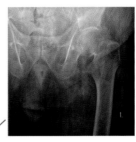

Figure 156.1 ECG shows third-degree heart block

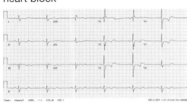

Vision test

Hearing impairment

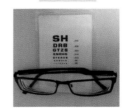
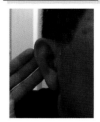

Figure 156.4 X-ray of the right wrist shows an impacted fracture of the distal radius with mild dorsal angulation: (a) lateral view; (b) posterior–anterior view

(a)   (b)

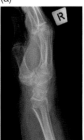
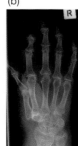

Hearing test

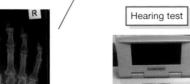

Box 156.1 Common drugs that can cause falls

- Antidepressants
- Antihypertensives
- Antipsychotics (typical and atypical)
- Benzodiazepines (short- and long-acting)
- Cholinesterase inhibitors
- Diuretics
- NSAIDs
- Sedatives and hypnotics

Clinical Investigations at a Glance, First Edition. Jonathan Gleadle, Jordan Li and Tuck Yong. © 2017 John Wiley & Sons, Ltd. Published 2017 by John Wiley & Sons, Ltd.

Falls are common in elderly people and are the leading cause of injury-related admissions to hospital, accounting for 14% of emergency admissions and 4% of all hospital admissions in people aged over 65 years. Falls are associated with increased morbidity and mortality, and nursing home placement.

Falls are often multifactorial in origin. The presence of the following factors is associated with falls and with greater probability of future falls:

- acute illness such as pneumonia and UTI;
- chronic underlying medical diseases such as Parkinson's disease and frailty;
- environmental hazards such as loose rugs;
- motor problems, such as gait disturbance and balance impairment, muscle weakness;
- sensory impairment, such as peripheral neuropathy, vestibular dysfunction, vision impairment;
- cognitive or mood impairment, such as dementia and depression;
- postural hypotension, dizziness, vertigo, syncope;
- polypharmacy or certain medicines such as psychotropic drugs (Box 156.1);
- urine incontinence;
- impairment of activities of daily living;
- age over 80 years.

Obtaining a detailed history of the fall and careful physical examination is the first step before the appropriate investigations. Postural hypotension and medications are common causes of fall. The 'Get up and go' test is a good test for functional status and fall risk. This is the time it takes for a person to stand up from a straight back chair, walk 3 m, and return and sit down: 10 seconds is normal; 11–20 seconds is normal for a frail or disabled patient; more than 20 seconds is abnormal and warrants further assessment. Identifying the circumstances and the symptoms associated with a fall will help to identify the risk factor(s) most likely to be contributing to falls.

Laboratory investigations (Box 156.2)

The role of laboratory and other investigations is to identify potentially treatable causes for falls. The recommended laboratory tests in patients with falls or at risk for falling include FBC, electrolytes, urea, creatinine, glucose, calcium, albumin, vitamin B_{12}, folate, and TFTs. These tests are relatively inexpensive, and abnormal results may suggest the presence of a treatable condition such as anaemia, dehydration, hypoglycaemia or hyperglycaemia. If the patient had been on the ground for more than 30 min, creatine kinase (CK) should be measured to ascertain if rhabdomyolysis is present that may warrant clinical intervention. CK and troponin may also be elevated if myocardial infarction is the cause of the syncope and fall. It is important to distinguish between fall and syncope (see Chapter 28).

ECG

ECG should be performed and followed by an echocardiogram if the fall is related to a syncopal episode or a cardiac-related problem is identified (Figure 156.1). A Holter monitor (24-hour ambulatory ECG) is not recommended unless there is clinical evidence of arrhythmia, such as a known history of cardiac events or an abnormal ECG. In elderly persons, this technique is associated with frequent false positives and false negatives.

Radiological investigations

CT of the head

Neuroimaging is indicated only if there is a head injury or new focal neurological findings on physical examination or if a central nervous system process is suspected on the basis of the history or examination. Occasionally, patients may sustain an intracranial haemorrhage or subdural haematoma (Figure 156.2) as a result of a head injury during the fall.

Plain X-ray

X-ray of the hip and/or wrist is indicated if injuries are suspected in those regions during the fall. Fractured neck of femur or pubic ramus (Figure 156.3) occurs quite commonly with falls among older people. Fracture of the distal radius (Figure 156.4) is another common site of injury following a fall especially if the patient had landed with an outstretched arm.

CXR

CXR is indicated if there is a cardiac or pulmonary condition that may have contributed to the fall. Another indication for CXR is to assess for rib fractures or aspiration pneumonia if the patient has vomited.

Bone densitometry and evaluation of osteoporosis

Low bone density increases the risk of hip and other fractures and should be identified and treated. Calcium and 25-hydroxyvitamin D levels should be checked (see Chapter 153).

Other investigations

EEG should be performed if a seizure is suspected. Formal vision and hearing assessments should be considered. Electromyography (EMG) is used for evaluation of peripheral neuropathy. Tilt table test is indicated in patients with recurrent falls due to syncope.

Urinary incontinence

The aim of investigation is to:
- Identify possible reversible causes leading to transient or acute incontinence
- Determine the type of incontinence
- Aid in treatment planning

Table 157.1 Common reversible causes of urinary incontinence

Mixed urinary incontinence
UTI
Constipation
Depression
Poorly controlled diabetes leading to polyuria
Drugs
Reduced mobility
Cognitive impairment
Delirium
Morbid obesity
Restricted mobility
Menopause, atrophic urethritis or vaginitis

Medications that can cause urinary incontinence
Antidepressants
Antipsychotics
Sedatives/hypnotics
Diuretics
Caffeine
Anticholinergics
Alcohol
Opioids
Beta-blockers
Calcium channel blockers

Patient presents with urinary incontinence
↓
Three-day bladder diary and cough test
↓
Urinary analysis and culture, measure post-void volume, consider renal and/or pelvic ultrasound, review medications
↓
- **Abnormal** Treat reversible causes
- **Normal** Further symptoms assessment
↓
Consider urodynamic and other investigations
↓
- Stress urinary incontinence
- Urgency urinary incontinence
- Mixed urinary incontinence
- Overflow incontinence

Key points

- Urinalysis and urine microscopy and culture should be performed to ascertain any UTI contributing to the incontinence.
- Ultrasound of the bladder to determine the post-void residual volume is a useful investigation of urinary incontinence. A high volume is indicative of incomplete bladder emptying and possible bladder outflow obstruction.
- Urodynamic testing aims to determine if there is an underlying abnormality of voiding or storage and make a definitive objective diagnosis.
- Impaired mobility and cognition may need to be investigated to determine if these factors are contributing to urinary incontinence.

Urinary incontinence is defined as involuntary loss of urine. The condition is common among older people. It affects more than 20% of people aged over 85 years though this is probably an underestimate. Although women report incontinence more often than men, after 80 years of age both sexes are affected equally. Urinary incontinence has both physical and psychological consequences, including damage to skin, UTIs, an increased risk of falls, depression, social embarrassment and dependence on caregivers.

Classification

Urinary incontinence can be classified as acute reversible incontinence and chronic incontinence, with the latter further classified as follows.
• *Stress urinary incontinence* (SUI): involuntary urinary leakage during physical exertion (sneezing, laugh or coughing) caused by sphincter weakness or in men after prostate surgery.
• *Urgency urinary incontinence* (UUI): involuntary leakage accompanied by or immediately preceded by urgency. It is a result of detrusor overactivity, and can be further divided into two subtypes: sensory (a result of local irritation, inflammation or infection within the bladder) or neurological (loss of cerebral inhibition of detrusor contractions).
• *Mixed urinary incontinence*: ageing increases the prevalence of SUI and UUI, and the two often coexist, leading to mixed incontinence that accounts for 30% of adult incontinence.
• *Overflow incontinence*: leakage caused by impaired detrusor contractility, bladder outlet obstruction or both, resulting in overdistension of the bladder.
• *Functional incontinence*: an inability to reach or use the toilet in time due to poor mobility or cognitive impairment.

Clinical evaluation

Initial history and physical examination are vital in attempting to identify reversible causes (Table 157.1). The number and type of pads used should be ascertained and nocturnal incontinence enquired about. A digital rectal examination will allow evaluation of prostate size, and a vaginal examination may find prolapse of pelvic organs or atrophic vaginitis.

Initial investigations

Voiding diary

This records the frequency of incontinence and the situations where episodes of incontinence occur. A 3-day diary is as reliable and informative as a longer-term assessment.

Cough stress test

When compared with more sophisticated multichannel urodynamic studies, the cough stress test demonstrates good sensitivity and specificity for stress incontinence, although it requires further confirmatory urodynamic evaluation if the results are inconclusive.

Urinalysis and urine culture

Urinalysis can be used to detect or rule out infection. If haematuria, proteinuria and glycosuria are present, it may require further investigation. A mid-stream urine specimen should be sent for culture and analysis of antibiotic sensitivities if urinalysis is suggestive of infection.

Laboratory investigations

Serum creatinine and glucose should be measured to exclude urinary obstruction leading to renal failure and diabetes leading to polyuria.

Post-void residual volume

The post-void residual volume can be measured using a portable ultrasound machine. In general a volume above 100 mL is considered abnormal and indicative of incomplete bladder emptying and possible bladder outflow obstruction. Renal and pelvic ultrasound can identify urinary tract obstruction, prostate enlargement and pelvic organ prolapse.

Urodynamic and other investigations

Urodynamic testing aims to determine if there is an underlying abnormality of voiding or storage and make a definitive objective diagnosis. This will assist in selecting the treatment most likely to be successful. However, the investigations are invasive and time-consuming. Urodynamic testing is not indicated for all patients because urinary incontinence can often be classified on the basis of history, examination and basic investigations. Urodynamic tests are not recommended before trial of conservative treatment but should be performed before surgery for SUI. In multichannel cystometry, catheters are inserted into the bladder and rectum or into the vagina to measure the detrusor pressure. The test replicates the patient's symptoms by filling the bladder and observing changes in pressure and urinary leakage with provocation tests such as jogging on the spot. To undergo the test, patients must be mobile and without advanced cognitive impairment.

Urodynamic testing is considered in women before surgery for stress incontinence if:
1 overactivity of the detrusor muscle is suspected;
2 symptoms of incomplete bladder emptying are present;
3 the patient has had previous surgery for SUI or prolapse.
Consider ambulatory urodynamic or video-urodynamic tests if the diagnosis is unclear after conventional urodynamic tests.

There is no role for cystoscopy in the initial assessment of urinary incontinence alone. Do not use imaging (MRI, CT and X-ray) for the routine assessment of urinary incontinence.

158 Allergy and anaphylaxis

The purpose of investigations is to:
- Establish that the presentation is an allergic reaction
- Identify the allergens which trigger the allergic reaction
- Detect and quantify mediators of anaphylaxis released by mast cells (e.g. tryptase)
- Assess disease activity

Key points

- Skin-prick tests are valuable when they are negative (NPV >95%).
- Intradermal testing has a higher false-positive rate and greater risk of adverse reactions; therefore, it should not be used for initial investigations.
- IgE concentration is a poor guide to allergic status. The normal range is very wide, and normal levels of IgE can be associated with very high levels of IgE to a single allergen.
- A positive skin test or serum food-specific IgE test result indicates sensitisation but not necessarily clinical allergy.

Figure 158.1
Positive skin-prick test

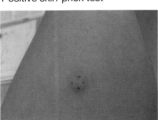

Table 158.1 Comparison of skin prick testing and specific IgE testing

Specific IgE testing	Skin-prick testing
Sensitive, safe, no risk for anaphylaxis, expensive	Often greater sensitivity than specific IgE
Widely available	Available in centres with appropriate reagents, equipment, and trained staff
Results can take days to weeks	Results in 15 min, visible to patients
No interference from drugs, suitable for patients with skin disease	Antihistamines, beta-blockers and some antidepressants can interfere with results
Standardised laboratory assay	Observer-dependent, experience/expertise required
Interference from high total IgE can cause positive results without clinical allergy	No interference from high total IgE

Allergic diseases are due to allergic inflammation as a result of an interaction between the environment and the patient's immune system, leading to the release of histamine and other proinflammatory mediators. Allergic reactions manifest as anaphylaxis, allergic asthma, urticaria, angioedema, allergic rhinitis, some types of drug reactions, and atopic dermatitis. These reactions are mediated by IgE, which differentiates them from pseudoallergic (formerly called anaphylactoid) reactions that involve IgE-independent mast cell and basophil degranulation. These pseudoallergic reactions can be caused by iodinated radiocontrast, opiates, NSAIDs and vancomycin and appear similar clinically to allergic reactions by resulting in urticaria or anaphylactoid reaction. Before allergy testing is carried out, a focused history is essential.

Non-specific markers of allergy

On FBC, an elevated eosinophil count may be observed in patients with atopic disease and serum IgE level is often raised. There are causes other than allergy of eosinophilia and elevated IgE. Conversely, significant allergic disease can occur in the absence of an elevated IgE or eosinophilia. Measuring serum tryptase level may be helpful (see next section).

Allergen-specific IgE *in-vitro* tests

These tests detect allergen-specific IgE in the serum. Patient serum is incubated with allergen or allergen mixtures bound to a solid material. Allergen-specific IgE is then detected using antibodies specific for human IgE that are labelled with either enzyme or a fluorescent compound. Detectable specific IgE does not necessarily imply a clinical allergy. Moreover, the level of specific IgE does not predict the severity of symptoms. Patients can be sensitised, meaning that they have raised serum concentrations of specific IgE to an allergen without associated immediate symptoms when exposed. The higher the specific IgE, the more likely it is that the test result will be clinically relevant. Incorrect use of specific IgE as a screening test, without a compatible history, can lead to food allergy being erroneously diagnosed, with the consequences of an unnecessarily restricted diet and patient anxiety. Requests for specific IgE testing must be tailored to the clinical history and with an appreciation of its limitations (Table 158.1).

Skin-prick testing

Skin-prick testing remains the gold standard for detection of allergen-specific IgE. This procedure requires experience for accurate interpretation and may rarely induce anaphylaxis. Therefore, it should be performed by trained practitioners with resuscitation facilities available. It involves the epicutaneous introduction of allergen extracts with a standardised lancet. Typically, the volar aspect of the forearm is used. The site is then inspected 15 min later and compared with suitable positive and negative controls. A weal more than 3 mm in diameter than the negative control is considered a positive test (Figure 158.1). Accurate interpretation requires an appropriate clinical history. Skin-prick tests may fail to show sensitisation when antihistamines are used concurrently. With fruits and vegetables, skin-prick testing with fresh allergen is desirable as the performance of the distilled extract is poor. The choice of specific IgE or skin-prick testing should be individualised to the patient and reflect the advantages and limitations of each test (Table 158.1).

In patients with suspected penicillin allergy, skin testing with benzylpenicilloyl polylysine can identify 93% of patients at risk. Penicillin skin testing, even when positive, does not predict risk of allergy with cephalosporins. In patients with penicillin allergy, the risk of adverse effects from cephalosporin therapy may be as high as 10% but anaphylaxis occurs in less than 0.02% of cases.

Oral food challenge testing

Food allergy is an adverse immune response to food proteins. Reactions may be IgE-mediated, non-IgE-mediated, or a mixture of both reactions. The gold standard test to confirm or refute the diagnosis of immediate food allergy is the double-blind placebo-controlled food challenge. Blinded challenges allow confident identification of clinical allergy and exclude asymptomatic sensitisation and functional symptoms. This approach is particularly important when the history and test results are ambiguous. In practice, most centres provide unblinded challenges by giving increasing amounts of suspected allergen over time under medical supervision. Direct mucosal exposure (allergen held to lip) is the first stage of of the challenge before titrated oral ingestion.

Anaphylaxis

Anaphylaxis is a severe life-threatening systemic allergic reaction involving the respiratory and/or cardiovascular systems, usually with additional cutaneous and/or gastrointestinal features. It usually occurs within half an hour of allergen exposure but may take up to 2 hours to develop. Allergy to medicines (57% of anaphylaxis-related deaths), insect stings (16%), food (6%) is the most frequent cause.

Characteristic reactions with urticaria accompanied by cardiovascular or respiratory distress are easy to recognise. However, some reactions can have atypical presentations. Sudden onset of symptoms affecting two or more organ systems or just hypotension on its own, or cardiac arrest even without cutaneous involvement, should prompt consideration of the diagnosis and investigation, especially if there is recent exposure to a potential allergen or stimulant.

Serum tryptase level

Measurement of mast cell tryptase may be useful where the diagnosis is uncertain but is not necessary when the diagnosis of anaphylaxis is definite. Serum samples should be taken as soon as possible after emergency treatment and a second sample ideally within 1–2 hours (but no later than 4 hours) from the onset of symptoms. Peak levels occur within 1–2 hours of reaction onset. Single measurements of tryptase have low sensitivity because the peak may be missed or occur within the reference interval. Serial measurements (arrival, 1 hour later, and then in convalescence) improve sensitivity by up to 75%. High tryptase may be due to mastocytosis and it is important to follow an elevated result with a convalescent sample to exclude this diagnosis. Tryptase is more useful in insect venom and medication-related anaphylaxis than in food-associated anaphylaxis.

Identifying triggers of anaphylaxis

Accurate identification of the causative allergen guides future avoidance. Following thorough history taking, skin-prick or blood allergen-specific IgE testing may be indicated. For skin-prick testing, appropriate safety precautions should be implemented. For food allergy, skin testing has a positive predictive value of less than 40% and a negative predictive value above 95%. If a causative food has not been identified but food allergy is suspected, a food challenge might be necessary as the specific food avoidance might be life-saving.

159 Primary immunodeficiency disorders

The purpose of investigations is to:
- Identify if an underlying immunodeficiency disorder explains the patient's presentation
- Diagnose the defect responsible for the immunodeficiency
- Diagnose and guide management of associated infective complications

Table 159.2 Investigations for primary immunodeficiency

FBC: lymphocyte, neutrophil and eosinophil numbers
Neutrophil function: respiratory burst, chemotaxis, CD18 expression
Lymphocyte subset analysis
Lymphocyte responses to mitogens and antigens in vivo
Measurements of T-cell effector cytokine production (including intracellular cytokine staining by flow cytometry and Elispot analysis)
Serum IgG, IgA, IgM and IgE levels
Serum IgG subclasses
IgG anti-vaccine levels: pneumococcus, tetanus, diphtheria
Total complement, CH50
A and B isohaemagglutinins

Table 159.1 Features suggestive of primary immunodeficiency disorders

Four or more episodes of infection within 12 months
Two or more serious sinus infections within 12 months
Two or more pneumonias within 12 months
Two or more deep-seated infections including septicaemia
Recurrent deep skin or organ abscesses
Persistent oral or skin fungal infections
Infection does not respond to >2 months of standard antibiotics
Intravenous antibiotics needed to clear infections
Failure to thrive or growth retardation
Family history of primary immunodeficiency disorders

Key points

- FBC and differential counts should be one of the initial investigations of primary immunodeficiency disorders.
- Immunophenotyping of lymphocyte subpopulations using flow cytometry can help to define both the presence and type of immunodeficiency, in particular cellular immunodeficiency.
- Quantitative serum immunoglobulin tests are used to detect abnormal levels of IgG, IgA and IgM and should be performed if a patient has symptoms suggestive of an immunoglobulin deficiency.
- Tests evaluating neutrophil function (e.g. oxidative burst assay) can be performed in the assessment of chronic granulomatous disease.

Clinical Investigations at a Glance, First Edition. Jonathan Gleadle, Jordan Li and Tuck Yong. © 2017 John Wiley & Sons, Ltd. Published 2017 by John Wiley & Sons, Ltd.

Primary immunodeficiency is a predisposition to infections associated with a deficiency of certain immune components, which are usually inherited. Secondary or acquired immunodeficiency may be caused by drug toxicities, infection or malignancy.

Primary immunodeficiency disorders can be classified as T-cell or T-cell-mediated deficiencies or as B-cell or B-cell antibody deficiencies, and as combined deficiencies, deficiencies affecting phagocytes, deficiencies of cytokine or complement pathways, and syndromic immunodeficiency.

Primary immunodeficiency tends to be associated with excessively frequent or severe infections, sometimes with organisms of low pathogenicity (Table 159.1). Disorders involving B cells result in antibody deficiency, with sinopulmonary infections caused by encapsulated organisms such as *Streptococcus pneumoniae* or *Haemophilus influenzae*. T-cell or combined immunodeficiency disorders may show a lack of antibody and display bacterial infections as well as an inability to mount an immune response against viral and fungal infections. Disorders of phagocytic function result in recurrent soft-tissue infections caused by pyogenic bacteria and/or fungi at multiple sites. Complement deficiencies may result in infections caused by encapsulated pyogenic bacteria, especially *Neisseria* species.

Haematological investigations

FBC may reveal lymphopenia (seen in combined immunodeficiency), neutropenia (congenital or acquired neutropenia) or thrombocytopenia.

Lymphocyte immunophenotyping

Immunophenotyping of lymphocyte subpopulations using flow cytometry can help to define both the presence and type of immunodeficiency, in particular cellular immunodeficiency. If a T-cell deficiency is suspected, then T-cell stimulation assays may be performed.

Immunoglobulin

Quantitative serum immunoglobulin tests are used to detect abnormal levels of IgG, IgA and IgM and should be performed if a patient has symptoms suggestive of an immunoglobulin deficiency, such as family history of immunodeficiency, recurrent or unusual bacterial infections, lack of response to antibiotics, unusual or recurrent viral infections and/or chronic unexplained diarrhoea. Patients with immunoglobulin deficiency are particularly predisposed to recurrent sinopulmonary infections, especially with polysaccharide-encapsulated organisms including *S. pneumoniae* and *H. influenzae*. Hypogammaglobulinaemia is more frequently due to secondary rather than primary causes.

Complement

Inherited deficiencies of the complement pathway cause sinopulmonary infections and, potentially, autoimmune disease and are best tested by measuring total classical and alternative complement pathway activity.

Other investigations

Tests evaluating neutrophil function (e.g. oxidative burst assay) can be performed in the assessment of chronic granulomatous disease. Specific antibody response to vaccines such as tetanus and pneumococcus provide a qualitative assessment of immunoglobulin function and can assist in the diagnosis of conditions such as specific antibody deficiency. Such patients have normal immunoglobulin levels but poor specific response to vaccines. Genetic testing may be available for some forms of primary immunodeficiency. The suggested investigations for primary immunodeficiency are summarised in Table 159.2.

160 Skin cancers

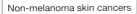

Non-melanoma skin cancers

Melanoma

Figure 160.1 Clinical evaluation: SCC on the lip

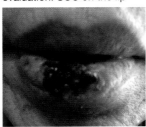

Figure 160.6 Clinical evaluation: a melanoma

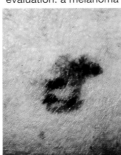

Box 160.1 ABCDE mnemonic for evaluating melanoma

- **A**symmetry: one half of lesion is different from the other half
- **B**order: irregular or poorly defined border
- **C**olour: varies from one area to another; different shades of tan, brown or black; sometimes red, white or blue within the same lesion
- **D**iameter: larger than 6 mm
- **E**volving: a mole that looks different compared with surrounding moles ('ugly duckling' sign) or the mole is changing in size, shape or colour

Figure 160.2 Dermoscopy examination

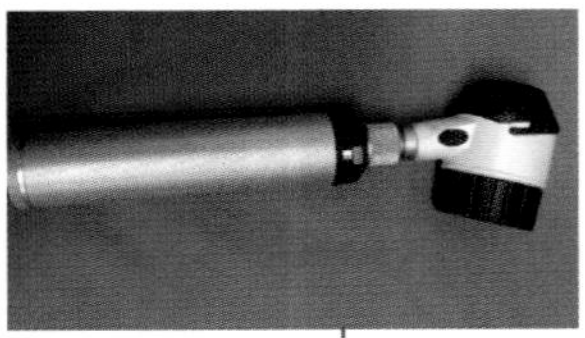

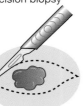

Figure 160.7 Excision biopsy for suspected melanoma

Figure 160.8 Histological examination shows a typical melanoma

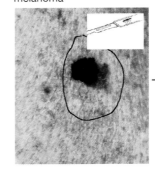
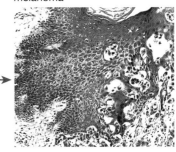

Figure 160.4 Punch biopsy

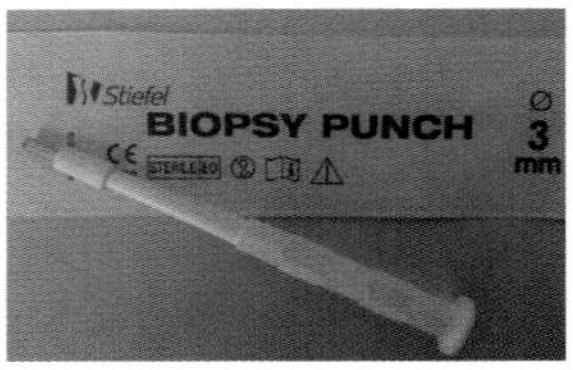

Figure 160.3 Excision biopsy

Figure 160.5 Shave biopsy

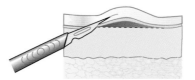

Box 160.2 Histological examination of melanoma

- Breslow thickness
- Margins of excision (microscopic)
- Mitotic rate/mm^2
- Level of invasion (Clark)
- Ulceration

Table 160.1 Factors associated with poor prognosis in non-melanoma skin cancer

	Basal-cell carcinoma	Squamous cell carcinoma
Tumour size	>5 cm	>2 cm
Tumour depth	—	>6 mm
Tumour site	Facial region	At sites of radiation, thermal damage, ulceration, sinuses, scars or Bowen's disease, non-sun exposed sites, ear, lip
Histological features	Morphoeic, infiltrative, micronodular, perineural or perivascular involvement	Poorly differential, spindle cell (carcinosarcomas), perineural involvement
Immunosuppression	+	+
Recurrent lesions	+	+
Lymph node involvement or distant metastases	Rarely	+

Key points

- Dermoscopy is a useful tool which increases the accuracy of a dermatologist in diagnosing melanoma.
- Any suspicious lesions should undergo full-thickness biopsy into the underlying subcutaneous tissue with a 2 mm border. Appropriate methods of biopsy can vary, including shave, punch and excisional biopsy. Shave biopsies should not be used if melanoma is suspected.
- It is important to obtain an adequate specimen that will allow a definitive diagnosis and measurement of the Breslow depth in melanoma.
- Sentinel node biopsy in patients with melanoma with a Breslow depth ≥1.0 mm is useful for staging and prognosis.

Clinical Investigations at a Glance, First Edition. Jonathan Gleadle, Jordan Li and Tuck Yong. © 2017 John Wiley & Sons, Ltd. Published 2017 by John Wiley & Sons, Ltd.

Skin cancers are the most common cancers and incidence is rising across the world. Early detection and treatment can reduce the morbidity and mortality associated with skin cancer. Skin cancers can be classified as follows.

- Non-melanoma skin cancers: basal cell carcinoma (BCC, 68%), squamous cell carcinoma (SCC, 28%) and rare tumours (e.g. Merkel cell carcinoma, 1%).
- Melanoma (3%).

Solar radiation is the most important risk factor for skin cancers. Human papillomaviruses are associated with non-melanoma skin cancers, especially in immunocompromised individuals. Long-term iatrogenic immunosuppression, as in organ transplantation, predisposes to skin cancers.

Non-melanoma skin cancers

Clinical evaluation

Early BCCs are usually small, translucent or pearly lesions and the majority occur on the head and neck regions. SCCs usually develops on sun-exposed areas (Figure 160.1). If a specific benign lesion can be diagnosed confidently, it may be left alone. However if there is uncertainty, excision biopsy should be performed. The clinical diagnostic accuracy of experienced dermatologists for BCC is 60% and for SCC is 40%.

Dermoscopy

Dermoscopy (Figure 160.2) with cross-polarised light, high-frequency (20–100 MHz) ultrasound, optical coherence tomography with infrared light, and *in vivo* confocal microscopy can be used for early detection of non-melanoma skin cancer but do not replace biopsy.

Excision biopsy

The gold standard for diagnosis and treatment is elliptical excision biopsy (Figure 160.3). If a lesion is too large or too difficult for simple elliptical excision, it should be biopsied or referred for specialist review. The choice of other biopsy technique can be determined by the site, size and shape of the lesion. For thicker lesions, a punch biopsy (Figure 160.4) is more appropriate so that deeper cells are included. For thin lesions, a partial shave biopsy (Figure 160.5) is better as it provides a larger surface area of malignant cells.

A well-defined cancer of 10 mm or less should be excised with a 2–3 mm margin. With larger and more poorly defined lesions, the excision margin should be 4–5 mm. Positive margins, or within 0.5 mm for an SCC, require re-excision (or referral) until clear margins are achieved.

Staging, prognosis and follow-up

The likelihood of metastases and recurrence of SCC and BCC depends on several prognostic indicators (Table 160.1). Metastasis rarely develops from BCC. Routine sentinel lymph node (SLN) biopsy is not justified in patients with high-risk SCC. If there is suspicion of regional lymph node spread, a regional CT should be performed with subsequent fine-needle aspiration. Open surgical biopsy should be avoided.

Excision with clear margins on histology gives a 96% cure rate. Patients who have had a non-melanoma skin cancer removed should have a yearly skin check to assess cancer site and draining lymph nodes and identify any new skin cancers. For patients with a high-risk SCC, follow-up should be every 3 months.

Melanoma

Melanoma risk depends on genetic and environmental factors. About 10% of cutaneous melanomas have familial predisposition. Melanoma develops from pre-existing naevi in about 20–40% of cases, with the remaining 60–80% of cases thought to occur *de novo*.

Clinical evaluation

Early visual detection of melanoma increases the cure rate. The 5-year survival from melanoma is 96% if localised, 63% if spread is regional, and only 34% with metastatic melanoma. Early identification of melanoma involves examination of the straightforward features of melanoma using the ABCDE rules of melanoma recognition (Figure 160.6 and Box 160.1). Total-body photography is used for patients who are under observation because of large numbers of atypical naevi. Population-based screening is not recommended but high-risk patients should undergo surveillance.

Dermoscopy

Dermoscopy or epiluminescence microscopy allows rapid and magnified (×10) *in vivo* observation of skin lesions with a hand-held instrument. The use of dermoscopy can decrease the number of unnecessary biopsies. Nodular or amelanotic melanomas are often difficult to diagnose.

Biopsy and histological diagnosis

Excision biopsy with 2-mm margins should be performed whenever possible in lesions suspected of melanoma (Figure 160.7). Histological examination (Figure 160.8 and Box 160.2) allows planning of definitive treatment and whether or not to recommend SLN biopsy.

Immediate wide excision with margins based on a clinical estimate of tumour thickness may result in inadequate or excessive tumour clearance. It may also compromise subsequent management by making it impossible to perform accurate lymphatic mapping to identify draining lymph node fields and SLNs within those fields. Punch biopsies, incision biopsies and shave biopsies are frequently unsatisfactory and result in misdiagnosis due to unrepresentative sampling.

Genetic screen

If there is a strong family history of melanoma, screening for a genetic mutation such as the *CDKN2A* gene can be considered, accompanied by genetic counselling. The major hereditary melanoma susceptibility gene, *CDKN2A*, is mutated in approximately 40% of families with three or more melanoma cases. Over half of the families with multiple cases of melanoma have no identified mutation.

Further investigation after the diagnosis of melanoma

- Following the diagnosis of primary cutaneous melanoma (stage I, II), routine investigations are not required for asymptomatic patients.
- The risk of metastasis to regional lymph nodes rises with increasing tumour thickness. SLN biopsy currently provides the most accurate prognostic information for melanomas of all thicknesses. Patients suspected of having lymph node metastasis or melanoma greater than 1 mm in thickness should have SLN biopsy under ultrasound guidance.
- Serum LDH, CT, MRI and/or PET are indicated for symptoms suggestive of metastatic melanoma.

161 Skin rashes

Figure 161.1
Maculopapular rash

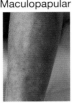

Figure 161.2
Vesicular-bullous rash

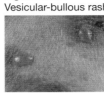

Figure 161.3
Pustular rash

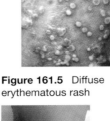

Figure 161.4
Exanthematous rash

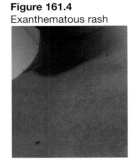

Figure 161.5 Diffuse erythematous rash

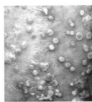

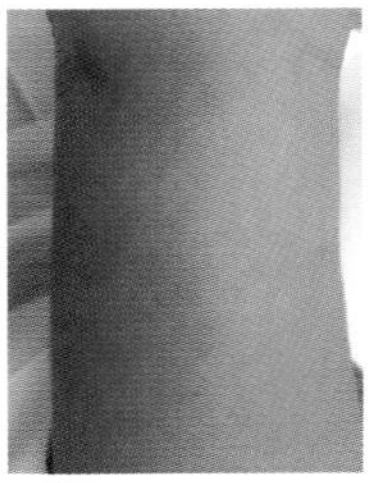

Figure 161.6
Purpuric/
vasculitic rash

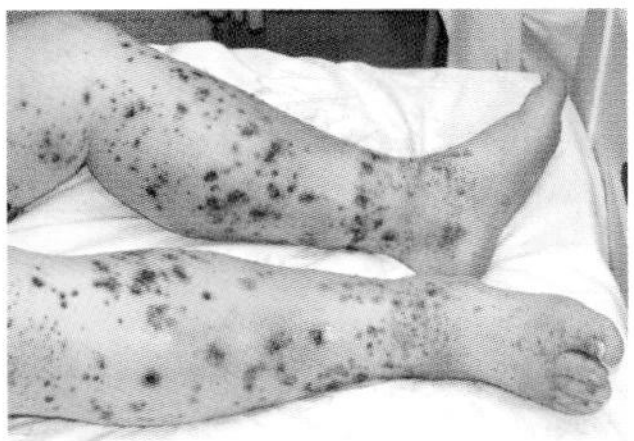

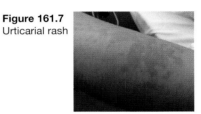

Figure 161.7
Urticarial rash

Box 161.1 Common causes for a rash

- Drug eruptions
- Viral exanthems
- Bacterial and other infections (including those toxin-mediated)
- Systemic diseases (acute graft-versus-host disease)
- Cutaneous vasculitis
- Autoimmune diseases: systemic lupus erythematosus (SLE)
- Dermatitis

Table 161.1 Diagnostic tests for rash related to infections

Disease	Pathogen	Tests
Chicken pox	Varicella zoster virus	Vesicle fluid PCR
Shingles (Herpes zoster)	Varicella zoster virus	Vesicle fluid PCR
Herpes simplex	HSV-1, HSV-2	Skin lesion swab PCR
Rubella	Rubella virus	Anti-rubella IgM antibodies detected within 4 days of onset of rash or a fourfold rise in anti-rubella IgG titre. Rubella RT-PCR is not widely available; samples from throat swab, urine or amniotic fluid for prenatal diagnosis of congenital infection
Hand foot and mouth disease	Coxsackievirus A and B5, enterovirus 71, echovirus 1 and 4	Clinical diagnosis; vesicle fluid, serum, faeces, respiratory tract and tissue samples for PCR
Fifth disease	Parvovius B19	Clinical diagnosis; confirmation by anti-B19 IgM antibody
Measles	Morbillivirus	Immunoassays for specific IgG and IgM antibody
Roseola	Human herpes virus 6 (HHV-6)	Detection of HHV-6 IgM antibody or a fourfold rise in anti-HHV-6 IgG titre
HIV infection	HIV	HIV antibodies, viral RNA PCR
Infectious mononucleosis	Epstein–Barr virus (EBV)	Detection of EBV IgM antibody or a fourfold rise in anti-EBV IgG titre
Scarlet fever	Group A Streptococcus	Bacterial culture of a throat swab to isolate group A Streptococcus; positive anti-streptolysin O titre
Rickettsial disease	Rickettsia species	PCR test from blood or rickettsial IgG and IgM antibody testing
Syphilis		See Chapter 116

Table 161.2 Common dermatological and systemic causes of pruritus

Dermatological conditions	Systemic conditions
• Skin xerosis • Atopic dermatitis • Contact dermatitis • Psoriasis • Lichen planus • Dermatophytes • Lice • Scabies • Insect bite • Urticaria	• Malignancy (paraneoplastic syndrome) • Advanced CKD • Chronic liver failure • Drug induced • Haematological disorders (polycythaemia vera, Hodgkin's lymphoma) • Schizophrenia • Depression • Infection (HIV, various parasite infections)

Table 161.3 Basic laboratory investigations for pruritus

Test	Systemic diseases
FBC	Iron-deficiency anaemia, polycythaemia vera
CRP	Inflammatory diseases
Iron study	Iron-deficiency anaemia
Serum biochemistry, creatinine	Advanced CKD
LFTs	Cholestatic pruritus
Fasting glucose	Diabetic neuropathy
TFTs	Hyperthyroidism and hypothyroidism

Key points

- Urinalysis should always be obtained in patient with cutaneous vasculitis; if normal, concomitant renal vasculitis is unlikely.
- Histological confirmation by skin biopsy is desirable in patients with suspected cutaneous vasculitis.
- Skin biopsy is useful in excluding or including many of the conditions in the differential diagnosis. An appropriate sample may be obtained using a large (>4 mm) punch biopsy or by deep shave biopsy technique.
- Skin biopsy with direct and indirect immunofluorescence is helpful in the diagnosis of bullous pemphigoid.

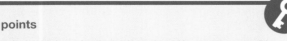

Clinical Investigations at a Glance, First Edition. Jonathan Gleadle, Jordan Li and Tuck Yong. © 2017 John Wiley & Sons, Ltd. Published 2017 by John Wiley & Sons, Ltd.

Skin rash

Generalised or local skin rashes are among the most common presentations. As for other disease, diagnosis of skin rashes starts with a detailed history and examination. Some rashes have distinctive features that allow immediate recognition, such as psoriasis and atopic dermatitis, without the need for further investigations. If a specific diagnosis is not immediately apparent, it is important to generate an inclusive differential diagnosis or at least a 'possible diagnostic pattern or label' for the type of disease process responsible in order to guide investigations and initial treatment. Mortality or significant morbidity can occur without prompt intervention, especially if the rashes are the manifestation of a systemic illness such as vasculitis. The common classifications and causes of rash are listed in Box 161.1.

Rash that requires urgent investigation

When rash, fever or signs of acute illness are present, the following diseases should be considered and investigated urgently if there is suspicion.

Meningococcaemia

See Chapter 32.

Anaphylactic reactions

See Chapter 158.

Toxic epidermal necrolysis and Stevens–Johnson syndrome

Toxic epidermal necrolysis is a clinical diagnosis, confirmed by histopathological analysis. No specific laboratory studies other than biopsy can definitively establish the diagnosis of Stevens–Johnson syndrome.

Staphylococcal scalded skin syndrome and toxic shock syndrome

The diagnosis of staphylococcal scalded skin syndrome is generally made clinically. Cultures and Gram stain from skin are negative, although *Staphylococcus aureus* may be cultured from the pharynx. Blister fluid is sterile. Toxic shock syndrome is also a clinical diagnosis, and the toxin involved may be isolated from serum.

Drug eruption

Drug eruptions can present with morbilliform, maculopapular, urticarial, pustular and bullous patterns. A drug reaction should be suspected when a symmetric cutaneous eruption begins within 4–12 days of commencement of a new medication. In a rash suspected to be caused by a drug, there are no laboratory tests to determine or confirm the responsible drug. FBC may show peripheral eosinophilia. Hepatic and renal function are usually normal.

Rash related to viral or bacterial infection

Accurate clinical diagnosis of rash related to viral infection (viral exanthem) may be difficult and laboratory confirmation should be encouraged if clinical diagnosis is in doubt (Table 161.1). This is especially true of rashes in pregnancy, where a laboratory-confirmed diagnosis is mandatory.

Cutaneous vasculitis

If there is suspicion of cutaneous vasculitis, the following blood tests may also be requested.
- FBC and CRP.
- Serum electrolytes, creatinine and LFTs.
- ANA and ENA: may indicate lupus or other autoimmune disorder.
- Hepatitis B and C serology.
- Immunoglobulin electrophoresis and light chain: detects lymphoma and multiple myeloma.
- Cryoglobulin: detects cryoglobulin-associated vasculitis.
- ANCA: may be present in vasculitis.

Laboratory investigations

Blood tests for FBC, serum electrolytes, creatinine and LFTs are used diagnostically and for assessing the impact of a skin disease or for monitoring systemic therapy. Many infective disorders or acute inflammatory disorders are associated with neutrophilia and raised CRP. Eosinophilia is also a feature of several dermatological conditions.

Skin biopsy

Skin biopsy is a key step in making a diagnosis in patients with a blistering disorder. The diagnosis of autoimmune blistering diseases requires detection of autoantibodies in the skin and mucous membranes. Skin direct immunofluorescence (DIF) is the diagnostic gold standard for detection of autoantibodies. Biopsy for DIF should be taken from perilesional (>1 cm from the lesion) uninvolved skin. The biopsy can be kept fresh in normal saline and taken straight to the laboratory or snap-frozen immediately and stored at −70°C. Indirect immunofluorescence (IIF) is a screening tool for circulating autoantibodies in autoimmune blistering diseases. IIF microscopy detects circulating autoantibodies. Skin biopsy should be considered in any patient who is systemically unwell or when the diagnosis is in doubt.

Pruritus

Severe itch can be debilitating and affect patients' quality of life. Pruritus can be a manifestation of an underlying dermatological condition or part of an underlying systemic disease (Table 161.2). Before investigating a patient with pruritus, a detailed history and full physical and dermatological examination are essential. The presence of a skin lesion/rash should raise the suspicion of an underlying dermatological disorder and the diagnosis is usually made based on clinical presentation and skin biopsy, and further investigation may not needed. Patients with healthy-looking skin or with scratch lesions require basic laboratory investigations as it may be caused by a systemic disease.

Laboratory investigations

Basic laboratory investigations are listed in Table 161.3. In suspected allergic dermatological conditions such as atopic dermatitis, the following investigations should be considered:
- total serum IgE level;
- allergen-specific IgE levels;
- prick tests with specific allergens (aeroallergens, food allergens, medications).

Microscopy of skin scrapings should be done to confirm scabies, and to exclude parasitic skin infestations. Stool microscopy should be performed in suspected parasitic infection.

Generally, a skin biopsy in the absence of any visible skin changes is unlikely to be helpful in the assessment of pruritus. A skin biopsy should be performed to confirm suspected lichen planus, dermatitis herpetiformis and bullous pemphigoid and to exclude subclinical dermatoses or skin conditions camouflaged by secondary scratch lesions.

Given the association with neoplasms, all patients should have up-to-date age-appropriate cancer screenings. Ultrasound of the abdomen is performed in evaluation of Hodgkin's lymphoma. Imaging in evaluation of paraneoplastic pruritus depends on the suspected malignancy and may include CT and MRI.

Urticaria and angioedema

Table 162.1 Common causes of urticaria/angioedema

Mechanism	Causes
Type I IgE-mediated hypersensitivity	Food allergy: shellfish, nut, milk Drug allergy: penicillin Insect bite: bee, wasp
Type III antigen–antibody mediated hypersensitivity	Infection: hepatitis B, respiratory tract viral infection Autoimmune disease: SLE Drugs: sulphonamides
Physical urticaria	Dermatographism, cold urticaria, solar urticaria, contact urticaria Exercise induced
Direct mast cell degranulation	Food chemicals, salicylates, tartrazine Drugs: NSAIDs, vancomycin, contrast

Table 162.2 Initial investigations for chronic urticaria

Test	Findings
FBC	Usually normal in chronic urticaria Anaemia due to chronic disease Lymphopenia due to SLE Eosinophilia due to parasitic infection
CRP	Usually normal in chronic urticaria Elevated in vasculitic urticaria
TFTs and thyroid autoantibodies	Autoimmune thyroiditis associated with urticaria
C3, C4	Decreased levels in urticarial vasculitis
ANA	Can be raised in patients with autoimmune diseases
LFTs, cryoglobulins, hepatitis B and C serology	If urticarial vasculitis suspected

Table 162.3 Indications for skin biopsy in a patient with wheals

Wheals persisting >48 hours
Painful urticarial lesions
Petechia or purpural lesions associated with urticaria
Systemic symptoms, raised CRP
Complete unresponsiveness to antihistamines
Features of mastocytosis (flushing, diarrhoea, syncope, abdominal cramping)

Table 162.4 Interpretation of complement results in angioedema

Condition	C1q	C4	C1-INH	C1-INH function
HAE type I	Normal	↓	↓	Normal
HAE type II	Normal	↓	N	↓
HAE type III	Normal	Normal	Normal	Normal
Acquired angioedema	↓	↓	↓	↓
ACE inhibitor-induced angioedema	Normal	Normal	Normal	Normal
Idiopathic angioedema	Normal	Normal	Normal	Normal

Key points

- If hereditary or acquired angioedema is suspected, levels of C4, C1-INH and C1q should be measured.
- Acquired C1-INH deficiency is often associated with underlying disease and frequently associated with C1-INH autoantibodies.
- Chronic urticaria initially requires laboratory work-up that includes FBC, biochemistry, LFTs and TSH.
- Skin biopsy should be done if there is any uncertainty as to the diagnosis or if wheals persist >48 hours to rule out urticarial vasculitis.

Urticaria

Urticaria is characterised by swelling of the skin and mucosa due to plasma leakage. It refers to a rash presenting with wheals, with or without angioedema. Urticaria can be divided into ordinary urticaria (acute or chronic), urticarial vasculitis or physical urticaria. The common causes of urticaria/angioedema are listed in Table 162.1. However, in half of cases of acute and chronic urticaria/angioedema, no cause is identified.

An urticaria that lasts for less than 6 weeks is an acute urticaria in which the characteristic wheals may persist for less than 24–48 hours. Chronic urticaria persists for longer than 6 weeks. If a patient describes individual lesions lasting for more than 48 hours, urticarial vasculitis should be considered.

Laboratory investigations

Urticaria is a clinical diagnosis. In physical urticarias, skin scratch test (dermatographism), ice cube test (cold urticaria) or sunlamp exposure test (solar urticaria) can be performed. In most patients with acute urticaria, no further investigation is required. However, laboratory investigations (Table 162.2) are indicated for chronic urticaria as it has been associated with many conditions such as SLE.

Autologous serum skin test

Autologous serum skin test is the most useful investigation for chronic urticaria and has a reported sensitivity and specificity of 81% and 78%, respectively. It is also used to determine whether a patient may have a good response to immunomodulatory treatments.

The procedure involves drawing a blood sample from the patient during a flare. The blood is separated by centrifugation to form serum and a small quantity of the serum is injected into an unaffected area of the forearm. At the same time equal amounts of normal saline and histamine are injected on the same forearm. The response at 30 min is then recorded. A positive response is recorded if a wheal of more than 1.5 mm is present at the site where the serum was injected or the wheal is larger than the saline-induced response. However, poor injecting techniques and administration in patients with dermatographism may elicit a false-positive result.

Skin-prick testing

Skin-prick testing is a procedure where a small sample of allergen is introduced into a patient's skin in order to induce an allergic response. It is indicated when an allergic cause for the urticaria is suspected and when confirmation would alter management, such as avoidance measures.

Skin biopsy

Skin biopsies are not usually performed in chronic urticaria unless urticarial vasculitis is suspected or the diagnosis is uncertain (Table 162.3).

Angioedema

Angioedema is the swelling of deep dermis, subcutaneous or submucosal tissue due to vascular leakage. It commonly affects the tongue, face, lips, throat and genital areas as well as abdominal organs. Angioedema can occur with or without urticaria (see above). Causes of angioedema without urticaria include the following.

- Angiotensin-converting enzyme (ACE) inhibitor-induced angioedema (prevalence of 1 in 1000 among ACE inhibitor users).
- Hereditary angioedema (HAE)
  - Type I: C1 esterase inhibitor (C1-INH) levels are reduced.
  - Type II: low functional C1-INH.
- Acquired C1-INH deficiency.

Most cases of angioedema can be diagnosed on the basis of the history and physical examination; it is important to obtain the drug history. Extensive diagnostic work-up and laboratory testing are not indicated in most cases of mild angioedema. Screening for suspected allergies to food, stinging insects, latex and antibiotics can be performed (see Chapter 158). In patients presenting with angioedema without urticaria (especially those with recurrent episodes), further investigations are required.

Complement level measurement

These should include the following:
- C4, CH50 levels
- C1-INH quantitative and functional measurements
- C1q level.

When the CH50 or C4 level is low, additional tests for C1-INH function and C1q level should be considered. These studies will help to establish or rule out C1-INH deficiency-associated angioedema, either hereditary or acquired (Table 162.4). HAE types I and II are characterised by low levels of C1-INH or elevated levels of dysfunctional C1-INH, as detected by an immune assay. Between attacks, low levels of C4 are noted. Elevated prothrombin fragment and D-dimer are associated with acute attacks in HAE.

Other laboratory investigations

General laboratory investigations have limited value in most cases. For chronic or recurrent angioedema without a clear trigger, the following tests can be considered:
- FBC
- CRP
- D-dimer level
- biochemistry
- ANA, rheumatoid factor, cryoglobulin levels
- TFTs, thyroid autoantibody (anti-microsomal or anti-thyroglobulin)
- urinalysis.

If the initial laboratory tests yield abnormal results or if a specific medical condition is suspected, additional tests may be needed. Chronic infection is a potential cause of unexplained angioedema (with or without urticaria). If suspected, consider the following tests:
- stool microscopy or PCR for ova and parasites;
- *Helicobacter pylori* investigations;
- hepatitis B and C serology.

Radiological investigations

Patients with angioedema do not need any imaging studies. When internal organ involvement is suspected during acute attacks, the following are used to exclude other pathology but not to confirm or rule out angioedema.
- Plain AXR may show a 'stacked coin' or 'thumbprint' appearance of the intestines due to small bowel wall oedema.
- Abdominal ultrasound may show ascites.
- CT abdomen may show oedema of the bowel wall.
- CXR may show pleural effusion.

Further reading

PART 2: COMMON PRESENTATIONS

Chapter 13: Chest pain
Cooper, A., Timmis, A. & Skinner, J. (2010) Assessment of recent onset chest pain or discomfort of suspected cardiac origin: summary of NICE guidance. *BMJ* 340, c1118.

Chapter 15: Headache
Stark, R. (2010) Investigation of headache. *Medicine Today* 11, 50–57.

Chapter 17: Diarrhoea
Thielman, N.M. & Guerrant, R.L. (2004) Acute infectious diarrhoea. *N Engl J Med* 350, 38–47.

Chapter 18: Constipation
Lembo, A. & Camilleri, M. (2003) Chronic constipation. *N Engl J Med* 349, 1360–1368.

Chapter 21: Dyspepsia
Bredenoord, A.J., Pandolfino, J.E. & Smout, A.J. (2013) Gastro-oesophageal reflux disease. *Lancet* 381, 1933–1942.

Chapter 22: Dysphagia
Bredenoord, A.J. & Smout, A.J. (2013) Advances in motility testing: current and novel approaches. *Nat Rev Gastroenterol Hepatol* 10, 463–472.

Chapter 23: Weight loss
McMinn, J., Steel, C. & Bowman, A. (2011) Investigation and management of unintentional weight loss in older adults. *BMJ* 342, d1732.

Chapter 24: Obesity
Haslam, D.W. & James, W.P. (2005) Obesity. *Lancet* 366, 1197–1209.

Chapter 25: Fatigue
Chronic Fatigue Syndrome Working Group (2002) Chronic fatigue syndrome: clinical practice guidelines 2002. *Med J Aust* 176, S21–S56.

Chapter 27: Preoperative investigations for elective surgery
Scott, I.A., Shohag, H.A., Kam, P.C. *et al.* (2013) Preoperative cardiac evaluation and management of patients undergoing elective non-cardiac surgery. *Med J Aust* 199, 667–673.

Chapter 28: Syncope
Task Force for the Diagnosis and Management of Syncope (2009) Guidelines for the diagnosis and management of syncope (version 2009). *Eur Heart J* 30, 2631–2671.

Chapter 29: Back pain
Downie, A., Williams, C.M., Henschke, N. *et al.* (2013) Red flags to screen for malignancy and fracture in patients with low back pain: systematic review. *BMJ* 347, f7095.

Chapter 28: Meningitis
van de Beek, D., de Gans, J., Tunkel, A.R. & Wijdicks, E.F. (2006) Community-acquired bacterial meningitis in adults. *N Engl J Med* 354, 44–53.

Chapter 33: Anaemia
Camaschella, C. (2015) Iron-deficiency anemia. *N Engl J Med* 372, 1832–1843.

Chapter 35: Cough
Irwin, R.S., Baumann, M.H., Bolser, D.C. *et al.* (2006) Diagnosis and management of cough. Executive summary: ACCP evidence-based practice guideline. *Chest* 129 (1 Suppl.), 1S–23S.

Chapter 37: Palpitations and cardiac arrhythmias
Link, M.S. (2012) Evaluation and initial treatment of supraventricular tachycardia. *N Engl J Med* 367, 1438–1448.

Chapter 39: Vertigo
Kim, J. & Zee, D.S. (2014) Benign paroxysmal positional vertigo. *N Engl J Med* 170, 1138–1147.

Chapter 40: Urinary tract infection
Hooton, T.M. (2012) Uncomplicated urinary tract infection. *N Engl J Med* 366, 1028–1037.

Chapter 49: Seizure
Angus-Leppan, H. (2014) First seizures in adults. *BMJ* 348, g2470.

PART 3: CONDITIONS

Cardiovascular disease

Chapter 53: Heart failure
Krum, H. & Abraham, W.T. (2009) Heart failure. *Lancet* 373, 941–955.

Chapter 56: Aortic disease
Gollege, J. & Eagle, K.A. (2008) Acute aortic dissection. *Lancet* 372, 55–66.

Chapter 58: Hyperlipidaemia
Viljoen, A. & Wierzbicki, A.S. (2011) Investigating mixed hyperlipidaemia. *BMJ* 343, d5146.

Respiratory disease and sleep disorders

Chapter 59: Pneumonia
Watkins, R.R. & Lemonovich, T.L. (2011) Diagnosis and management of community-acquired pneumonia in adults. *Am Fam Physician* 83, 1299–1306.

Chapter 61: Chronic obstructive pulmonary disease
Niewoehner, D.E. (2010) Outpatient management of severe COPD. *N Engl J Med* 362, 1407–1416.

Chapter 65: Pulmonary hypertension
Kiely, D.G., Elliot, C.A., Sabroe, I. *et al.* (2013) Pulmonary hypertension: diagnosis and management. *BMJ* 346, f2026.

Chapter 68: Sleep disorders
Usmani, Z.A., Chai-Coetzer, C.L., Antic, N.A. & McEvoy, R.D. (2013) Obstructive sleep apnoea in adults. *Postgrad Med J* 89, 148–156.

Gastroenterology and hepatology

Chapter 71: Malabsorption
Green, P.H. & Jabri, B. (2003) Coeliac disease. *Lancet* 362, 383–391.

Chapter 72: Inflammatory bowel disease
Baumgart, D. C. & Sandborn, W.J. (2012) Crohn's disease. *Lancet* 380, 1590–1605.
Danese, S. & Fiocchi, C. (2011) Ulcerative colitis. *N Engl J Med* 365, 1713–1725.

Chapter 73: Irritable bowel syndrome
Mayer, E.A. (2008) Irritable bowel syndrome. *N Engl J Med* 358, 1692–1699.

Chapter 74: Colorectal cancer
Brenner, H., Kloor, M. & Pox, C.P. (2014) Colorectal cancer. *Lancet* 383, 1490–1502.
Meyerhardt, JA, Mangu, P.B., Flynn, P.J., et al. (2013) Follow-up care, surveillance protocol, and secondary prevention measures for survivors of colorectal cancer: American Society of Clinical Oncology clinical practice guideline endorsement. *J Clin Oncol* 31, 4465-4470.

Chapter 75: Liver mass
El-Serag, H.B. (2011) Hepatocellular carcinoma. *N Engl J Med* 365, 1118–1127.

Chapter 76: Cirrhosis
Schuppen, D. & Afdhal, N.H. (2008) Liver cirrhosis. *Lancet* 371, 838–851.

Chapter 77: Liver function tests
Mieli-Vergani, G. & Vergani, D. (2011) Autoimmune hepatitis. *Nat Rev Gastroenterol Hepatol* 8, 320–329.

Nephrology and urology

Chapter 80: Chronic kidney disease
Levey, A.S. & Coresh J. (2012) Chronic kidney disease. *Lancet* 379, 165–180.

Chapter 82: Potassium disorders
Oram, R.A., McDonald, T.J. & Valdya, B. (2013) Investigating hypokalaemia. *BMJ* 347, f5137.

Chapter 83: Sodium disorders
Ellison, D.H. & Berl, T. (2007) The syndrome of inappropriate antidiuresis. *N Engl J Med* 356, 2064–2072.

Chapter 85: Proteinuria
Hull, R.P. & Goldsmith, D.J.A. (2008) Nephrotic syndrome in adults. *BMJ* 336, 1185–1189.

Chapter 86: Renal mass
Gill, I.S., Aron, M., Gervais, D.A. & Jewett, M.A. (2010) Small renal mass. *N Engl J Med* 362, 624–634.

Chapter 87: Kidney stones
Worcester, E.M. & Coe, F.L. (2010) Calcium kidney stones. *N Engl J Med* 363, 954–963.

Chapter 88: Renal artery stenosis
Dworkin, L.D. & Cooper, C.J. (2009) Renal-artery stenosis. *N Engl J Med* 361, 1972–1978.

Endocrinology

Chapter 92: Thyroid disorders
Brent, G.A. (2008) Graves' disease. *N Engl J Med* 358, 2594–2605.

Chapter 97: Adrenal insufficiency
Arlt, W. (2009) The approach to the adult with newly diagnosed adrenal insufficiency. *J Clin Endocrinol Metab* 94, 1059–1067.

Chapter 99: Cushing's syndrome
Newell-Price, J., Grossman, A.B. & Nieman, L.K. (2006) Cushing's syndrome. *Lancet* 367, 1605–1617.

Chapter 100: Phaeochromocytoma
Clifton-Bligh, R. (2013) Diagnosis of silent pheochromocytoma and paraganglioma. *Expert Rev Endocrinol Metab* 8, 47–57.

Reproductive and obstetric medicine

Chapter 102: Male hypogonadism
Basaria, S. (2014) Male hypogonadism. *Lancet* 383, 1250–1263.

Chapter 104: Erectile dysfunction
McMahon, C.G. (2014) Erectile dysfunction. *Intern Med J* 44, 18–26.

Chapter 106: Hirsutism
Rosenfield, R.L. (2005) Hirsutism. *N Engl J Med* 353, 2578–2588.

Chapter 107: Polycystic ovary syndrome
Teede, H.J., Misso, M.L., Deeks, A.A. *et al.* on behalf of the Guideline Development Groups (2011) Assessment and management of polycystic ovary syndrome: summary of an evidence-based guideline. *Med J Aust* 195, 65.

Infectious diseases

Chapter 111: Leucopenia and febrile neutropenia

Tam, C.S., O'Reilly, M., Andresen, D. *et al.* (2011) Use of empiric antimicrobial therapy in neutropenic fever. *Intern Med J* 41 (Suppl. 1), 90–101.

Chapter 112: Illness in returned travellers

Johnston, V., Stockley, J.M., Dockrell, D. *et al.* (2009) Fever in returned travellers presenting in the United Kingdom: recommendations for investigation and initial management. *J Infect* 59, 1–18.

Zwar, N.A. & Torda, A. (2011) Investigation of diarrhoea in a traveller just returned from India. *BMJ* 342, d2978.

Chapter 115: Osteomyelitis

Lew, D.P. & Waldvogel, F.A. (2004) Osteomyelitis. *Lancet* 364, 369–379.

Chapter 117: Tuberculosis

Zumla, A., Raviglione, M., Hafner, R. *et al.* (2013) Tuberculosis. *N Engl J Med* 368, 745–755.

Haematology

Chapter 120: Myelodysplastic syndromes

Adès, L., Itzykson, R. & Fenaux, P. (2014) Myelodysplastic syndromes. *Lancet* 383, 2239–2252.

Chapter 121: Erythrocytosis

Keohane, C., McMullin, M.F. & Harrison, C. (2013) The diagnosis and management of erythrocytosis. *BMJ* 347, f6667.

Chapter 123: Leukaemia

Grigoropoulos, N.F., Petter, R., Van't Veer, M.B. *et al.* (2013) Leukaemia update. Part 1: diagnosis and management. *BMJ* 346, f1660.

Chapter 124: Lymphoma

Shankland, K.R., Armitage, J.O. & Hancock, B.W. (2012) Non-Hodgkin lymphoma. *Lancet* 380, 848–857.

Townsend, W. & Linch, D. (2012) Hodgkin's lymphoma. *Lancet* 380, 836–847.

Chapter 125: Multiple myeloma

Smith, D. & Yong, K. (2013) Multiple myeloma. *BMJ* 346, f3863.

Chapter 126: Platelet disorders

Schafer, A.I. (2004) Thrombocytosis. *N Engl J Med* 350, 211–219.

Stasi, R. (2012) How to approach thrombocytopenia. *Hematology Am Soc Hematol Educ Program* 2012,153–158.

Oncology

Chapter 129: Breast cancer

Benson, J.R., Jatoi, I., Keisch, M. *et al.* (2009) Early breast cancer. *Lancet* 373, 1463–1479.

Warner, E. (2011) Breast-cancer screening. *N Engl J Med* 365, 1025–1032.

Chapter 132: Tumour markers

Sturgeon, C.M., Lai, L.C. & Duffy, M.J. (2009) Serum tumour markers: how to order and interpret them. *BMJ* 339, b3527.

Chapter 133: Ovarian cancer

Jayson, G.C., Kohn, E.C., Kitchener, H.C. *et al.* (2014) Ovarian cancer. *Lancet* 384, 1376–1388.

Neurology

Chapter 135: Stroke

van der Worp, H.B. & van Gijn, J. (2007) Acute ischemic stroke. *N Engl J Med* 357, 572–579.

Chapter 136: Haemorrhagic stroke

van Gijn, J., Kerr, R.S. & Rinkel, G.J. (2007) Subarachnoid haemorrhage. *Lancet* 369, 306–318.

Chapter 139: Brain tumours

Louis, D.N., Ohgaki, H., Wiestler, O.D. *et al.* (2007) The 2007 WHO classification of tumours of the central nervous system. *Acta Neuropathol* 114, 97–109.

Chapter 140: Multiple sclerosis

Compston, A. & Coles, A. (2008) Multiple sclerosis. *Lancet* 372, 1502–1517.

Chapter 142: Peripheral neuropathy

Fuller, G. (2005) How to get the most out of nerve conduction studies and electromyography. *J Neurol Neurosurg Psychiatry* 76 (Suppl. 2), 41–46.

Chapter 143: Movement disorders

Mehanna, R. & Jankovic, J. (2013) Movement disorders in cerebrovascular diseases. *Lancet Neurol* 12, 597–608.

Rheumatology

Chapter 144: Septic and crystal arthropathies

Mathews, C.J. (2010) Bacterial septic arthritis in adults. *Lancet* 375, 846–855.

Neogi, T. (2011) Gout. *N Engl J Med* 364, 443–452.

Chapter 145: Osteoarthritis

Felson, D.T. (2006) Osteoarthritis of the knee. *N Engl J Med* 354, 841–848.

Lane, N.E. (2007) Osteoarthritis of the hip. *N Engl J Med* 354, 1413–1421.

Chapter 147: Rheumatoid arthritis

Scott, D.L., Wolfe, F. & Huizinga, T.W. (2010) Rheumatoid arthritis. *Lancet* 376, 1094–1108.

Chapter 148: Systemic lupus erythematosus

Binder, A. & Ellis, S. (2013) When to order an antinuclear antibody test. *BMJ* 347, f5060.

Chapter 150: Sjögren's syndrome

Ramos-Casals, M., Brito-Zeron, P., Siso-Amirall, A. *et al.* (2012) Primary Sjögren's syndrome. *BMJ* 344, e3821.

Chapter 151: Vasculitis

Bosch, X., Guilabert, A. & Font, J. (2006) Antineutrophil cytoplasmic antibodies. *Lancet* 368, 404–418.

Chapter 152: Polymalgia rheumatica and giant cell arteritis

Salvarani, C., Cantini, E. & Hunder, G.G. (2008) Polymyalgia rheumatica and giant-cell arteritis. *Lancet* 372, 234–245.

Chapter 153: Osteoporosis

Raisz, L.G. (2005) Screening for osteoporosis. *N Engl J Med* 353, 164–171.

Geriatric and general medicine

Chapter 154: Dementia

Blennow, K., de Leon, M.J. & Zetterberg, H. (2006) Alzheimer's disease. *Lancet* 368, 387–403.

Petersen, R.C. (2011) Mild cognitive impairment. *N Engl J Med* 364, 2227–2234.

Yesavage, J.A. (1988) Geriatric Depression Scale. *Psychopharmacol Bull* 24, 709–711.

Chapter 157: Urinary incontinence

Thirugnanasothy, S. (2010) Managing urinary incontinence in older people. *BMJ* 341, c3835.

Clinical immunology and allergy

Chapter 158: Allergy and anaphylaxis

Steele, C., Conlon, N. & Edgar, J.D. (2014) Diagnosis of immediate food allergy. *BMJ* 349, g3695.

Dermatology

Chapter 160: Skin cancers

Eggermont, A.M.M., Spatz, A. & Robert, C. (2010) Cutaneous melanoma. *Lancet* 383, 816–827.

Madan, V., Lear, J.T. & Szeimies, R.M. (2010) Non-melanoma skin cancer. *Lancet* 375, 673–685.

Chapter 161: Skin rashes

Stein, R.S. (2012) Exanthematous drug eruptions. *N Engl J Med* 366, 2492–2501.

Index

Page numbers in *italics* refer to figures. Those in **bold** refer to tables.

Clinical Investigations at a Glance, First Edition. Jonathan Gleadle, Jordan Li and Tuck Yong. © 2017 John Wiley & Sons, Ltd. Published 2017 by John Wiley & Sons, Ltd.

target cells **72**, *73*
target organ damage, hypertension **126**, 127
TBW (total body water) 181
^{99}Tc-iminodiacetic acid 33
temporal arteritis 35, **112**, 326–7
tension pneumothorax **96**, *138*, 139
terminal ileum, malabsorption **156**
testosterone 220, 221
  amenorrhoea 227
  erectile dysfunction 225
  hirsutism 228, 229
  polycystic ovarian syndrome 231
  replacement therapy 221
thalassaemias 73, 261
therapeutic drug monitoring 20–1
third world 22–3
thoracentesis 137
thoracic trauma **98**, 99, 100–1
thoraco-lumbar spine, trauma 102, 103
thoracoscopy 137, 149
thrombocytopenia 268, 269
thrombocytosis **268**, 269
thromboembolism (venous) 143, 272, 273
thrombophilia **10**, 272–3
thrombophilia screen
  ascites 153
  peripheral artery disease 120, 121
  pulmonary hypertension 145
thrombotic thrombocytopenic purpura (TTP) 268, 269
thumbprinting *44*
thunderclap headache 34
thymoma 111
thyroglobulin 201, **280**
thyroid carcinoma 198, 201
thyroid disease 198–203
  coma **58**
  heart failure 119
  hypertension **126**
  potassium disorders 179
  treatment monitoring 203
thyroid function tests 202–3
thyroid peroxidase, antibodies 199
thyroiditis *200*
thyroid-stimulating hormone 199, 201, 202, 203
thyroxine 199, **202**, 203
tilt tables *62*, 63
tissue transglutaminase antibodies 161
total body water (TBW) 181
total iron binding capacity 73
toxic multinodular goitre *200*
toxicology 91
toxins *see* poisoning
toxoplasmosis 74, 291, 293
TP53 gene 267
traffic accidents, computed tomography **98**
transbronchial lung biopsy 148, 149
transferrin **72**
transient elastography 167
transient ischaemic attacks 287
transient proteinuria 185
transit studies (intestinal) *40*, 41
transitional cell carcinoma (TCC) *88*, 89
transketolase **104**
transoesophageal echocardiography (TOE) 122, 123
transplantation (organs), infections **92**, 93
transport of patients 19
transudates, pleural effusions 136, 137

trauma 98–103
  eye 83
travellers, illnesses 240–1
tremor 304, 305
trichomoniasis 249
tricuspid valve, infective endocarditis 123
triglycerides 129
triiodothyronine 199, 203
triple faeces test 241
triple phase CT, liver 164
troponins
  chest pain 28, 29
  heart failure 119
  point-of-care tests 23
  pulmonary embolism 141
  subarachnoid haemorrhage 289
  trauma 101
trough concentrations 21
trypsinogen, malabsorption 157
tryptase 339
T-score, osteoporosis 329
tubal patency 223
tuberculin skin testing (TST) 250, 251
tuberculosis 250–1
  cerebrospinal fluid 70, 71
  lymphadenopathy **74**
  pleural effusions 137
tumour markers 279, 280–1
tumour necrosis factor, drugs *vs* 93
tuning fork tests 115
24-hour ECG monitoring 63, 81, 335
24-hour urine collection
  calcium 183
  free cortisol 215
  hypertension 126
  kidney stones 189
  phaeochromocytoma 217
  protein 185
twin pregnancy *234*
tympanometry 114
typhoid 241

ulcerative colitis *82*, 158–9
ultrasound 12, 13
  abdominal aortic aneurysm 125
  abdominal pain *31*, 32
  appendicitis 33
  ascites 153
  breast cancer 275
  female pelvis 226, *228, 230*
  haematuria 89
  inflammatory bowel disease 159
  jaundice 69
  kidney 173, 175, 183, *186*, 187, 189
  liver 152, 164, 165, 167
  lower extremity venous 143
  ovary 223, *230*, 231, 283
  pancreatitis 170, 171
  penis 225
  peripheral artery disease 120, 121
  peripheral oedema 67
  pleural effusions 137
  pneumothorax 139
  pregnancy 33, 234, 235
  renal artery stenosis 190, 191
  sepsis 243
  thyroid disease 201
  trauma 99, 103
  vision loss 113
  weight loss 53
upper gastrointestinal bleeding (UGIB) 42–3
urea, acute kidney injury 173
urea breath tests **46**, 48
urea/creatinine ratio 43

urease test, endoscopy **46**
ureter, stone *31*, 33, *86*, *172*
urgency urinary incontinence 337
uric acid
  gout 308
  urine crystals *188*
urinary incontinence 336–7
urinary tract infections 86–7
urine
  abdominal pain 32
  acute kidney injury *172*, 173
  antigen tests 131
  attempted suicide 90
  β-hCG 235
  chronic kidney disease 175
  diabetes insipidus 197
  haematuria 88, 89
  haemolytic anaemia 260
  haemoptysis 79
  hypertension 126
  jaundice 68, 69
  kidney stones 189
  osmolality 181, 197
  pH 177
  phaeochromocytoma 217
  potassium disorders 179
  preoperative 61
  proteinuria 184, 185
  sodium 181
  urinary tract infections 87
  see also specific substances
urobilinogen, urine 68, 69
urodynamics 337
urography (CT; MRI) 89, *188*, 189
usual interstitial pneumonia *148*
uterus, absence 227
uveitis 82, 83, 295

valproate **20**
Valsalva manoeuvre, headache 35
valvular heart disease 122–3
vancomycin **20**
vanillylmandelic acid **216**
varices, oesophagus *152*
vas deferens, congenital absence 223
vascular dementia **330**
vascular surgery, blood loss **60**
vascular trauma **99**, 101
vasculitis 324–5
  cerebral *320*
vasovagal syncope 63
vegetations, mitral valve *122*
venepuncture 9
Venereal Disease Research Laboratory test 249
venous sinus thrombosis 35
venous thromboembolism 143, 272, 273
ventilation–perfusion mismatch 135
ventilation–perfusion scan
  PE **140**, 142, 143, *144*
  pulmonary hypertension 145
ventricular tachycardia *80*
vertebrae
  crush fractures *64*
  osteomyelitis 247
vertigo 84–5
very low density lipoprotein **128**
vestibular function 85
video capsule endoscopy 159
video-assisted thoracoscopy 149
video-EEG monitoring 109
video-fluoroscopic swallowing study 50, 51
villous atrophy 157
viral infections **244**
  encephalitis 292

hepatitis **166**
meningitis, cerebrospinal fluid 70, 71
pneumonia 131
sexually transmitted diseases 248, 249
virilisation 229
virtual colonoscopy 45
vision loss 112–13, 195
visual evoked potentials, MS 297
visual fields
  acromegaly 207
  hyperprolactinaemia *208*, 209
visual impairment, defined 113
vitamin B12 deficiency 73
vitamin D 183, 329
vitamin K deficiency **270**
vitreous-body biopsy 295
voiding diaries 337
volvulus, sigmoid 155
vomiting 36–7
von Willebrand disease (VWD) 270, 271

waist-to-hip ratio 55
walking tests
  COPD 135
  interstitial lung disease 148, 149
  pulmonary hypertension 145
warm haemolysis 260
watchful waiting, weight loss 53
water deprivation test 196, 197
water loss 180, 181
water-swallow test 50, 51
Weber test 115
Wegener's granulomatosis (GPA) *324*, 325
weight
  peripheral oedema 67
  WHO classification **54**, 55
weight loss 52–3
Wells score, pulmonary embolism **140**, 141
Western blot test, HIV 253
Whipple's disease **156**, 157
white blood cell-labelled radionuclide imaging, osteomyelitis 246, 247
white blood cells, synovial fluid 307
white coat hypertension 127
WHO classification, weight **54**, 55
whole-body CT, weight loss 53
wide-field microscopy, nailfold capillary bed 314
Wilson's disease **166**, **304**, 305
Wolff–Parkinson–White syndrome *62*, *80*
wrist, trauma 102, 103, *334*
written consent 7

xanthochromia 290
xanthomas 129
X-ray imaging 12, 13
  abdominal pain *31*, 32
  back pain 65
  chest pain 29
  intensive care 24, 25
  intestinal obstruction 154, 155
  kidney stones 188, 189
  myeloma 266, 267
  osteomyelitis 246, 247
  rheumatoid arthritis 317
  skull 35, 100
  trauma 100, 101, 102
  see also chest X-rays

Ziehl–Neelsen stain 14, 251
Z-score, osteoporosis 329